Board Review Seri

General Surgery

Board Review Series

General Surgery

Traves D. Crabtree, M.D.
Resident in General Surgery
Department of Surgery
University of Virginia
Charlottesville, Virginia

Associate Editors:

Eugene F. Foley, M.D.
Associate Professor of Surgery
Director of Colon & Rectal Surgery
Department of Surgery
University of Virginia
Charlottesville, Virginia

Robert G. Sawyer, M.D.
Assistant Professor of Surgery
Department of Surgery
University of Virginia
Charlottesville, Virginia

LIPPINCOTT WILLIAMS & WILKINS
A **Wolters Kluwer** Company
Philadelphia • Baltimore • New York • London
Buenos Aires • Hong Kong • Sydney • Tokyo

Editor: Elizabeth Nieginski
Editorial Director: Julie P. Martinez
Development Editors: Bridget Blatteau, Dvora Konstant
Marketing Manager: Aimee Sirmon
Managing Editor: Darrin Kiessling

351 West Camden Street
Baltimore, Maryland 21201-2436 USA

530 Walnut Street
Philadelphia, Pennsylvania 19106 USA

Printed in the United States of America

Library of Congress Cataloging-in-Publication Data

General surgery / [edited by] Traves D. Crabtree ; associate editors, Eugene F. Foley, Robert G. Sawyer.
p. ; cm. — (Board review series)
Includes bibliographical references and index.
ISBN 0-683-30636-7
1. Surgery—Examinations, questions, etc. I. Crabtree, Traves D. II. Foley, Eugene F. III. Sawyer, Robert G. IV. Series.
[DNLM: 1. Surgical Procedures, Operative—Examination Questions. WO 18.2 G3256 2000]
RD37.2.G4598 2000
617′.0076—dc21

00-025009

To purchase additional copies of this book call our customer service department at **(800) 638-3030** or fax orders to **(301) 824-7390.** International customers should call **(301) 714-2324.**

00 01 02
1 2 3 4 5 6 7 8 9

Dedication

This book is dedicated to my two little girls, Abby and Ellie, and to my wife, Faye, for her unconditional support, patience, and love, and understanding that "I'll be home soon" is very much a relative term during a surgical residency.

Traves D. Crabtree

Contents

Preface

With continued advances in the field of surgery, a comprehensive textbook covering all aspects of surgery, though important as a reference guide, can be overwhelming to the medical student or junior resident seeking a general review of the entire field. *BRS General Surgery* represents a concerted effort on the part of the faculty and resident staff at the University of Virginia and Southern Illinois University to provide a concise review of surgery for medical students and junior residents, specifically for the surgical section of the United States Medical Licensing Examination (USMLE Step 2).

This text covers the background principles of surgery, in addition to major topics in general surgery, with essential information on epidemiology, pathogenesis, diagnosis, and treatment. It is designed to provide an understanding of the details of each disease process, but intentionally focuses on the practical clinical approach to diagnosis and management of surgical problems. To this end, we have heavily relied on outlines, tables, figures, and clinical questions with explanations, instead of depending solely on standard text.

This book incorporates input from a large number of faculty and residents from two separate institutions. Recognizing that no one style of presentation is appropriate for all students or all topics, we hope to have combined the best aspects of the teaching skills from this diverse group of "experts." We are hopeful that this text will provide an interesting, effective, and enjoyable clinical review for students of surgery at this critical and exciting point in their careers.

Eugene F. Foley, M.D.

Acknowledgment

I would like to especially thank Dr. Kristen M. Jacobs and Dr. James Thiele for their valuable input and assistance during the writing of this book.

Contributors

Laurence H. Brinckerhoff, M.D.
Resident in General Surgery
University of Virginia Health System
Charlottesville, Virginia

James Forrest Calland, M.D.
Resident in General Surgery
University of Virginia Health System
Charlottesville, Virginia

Gerald A Cephas, M.D.
Resident in General Surgery
University of Virginia Health System
Charlottesville, Virginia

Jeffrey A. Claridge, M.D.
Resident in General Surgery
University of Virginia Health System
Charlottesville, Virginia

Traves D. Crabtree, M.D.
Resident in General Surgery
University of Virginia Health System
Charlottesville, Virginia

Steven M. Fiser, M.D.
Resident in General Surgery
University of Virginia Health System
Charlottesville, Virginia

James J. Gangemi, M.D.
Resident in General Surgery
University of Virginia Health System
Charlottesville, Virginia

Thomas G. Gleason, M.D.
Resident in General Surgery
University of Virginia Health System
Charlottesville, Virginia

Santosh N. Krishnan, Ph.D., M.D.
Resident in General Surgery
University of Virginia Health System
Charlottesville, Virginia

Steward M. Long III, M.D.
Resident in General Surgery
University of Virginia Health System
Charlottesville, Virginia

Patrick J. O'Neill, Ph.D., M.D.
Resident in General Surgery
University of Virginia Health System
Charlottesville, Virginia

Allan J. Parungao, M.S., M.D.
Resident in Plastic Surgery
Southern Illinois University School of Medicine
Springfield, Illinois

Shawn J. Pelletier, M.D.
Resident in General Surgery
University of Virginia Health System
Charlottesville, Virginia

Daniel P. Raymond, M.D.
Resident in General Surgery
University of Virginia Health System
Charlottesville, Virginia

P. James Renz III, M.D.
Resident in General Surgery
Southern Illinois University School of Medicine
Springfield, Illinois

Craig L. Slingluff Jr., M.D.
Associate Professor of Surgery
Division of Surgical Oncology
University of Virginia Health System
Charlottesville, Virginia

Lisa M. Sullivan, M.D.
Resident in Anesthesiology
University of Virginia Health System
Charlottesville, Virginia

Robert D. Sullivan, M.D.
Resident in Anesthesiology
University of Virginia Health System
Charlottesville, Virginia

James W. Thiele, M.D.
Resident in General Surgery
Southern Illinois University School of Medicine
Springfield, Illinois

Lee W. Thompson, M.D.
Resident in General Surgery
University of Virginia Health System
Charlottesville, Virginia

I

Background Principles of Surgery

1

Anesthesiology

Robert D. Sullivan and Lisa M. Sullivan

I. Initial Assessment and Monitoring

A. Preoperative assessment of the surgical patient

1. The American Society of Anesthesiologists (ASA) Classification

—is part of the physical evaluation of the patient (**Table 1-1**).

2. The classification system

—is graded as classes 1–6 in order of increasing risk of mortality.

B. Blood pressure

1. Noninvasive blood pressure monitoring

a. An appropriate size cuff

—is most often placed on the arm, avoiding limbs with arterial-venous shunts or intravenous (IV) sites.

b. A cuff that is too narrow

—relative to patient size may give a **falsely elevated blood pressure.**

2. Intra-arterial blood pressure monitoring

a. Indications for intra-arterial monitoring include

—elective hypotension.

—anticipation of wide blood pressure variation.

—the need for frequent blood sampling.

b. The most common sites of measurement

—are the radial and femoral arteries.

C. Electrocardiogram (ECG)

1. The ECG is used for detection of

—cardiac dysrhythmias.

—myocardial ischemia.

Table 1-1. American Society of Anesthesiologists (ASA) Physical Status Classification

Class 1:	Healthy
Class 2:	Mild systemic disease without functional limitation
Class 3:	Moderate to severe systemic disease with functional limitation
Class 4:	Severe systemic disease that is constantly life-threatening and functionally incapacitating
Class 5:	Not expected to survive 24 hours with or without surgery
Class 6:	Organ donor
E:	Added to classification if procedure is an emergency

—electrolyte abnormalities, which are not uncommon under anesthesia.

2. Leads V2 and V5

—together can detect **95%** of intraoperative ischemia, allowing for early intervention.

D. Pulse oximetry

1. An oximeter

—is placed on any **perfused tissue** that can be transilluminated.

2. This provides

—an estimate of the level of **oxygen binding by hemoglobin** in the blood, providing an early warning of hypoxia.

3. Arterial oxygen saturation (SaO_2)

—of **70%, 80%, and 90%** corresponds to arterial oxygen tensions (PaO_2) of **40, 50, and 60,** respectively.

4. In the presence of severe anemia

—oximeter readings may be normal even when tissue hypoxia is present.

E. Temperature

1. Monitoring sites include

—esophagus.

—nasal pharynx.

—axilla.

—bladder.

2. Maintenance of normothermia

—can improve tissue perfusion and limit coagulopathies.

3. Elective hypothermia

—is used to decrease tissue oxygen demand, particularly for some cardiac and neurosurgical procedures.

F. Urine output (UOP)

1. Monitoring UOP

—via a Foley catheter provides an **estimate of end-organ perfusion and fluid status.**

2. This is generally used

—for all surgeries over 2 hours.

—to **decompress the bladder** to avoid injury during laparoscopic procedures and cesarean sections.

G. Swan-Ganz catheter

1. The tip of this catheter

—lies in the pulmonary arterial system.

2. The pressure changes

—observed during initial placement of a Swan-Ganz catheter are demonstrated in **Figure 1.1.**

3. This catheter is used to monitor

—left ventricular filling pressures.

—cardiac output.

—systemic vascular resistance.

H. Capnography

1. This method

—provides measurement of **end-tidal carbon dioxide (CO_2) tension.**

—confirms adequacy of ventilation and thus endotracheal tube (ETT) placement.

2. This measurement is an estimate of $PaCO_2$

3. The same device also measures inspiratory and expiratory anesthetic gas concentrations, confirming anesthetic gas delivery.

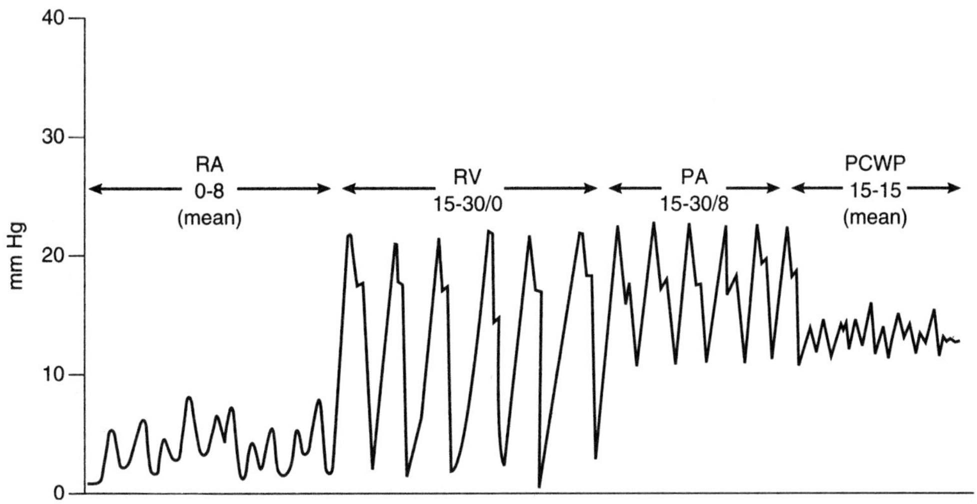

Figure 1.1. Swan-Ganz catheter placement. A pressure tracing during passage of a Swan-Ganz catheter from the right atrium (RA) to the point where the catheter tip is wedged within a branch of the pulmonary artery (PCWP). Passage into the right ventricle (RV) is marked by a sudden increase in systolic pressure, the pulmonary artery (PA) by an increase in diastolic pressure, and PCWP by a decrease in pressure. (Reprinted with permission from Morgan E, Mikhail N: *Clinical Anesthesiology,* 2nd ed. Stamford, CT, Appleton & Lange, 1996, p 89.)

—Unexpected severe hypercapnia can also be a sensitive indicator of **malignant hyperthermia.**

I. Transesophageal echocardiogram (TEE)
—may be used to monitor cardiac function, particularly during cardiac or aortic procedures.

II. Induction of Anesthesia

A. Methods

1. **IV or mask induction**
   —of **general anesthesia** may be used.
2. **Children** frequently undergo a mask induction with volatile anesthetic gas before placement of an IV, whereas **adults** most often undergo an IV induction.
3. **A variable combination of agents** is based on patient characteristics and the surgical procedure.
   —These include **an amnestic, analgesic, hypnotic, muscle relaxant,** and **volatile agent.**
4. **A "rapid sequence" induction**
   —is performed by sequential IV administration of fast-acting agents with rapid endotracheal intubation.
   a. **Pre-oxygenation with 100% oxygen**
      —allows de-nitrogenation of the patient's functional residual volume.
      —provides extra time for airway management before arterial oxygen desaturation occurs.
   b. **Indications for rapid sequence induction include**
      —**recent oral intake.**
      —**symptomatic gastroesophageal reflux disease (GERD).**
      —delayed gastric emptying (e.g., gastroparesis) or previous gastrectomy.
      —pregnancy.
      —**bowel obstruction.**

B. Analgesic agents

1. **Analgesic agents are generally administered**
   —in boluses at induction and before surgical incision, then in maintenance doses as needed.
2. **Additional doses may be administered**
   —based upon signs of the **sympathetic response to pain,** such as increasing heart rate and blood pressure.
3. **Fentanyl**
   —is a synthetic narcotic.

—has an onset of action in 2 minutes and peak effect in 5 minutes.

a. **This drug is metabolized**

—by the **liver.**

b. **Airway reflexes are blunted** with minimal cardiac depression.

—Like other narcotics, this may induce **respiratory arrest.**

4. **Morphine sulfate**

—is a narcotic.

—has a 5-minute onset of action and 20 minutes to peak effect.

a. **The active metabolites are cleared** by the **kidney.**

—Therefore morphine should be used cautiously in patients with impaired renal function.

b. **This may cause histamine release**

—and associated mild hypotension.

5. **Alfentanil, sufentanil, and remifentanil**

—are synthetic narcotics.

—have very fast onset and progressively shorter durations of action.

6. **Ketamine**

—is a phencyclidine (PCP) analog.

a. **This drug provides intense**

—analgesia.

—amnesia.

—**dissociative anesthesia.**

b. **It also**

—generally increases heart rate and blood pressure.

—**maintains spontaneous ventilation.**

—is an excellent **bronchodilator.**

c. **Illusions and dysphoria are common**

—but can be limited by premedicating with a benzodiazepine.

d. **Ketamine**

—is not a respiratory depressant.

—may be given as the sole anesthetic agent.

—is one of several agents used for induction of anesthesia (**Table 1-2**).

C. **Sedative–hypnotic agents**

1. **Sodium thiopental** (see Table 1–2)

—is a barbiturate.

—induces unconsciousness within 30 seconds without providing analgesia.

—reduces cerebral oxygen demand and is an excellent **anticonvulsant.**

a. **After a single dose,** drug redistribution into muscle may result in rapid awakening.

—Therefore frequent repeated dosing is necessary.

b. **Side effects include**

—**hypotension** that may be profound in the setting of hypovolemia.

—heart failure.

—beta-blockade.

c. **Thiopental may also cause**

—**respiratory arrest.**

2. **Propofol** (see Table 1–2)

—is also a fast-acting agent.

—does not produce a "hangover" effect, thus it is ideal for outpatient surgeries.

—possesses antipyretic and **antiemetic properties.**

a. **Rapid metabolism**

—occurs via the **liver** and plasma esterases.

b. **Side effects include**

—**hypotension.**

—blunting of airway reflexes facilitating intubation.

—respiratory arrest.

c. **This drug may be used**

—to maintain anesthesia.

—in the intensive care unit to provide sedation.

d. **Propofol**

—is suspended in a 10% lipid solution providing 1.1 kCal/mL.

3. **Etomidate** (see Table 1-2)

—is a fast-acting hypnotic agent.

—is commonly used for induction when hypotension must be minimized.

a. **Rapid metabolism**

—is via the **liver** and plasma esterases.

b. **Continuous infusions**

—are avoided because of the risk of **adrenocortical suppression.**

c. **Other side effects**

—include **myoclonus.**

4. **Benzodiazepines**

a. **These drugs provide**

Table 1-2. Anesthetic Induction Agents

Agent	Blood Pressure	Metabolism	Analgesia	Onset	Actions and Effects
Ketamine	Stable	Liver	Potent	Fast	Illusions and dysphoria
Sodium thiopental	Decreased	Liver	None	Fast	Antiseizure
Propofol	Decreased	Liver and plasma esterases	Mild	Fast	Antiseizure, infusions
Etomidate	Stable	Liver and plasma esterases	None	Fast	Adrenocortico depressant

—anxiolysis.
—hypnosis.
—amnesia.
—anticonvulsant effects.
—some skeletal muscle relaxation.

b. **They do not provide**
—analgesic properties.

c. **The most commonly used benzodiazepine**
—is the short-acting agent, **midazolam.**

d. **These agents**
—are hepatically metabolized.
—may have prolonged activity in geriatric patients and patients with liver failure.

e. **Morphine agents may cause**
—**respiratory arrest,** especially when combined with a narcotic.

f. **Flumazenil** is a **benzodiazepine antagonist** used to treat overdoses.
—However, this agent may be associated with seizure development.

D. Muscle relaxants (Table 1–3)

1. **Muscle relaxation is often used**
—to facilitate **endotracheal intubation.**
—during abdominal surgery.
—when movement could be devastating (neurosurgery).

2. These drugs do not posses properties of analgesia, hypnosis, or amnesia.
—Patients are paralyzed, but will still feel and remember the surgery.

3. **Relaxants** are divided into **depolarizing** and **nondepolarizing** agents.
—**Depolarizing** agents cause an initial transient muscle fiber activation before relaxation occurs.

4. **Succinylcholine**

Table 1-3. Neuromuscular Blocking Agents

Agent	Depolarizing Blockade Fasiculations	Metabolism	Increased Serum Potassium	Activity
Succinylcholine	+	Pseudocholinesterase	+	**Fastest onset and shortest duration**
Rocuronium	–	Liver	–	Fastest onset of nondepolarizers
Pancuronium	–	Renal	–	Longest acting
Cis-atracurium	–	Nonenzymatic breakdown	–	**Action not prolonged in renal or liver disease**
Mivacurium	–	Pseudocholinesterase	–	Brief duration

—provides rapid **depolarizing** neuromuscular blockade.

a. **This agent**

—mimics acetylcholine.

—has a rapid onset of **30 seconds.**

—has a short duration of action (5–10 minutes).

b. **It is rapidly metabolized**

—by **plasma pseudocholinesterase.**

c. **Patients with abnormal pseudocholinesterase**

—may have prolonged paralysis after administration of succinylcholine.

(1) About 1 in 3000 patients are homozygous for this trait.

(2) The onset of this effect is heralded by muscle **fasciculations.**

d. Cellular potassium release from initial muscle fiber activation causes an **increase in serum potassium** that can be dangerous in some patients.

—Patients with the potential for a greatly exaggerated increase in serum potassium are at risk for **hyperkalemic cardiac arrest.**

e. **Conditions where this agent is contraindicated include**

—**denervation injuries** (e.g., stroke).

—**myopathy.**

—major burn injuries.

—severe trauma.

—potentially undiagnosed myopathy (i.e., children).

—bedridden states.

f. **Malignant hyperthermia**

—is a rare complication associated with succinylcholine administration.

—is an **autosomal dominant hypermetabolic disorder of skeletal muscle.**

(1) **The combination**

—of volatile anesthetics and succinylcholine most frequently triggers this disorder.

(2) **Manifestations** may include

—acidosis.

—trismus/masseter **muscle spasm.**

—**hypercapnia.**

—**tachycardia.**

—**rapid temperature elevation.**

—hypertension.

—arrhythmias.

—hypoxemia.

—hyperkalemia.

—myoglobinuria.

(3) **Treatment** involves

—discontinuing the volatile agent.

—cooling the patient.

—IV **dantrolene.**

5. **The nondepolarizing neuromuscular blocking agents** include

—rocuronium.

—pancuronium.

—vecuronium.

—atracurium.

—mivacurium.

a. **These agents**

—competitively **inhibit acetylcholine** at the neuromuscular junction.

b. **These agents do not cause**

—fasciculations.

—an increase in serum potassium.

c. **Rocuronium**

—has the fastest onset (45–60 seconds).

—is often substituted for rapid sequence induction when succinylcholine is contraindicated.

d. **Pancuronium**

—is inexpensive and used when prolonged paralysis is needed.

(1) This agent blocks autonomic ganglia, resulting in a mild **tachycardia.**

(2) Clearance is dramatically prolonged in renal failure.

e. **Atracurium**

—undergoes **esterase elimination.**

—does not require the kidney or liver for metabolism.

f. **Mivacurium** metabolism is dependent on **pseudocholinesterase.**

g. **All agents are potentiated by**

—hypokalemia.

—hypocalcemia.

—hypermagnesemia.

h. **The degree of neuromuscular blockade**

—can be monitored by **peripheral nerve stimulation.**

i. **To reverse neuromuscular blockade**

—**acetylcholinesterase inhibitors** (e.g., neostigmine) given with an **anticholinergic** (e.g., glycopyrrolate) to counteract bradycardia are often administered at the end of a surgery.

III. Airway

A. Mask ventilation

—is used at the time of induction.

—can be the sole means of airway management in a patient with minimal risk of aspiration.

1. **The head and jaw**

   —must be positioned appropriately to open the airway and to avoid collapse of soft tissues.

2. **Ventilation can also be facilitated**

   —by either **an oral or a nasal airway device (Figure 1.2).**

   a. **Oral airway devices**

      —**prevent the tongue from obstructing the oropharynx.**

   b. **Insertion of nasal airway devices**

      —may be tolerated by an awake patient.

B. A laryngeal mask airway (LMA) device

—is designed to lodge in the hypopharynx superior to the larynx.

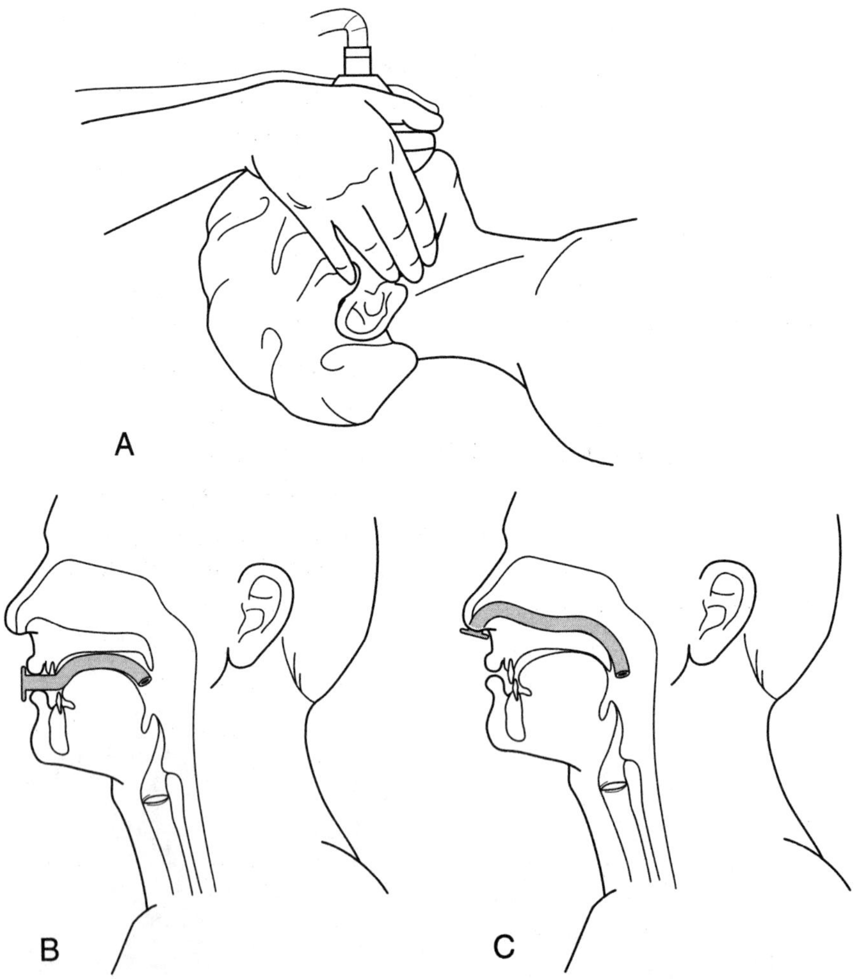

Figure 1.2. Interventions providing airway patency without endotracheal intubation. All of these measures alleviate obstruction often caused by the tongue allowing for ventilation, but these do not protect against aspiration. *(A)* Mask ventilation with jaw thrust. *(B)* Oropharyngeal airway device. *(C)* Nasopharyngeal airway device. (Adapted with permission from Dorsch JA, Dorsch SE: *Understanding Anesthesia Equipment: Construction, Care, and Complications.* Baltimore, Williams & Wilkins, 1994, p 371.)

—prevents soft tissue obstruction of the airway.

1. **The LMA can be used**

   —to ventilate a patient with up to 20 cm H_20 pressure (the competency of the upper esophageal sphincter).

2. **This device is contraindicated**

   —in patients at risk for aspiration.

   —in cases where paralysis, controlled ventilation, or both, are necessary.

C. Endotracheal intubation

—involves placement of a tube through the vocal cords into the trachea under direct visualization.

1. **Placement of an ETT allows for**

   —ventilatory support.

   —oxygenation.

   —relative protection of the airway from aspiration.

2. **Tube position may be confirmed by**

   —observing bilateral chest rising with ventilation.

   —looking for condensation of breaths within the ETT.

3. **Continuous measurement of end-tidal CO_2**

   —may also confirm appropriate placement of the tube within the trachea.

4. **If a patient appears difficult to intubate**

   —the safest option is to allow for spontaneous ventilation and intubate with topical airway anesthetics and minimal sedation.

5. **Fiberoptic laryngoscopy**

   —can aid in the intubation of the difficult airway, especially in patients with head and neck injuries.

IV. Inhalational Anesthetics

A. After induction

—anesthesia is maintained with a **volatile anesthetic.**

B. The volatile anesthetics provide

—hypnosis.

—amnesia.

—some degree of analgesia and muscle relaxation.

C. The agents differ in

—blood solubility.

—potency.

—side effect profiles.

1. **The minimum alveolar concentration (MAC)**

—is the smallest concentration of anesthetic at which 50% of patients will not move in response to surgical incision.

2. **The MAC of the agents**

—are generally additive, while the side effects are not.

—Combining different agents to optimize the MAC while minimizing potential side effects is referred to as **balanced anesthesia.**

3. **The solubility of the agent**

—within the blood correlates with **speed of induction.**

—Thus **insoluble agents** provide the quickest onset.

D. **The volatile agents commonly used today** include

—**halothane.**

—**isoflurane.**

—**sevoflurane.**

—**desflurane** (Table 1-4).

E. **Side effects**

1. **Cardiovascular**

a. **All of these agents cause hypotension**

—either through depression of myocardial contractility (e.g., halothane) or via vasodilation.

b. **These agents, particularly halothane**

—tend to be **arrhythmogenic,** an effect potentiated in many cases by epinephrine.

c. **Isoflurane is often preferred**

—for patients with cardiac disease because it causes the least cardiac depression and the most coronary artery dilation.

Table 1-4. Inhalational Anesthetic Agents

Agent*	**Blood Pressure**	**Muscle Relaxation**	**Broncho-dilatation**	**Expands Air Cavities**	**Misc.**
Halothane	Decreased cardiac output	+	+	−	Rarely causes **hepatitis**
Isoflurane	Decreased vascular resistance	+	+	−	Used in cardiac and CNS surgery
Sevoflurane	Decreased vascular resistance	+	+	−	Used in mask inductions
Desflurane	Decreased vascular resistance	+	+	−	Irritating to airway
Nitrous oxide (N_2O)	Stable	−	−	+	Mask analgesia

CNS = central nervous system.
*The agents are listed in order of **decreasing blood solubility (faster induction and emergence)** and also in order of **decreasing potency (higher percentage of inhaled gas required for effect).**

2. **Respiratory**
   a. **Volatile agents cause**
      —rapid shallow breathing, resulting in a net **decrease in minute ventilation.**
      —**bronchodilation.**
   b. **All agents severely blunt hypoxic drive**
      —and to a lesser degree, blunt hypercapnic drive, in subanesthetic concentrations.
3. **Central nervous system**
   a. **These agents**
      —**impair cerebral autoregulation,** or the ability of the brain vasculature to control blood flow over a wide range of blood pressures.
   b. **Isoflurane**
      —used in conjunction with hyperventilation minimizes the impaired autoregulation.
      —is used in patients with **increased intracranial pressure.**
4. **Halothane**
   —can rarely cause a chemical **hepatitis.**
5. **All volatile agents cause**
   —**significant muscle relaxation** independent of paralytic agents.

F. **Nitrous oxide (N_2O)**

—requires high inhalational concentrations (not potent).

—is **insoluble in blood.**

1. **Cardiac effects**
   —N_20 causes **minimal cardiac depression.**
   —It generally does not alter blood pressure.
2. **Respiratory effects**
   —This agent shares many of the respiratory effects of the volatile agents.
   —However, it is not bronchodilatory and causes an increase in pulmonary vascular resistance.
3. **This agent does not**
   —provide muscle relaxation.
4. **Administration of N_20 may expand air cavities**
   —by diffusing in faster than nitrogen diffuses out.
5. This agent should be avoided in patients with
   —a **pneumothorax.**
   —intracranial air.
   —**intestinal obstruction.**
   —middle ear occlusion.

V. Regional Anesthesia

A. Overview

1. **Many surgeries can be successfully performed**
   —with neuraxial or peripheral application of local anesthetics.
2. **Regional anesthesia may also be used**
   —for **postoperative pain relief.**
3. **Upper extremity regional blocks** include
   —intrascalene.
   —supraclavicular.
   —**axillary nerve blocks.**
4. **A femoral nerve block** can be used for lower extremity anesthesia.
5. **A Bier block** involves **IV injection of local anesthetic** for upper and occasionally lower extremity anesthesia.
   —Before IV injection of anesthetic into the designated extremity, the venous system is emptied by compression with elastic wraps and a tourniquet is placed to block arterial inflow.
6. **Neuraxial blockade** involves
   —injection of anesthetic into either the **epidural or subarachnoid spaces.**
7. **Contraindications shared by the Bier and neuraxial blocks** include
   —local or systemic infection.
   —coagulopathy.
   —hypotension.
8. **Complications** include
   —headache.
   —urinary retention.
   —rarely, epidural or intraspinal hematomas or infection.
   a. **Postpuncture dural headaches**
      —are positional, being much worse when the patient is upright.
   b. **Treatment of these headaches** includes
      —bedrest.
      —hydration.
      —analgesics.
      —caffeine.
      —epidural blood patching.
   c. For an **epidural blood patch,** peripherally drawn blood is injected into the epidural space at the dural puncture site to seal the injured dura.

B. Spinal anesthesia (Figure 1.3)

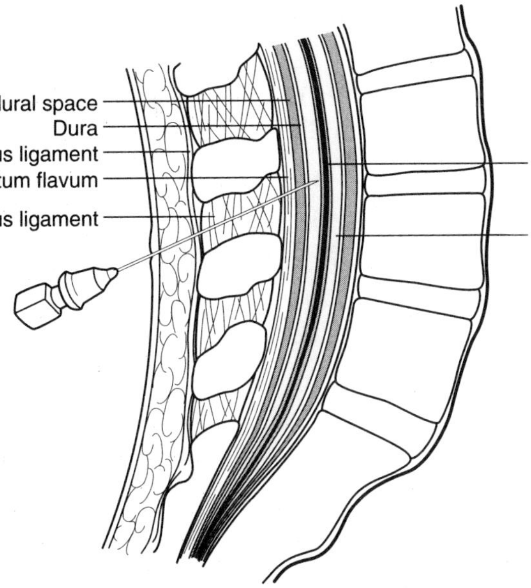

Figure 1-3. Lumbar spinal versus epidural anesthesia. (Reprinted with permission from Morgan E, Mikhail N: *Clinical Anesthesiology,* 2nd ed. Stamford, CT, Appleton & Lange, 1996, p 222.)

1. **A small gauge needle (e.g., < 22 gauge)**

   —designed to minimize dural trauma is usually inserted midline in the **L3–L4 interspace.**

2. **Free flow of cerebrospinal fluid (CSF)**

   —confirms **subarachnoid placement** where local anesthetic is injected.

3. **Anesthesia**

   —**onset occurs within minutes.**

   —**can last up to 2 hours** depending on the agent and dosage.

4. **The level of sympathetic blockade**

   —**is typically higher** than the level of sensory block.

   a. This is, in turn, above the level of motor block.

   b. These differences are caused by variations in nerve size and myelination.

5. **Sympathetic blockade results** in **hypotension** that may be profound.

6. **Excessively high spinal anesthesia** may cause **respiratory depression.**

7. **Motor function** typically recovers before sensation.

8. **Small doses of narcotics**

   —can also be injected intrathecally to provide analgesia or to augment local anesthetic action.

9. **A "saddle block"**

   —provides anesthesia to the perineum by using hyperbaric solutions (solutions more dense than CSF) to block the sacral dermatomes.

C. **Epidural anesthesia**

1. **A catheter**

—**may be placed** in the **epidural space,** allowing for continuous infusion of anesthetic agent to relieve perioperative pain or labor pain.

2. **Dilute concentrations of anesthetic**

—allow for **sparing of motor function.**

3. **The final level of sensory blockade**

—is related to the **volume injected,** which is in contrast to spinal anesthesia, where it is related to dosage.

4. **The onset of blockade**

—occurs more slowly than with spinal anesthesia.

5. **A caudal block**

—involves placement of anesthetic into the epidural space through the **sacral hiatus.**

D. **Local anesthetics**

—may be infiltrated in a wound to provide local pain relief.

1. **The most common agents are**

—**lidocaine.**

—**ropivacaine.**

—**bupivacaine.**

a. **These agents may be associated with**

—**seizures and severe refractory arrhythmias** if injected intravascularly, particularly **bupivacaine.**

b. **Early manifestations may include**

—perioral numbness.

—visual and hearing disturbances.

—sedation.

2. **Epinephrine-induced local vasoconstriction** may prolong the anesthetic effects of these agents.

—Epinephrine with local anesthetics should be used cautiously in patients with **cardiac disease,** uncontrolled hypertension, or when infiltrating tissues with minimal collateral blood flow (e.g., **digits, ears, nose, penis**).

VI. Pain Management

A. **Patient controlled analgesia (PCA)**

—is often used for postoperative pain relief.

1. **Narcotics**

—are self-administered by the patient through a device that allows a **selected dose** to be delivered at specific time intervals to a **preset maximum.**

2. **The pump can also be set**
   —to deliver a **basal rate** of medication per hour.
3. **PCA is designed to**
   —provide better pain control.
   —avoid over-medication of the patient.

B. Pain management clinics

—specialize in the treatment of **chronic pain.**

1. **Components of treatment of chronic pain**
   —routinely include **psychological evaluation and therapy.**
2. **Narcotics are avoided when possible in favor of other agents including**
   —nonsteroidal anti-inflammatory agents.
   —antiseizure medications (e.g., gabapentin).
   —antidepressant medications (e.g., amitriptyline).
3. **Regional anesthetic techniques**
   —are also frequently used.

Review Test

Directions: Each of the numbered items or incomplete statements in this section is followed by answers or by completions of the statement. Select the ONE lettered answer or completion that is BEST in each case.

1. At emergence from an uncomplicated general anesthetic for a laparoscopic appendectomy, an otherwise healthy 19-year-old male smoker develops a severe cough. Intravenous lidocaine is administered and the endotracheal tube is pulled before the patient is responsive to verbal commands. The patient becomes cyanotic and the SaO_2 is 75%. The anesthesiologist is unable to administer positive pressure mask ventilation. What is the most appropriate initial step in the management of this patient?

(A) Intravenous naloxone
(B) Deepen anesthetic depth
(C) Re-intubate the patient
(D) Intravenous succinylcholine
(E) Intravenous fentanyl

2. A 27-year-old woman with gastroesophageal reflux disease (GERD) undergoes a rapid sequence anesthetic induction for an anterior cruciate ligament repair. She is pre-oxygenated with 100% oxygen (4 deep breaths) and induced with propofol, lidocaine, and fentanyl. Succinylcholine is administered and cricoid pressure applied. The endotracheal tube (ETT) is placed with direct laryngoscopy to 20 cm at the teeth and the SaO_2 is 100%. What is the most reliable indication of ETT placement in the trachea?

(A) Persistent $ETCO_2$ measurement with ventilation
(B) Bilateral breath sounds with ventilation
(C) Breath condensation in the ETT
(D) Absence of sound over the epigastrium with ventilation
(E) SaO_2 of 100% immediately after intubation

3. A 40-year-old woman with Type I diabetes mellitus and end-stage renal disease is scheduled for an arteriovenous fistula repair. She refuses a regional anesthetic technique (axillary block). She undergoes a rapid-sequence induction with cricoid pressure to lessen the chance of gastric content aspiration, and after much difficulty an endotracheal tube is correctly placed and the cuff inflated. Two hours after an uneventful anesthetic the patient remains somnolent and intubated in the postanesthetic care unit with a respiration rate of 10/min. An arterial blood gas reveals hypercapnia ($PaCO_2$ of 65) and an acidosis (pH 7.2). What anesthetic agent is most likely responsible for this patient's prolonged anesthesia?

(A) Pancuronium
(B) Morphine
(C) Fentanyl
(D) Isoflurane
(E) Midazolam

4. A surgeon is performing a laparoscopic cholecystectomy on an obese 35-year-old woman under general anesthesia with endotracheal intubation. The anesthetic is maintained with isoflurane, fentanyl, and rocuronium. The surgeon repetitively asks for more "relaxation" to better visualize the field. The patient has no response to peripheral nerve stimulation and is hemodynamically stable. Which of the following may provide additional relaxation in this setting?

(A) Additional fentanyl
(B) Adding nitrous oxide to anesthetic
(C) Increasing isoflurane concentration
(D) Additional rocuronium
(E) Administering intravenous thiopental

5. During intubation, a 21-year-old paraplegic patient is given succinylcholine. The patient demonstrates fasciculations and the vocal cords are easily visualized with a laryngoscope with subsequent placement of the endotracheal tube. Peaked T waves and intermittent ectopy are then noted on the electrocardiogram. What is the most appropriate first step in this patient's management?

(A) Administration of a beta-agonist
(B) Administration of insulin and glucose
(C) Oral exchange resin
(D) Administration of calcium chloride
(E) Administration of sodium bicarbonate

6. A 40-year-old man with epiglottitis is intubated at an outside hospital and sent to the emergency room for evaluation. The transport team states that the patient became combative during the trip and was given more "sedative" and strapped more securely to the stretcher. During your examination you notice that the patient can blink his eyes to command but is unable to move any extremities nor make respiratory effort. He blinks affirmatively to your query if he is in pain. You administer a narcotic and a benzodiazapine. What is the most likely cause of paralysis?

(A) A C2 cord lesion
(B) Meningitis
(C) Guillain-Barré syndrome
(D) Subarachnoid hemorrhage
(E) Muscle relaxant

Questions 7–8

A 24-year-old man is transported to the emergency room after a motor vehicle accident. He is alert and hemodynamically stable, but has an obvious right femur fracture. He is brought to the operating room for an open reduction of the fracture. He undergoes a rapid sequence induction with sodium thiopental, fentanyl, and succinylcholine; the anesthetic is maintained with nitrous oxide and isoflurane. During surgery the ventilation pressures begin to rise while the blood pressure begins to fall. Auscultation reveals decreased breath sounds on the right. A right thoracostomy tube is placed, relieving a tension pneumothorax.

7. Which agent most likely contributed to the pneumothorax?

(A) Fentanyl
(B) Sodium thiopental
(C) Nitrous oxide
(D) Isoflurane
(E) Succinylcholine

8. The N_20 is discontinued, the isoflurane inspired concentration increased, and the newly inserted chest tube is left to water seal while the patient continues to receive positive pressure ventilation. The surgery continues and the femoral artery is found to be lacerated. The patient suffers severe hemorrhage and becomes hypotensive. Isoflurane is discontinued and a small dose of midazolam is given for amnesia. Which of the following is the most appropriate muscle relaxant to administer at this time to avoid excessive hypotension?

(A) Pancuronium
(B) Succinylcholine
(C) Atracurium
(D) Rocuronium
(E) Mivacurium

Answers and Explanations

1–D. The anesthesiologist is probably unable to ventilate the patient because the patient is in laryngospasm. Intravenous (IV) lidocaine is effective at preventing and treating laryngospasm but smokers have particularly reactive airways that predispose to coughing and laryngospasm at emergence. IV or intramuscular succinylcholine can rapidly relieve the spasm. Partial laryngospasm (stridor) often responds to gentle positive pressure ventilation, deepening the anesthetic volatile agent, or both. An initial attempt at intubation would likely be unsuccessful and can worsen the spasm. Neither naloxone nor fentanyl is likely to have much effect. Healthy adults can generate enough negative intrathoracic pressure against a closed glottis that they can suffer postobstructive pulmonary edema.

2–A. Esophageal intubation is only a disaster if unrecognized. Ideally, the endotracheal tube (ETT) is placed through the vocal cords under direct vision. Bilateral breath sounds and ETT condensation can sometimes occur with esophageal intubation. Persistent $ETCO_2$ tracings with ventilation confirms tube placement in the trachea. Tracheal breath sounds can radiate to the epigastrium. One-sided breath sounds represent mainstem intubation, usually right-sided. With optimal pre-oxygenation a healthy individual can take over 5 minutes to desaturate.

3–B. The metabolites of morphine accumulate in renal failure and can produce prolonged narcosis, evidenced by somnolence, a slow respiratory rate, hypercapnia, and a corresponding respiratory acidosis. Pancuronium clearance is also prolonged in renal failure but does not produce somnolence. Fentanyl and midazolam provide analgesia and sedation, respectively, but do not accumulate in renal failure. Isoflurane elimination is dependent on ventilation.

4–C. Additional paralytic agents provide no further clinical relaxation effect after abolishing neuromuscular stimulation, but do make reversal of paralysis impossible until a response returns as the paralytic agent is eliminated. The volatile agents (isoflurane), unlike nitrous oxide, barbiturate (thiopental), or narcotics (fentanyl), do provide muscle relaxation independently of neuromuscular blockers (rocuronium), but it is unclear if they would have much additional effect in this scenario.

5–D. Calcium is thought to play a cardioprotective role in the event of hyperkalemia by preventing life-threatening arrhythmias. Additionally, hyperventilation can be started immediately if the patient is intubated because the respiratory alkalosis will lower serum potassium. The other agents listed should also be administered as quickly as possible to decrease serum potassium, however, none of them provide the immediate cardioprotective effect seen with calcium.

6–E. Muscle relaxants are successful in making a restless patient remain still, and thus are mistakenly thought by some to possess sedative or analgesic properties. They do not impair consciousness or memory, and most importantly, they do not provide any analgesia. The history and initial physical findings are inconsistent with a C2 cord lesion or a subarachnoid hemorrhage. Meningitis is unlikely to be associated with such paralysis without significant depression of the level of consciousness. Guillain-Barré syndrome would not present in such an acute fashion.

7–C. Nitrous oxide (N_20) diffuses into air cavities faster than nitrogen can diffuse out. Therefore, expansion of such potential spaces will continue until the concentration of N_20 in the cavity approaches the inspired N_20 concentration. Other volatile anesthetic agents such as isoflurane and the other agents mentioned are not associated with expansion of air cavities.

8–A. Pancuronium provides a mild vasoconstrictive effect that is useful when the patient is initially hypotensive and thus prone to worsening hypotension with many other anesthetics. In addition, pancuronium also provides long-lasting muscle relaxation that is important for preventing sudden movement in response to surgical stimulation during long delicate operations. The other agents listed may augment the hypotension.

2

Surgical Complications

Patrick J. O'Neill

I. General Principles

—Surgical complications may be defined as any deviation from the normal expected postoperative recovery.

A. Most complications result from

—poor operative technique.

—magnitude of the operation.

—general medical condition of the patient.

—chronic medications taken by the patient.

B. One complication may follow another.

—For example, myocardial infarction may occur secondary to anemia from acute hemorrhage.

C. Surgical care

—**should be well planned** at the preoperative, intraoperative, and postoperative level (Table 2-1).

D. Prevention of complications

—remains the best form of management.

1. Nutritional care

a. Optimizing the patient's preoperative nutritional status

—will help decrease the rate of many postoperative complications.

b. Weight loss

—in obese patients decreases the risk of wound and pulmonary complications.

2. Pulmonary care

a. Cessation of smoking

Table 2-1. The Stages of Complete Surgical Care

Preoperative	Understand all surgical and anesthetic options and risks Understand the patient's general medical condition and potential dangers Try to improve general health of the patient (e.g., nutrition, smoking cessation) Have a thorough knowledge of the patient's current medications
Intraoperative	Use meticulous surgical technique and minimize time under anesthesia Optimize the patient's physiological condition and vital signs Use appropriate antithromboembolic and anti-infective measures
Postoperative	Frequently examine and closely monitor the patient Detect and correct any abnormalities early Normalize the patient as soon as possible (e.g., early ambulation, enteral feeding when possible) Remove surgical tubes as quickly as possible Administer appropriate postoperative pain control

—6 weeks before surgery will decrease the incidence of pulmonary complications from 50% to 10%.

b. Early postoperative ambulation and aggressive respiratory therapy

—may help prevent pulmonary complications.

II. Complications Specifically Related to Surgery

A. Bleeding

1. Postsurgical bleeding is most often caused by the **lack of adequate hemostasis** at the time of surgery.

—The absence of bleeding from other sites suggests surgical bleeding rather than an underlying coagulopathy.

2. Risk factors include

—perioperative anticoagulant therapy.

—vigorous coughing or excess activity.

—poor blood pressure control.

—an **underlying coagulopathy.**

3. Forms of surgical bleeding

a. Hematoma formation

(1) Small hematomas

—may be observed because they may resorb without complication.

(2) Large hematomas

—and those in compromising locations (e.g., neck, mediastinum) require operative evacuation.

b. Hemoperitoneum

—is defined as a collection of blood within the abdominal cavity.

—is the **most common cause of hypovolemic shock** in the first 24 hours after abdominal surgery.

(1) **Signs and symptoms** include
—low-grade fever.
—tachycardia.
—hypotension.
—oliguria.
—peripheral vasoconstriction.

(2) **Diagnosis**
—Worsening anemia or persistent anemia despite blood transfusion is suggestive of the diagnosis.
—Computed tomography (CT) scanning can confirm the diagnosis when it is suspected.
—CT scanning should not be performed in a hemodynamically unstable patient.

(3) **Treatment** consists of
—appropriate **volume resuscitation.**
—**correction of coagulopathy** if one exists.
—**re-operation** to obtain hemostasis.

4. **Underlying coagulopathies**
—can frequently contribute to perioperative bleeding.
—require treatment specific for the disorder (Table 2-2).

a. **Preoperative history**
—is the most reliable measure for determining the presence of a coagulopathy.

b. **Risk factors** include
—**positive family history** for inherited coagulopathies.
—**abnormal bleeding** with normal activities (e.g., brushing teeth) or abnormal menstrual bleeding.
—**abnormal bleeding** after minor procedures or trauma.
—**medications** (e.g., aspirin, dipyridamole, warfarin, heparin).
—**positive medical/surgical history** of conditions predisposing to coagulopathies.

c. **Appropriate treatment measures**
—for managing coagulopathies are also included in Table 2-2.

B. **Wound problems**

1. **Hematoma formation** (see section II A 3 a)

2. **Seroma**
—Seroma is a collection of fluid in the wound usually secondary to **liquefaction of necrotic fat** or disruption of lymphatic drainage.
—**Large seromas** may **delay wound healing** and **increase the risk of infection.**

a. **Risk factors** include
—skin flap formation.
—inadequate wound closure.

Table 2-2. Characteristics and Treatment of Coagulopathies in Surgical Patients

Disease	Etiology	Signs and Symptoms	Treatment
Congenital coagulopathy			
Hemophilia A (classic hemophilia)	X-linked factor VIII deficiency	Elevated PTT, hemarthrosis	Cryoprecipitate, factor VIII
Hemophilia B (Christmas disease)	X-linked factor IX deficiency	Elevated PTT	Cryoprecipitate
Von Willebrand's (vW) disease	Factor VIII: vW deficiency	Increased bleeding time, with or without elevated PTT	Cryoprecipitate, DDAVP
Acquired coagulopathy			
Vitamin K deficiency	Dietary deficiency, malabsorption	Elevated PT	Vitamin K, FFP
Liver failure	Decreased factor production	Elevated PT/PTT	Vitamin K, FFP
Hypothermia	Impaired factor	Elevated PT/PTT	Rewarming, FFP
Heparin therapy	Promotes antithrombin III activity function	Elevated PTT	Protamine
Warfarin therapy	Vitamin K antagonism	Elevated PT	Vitamin K, FFP
Dilutional	Massive crystalloid or blood transfusion	Elevated PT/PTT, thrombocytopenia	Platelets, FFP
DIC	Trauma, sepsis, burns, malignancy, obstetrical complications, anaphylaxis	Diffuse bleeding, elevated PT/PTT, decreased fibrinogen, increased FDP and D-dimers, thrombocytopenia	Treat primary cause, supportive care, cryoprecipitate, vitamin K, FFP, platelets, antithrombin III
Platelet disorders			
Thrombocytopenia	Platelet counts >40,000 typically ensure hemostasis	Petechiae, mucocutaneous bleeding, prolonged bleeding time	Platelets
Poor function (uremia, aspirin)	Variable	Petechiae, mucocutaneous bleeding, prolonged bleeding time	Dialysis, DDAVP, cryoprecipitate, conjugated estrogens

DDAVP = 1-deamino-8-D-arginine vasopressin; DIC = disseminated intravascular coagulation; FDP = fibrin degradation products; FFP = fresh frozen plasma; PT = prothrombin time; PTT = partial thromboplastin time.

—lymphatic disruption.

b. Treatment

—Generally, treatment involves **observation** because attempted drainage further increases the possibility of infection.

—**Persistent seromas** may represent a **lymphocele,** requiring surgical exploration and ligation of the injured lymphatic vessels.

3. Wound infection (see Chapter 4)

4. Dehiscence

—involves a partial or total **disruption of fascial layers** after surgical closure.

—occurs most commonly between postoperative days 5 and 8.

a. **Risk factors** include
   - —poor surgical technique (e.g., devascularization of tissue, inadequate closure).
   - —**increased intra-abdominal pressure** (e.g., obesity, bowel obstruction, ascites).
   - —**factors associated with deficient wound healing** (see Chapter 5).
   - —**advanced age.**
   - —**diabetes.**
   - —**renal failure.**
   - —**immunosuppression** (e.g., cancer, chronic steroid use).
   - —**hepatic failure.**

b. Dehiscence may frequently be **associated with**
   - —coughing.
   - —excessive activity.
   - —retching.

c. A **common sign** of dehiscence is
   - —sudden discharge **of serosanguinous fluid from the incision.**

d. **Evisceration**
   - —Evisceration is wound **dehiscence** with the **extrusion of abdominal contents.**
   - —Mortality with evisceration is greater than 10%.

e. **Treatment**
   - —of **partial dehiscence** generally involves elective fascial repair. Delayed repair is generally performed when a wound infection is present.
   - —of **evisceration** consists of **immediate wound coverage** with sterile, moist towels and **emergent surgical exploration and fascial repair.**

C. Postoperative pain

1. Normal postoperative pain

—should subside within 4–6 days.

2. Extraordinary pain may be associated with

—excessive **repetitive motion.**

—**wound infection.**

—occult dehiscence.

—granuloma or neuroma formation (rare).

3. Treatment involves

—early identification.

—management of the cause of persistent, severe pain.

III. System-Specific Complications

A. Central nervous system complications

1. **Focal neurologic signs noted postoperatively may be secondary to**
   —direct injury to the brain, spinal cord, or peripheral nerves.
   —complications of spinal, epidural, or regional anesthesia.
   —**focal ischemia or infarction** from an embolic or thrombotic source.
2. **Prolonged altered consciousness**
   —after general anesthesia may also result from poor metabolism of anesthetic agents.
   a. **Risk factors** include
      —advanced age.
      —renal or hepatic insufficiency.
      —obesity.
   b. **Differential diagnosis includes**
      —**hypoxic brain injury** or cerebral hypoperfusion.
      —diabetic coma or **hypoglycemic episodes.**
      —**strokes,** caused by hypertensive, embolic, or thrombotic injury.
3. **Postoperative seizures** may be secondary to
   —cerebral injury.
   —pre-existing seizure disorder.
   —metabolic abnormalities.
   —adverse medicine reactions.
   —delirium tremens.
   a. **Evaluation** includes
      —complete laboratory studies [complete blood count (CBC), electrolytes, liver function studies].
      —review of potential medicine interactions.
      —a CT scan of the head.
   b. **Treatment** includes
      —close observation with supplemental oxygen.
      —intravenous (IV) fluids.
      —correction of any metabolic abnormalities.
      —**anticonvulsants or benzodiazepines,** if seizures persist.
4. **Psychosis or delirium may be precipitated by**
   —anxiety.
   —sleep deprivation.
   —certain drugs (e.g., pain medications).
   —hypoxia.
   —electrolyte abnormalities.
   —alterations in body image as a result of surgery.
   a. The **incidence is higher**
      —**after cardiac surgery.**
      —in the **elderly.**
      —in those with **chronic disease.**

b. It generally occurs

—after postoperative day 3 and is frequently **preceded by a lucid interval.**

c. Characteristics include

—disorientation.

—memory impairment.

—disturbed speech, sleep, or psychomotor activity.

—**rapid onset, often at night.**

—signs or symptoms unrelated to a specific organic factor.

d. Treatment consists of

—identification and management of factors contributing to the psychosis or delirium as outlined in Table 2-3.

5. Withdrawal symptoms

—occurring after stopping mood-altering substances occur in patients at risk for substance dependence.

a. Signs and symptoms include

—personality changes.

—anxiety.

—diaphoresis.

—tachycardia.

—hypertension.

—tremor.

b. Time of onset depends on

—the half-life of the abused substance.

6. Delirium tremens

—is defined as a severe withdrawal syndrome precipitated by **sudden abstinence in an alcohol-dependent person.**

a. Findings include

—**hyperventilation.**

—**agitation.**

—overactivity.

—**confusion.**

—metabolic alkalosis.

—hypomagnesemia.

—hypokalemia.

—hallucinations and seizures (occur in the later stages).

Table 2-3. Risk Factors for Postoperative Psychosis or Delirium

- Surgery-associated effects (e.g., hypoxia, hypercapnia, hypotension, sepsis)
- Advanced age or baseline dementia
- Chronic drug or alcohol abuse
- Central nervous system lesions
- Metabolic disorders (e.g., uremia, heptic failure, acidosis)
- Medication side effects (e.g., meperidine, cimetidine, and corticosteroids)
- Sleep deprivation and loss of normal circadian rhythm

b. Treatment

(1) With proper treatment, the syndrome usually improves within 72 hours.

(2) Treatment includes

—**thiamine** (vitamin B_1).

—**magnesium.**

—**benzodiazepines.**

—**correction of nutritional deficiencies** or other **metabolic abnormalities.**

B. Pulmonary complications

—are the largest single cause of postoperative **morbidity.**

—are associated with the risk factors in Table 2-4.

1. Atelectasis

—represents a **partial collapse of alveoli.**

—accounts for 90% of postoperative pulmonary complications.

—occurs most frequently in the **first 48 hours** after surgery.

a. Ventilation/perfusion (V/Q) mismatches result in **relative hypoxemia.**

b. A **coexisting fever** is usually low-grade and self-limited.

c. Diagnosis is made by

—radiographic signs (e.g. characteristic discoid infiltrate, elevated hemidiaphragm).

—physical examination signs (e.g., **basilar crackles, decreased breath sounds**).

d. Preventive and therapeutic measures include

—**early mobilization.**

—**pulmonary therapy** (e.g., cough, deep breathing, incentive spirometry).

—**adequate pain control.**

Table 2-4. Risk Factors for Postoperative Pulmonary Complications

Patient co-morbidities	Advanced age Obesity Pre-existing chronic lung disease (e.g., COPD) History of smoking Poor cough effort postoperatively
Surgery-related factors	Long duration of anesthesia Prolonged mechanical ventilation Chest or upper abdominal surgery Abdominal distention Inadequate pain control
Iatrogenic factors	Oversedation or excessive narcotic analgesic use Endotracheal tube malposition

COPD = chronic obstructive pulmonary disease.

2. **Pneumonia** (see Chapter 4)

3. **Aspiration**

a. **Gastric secretions**

—are the usual source.

—result in a **chemical pneumonitis (Mendelson's syndrome).**

b. **Minor amounts of aspiration during surgery**

—are frequent and well tolerated.

c. **Significant aspiration**

—is normally prevented by the esophageal sphincters and the epiglottis.

d. **The magnitude of injury** is proportional to the

—volume of aspirate.

—frequency of aspiration.

—pH of aspirates.

e. **Aspiration pneumonia**

—is associated with a **high mortality.**

f. **Risk factors for aspiration** include

—decreased sensorium (e.g., head injury, narcosis).

—**nasogastric tube placement.**

—**intestinal obstruction.**

—**pregnancy** (caused by increased abdominal pressure and decreased lower esophageal sphincter tone secondary to progesterone).

g. **The lobes most frequently affected** include the

—posterior right upper lobe.

—superior right lower lobe because of the orientation of the right bronchus.

h. **Common signs** include

—tachypnea.

—crackles on examination.

—hypoxia.

i. **Treatment** involves

—appropriate airway control.

—aggressive airway hygiene.

—adequate fluid resuscitation.

(1) **Bronchoscopy**

—may be necessary to remove solid material.

(2) **Antibiotics**

—The use of antibiotics is controversial.

—Antibiotics should only be used for aspiration resulting in pneumonia and not for aspiration alone.

—The choice of agents should be based on culture results, although initial empiric therapy is often used to treat potential causative organisms (e.g., gastrointestinal or oral flora).

(3) **Prevention remains the most important strategy,** including

—preoperative fasting.
—proper patient positioning.
—careful intubation.

4. Pleural effusion

—is a collection of fluid in the pleural space.

a. Transudates versus exudates

(1) Properties and associated diseases

—are listed in Table 2-5.

(2) Gross blood in pleural fluid may represent

—iatrogenic vascular injuries.
—trauma.
—malignancy.
—pulmonary infarction.

b. Findings include

—dyspnea.
—decreased breath sounds.
—dullness to percussion on examination.
—radiographic evidence of pleural fluid.

c. Treatment options include

—**observation** of small asymptomatic effusions.
—**drainage** (e.g., thoracentesis, tube thoracostomy) for symptomatic cases (e.g., respiratory compromise).

C. Cardiac complications

1. Arrhythmias

—usually appear either intraoperatively or within 1–3 days postoperatively.

a. Intraoperative arrhythmias

—usually occur during **induction of anesthesia.**

(1) Risk factors include

—**type of anesthesia** (especially halothane).

Table 2-5. Properties of Pleural Effusion Fluid

Components	Transudate*	Exudate†
Protein	< 3 g/dL	> 3 g/dL
Specific gravity	< 1.016	> 1.016
LDH (effusion:serum)	< 0.5	> 0.6
Glucose	60% of serum level	Low
Amylase	Low	> 500 units/ml
RBC count	< 10,000 cells/mm^3	> 100,000 cells/mm^3
WBC count	< 1000 cells/mm^3	> 1000 cells/mm^3

LDH = lactate dehydrogenase; RBC = red blood cell; WBC = white blood cell.
*Transudates can be found in hepatic failure, nephrotic syndrome, congestive heart failure, viral infection, and severe lobar atelectasis.
†Exudates can be found in malignancy, empyema, abdominal infection, pancreatitis, trauma, pulmonary infarction, chylothorax, and tuberculosis.

—use of **sympathomimetics.**

—**digoxin toxicity.**

—**hypercapnia.**

—electrolyte abnormalities.

(2) **Treatment** involves

—correction of underlying abnormalities.

—occasional administration of antiarrhythmic agents.

b. **Postoperative arrhythmias may be associated with**

—hypokalemia.

—hypoxia.

—alkalosis.

—digoxin toxicity.

—sympathetic stimulation (i.e., pain).

—myocardial ischemia.

—invasive cardiac monitoring.

c. **Most patients are asymptomatic;** however, any patient with chest pain, palpitations, or dyspnea must be evaluated for a cardiac event.

2. **Postoperative hypertension**

—Postoperative hypertension may result from an exacerbation of underlying disease or may be secondary to **poor pain control.**

—**Treatment** involves resumption of home antihypertensive medications and adequate pain control.

3. **Myocardial infarction**

a. **The incidence is**

—0.4% in all patients undergoing surgery.

—5%–12% in patients having operations related to vascular disease (e.g., aortic aneurysm).

b. **Risk factors** include

—congestive heart failure.

—ischemic heart disease.

—age older than 70 years.

—significant atherosclerotic disease.

c. **Postoperative factors** include

—hypotension.

—anemia.

—hypoxemia.

d. **To decrease the risk for developing myocardial infarction**

—avoid hypotension and hypoxemia.

—administer perioperative beta-blockers.

e. **Signs and symptoms**

(1) Most patients are **initially asymptomatic** owing to residual anesthesia and analgesia.

(2) The signs and symptoms of myocardial infarction include

—**chest pain.**

—**hypotension.**

—a **new arrhythmia** associated with electrocardiogram (ECG) changes and elevated cardiac enzyme levels.

4. **Cardiac failure**

—may occur perioperatively in patients with marginal cardiac function.

a. **Risk factors** include

—volume overload.

—postoperative myocardial infarction.

—arrhythmias.

b. **Prevention and treatment** involves

—appropriate management of underlying cardiac disease.

—careful monitoring of the patient's volume status.

D. **Pancreatitis**

—occurs infrequently, however, approximately **10% of all pancreatitis cases are related to surgery.**

1. **The incidence is**

—1%–3% when the operative procedure is in the vicinity of the pancreas.

—greater than 1%–3% when the biliary tract is manipulated.

2. **Risk factors** include

—a history of pancreatitis.

—parathyroid surgery (i.e., acute changes in serum calcium levels).

—cardiopulmonary bypass.

—renal transplantation.

3. **Signs and symptoms** include

—fever.

—epigastric pain.

—hyperamylasemia.

—hypocalcemia.

—unexplained renal or respiratory compromise in a postoperative patient.

E. **Gastrointestinal complications**

1. **Acute gastritis and duodenitis**

—may occur in postoperative patients, particularly in the critically ill.

a. **Significant bleeding** may occur.

b. **Prevention involves**

—postoperative administration of agents that **inhibit acid production** (e.g., famotidine) or **augment the mucosal barrier** (e.g., sucralfate).

2. **Intestinal ileus**

—is a depression in the normal propulsive activity of the intestine by the enteric nervous system.

—frequently occurs after abdominal operations (see Chapter 13).

a. A slightly **distended abdomen** and **absent or hypoactive bowel sounds** are frequently present.

b. **Potential factors contributing to persistent ileus include**
—electrolyte abnormalities (hypokalemia).
—coexisting infection.
—excessive narcotic use.

c. **Treatment includes**
—correction of any contributing abnormality and patience.

3. **Anastomotic leaks**
—may result in **abscess formation, enterocutaneous fistulae** (see Chapter 13), or **diffuse peritonitis.**

a. **Risk factors include**
—**poor intestinal perfusion** (colonic anastomoses are at higher risk because of their more tenuous blood supply).
—**technical failure** (e.g., excessive tension, devascularization during repair).
—**concurrent infection or inflammation.**
—**distal obstruction.**

b. **Some large bowel anastomotic leaks**
—are well localized.
—can be managed with percutaneous drainage of potential fluid collections without the need for surgery.

c. **Other leaks**
—are not well localized.
—require reoperation for prevention and treatment of potential sequelae of anastomotic breakdown.

4. **Other gastrointestinal complications may include**
—postoperative colitis (see Chapter 4).
—mechanical obstruction.
—intussusception.
—colonic pseudo-obstruction (Ogilvie's syndrome) [see Chapter 13].

F. **Acute renal failure (ARF)**
—is generally defined as an **abrupt impairment in renal function** associated with elevations in plasma creatinine (Cr) and urea.

1. **Low urine output is frequently present**
—**oliguria** (defined as less than 0.5 mL/kg urine output per hour) or **anuria.**

2. **Characteristics of ARF**
—in surgical patients are outlined in **Table 2-6.**

3. **Hypovolemia**
—is the most common cause of ARF in surgical patients.

a. **The fractional excretion of Na^+ (FE_{Na})**
—may help differentiate prerenal causes of renal failure from other causes.

b. **The formula for determining FE_{Na} is**

Table 2-6. Causes, Diagnosis, and Treatment of Acute Renal Failure in Surgical Patients

Causes	Diagnosis	Treatment
Prerenal causes [hypovolemia, decreased renal blood flow (congestive heart failure, cirrhosis, NSAIDs, ACE inhibitors)]	BUN:creatinine > 20, FE_{Na} < 1%	Volume replacement, correct underlying abnormality
Renal causes [acute tubular necrosis, toxins (contrast agents, aminoglycosides), rhabdomyolysis, hemolysis]	Tubular cells on urinalysis, FE_{Na} > 2%, hemoglobinuria, myoglobinuria	Remove offending agent, restore intravascular volume, treat associated abnormalities
Postrenal causes [cancer (prostate, cervix), bladder outlet obstruction (BPH, urethral stricture, clogged urinary bladder, neurogenic bladder), accidental ureteral ligation or injury, pelvic abscess]	Ultrasound, signs of obstruction	Treat cause of obstruction

ACE = angiotensin-converting enzyme; BPH = benign prostatic hypertrophy; BUN = blood urea nitrogen; FE_{Na} = fractional excretion of Na; NSAIDs = nonsteroidal anti-inflammatory drugs.

$$FE_{Na} = \frac{\text{Urine Na}^+ / \text{Plasma Na}^+}{\text{Urine Cr} / \text{Plasma Cr}} \times 100\%$$

c. **FE_{Na}**

—of less than 1% suggests a prerenal source.

—of greater than 2% suggests a primary renal source.

4. **Inadequately treated ARF leads to**

—progressive metabolic acidosis.

—hyperkalemia.

—severe uremia.

—volume overload.

5. **Hemodialysis**

—may be necessary as a bridge until renal function returns to normal.

G. **Genitourinary complications**

1. **Postoperative urinary retention**

a. Postoperative urinary retention **may occur** after any surgery, but especially after **pelvic and perineal procedures** or **after epidural** or **spinal anesthesia.**

b. **Prevention includes**

—catheterizing the bladder for long cases or for those where large volumes of IV fluids are used.

—removing the bladder catheter and encouraging early postoperative voiding.

2. **Urinary tract infection** (see Chapter 4)

H. Vascular complications

1. Iatrogenic IV catheter complications

a. Pneumothorax

—represents the presence of air in the pleural cavity with collapse of the lung.

(1) Risk factors include

—central line placement.

—recent thoracotomy.

—trauma to the chest.

—underlying severe pulmonary disease.

(2) Diagnosis

—is made on examination by decreased breath sounds and hyperresonance to percussion.

(3) Confirmation

—A **chest radiograph** usually confirms the diagnosis.

(4) Treatment includes

—**tube thoracostomy.**

—evacuation of air from the pleural space.

b. Catheter sepsis may occur from

—local infection.

—hematoma.

—a break in sterile technique.

c. Other complications include

—**hemothorax.**

—**cardiac puncture** and **tamponade.**

—**arterial injury, embolization,** and **air emboli.**

(1) Air can enter the venous system

—when a catheter is left open, exposing air at atmospheric pressure to low or negative intrathoracic pressure.

(2) With a large embolus

—**air lodges in the right atrium** and prevents adequate right ventricular filling.

(3) Symptoms include

—hypotension.

—jugular venous distention.

—tachycardia.

(4) Treatment

—Placing the patient in the left lateral decubitus and Trendelenburg positions can help to dislodge air from the right atrium and trap it in the right ventricle.

—The best treatment involves prevention with careful technique in placement of the catheter.

d. Iatrogenic cardiac tamponade

(1) This may occur

—with **placement** of a **central venous catheter.**

—after **coronary artery bypass grafting** (CABG).

(2) **Diagnosis classically is made clinically**

—by Beck's triad (i.e., **hypotension, jugular venous distension,** and **muffled heart sounds),** in addition to equalization of pulmonary and systemic blood pressures.

(3) **Confirmation**

—An **echocardiogram** may be used to confirm the diagnosis in some cases; however, the diagnosis is primarily based on examination.

(4) **Treatment involves**

—**decompression of the pericardial space** with pericardiocentesis.

—surgical drainage and repair of the injured site.

2. **Deep venous thrombosis (DVT)**

a. **DVTs may be present**

—in approximately 40% of postoperative patients.

b. **Most thrombi originate**

—in the **deep venous system of the lower extremities.**

c. **Clot may propagate cephalad into**

—the popliteal, femoral, and iliac systems.

d. **Most (more than 80%) pulmonary emboli originate**

—from above the knee.

e. **Risk factors include Virchow's triad**

—**vascular stasis** (e.g., venous insufficiency, obesity)

—**abnormal vessel walls** (e.g., fractures)

—**hypercoagulability** (e.g., estrogen therapy, pregnancy, cancer).

f. **Diagnosis is difficult**

—because 50% of patients are asymptomatic.

g. **Possible signs and symptoms include**

—lower extremity swelling.

—fever.

—pain.

—Homan's sign (calf pain with foot dorsiflexion).

h. **Confirmation is made either with**

—lower extremity duplex ultrasound examination.

—angiographic evaluation of the venous system.

i. **Treatment includes anticoagulation therapy** (e.g., heparin).

—If anticoagulation is contraindicated, some patients may benefit from placement of a filter within the inferior vena cava (Figure 2.1) to prevent pulmonary embolization.

j. **Preventive measures include**

—**early mobilization.**

—the use of support hose or sequential compression devices.

—subcutaneous **administration of heparin.**

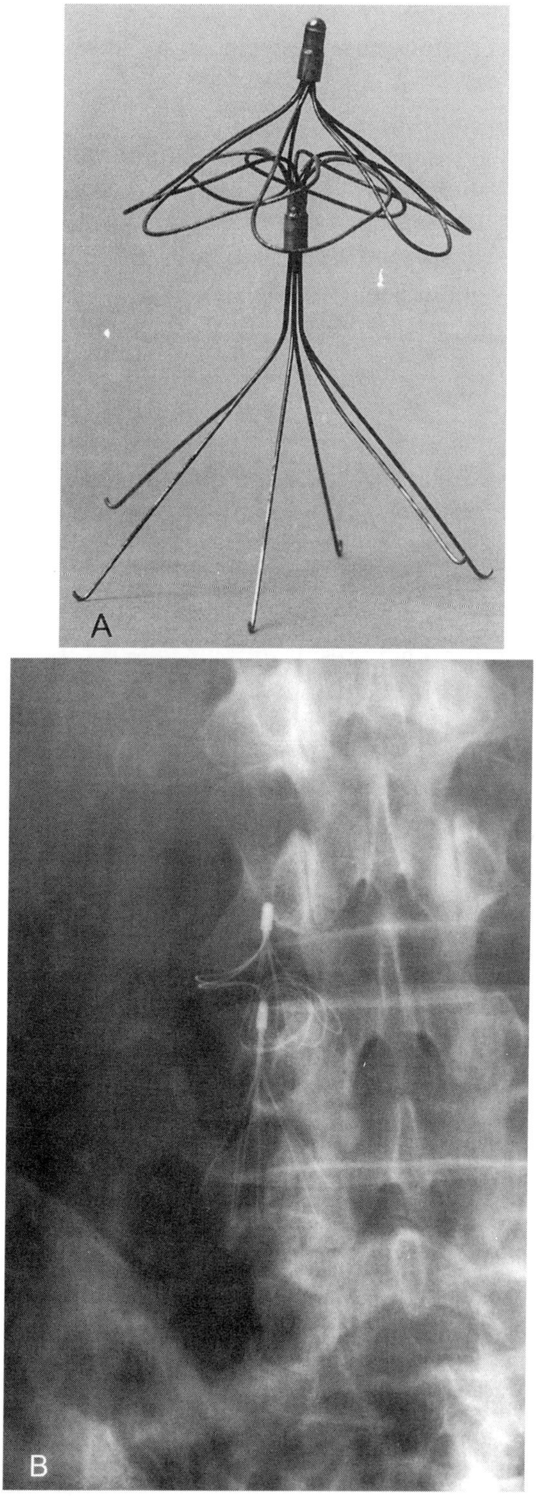

Figure 2-1. Inferior vena cava filter. *(A)* Simon-Notinol filter. *(B)* Abdominal radiograph showing deployment of the filter from a catheter passed percutaneously. (Reprinted with permission from Daffner RH: *Clinical Radiology: The Essentials,* 2nd ed. Baltimore, Williams & Wilkins, 1999, p 66.)

3. **Pulmonary embolus**

—is one of the **most common causes of sudden death in hospitalized patients.**

a. **Thromboemboli**

—from the deep venous system of the lower extremities and pelvis lead to **mechanical obstruction of the pulmonary arterial system.**

b. **Risk factors include**

—history of pulmonary embolism.

—older age.

—heart disease.

—obesity.

—malignancy.

—major trauma (especially spinal cord injury and pelvic or femoral shaft fractures).

—varicose veins.

—women who are pregnant or postpartum or receiving estrogen therapy.

c. **Large emboli** may result in

—decreased cardiac output.

—hypotension.

—impaired oxygenation caused by bronchospasm and vasospasm.

d. **Other signs include**

—hemoptysis.

—pleural friction rub.

—new cardiac gallop.

—ECG changes (e.g., diffuse ST elevation).

e. **Possible radiographic findings include**

—diminished pulmonary vascular markings (Westermark's sign).

—pleural effusion.

—a new pulmonary infiltrate.

f. **Key for management of pulmonary emboli includes**

—**early recognition** of suspicious signs and symptoms.

—**prompt diagnosis** and treatment.

g. **Confirmation is possible with**

—**V/Q scan.**

—**pulmonary arteriogram.**

h. **Treatment involves**

—appropriate airway management.

—cardiovascular support (e.g., mechanical ventilation, volume resuscitation).

—**anticoagulation therapy (heparin).**

—**thrombolytic therapy** or **pulmonary embolectomy** for severe cases.

4. **Superficial thrombophlebitis**
   —is frequently associated with infected or infiltrated peripheral IV catheters.
   a. **Prevention is possible**
      —with meticulous placement and care of these catheters.
   b. **Diagnosis is made by clinical findings of**
      —a swollen, tender, red, warm, indurated, palpable cord along a vein.
   c. **Treatment involves**
      —**removal of the intravenous catheter.**
      —elevation and local moist heat for pain relief.
      —nonsteroidal anti-inflammatory drugs (NSAIDs).
   d. **Surgical removal**
      —of the infected vein may be necessary in some cases.
5. **Fat emboli**
   —**originate from bone marrow.**
   —enter the circulation through **torn venules.**
   a. **This may be associated with**
      —long-bone fractures.
      —joint replacement surgery.
   b. **These cause**
      —**direct occlusion of small blood vessels** in the lung, brain, and skin.
   c. **The embolic plugs generate**
      —toxic free-fatty acids and cause platelets to release serotonin.
   d. Fat emboli syndrome results from severe cases of fat embolization.
      (1) **This syndrome typically arises**
         —within **12–72 hours after injury.**
      (2) **Signs and symptoms include**
         (a) **Bergman's triad**
            —**neurodysfunction** (mild confusion with or without focal deficits)
            —**respiratory insufficiency** (i.e., dyspnea and hyperoxemia)
            —**petechiae** (on the axilla, chest, and proximal arms).
         (b) **Fever and tachycardia**
      (3) **Laboratory studies may show**
         —**fat droplets** in blood, urine, or sputum.
         —elevated serum lipase or fatty acid levels.
         —leukopenia and thrombocytopenia.
         —hypoalbuminemia.
         —hypocalcemia.
      (4) **Treatment** is predominantly supportive (i.e., ABC's).
         —**Early fixation of long-bone fractures** is most important.

(5) Prognosis

—is proportional to the degree of pulmonary insufficiency.

I. Pressure sores and decubitus ulcers

1. Patients at high risk for developing pressure ulcers are

—critically ill.

—obese.

—immobile.

2. Ulcers occur most often

—near the sacrum in these patients.

3. Prevention

a. Early mobilization and frequent position changes

b. Adequate nutrition and proper hygiene

IV. Global Complications

A. Fever

—is frequently present postoperatively.

—can represent an early sign of postoperative complications.

1. Body temperature

—higher than 38.5°C is common (40% of patients after major surgery).

2. The temporal relationship to the time of surgery

—is important (e.g., at $\leq$ 24 hours, a specific cause is found only 20% of the time).

3. The differential diagnosis

—of postoperative fever is found in **Table 2-7.**

4. Most fevers spontaneously resolve without treatment.

5. Risk factors that suggest an infectious cause for fever include

—preoperative history of trauma.

—American Society of Anesthesiologists (ASA) score higher than 2.

—fever after postoperative day 2.

—white blood cell count higher than 10,000 cells/dL.

—blood urea nitrogen (BUN) greater than 15 mg/dL.

—systemic manifestations (e.g., chills, rigors, erythema, induration).

6. Evaluation includes

—a thorough physical examination.

—laboratory studies.

—review of medicines for possible interactions.

B. Abnormalities of fluid balance, electrolytes, and acid-base disorders (see Chapter 7)

Table 2-7. Differential Diagnosis of Postoperative Fever

Wind (pulmonary)	Atelectasis, pneumonia, pulmonary emboli, sinusitis
Water (urinary tract)	Cystitis, pyelonephritis
Walking	Deep venous thrombosis
Wonder drug (drug fever)	β-Lactams (e.g., penicillins), sulfa derivatives, amphotericin B, phenytoin/barbiturates
Wound	Infections, abscess, anastomotic leaks, peritoneal hematoma
Other	Thrombophlebitis, adrenal insufficiency, thyroid storm/thyrotoxicosis, parotitis, intravenous catheter infection, pancreatitis, malignant hyperthermia, transfusion reaction, perirectal abscess

V. Complications of Minimal Access Surgery (Laparoscopy or Thoracoscopy)

A. Technique failures

1. Needle or trocar injury to a

—solid organ.

—hollow viscus.

—blood vessel.

—nerve.

2. Hypotension

—secondary to decreased venous return because of increased pressure within the abdomen.

—vena caval compression after insufflation of air.

3. Damage to adjacent organs

—when using **heat-producing instruments** (e.g., electrocautery, harmonic scalpel, lasers).

4. Extraperitoneal insufflation

—during attempted injection of air (e.g., CO_2 or helium) into the peritoneal space.

5. Trocar site herniation or wound infection.

6. Rarely, an air embolus can occur

—if the pneumoperitoneum is inadvertently exposed to venous blood flow (i.e., large venous injury during the operation).

B. Pneumothorax

—can occur with insufflation of air into the peritoneal space especially with surgery near the diaphragmatic hiatus (e.g., Nissen fundoplication) [see Chapter 11].

C. A laparoscopic procedure

—should be **converted to an open procedure** if it cannot be completed safely or if a significant technique failure has occurred.

Review Test

Directions: Each of the numbered items or incomplete statements in this section is followed by answers or by completions of the statement. Select the ONE lettered answer or completion that is BEST in each case.

1. A 28-year-old man was involved in a high-speed motor vehicle accident where he sustained a closed comminuted left femur fracture. He subsequently underwent operative fixation by placement of an intramedullary nail. On postoperative day 2, the patient was noted to have dyspnea and fever (39.5°C). Other vital signs were a blood pressure of 136/74 mm Hg, pulse of 120 beats/min, respiration of 32/min. Oxygen saturations were 100% using a 40% face tent. The physical examination was significant for the patient being minimally arousable, having diffusc fine crackles on pulmonary auscultation, and widespread petechiae involving the axilla, chest, and upper arms. Which of the following statements most closely describes the above condition?

(A) An immediate pulmonary angiogram is both diagnostic and therapeutic for this condition
(B) Treatment of this condition requires rapid administration of cyclo-oxygenase inhibitors, fresh frozen plasma, and platelets
(C) Microscopic examination of blood, urine, and sputum may be helpful in making the diagnosis
(D) Early long-bone fracture fixation has little influence on the development of this condition
(E) The prognosis of this condition is proportional to the degree of renal insufficiency

2. A 32-year-old man was recovering from acute necrotizing pancreatitis, which required operative débridement. On postoperative day 9 he had a large, melenic stool. Routine hematologic studies showed a drop in hematocrit from 32% to 26%. A nasogastric tube was placed, which returned minimal "coffee ground" residue (guaiac-positive) with a pH of 4.5. Which of the following statements is true regarding this patient's condition?

(A) Gastrointestinal protection should not routinely be instituted because of the side effects of mucosal-protective drugs
(B) Emergent exploratory laparotomy is indicated to quickly identify the source of bleeding
(C) Gastric ulcers are most likely present, necessitating immediate treatment for *Helicobacter pylori*
(D) Proton pump inhibition is an effective method for preventing this condition
(E) Upper and lower endoscopy have little role in identifying the source of bleeding

3. A 65-year-old man underwent an uneventful open inguinal herniorrhaphy, but during overnight observation was found to have vomited while he slept. He received aggressive suctioning but later that day he displayed a fever of 39.0°C. Other vital signs were a blood pressure of 140/70 mm Hg, pulse of 90 beats/min, and respiration of 24/min. Oxygen saturations were 92% with a 40% face tent. There were thick crackles on auscultation of the lungs. Chest radiograph was significant for bilateral infiltrates. Which of the following statements most accurately reflects the patient's current clinical condition?

(A) Cefazolin is the antibiotic of choice for treatment of this condition because of its activity against oral flora
(B) Pneumonias resulting from this condition are associated with minimal morbidity and mortality
(C) The left upper lobe is the most frequently involved pulmonary segment
(D) Nasogastric suction tubes and endotracheal tubes do not uniformly prevent this complication
(E) Bronchoscopy has little role in the diagnosis or treatment of this condition

4. During a routine postoperative check, a 67-year-old woman who had undergone resection of an infrarenal, abdominal aortic aneurysm complained of peri-incisional tenderness and some light-headedness. Her vital signs were a blood pressure of 110/40 mm Hg, pulse of 130 beats/min, respiration of 24/min, and temperature of 37.9°C. She had 25 mL urine output for the last 2 hours. On examination, she had dry mucus membranes, there were faint bibasilar crackles on pulmonary auscultation, her abdomen was mildly distended, the incisional dressing was clean and dry, and her feet were cool to the touch. Hematocrit dropped from 43% to 27%. Which of the following statements is true of her condition?

(A) These findings are suggestive of acute myocardial infarction with congestive heart failure
(B) Plain radiographs are the most sensitive imaging modality for determining the cause of abdominal pathology
(C) More potent narcotic analgesics may be helpful because her examination suggests a sympathetic nervous system response to poor postoperative pain control
(D) The presence of infection and sepsis is sufficient to explain all of the physical signs
(E) Operative exploration may be necessary if nonoperative measures fail to correct this condition

5. A 45-year-old, obese man was involved in a high-speed motor vehicle accident. He was hypotensive at the scene and was noted to have a distended abdomen upon presentation. He was quickly evaluated and taken to the operating room for an exploratory laparotomy. Which of the following is true with regard to adequate closure of the abdomen after this procedure?

(A) Permanent suture materials should not be used for closing the fascial layers because of the increased risk of local inflammation
(B) The instability of wound closure is decreased by the removal of devitalized tissue
(C) Body habitus and nutritional status are not important factors influencing wound stability
(D) Wound dehiscence is uncommon, although when it does occur it is usually during the first or second postoperative day
(E) Evisceration of the abdominal contents is a uniformly fatal event

6. A 53-year-old, obese woman with a history of Type II diabetes and chronic obstructive pulmonary disease (COPD) underwent mesh closure of an abdominal incisional hernia. She tolerated the procedure well and was discharged from the hospital the following morning. Which of the following factors would LEAST likely contribute to the incidence of postoperative complications in this patient?

(A) A small enterotomy made while dissecting the fascial layers was closed with dissolvable suture after minimal spillage of intestinal contents
(B) Her last hemoglobin A_1C was 11.7 and she has a history of an anaphylactic reaction to penicillin
(C) She is morbidly obese and has significant lower extremity claudication when attempting exercise
(D) She has end-stage COPD and her medications include prednisone 20 mg per day
(E) She had previously smoked 2 packs of cigarettes per day for 40 years, but has not smoked for the last 5 years

7. After an uneventful laparoscopic inguinal herniorrhaphy, a 58-year-old man had the urinary catheter removed and began to ambulate. During routine vital sign checks, he was noted to have had no urine output over the previous 8 hours. An intravenous bolus of saline (500 mL) did not stimulate voiding. Straight catheterization revealed 1000 mL of urine. Urinalysis showed a specific gravity of 1.018, a pH of 6, moderate blood, and negative leukocyte esterase and nitrites. There were 23 red blood cells/high power field (hpf) and 2 white blood cells/hpf. What is the most appropriate treatment for his failure to void?

(A) Catheterization and initiation of hemodialysis
(B) Catheterization and antibiotic administration
(C) Catheterization and administration of furosemide
(D) Catheterization and administration of mannitol
(E) Catheterization alone with continued observation

8. A 75-year-old, obese woman with a history of insulin-dependent Type II diabetes mellitus underwent an uneventful laparoscopic cholecystectomy. She was slow to wake after the operation and was taken to the postoperative recovery unit intubated but breathing on her own. Vital signs were stable and all laboratory studies were within normal limits. Head computed tomography (CT) scan was interpreted as age-appropriate atrophy with no mass lesions or midline shift. She was taken to the intensive care unit where she slowly began to awaken over the next 48 hours. Which of the following most likely contributed to this patient's depressed level of consciousness postoperatively?

(A) Cerebrovascular accident
(B) Poor metabolism of anesthetics
(C) Acute myocardial infarction
(D) Hypoxic brain injury
(E) Hypoglycemic coma

9. A 65-year-old woman with an open tibia/fibula fracture of her left lower extremity underwent uneventful débridement and external fixation. Her initial postoperative course was uneventful. On postoperative day 4, she was noted to have mild swelling of her left ankle and a fever of 38.6°C. Her wounds were without signs of infection and there were no palpable cords. Which of the following is the most likely cause of this patient's findings?

(A) Fat emboli
(B) Iatrogenic lymphatic disruption
(C) Thrombophlebitis
(D) Deep venous thrombosis
(E) Ascending lymphangitis

Directions: Each set of matching questions in this section consists of a list of four to twenty-six lettered options followed by several numbered items. For each numbered item, select the appropriate lettered option(s). Each lettered option may be selected once, more than once, or not at all.

Questions 10–12

(A) Pneumonia
(B) Pulmonary atelectasis
(C) Fat emboli
(D) Adult respiratory distress syndrome
(E) Pneumothorax
(F) Hemothorax
(G) Pulmonary embolism
(H) Air emboli

Select the most likely source of each patient's clinical problem.

10. A 16-year-old boy was diagnosed with acute appendicitis and subsequently underwent an uneventful laparoscopic appendectomy. He was admitted to the hospital overnight for observation. At 3:00 am, he was found to have a fever of 38.7°C. His examination was significant for bibasilar crackles and cough on deep inspiration. The surgical wounds were clean without signs of infection. (SELECT 1 SOURCE)

11. A 52-year-old man underwent an orthotopic liver transplantation for cirrhosis secondary to hepatitis C. On postoperative day 4 the patient developed rapidly worsening respiratory failure secondary to presumed aspiration with diffuse airspace disease noted bilaterally on chest radiograph. On postoperative day 5 the patient underwent a liver biopsy for worsening liver function as well. The patient continues to deteriorate and rapidly develops hypotension refractory to volume resuscitation and pressors. On examination the patient is noted to have significantly decreased breath sounds on the right compared with the left, with hyperresonance to percussion. Diffuse crackles are noted on the left. (SELECT 1 SOURCE)

12. A 32-year-old woman had a postgastric bypass for morbid obesity 6 days ago. Because of significant incisional pain, she was slow to ambulate. At 2:00 pm, while walking to the bathroom, she experienced sharp chest pain, cough, wheezing, hemoptysis, and syncope. Physical examination was significant for a pleural friction rub. Electrocardiogram was unchanged, but there was a wedge-shaped area of diminished pulmonary vascular markings at the periphery of her left lung. (SELECT 1 SOURCE)

Answers and Explanations

1–C. Fat emboli originate from bone marrow and enter the circulation through torn venules, causing direct occlusion of small blood vessels in the lung, brain, and skin. The embolic plugs generate toxic free-fatty acids and cause platelets to release serotonin. Severe cases cause fat emboli syndrome, which has been described in trauma victims 12–72 hours after injury. Bergman's triad—neurodysfunction (mild confusion with or without focal deficits), respiratory insufficiency (dyspnea, hyperoxemia), and petechiae (axilla, chest, proximal arms)—as well as fever and tachycardia are seen. Fat droplets in the blood, urine, or sputum; elevated serum lipase or fatty acid levels; leukopenia or thrombocytopenia; and decreased serum albumin and calcium confirm the diagnosis. Treatment is predominantly supportive (e.g., positive pressure ventilation, increasing albumin, calcium), however early fixation of long-bone fractures is paramount. Prognosis is proportional to the degree of pulmonary insufficiency.

2–D. Mucosal inflammation and hemorrhage occurs frequently in severely ill and septic patients. Diffuse gastritis, duodenitis, and shallow ulcerations are often seen with endoscopy. If the ulceration involves large blood vessels, however, significant bleeding may occur. This is most likely caused by a breakdown of the protective mucosal barrier, rendering the intestinal lining susceptible to the corrosive acidic environment. Effective preventative measures include inhibiting acid production (e.g., histamine receptor antagonists, proton pump inhibitors) or augmenting the mucosal barrier (e.g., misoprostol, sucralfate [Carafate], antacids) because these agents have few side effects. Emergent laparotomy is not indicated unless medical management fails and the source of bleeding cannot be stopped by any other means (e.g., endoscopy, angiography). Although *Helicobacter pylori* is a known cause of gastrointestinal ulcer disease and bleeding, it has little influence on stress gastritis or duodenitis.

3–D. Aspiration of abdominal contents into the lungs can be a serious complication associated with significant morbidity and mortality. The magnitude of lung injury is proportional to the volume, the frequency, and the pH of the aspirate. Risk factors include decreased sensorium (i.e., narcosis, stroke), nasogastric tube placement, intestinal obstruction, and pregnancy. The most commonly affected segments include the posterior right upper lobe, superior right lower lobe, or superior and posterior basal left lower lobes. Treatment involves re-establishment of the airway (if necessary), aggressive airway hygiene, and adequate fluid resuscitation. Although intubation is helpful, aspiration into the airway can still occur. Antibiotic use for large volume aspiration is controversial. However, pneumonia resulting from aspiration can be secondary to a variety of organisms and ideal antibiotic selection should be based on culture results. Bronchoscopy is an important tool for pulmonary hygiene and may be used if necessary.

4–E. Hemoperitoneum is the most common cause of hypovolemic shock in the first 24 hours after abdominal surgery. Signs include low-grade fever, tachycardia, hypotension, oliguria, and peripheral vasoconstriction. The diagnosis is confirmed by demonstrating increasing anemia on routine hematologic tests. A computed tomography (CT) scan showing fluid in the abdomen consistent with blood may also be used if the clinical picture is questionable. Treatment consists of volume resuscitation, possible blood transfusion, correction of coagulopathy (if one exists), and re-operation with meticulous hemostasis if other measures fail. Although tachycardia is sometimes an indication of poor pain control, or infection and sepsis, there are enough other signs to quickly rule these out as the source of the current problem.

5–B. Inadequate closure of fascial layers is the most important factor in determining the likelihood of dehiscence. Other important factors contributing to dehiscence events include increased intra-abdominal pressure (e.g., obesity, severe pulmonary disease, excess postoperative coughing, bowel obstruction, and cirrhosis with ascites formation) and deficient wound healing (e.g., infection, seroma or hematoma formation, drain placement, chronic disease, malnutrition, or chronic steroid use). Suture material for fascial closure should not be rapidly dissolvable because these layers are so important to wound integrity. Devitalized tissue predisposes to wound infection and should be eliminated. Dehiscence is a partial or total disruption of anatomic layers after surgical closure. Evisceration is wound dehiscence with the extrusion of abdominal contents. This is a highly morbid event, however not uniformly fatal. Treatment would consist of rapid wound coverage with sterile, moist towels, and emergent surgical exploration and repair.

6–E. Factors contributing to most postoperative complications include the failure of operative techniques, the magnitude of the operation, the general medical condition of the patient, or chronic medications taken by the patient. The high hemoglobin A_1C level signifies poorly controlled diabetes. This may lead to poor wound healing. Obesity and peripheral vascular disease may be associated with cardiovascular complications and poor wound healing. Chronic steroid use may also lead to problems with wound healing, adrenal insufficiency, and immunosuppression. Moreover, COPD may predispose the patient to pulmonary complications. Smoking is a significant risk factor for postoperative complications, however not having smoked for over 5 years will significantly decrease the incidence of all complications, including pulmonary problems.

7–E. Postoperative urinary retention is a common problem especially after pelvic and perineal procedures or after spinal anesthesia. The causes in those cases appear to be interference with the normal autonomically mediated bladder emptying and overdistention of the bladder that inhibits contraction of the smooth muscle. Prevention of this includes catheterization of the bladder for long cases or for those where large volumes of intravenous fluids are used. Removing the bladder catheter and encouraging early postoperative voiding is also useful. If this is unsuccessful, in and out catheterization to decompress the bladder is used. The catheter should be left in place if the volume obtained is over 1000 mL. An indwelling catheter left for 4–5 days should be used if prior insertions were traumatic or if there is a continued inability to void. Formal urologic follow-up may be necessary.

8–B. Prolonged altered consciousness after general anesthesia may result from poor metabolism of anesthetic agents by the patient. Risk factors include advanced age, renal or hepatic insufficiency, and obesity. Other more serious events (e.g., hypoxic brain injury, diabetic coma, hypoglycemia) must be ruled out. Cerebral vascular accidents (e.g., strokes) may occur secondary to hypertensive, embolic, or thrombotic injury. After a cerebrovascular accident, patients may remain obtunded for up to 72 hours and then recover without neurologic deficits. Those with deficits, however, may have paralysis, abnormal reflexes, posturing, or convulsions. Treatment includes aspirin and anticoagulation if not contraindicated.

9–D. Deep venous thrombosis remains an important cause of postoperative morbidity because of the high prevalence and the potentially life-threatening consequences. Clot may propagate from the deep venous system of the lower leg into the femoral and iliac systems. Most pulmonary emboli originate from above the knee. Risk factors include Virchow's triad: vascular stasis (e.g., venous insufficiency, obesity), abnormal vessel walls (e.g., fractures), and hypercoagulability (e.g., estrogen therapy, pregnancy, cancer). Diagnosis is sometimes difficult because 50% of patients have no symptoms; the remainder have lower extremity swelling, fever, and pain as well as the classic positive Homan's sign characterized by calf pain with foot dorsiflexion. Fat emboli are not associated with ankle swelling. Iatrogenic lymphatic disruption is rare except with extensive resections of nodal groups. Thrombophlebitis typically presents with erythema, tenderness, and a palpable cord over the affected vein.

10–B. Atelectasis, or the partial collapse of alveoli, accounts for 90% of postoperative pulmonary complications and occurs most frequently in the first 48 hours after surgery. Closure of small (smaller than 1 mm) bronchioles leads to a ventilation/perfusion (V/Q) mismatch and subsequent hypoxemia. The mechanism of the febrile response remains unknown, however, but is usually self-limited. The diagnosis is made by both radiographic (e.g., characteristic discoid infiltrate, elevated hemidiaphragm) and physical examination signs, including scattered basilar crackles and decreased breath sounds.

11–E. In critically ill patients all of these conditions can contribute to respiratory compromise and even hypotension. In patients with refractory hypotension in this setting, one should always consider tension pneumothorax as a potential cause. Pneumothorax is a potential complication of a liver biopsy because of the proximity of the lung and pleural space when passing the biopsy needle. Although a hemothorax can also occur, hyperresonance to percussion is suggestive of a pneumothorax.

12–G. Pulmonary embolism remains one of the most common causes of sudden death in hospitalized patients. Mechanical obstruction of the pulmonary arterial system occurs secondary to migration of a thromboembolus, usually from the deep venous system of the lower extremities. If the blockage is large enough, decreased cardiac output, hypotension, and impaired oxygenation caused by bronchospasm and vasospasm occur. Other signs include hemoptysis, pleural friction rub, new cardiac gallop, and electrocardiogram changes. Radiographically, diminished pulmonary vascular markings (Westermark's sign), pleural effusion, and a new pulmonary infiltrate may be present. Confirmation is possible with a ventilation/perfusion (V/Q) scan or pulmonary arteriogram.

3

Surgical Nutrition

Gerald A. Cephas and Traves D. Crabtree

I. Assessment of Nutritional Status

A. History and physical examination

1. **Weight loss**
   —is a significant indicator of **malnutrition.**
   a. **More than 10% unintentional weight loss**
      —in a 6 month period is significant.
   b. **A 5% unintentional weight loss**
      —in 1 month is also significant.
2. **Other suggestive findings** in the history include
   —**anorexia.**
   —persistent nausea.
   —vomiting.
   —diarrhea.
   —generalized malaise.
3. **Significant physical findings** include
   —loss of subcutaneous fat.
   —**muscle wasting.**
   —**edema.**
   —ascites (late finding).
4. Signs suggestive of **specific nutrient deficiencies** include
   —skin rash.
   —pallor.
   —cheilosis.
   —glossitis.

—gingival lesions.

—hepatomegaly.

—neuropathy.

—dementia.

B. Evaluation of body composition

1. Estimates of **ideal body weight (IBW)** are:

   a. **Men:** 106 lb + 6 lb for each inch over 5 feet (height).

   b. **Women:** 100 lb + 5 lb for each inch over 5 feet.

   —The IBW also depends on patient age and overall body habitus.

2. **Other measures include**

   —anthropometric measurements, including **triceps skin fold** or mid-arm muscle circumference.

   —densitometry.

3. **The body mass index (BMI)**

   —is used to characterize the degree of **obesity.**

   —BMI = weight (kg)/total body surface area (m^2).

   a. Patients with a **BMI higher than 40 or over 35 with other co-morbid conditions**

   —are considered candidates for surgical treatment of morbid obesity.

   b. **Severe obesity**

   —is associated with a significant **increase in overall morbidity and mortality.**

C. Laboratory markers of nutritional status

1. **Several serum proteins**

   —are used to evaluate nutritional status (**Table 3-1**).

   a. **Severe hypoalbuminemia**

   —is associated with poor outcome in surgical patients.

   b. **Serum albumin**

   —has a long half-life, and as such, it is not a reliable short-term marker for nutritional assessment during nutritional support.

   c. **Serial measurements of transferrin as well as prealbumin, and retinol-binding protein**

   —are useful in monitoring the impact of nutritional support.

2. **Energy expenditure**

   —can be measured by the **respiratory quotient (RQ).**

Table 3-1. Serum Proteins Used as Markers of Nutritional Status

Protein	Half-life (days)
Albumin	20
Transferrin	8.5
Prealbumin	1.3
Retinol-binding protein	0.4

a. **RQ** = carbon dioxide production (**VCO_2**)/oxygen consumption (**VO_2**).

b. Indirect calorimetry (metabolic cart)
—allows for gas analysis and subsequent calculation of the RQ.

c. An **RQ value**
—**of 1.0** is consistent with predominant glucose utilization.
—**of 0.7 and 0.8** is consistent with **fat and protein utilization, respectively.**
—**higher than 1.0** suggest the presence of lipogenesis or overfeeding.

d. **These values are used**
—to estimate the adequacy of nutritional support.

3. **Measures of immune function**
—have also been used to assess nutritional status.

a. **Skin anergy tests** to assess the delayed type hypersensitivity response to antigens (e.g., mumps, tuberculosis, *Candida*) have been used as such markers.

b. Although a poor response may be found in malnourished states, these markers have been relatively unreliable in assessing nutritional status.

II. Nutritional Requirements

A. **The basic assessment of patients' nutritional needs** includes
—total energy (kcal) requirements.
—total protein requirements.
—the relative distribution of calories between carbohydrates, fats, and protein.

B. **Energy requirements**

1. **The Harris-Benedict equation**
—estimates the **basal energy expenditure (BEE)** or basic energy requirements at rest in kcal/day.

a. **Men:** 66 + (13.7 × weight [kg]) + (5 × height [cm]) – (6.8 × age [years]).

b. **Women:** 655 + (9.6 × weight [kg]) + (1.7 × height [cm]) – (4.7 × age [years]).

2. Most patients **at rest** require **25–35 kcal/kg/day.**

a. **Stress** significantly increases these values.
—Low stress: 1.2 × BEE.
—Moderate stress: 1.2–1.3 × BEE.
—Severe stress: 1.3–1.5 × BEE.
—**Major burn injury: 1.5–2.0 × BEE.**

b. **Energy requirements are increased by**
—fever.

—infection.
—activity.
—burns.
—head injury.
—trauma.
—renal failure.
—surgery.

c. **Energy requirements are decreased by**
—sedation.
—paralysis.
—β blockers.

3. **Differing amounts of kcal/g are produced by**
—carbohydrates, proteins, and lipids.

a. **Carbohydrates**
—generally provide **4 kcal/g.**
—Dextrose provides 3.4 kcal/g.

b. **Proteins**
—generally provide **4–5 kcal/g,** depending on the amino acid composition.

c. **Lipids**
—generally provide **9 kcal/g.**

C. **Carbohydrates**

—should generally account for **30%–60% of total calories.**

1. A **minimum of 100–150 g/day**
—is necessary to provide the minimum needs of the brain and red blood cells, which prefer glucose as an energy source.

2. **Glucose is stored**
—**as glycogen** in the liver (40%) and in muscle (60%).

a. **The body stores** 300–500 g of glycogen.

b. **These stores are depleted**
—**within 48 hours** during starvation.
—in as little as 12–24 hours in the stressed patient.

D. **Proteins**

1. **Most healthy individuals** require **0.8–1.0 g protein/kg/day.**

2. **Stress** increases these requirements:
—Mild stress: 1.0–1.2 g/kg/day.
—Moderate stress: 1.3–1.5 g/kg/day.
—**Severe stress: 1.5–2.5 g/kg/day.**

3. **Patients with renal failure**
—may also have a higher protein requirement compared with baseline.

4. **Patients with hepatic encephalopathy**

—may require less protein (0.8 g/kg/day) to avoid additional encephalopathy.

5. **Nitrogen balance**

—is a crude measure of protein consumption.

—is calculated by determining the **difference between net nitrogen intake and excretion.**

a. **Positive nitrogen balance**

—indicates more protein ingested than excreted (**net protein anabolism**).

b. **Negative nitrogen balance**

—indicates more protein is excreted than ingested (**net protein catabolism**).

c. **Protein excreted in the urine**

—can be measured over 12–24 hours:

protein (g) = nitrogen (g) × 6.25.

d. **Neutral nitrogen balance**

—is the goal, although positive nitrogen balance is frequently present during the recovery phase of illness.

6. **Amino acids** (Table 3-2)

a. **Essential amino acids**

—cannot be produced by the body, but **nonessential** amino acids can.

b. **Amino acid metabolism**

—Most amino acids are metabolized by the liver.

—The **branched-chain amino acids are metabolized by muscle.**

c. **Patients require**

—at least 20% of their protein intake as essential amino acids.

d. Generally, **protein metabolism** in muscle

—is regulated by insulin.

7. **Glutamine**

—is the most abundant amino acid in the blood.

a. It is the **principal fuel for enterocytes**

Table 3-2. Essential and Nonessential Amino Acids

Essential	Semiessential	Nonessential
Leucine*		Glycine
Isoleucine*		Arginine
Valine*		Proline
Lysine		Glutamic acid
Tryptophan		Aspartic acid
Histidine		Serine
Methionine↔	Cystine†	Alanine
Phenylalanine↔	Tyrosine†	

*Branched-chain amino acids.
†Cystine and tyrosine are considered semiessential because when methionine and phenylalanine are supplied in adequate amounts, their requirement can be satisfied.

—and may play an essential role in maintaining mucosal integrity during times of stress.

b. **Glutamine**

—may also be required for lymphocyte and macrophage proliferation.

E. Lipids

1. **Lipids should provide**

—**25%–40%** of total calorie requirements during nutritional supplementation.

2. **Fatty acids**

—are a major fuel for the heart, liver, and skeletal muscle.

3. **Liver oxidation of fatty acids** forms **ketone bodies** (e.g., β-hydroxybuturate).

—These ketone bodies are used by the **heart, skeletal muscle, and the brain** specifically during times of starvation.

4. **During the fed state, insulin**

—stimulates lipogenesis and fat storage and inhibits lipolysis in adipocytes.

5. **Triglycerides**

a. **Long chain triglycerides**

—must be emulsified by **bile salts** to form micelles.

—must be hydrolyzed by **pancreatic lipase** in the proximal small bowel before absorption can occur.

b. **Medium chain triglycerides**

—**are absorbed directly by the enterocytes.**

—are transported through the portal venous system to the liver.

—may be readily absorbed despite significant deficiencies in pancreatic function (i.e., severe pancreatitis).

6. **During intravenous (IV) nutritional supplementation**

—a minimum of 3%–5% of the total calories as fat is necessary to prevent essential fatty acid deficiency.

a. **The essential fatty acids**

—are **linoleic** and **linolenic acid.**

—act as precursors for prostaglandins and eicosanoids.

b. **Essential fatty acid deficiency** may result in

—dermatitis.

—ecchymoses.

—alopecia.

—anemia.

—edema.

—thrombocytopenia.

—respiratory distress.

c. The **manifestations** of fatty acid deficiency may occur within 4–6 weeks if nutritional support does not include lipids.

F. Other requirements

1. **Vitamins**

   a. **Potential vitamin deficiencies can occur**

   —in severely malnourished patients.

   —in patients receiving chronic nutritional support.

   b. **Characteristics of several vitamins** as well as implications of deficiency are outlined in **Table 3-3.**

   —Of note, **impaired wound healing** may be a direct result of **deficiencies in vitamin A, vitamin C,** and the mineral **zinc.**

2. **Minerals**

   —**Characteristics of several essential minerals** as well as implications of deficiency are outlined in **Table 3-4.**

III. Alterations During Stress

A. Carbohydrates

1. The **major hormones** that play an active role in metabolism in the presence of stress or sepsis include

   —**adrenocorticotropic hormone (ACTH).**

   —**cortisol.**

   —**catecholamines.**

   —**glucagon.**

2. **Hyperglycemia**

   —is frequently present during stress secondary to a relatively low insulin level and peripheral insulin resistance.

   a. **Insulin secretion may be inhibited by**

   —catecholamines.

   —sympathetic nervous system activation.

   —somatostatin.

   b. **Catecholamines and cortisol**

   —also contribute to a relative **resistance of peripheral tissues to the effects of insulin.**

   —Despite this relative insulin resistance, there is still an overall increase in peripheral glucose utilization.

3. **Liver glycogenolysis and gluconeogenesis** are stimulated by

   —catecholamines.

   —cortisol.

   —glucagon.

4. The **glucose** produced from these processes is **essential for** certain tissues, including

   —red blood cells.

   —white blood cells.

Table 3-3. Vitamins and Vitamin Deficiencies

Vitamin	RDA	Function	Characteristics of Deficiency
Vitamin A (retinol)	800–1000 μg	Active site of rhodopsin (retinal pigmentation), glycoprotein synthesis, soft tissue and bone growth	**Night blindness,** xerophthalmia, keratomalacia, **impaired wound healing,** hypogonadism
Vitamin D (cholecalciferol)	5–7.5 μg	Calcium absorption from the gut, calcium homeostasis	Rickets (children), osteomalacia (adults)
Vitamin E (α-tocopherol)	8–10 mg	Antioxidant	Hemolytic anemia, ataxia, nystagmus, loss of DTR's, myopathy, edema, infertility
Vitamin K	70–140 μg	δ-carboxylation of glutamic acid in clotting factors II, VII, IX, X, protein C & S	**Coagulopathy**
Vitamin C	60 mg	Antioxidant, proline hydroxylation in collagen synthesis and cross-linking	**Poor wound healing,** scurvy, gingivitis
Thiamine (B_1)	1.2–1.7 mg	Decarboxylation of α-keto acids involved in carbohydrate metabolism	**Wernicke's encephalopathy,** peripheral neuropathy (dry beriberi) ± cardiomyopathy and high output heart failure (wet beriberi)
Pyridoxine (B_6)	2.0–2.2 mg	Coenzyme for amino acid deamination, transamination, and carboxylation; involved in synthesis of niacin from tryptophan, DOPA decarboxylase activity, and glucose metabolism	Sideroblastic anemia, weakness, cheilosis, glossitis, peripheral neuropathy
Cobalamin (B_{12})	2–4 mg	Coenzyme for demethylation involved in purine and pyrimidine synthesis	**Megaloblastic anemia,** peripheral neuropathy
Biotin (B_2 Complex)	100–200 μg	Coenzyme for carboxyl transfer in carbohydrates, lipids, and amino acids	Dermatitis, mucositis, atrophy of lingual papilla, paresthesia
Niacin	13–19 mg	Coenzyme for oxidation-reduction reactions and energy metabolism. Active forms: NAD^+ and $NADP^+$	**Pellagra (dermatitis, diarrhea, dementia)**
Riboflavin	1.2–1.7 mg	Oxidation-reduction reactions, flavoprotein enzymes	Dermatitis, glossitis (magenta tongue), mucositis, angular stomatitis
Folate	–	Involved in purine and thymine synthesis for DNA	**Leukopenia, megaloblastic anemia,** glossitis
Pantothenic acid	4 mg	Involved in synthesis of Coenzyme A; used for acyl transfer in amino acid, carbohydrate, and fat metabolism	Heel tenderness, altered mental status, gastrointestinal complaints

RDA = Recommended dietary allowance; DTR's = deep tendon reflexes; NAD^+ = nicotinamide adenine dinucleotide (oxidized form); $NADP^+$ = nicotinamide adenine dinucleotide phosphate (oxidized form).

Table 3-4. Minerals and Trace Element Deficiencies

Nutrient	RDA	Function	Characteristics of Deficiency
Iron	10–18 mg	Component of hemoglobin, myoglobin, and cytochromes	Hypochromic **anemia**
Zinc	15 mg	Metalloenzymes involved in carbohydrate, protein, and nucleic acid synthesis	**Impaired wound healing,** acrodermatitis enteropathica (bullous skin lesions of the face), hypogonadism
Iodine	150 mg	Thyroid hormone synthesis	Hypothyroidism, **goiter**
Copper	2.0–3.0 mg	Metalloenzymes, iron uptake in hemoglobin	Menkes' syndrome, anemia, leukopenia
Manganese	2.5–5.0 mg	Enzyme cofactor in protein and energy metabolism	Unknown
Fluoride	1.5–4.0 mg	Found in bone and tooth apatite	Increased caries
Chromium	0.05–0.2 mg	Insulin cofactor	Glucose intolerance, hyperlipidemia
Selenium	0.05–0.2 mg	Enzyme cofactor in hydrogen peroxide detoxification	Keshan disease (cardiomyopathy), anergy
Molybdenum	0.15–0.5 mg	Bioelement in a number of proteins	Unknown

RDA = Recommended dietary allowance.

—the **renal medulla.**

—**neural tissue.**

—**wound tissue.**

B. Proteins

1. **Protein synthesis** increases during stress.

   —Net proteolysis and **negative nitrogen balance,** however, are characteristic of **severe stress.**

2. **Alanine release**

   —from peripheral tissues increases during stress because it is the major source of amino acid substrate for gluconeogenesis in the liver (**Figure 3.1**).

3. **During severe sepsis,** muscle protein loss may occur at 240 g protein/day.

   —Interleukin (IL)-1 may play a role in stimulating proteolysis in this setting.

C. Lipids

1. During severe stress, **lipolysis is stimulated** by increased

   —cortisol.

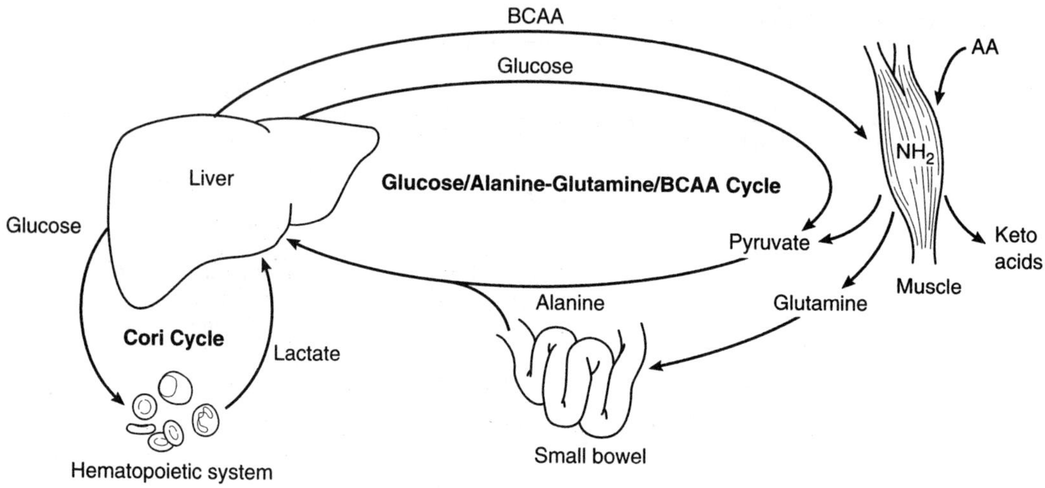

Figure 3-1. Recycling of metabolites to produce glucose during stress: gluconeogenesis and the Cori cycle. BCAA = branched-chain amino acids; AA = amino acid. (Adapted with permission from Way LW: *Current Surgical Diagnosis and Treatment,* 10th ed. Stamford, CT, Appleton & Lange, 1996, p 151.)

—catecholamines.

—glucagon.

—growth hormone.

—ACTH.

—sympathetic activity.

2. **This increased lipolysis** occurring during stress is often characterized by an RQ of 0.7.

IV. Nutritional Supplementation

A. Nutritional supplementation

—has been shown to improve overall outcome in selected patients.

1. **This has benefited** high-risk patients who

   —are **severely malnourished.**

   —are **critically ill.**

   —have **massive burn injury.**

   —have incurred **severe trauma.**

2. **Other patients who may benefit** include those in whom an illness or operative procedure may **delay oral intake for at least 7–10 days.**

   —Nutritional support should be initiated early in these settings because it is more effective at preservation of body mass than for repletion.

3. **Normally nourished patients**

   —undergoing surgical procedures where oral intake will be delayed for fewer than 7 days generally do not require nutritional support beyond fluid and electrolyte administration with dextrose.

B. Enteral nutritional support

1. **When a patient requires nutritional support**
   —the enteral route is indicated in **all patients with an intact, functional gastrointestinal (GI) tract.**
2. Well-nourished patients with an anticipated inability to eat **who may benefit from enteral feeding** include those with
   —severe facial or oropharyngeal trauma.
   —swallowing abnormalities.
   —oral or upper GI obstruction/dysfunction.
3. **Potential benefits include**
   —prevention of intestinal mucosal atrophy.
   —preservation of intrinsic gut immune function.
   —inhibition of stress-associated increases in intestinal permeability.
4. **Enteral nutritional support may be provided**
   —via oro-enteric or nasoenteric routes or by direct enteric routes (e.g., gastrostomy or jejunostomy).
   a. **Small-bore nasoenteric feeding tubes**
      —may be used for **short-term and intermediate-term** nutritional support.
   b. **Nasoduodenal tubes**
      —are preferred in most patients because of the potential increased risk of aspiration with nasogastric tubes.
   c. A **gastrostomy or jejunostomy tube**
      —may be indicated for direct enteral feeding for patients who require **long-term nutritional support.**
   d. **Potential complications**
      —of these routes of nutritional support are outlined in **Table 3-5.**
5. Relative **contraindications to enteral feeding** include
   —mesenteric ischemia.
   —bowel obstruction.
   —intra-abdominal sepsis.
   —necrotizing pancreatitis.
   —high-output GI fistula.
   —short bowel syndrome (see Chapter 13).
6. **The most frequently cited advantage** of enteral feeding versus parenteral feeding is the relative **decreased infection rate in critically ill patients fed enterally.**
   —**Table 3-6** outlines the comparison between enteral and parenteral nutrition.
7. A variety of commercially available formulas are used for enteral feeding.
   —They provide varying amounts of calories, carbohydrates, protein, and lipids.

Table 3-5. Complications Associated with Enteral Nutritional Support

Complication	Prevention and Management
Inadvertent placement of nasoenteric tube into trachea or bronchus	Careful attention to proper tube placement
Inadvertent intra-abdominal injury during placement of gastrostomy or jejunostomy tube (e.g., liver injury, colon injury, adhesions)	Careful surgical technique
Aspiration	Elevate head of bed ≥ 30°, avoid large gastric residuals (>150 mL), tube placement beyond pylorus, correction of ilius (i.e., electrolyte abnormalities)
Obstruction of feeding tube	Flush tube frequently with water, avoid insertion of large particles (e.g., pills)
Tube rupture or malfunction	Handle feeding tube carefully
Ulceration of external nares with nasoenteric tube	Secure tube appropriately with frequent skin care and monitoring
Leakage or irritation around gastrostomy or jejunostomy tube site	Appropriate initial tube placement, close wound monitoring, and local wound care techniques
Sinusitis or otitis media or parotitis	Avoid long-term use of nasoenteric tubes
Nausea, vomiting	Reduce flow rate, increase time interval between intermittent feedings
Esophageal erosion	
Diarrhea	Reduce flow rate, reduce formula concentration, appropriate formula selection
Metabolic abnormalities (e.g., hyperglycemia, electrolyte abnormalities, dehydration, overhydration)	Monitor blood glucose, electrolytes, and fluid status

a. Some **specialized formulas** are marketed as having an **immune-enhancing function** because of the addition of certain substrates.

(1) **Glutamine**

—may play a role in maintaining intestinal mucosal integrity and immune function.

—levels fall significantly during severe stress and sepsis, therefore repletion may potentially benefit such patients.

(2) **Arginine** may

—improve nitrogen balance.

—improve wound healing.

—stimulate T-cell responsiveness.

—act as a precursor to nitric oxide synthesis.

—reduce overall infectious complications.

(3) **Omega-3 fatty acids** found in fish oils

—act as precursors for eicosanoids.

—may also potentially play an immunoregulatory role.

(4) **Nucleotide supplementation** may improve T lymphocyte function.

—T lymphocytes depend on hepatic synthesis of nucleotides, which is significantly decreased during severe stress and sepsis.

Table 3-6. Enteral Versus Parenteral Nutritional Support

Enteral	Parenteral
Advantages	**Advantages**
Maintains mucosal integrity	Useful when gut unavailable or nonfunctional
Decreased infectious complications	Avoids inherent risks of enteral tube placement
No IV access required	
Less expensive	
Disadvantages	**Disadvantages**
Risk of aspiration	Increased risk of catheter infection
Inherent risks of enteral tube placement	Complications of central venous catheterization (pneumothorax, arterial injury)
Intolerance of GI tract to enteral feeds	Rapid metabolic abnormalities (e.g., hyperglycemia, hypoglycemia, dehydration)
	Very expensive

IV = intravenous; GI = gastrointestinal.

b. The potential benefit of decreasing infectious complications

—is suggested by early studies, although the impact of these formulas on improving mortality and overall outcome is still uncertain.

c. These new immune-enhancing formulas contribute to a significant cost increase.

8. Complications of enteral feeding

—are generally related to tube placement and function, although other factors may play a role.

C. Parenteral nutrition

1. Total parenteral nutrition (TPN)

—is indicated in patients who require nutritional support when the **GI tract is unavailable or nonfunctional.**

2. TPN must be administered

—via a central venous catheter placed in a large central vein (e.g., subclavian vein).

a. The **hyperosmolarity** of the solutions

—precludes administration through smaller veins.

b. Complications

—associated with central venous catheter placement are a frequent source of morbidity associated with parenteral nutrition.

3. Several metabolic complications

—may occur in association with parenteral nutrition (**Table 3–7**).

4. Refeeding syndrome

—may develop rapidly in severely malnourished patients started on parenteral nutritional support.

a. This is most **frequently associated** with

Table 3-7. Complications Associated with Parenteral Nutrition

Complication	Prevention and Management
Complications associated with **central venous catheter placement** (e.g., **pneumothorax, arterial injury, air embolism)**	Careful attention to catheter placement (see Chapter 2)
Catheter-associated infection and sepsis	Attentive catheter maintenance care, prompt replacement of catheter (i.e., over guidewire or removal and placement at alternative site) as indicated if infection presents
Hyperglycemia	Insulin supplementation, decrease rate of infusion, supplement caloric intake with relatively higher percentage of lipids
Hypoglycemia (often seen with sudden discontinuation of parenteral nutrition)	Glucose administration, slowly wean parenteral therapy over 24 hour period as oral intake increases
Electrolyte depletion (e.g., hyponatremia, hypokalemia, hypocalcemia, hypomagnesemia, hypophosphatemia)	**Monitor serum electrolytes,** appropriate IV electrolyte supplementation acutely, supplementation of parenteral solutions with additional electrolytes as needed
Electrolyte excess (e.g., hyperkalemia, hyperphosphatemia, hypercalcemia)	Immediate **discontinuation of current parenteral solution,** administration of crystalloid, treatment of specific excess as needed (see Chapter 7)
Hyperchloremic metabolic acidosis	Decrease chloride supplementation, replace with sodium acetate and potassium acetate salts instead of NaCl and KCl
Refeeding syndrome	Slowly increase initial rate of administration over 24-hour period, monitor blood glucose and electrolytes, aggressive **replacement of PO_4^- salts as needed for hypophosphatemia**
Dehydration	Monitor fluid status closely, **administer crystalloid separate from parenteral solutions as needed**
Overhydration	Concentrate parenteral solutions, provide higher percentage of calories with lipid solutions versus carbohydrates
Essential fatty acid deficiency	Co-administration of **lipid emulsions**

IV = intravenous.

—administration of **high-calorie supplements and supplements high in carbohydrates.**

b. **Abrupt administration**

—of high energy supplements results in massive cellular utilization of glucose and intracellular **phosphate** substrates.

c. This can result in significant **hypophosphatemia** with

—malaise.

—lethargy.

—perioral paresthesias.

—tremors.

—dysarthrias.

—coma.

—even death.

d. **Phosphorus supplementation**

—can be used in the treatment and prevention of this syndrome.

5. **Co-administration of lipid solutions** with standard parenteral nutrition solutions

—help to **prevent essential fatty acid deficiency.**

—provide a relatively high density source of calories compared with carbohydrates.

a. **Lipid solutions**

—**provide more calories in a smaller volume** than carbohydrate solutions, which is important in patients at risk for fluid overload.

b. A 10% solution of IV lipids supplies 1.1 kcal/mL.

c. A 20% lipid solution supplies 2 kcal/mL.

6. **Vitamin and mineral supplements**

—are also available to avoid deficiencies of these nutrients during parenteral nutritional support.

7. **Guidelines for placing TPN orders**

a. **Calculate volume requirements**

—over 24 hours (see Chapter 7).

b. **Determine protein requirements**

—as g/kg/day (see II D).

c. **Calculate total daily caloric need**

—as kcal/kg/day (see II B).

d. **Determine percentage of calories**

—to be given as protein, carbohydrates, and fat (see II C 1 and II E 1).

e. **Add electrolytes** and **trace elements.**

8. **Peripheral parenteral nutrition (PPN)**

a. PPN involves infusion of lower-concentration solutions (carbohydrates, protein, and lipids) into peripheral veins.

b. Indications for PPN are very limited and there are little data demonstrating a benefit from PPN therapy versus other modes of nutritional support.

D. **Specialized formulas**

1. **Specialized formulas**

—for patients with **renal insufficiency and azotemia** are **high in carbohydrates with limited protein.**

a. A large percentage of **protein**

—is administered as **essential amino acids** to avoid unnecessary excessive protein administration.

b. This helps to **improve nitrogen balance**

—and contribute to reduction of blood urea nitrogen levels.

2. Patients with severe **liver disease** may benefit from formulas

—**high in branched-chain amino acids** (metabolized by skeletal muscle).

—**low in aromatic amino acids and methionine** (metabolized by the liver).

a. **The amino acids metabolized by the liver**

—are theoretically thought to contribute to encephalopathy of liver failure.

b. **Early clinical studies suggest**

—these formulas may benefit encephalopathy, but further studies are ongoing to assess their impact on overall outcome.

Review Test

Directions: Each of the numbered items or incomplete statements in this section is followed by answers or by completions of the statement. Select the ONE lettered answer or completion that is BEST in each case.

1. A 52-year-old, alcoholic man with a 4–5 day history of vomiting and epigastric abdominal pain is admitted to the hospital with a diagnosis of acute pancreatitis. The patient states that he has not eaten a meal in over 1 month and has been binge drinking during that time. He refuses to eat because of persistent vomiting and is started on enteral tube feeds containing medium chain triglycerides. Which of the following statements is appropriate regarding administration of medium chain triglycerides?

(A) They are converted to chylomicrons within the enterocyte.
(B) They require pancreatic lipase for absorption.
(C) They are transported to the liver via lymphatic channels.
(D) They may prevent steatorrhea associated with enteral feeding.
(E) They form micelles in the presence of bile salts.

2. A 66-year-old, 70-kg man undergoes extensive small bowel resection for mesenteric ischemia and receives parenteral nutritional support. He is receiving 5 g/kg/day of carbohydrates, 0.2 g/kg/day of nitrogen, and 0.6 g/kg/day of lipids. Which of the following most closely approximates the number of calories this patient is receiving each day?

(A) 2850
(B) 1800
(C) 2450
(D) 3500
(E) 2100

3. A 65-year-old man undergoes an emergent sigmoid colectomy with colostomy for a perforated diverticulum. On postoperative day 3 the patient develops persistent fever with a white blood cell count of 24,000. An abdominal computed tomography (CT) scan reveals a large fluid collection in the left lower quadrant. The patient's heart rate is 130, with a blood pressure of 90/60. Which of the following statements is true regarding this patient's metabolic state?

(A) The insulin/glucose ratio is probably high compared to normal.
(B) This patient is probably in positive nitrogen balance.
(C) Glutamine levels are probably increased in this patient.
(D) Alanine levels are probably increased in this patient.
(E) The respiratory quotient (RQ) value in this patient is probably ≥ 1.0.

4. A 55-year-old man with metastatic carcinoid disease presents to the office complaining of persistent diarrhea for 2–3 weeks. He denies any other symptoms although his wife states that he seems "confused" at times. He states that he has been eating well although his wife states his appetite has been very poor for the past few months. He is currently only taking a topical steroid prescribed by his family physician for a persistent rash. Which of the following is the most appropriate definitive therapy for this patient's condition?

(A) Administer loperamide.
(B) Supplement his diet with vitamins.
(C) Administer somatostatin.
(D) Supplement his diet with zinc.
(E) Administer octreotide.

5. A 72-year-old man has recently undergone extensive resection of a primary squamous cell carcinoma of the tongue with radical neck dissection. Postoperatively he is found to have extensive esophageal candidiasis with severe diffuse ulceration. His past medical history is significant for a previous sigmoid resection for diverticular disease and he has had intermittent symptoms of nausea and vomiting over the past several months which seem to resolve on their own. Which of the following would be the most appropriate reason for parenteral versus enteral nutritional support?

(A) Severe esophageal ulceration
(B) Extensive oropharyngeal resection
(C) Severe sepsis
(D) Small bowel obstruction secondary to adhesions
(E) Previous abdominal surgery precludes percutaneous placement of gastrostomy tube

6. A 68-year-old woman is transferred to a tertiary care hospital after a recent extensive small bowel resection at an outside hospital. She has been diagnosed with short bowel syndrome following the surgery and has received parenteral nutritional support for approximately 3 months. The patient cannot remember exactly what she is taking but she states that she hangs 1 large bag of clear-yellow fluid 3 times a day at home administered through a central venous catheter. She presents with complaints of worsening fatigue and hair loss. Her hematocrit is 34%, white blood cell count 6,000, and platelets 45,000. For managing this patient it would be most appropriate to administer

(A) Niacin
(B) Vitamin C
(C) Zinc
(D) Iron
(E) Lipids

7. A 37-year-old woman sustains 50% full-thickness burn injury to her torso, neck, and upper extremities. Upon admission appropriate fluid resuscitation and local burn wound care are initiated. She is also intubated and receiving 100% oxygen for significant inhalational injury with significant burns to the face and oropharynx. Which of the following is an appropriate statement regarding nutritional supplementation in this patient?

(A) Parenteral nutritional support should be initiated immediately because of the facial and oropharyngeal burn injuries.
(B) Parenteral nutritional support should be initiated immediately because of the risk of aspiration associated with burn injury-induced gastric ileus.
(C) Enteral nutritional support should be initiated immediately despite the oropharyngeal burns and potential risk of aspiration.
(D) Enteral nutritional support should be initiated within 48–72 hours of the initial injury to allow for adequate volume resuscitation.
(E) Enteral nutritional support should be initiated only if there are no sites available for central venous catheter placement for total parenteral nutrition secondary to burn injury.

8. A 25-year-old man sustains a 45% full-thickness burn injury to his lower extremities and torso. After adequate initial fluid resuscitation and local wound care he is awake and alert. On hospital day 3, his heart rate is 130, blood pressure is 130/80, and respiration rate is 24. He is also noted to have a blood glucose of 300 despite administration of 12 units of regular insulin. His blood urea nitrogen is 45 and his creatinine is 1.8. Which of the following statements is appropriate with regard to this patient's metabolic state?

(A) The major source of glucose for the burn wound is probably via glycogenolysis.
(B) Protein requirements are 1 g/kg/day to avoid excessive azotemia with associated renal insufficiency.
(C) Insulin stimulation of lipolysis plays a critical role in providing glucose for peripheral tissues.
(D) Catecholamines and glucagon play a critical role in stimulating glucose production via hepatic gluconeogenesis.
(E) Cortisol, catecholamines, and glucagon play a critical role in stimulating net protein anabolism in this setting.

9. A 65-year-old man undergoes pancreatic débridement for alcohol-induced necrotizing pancreatitis. He is noted to be malnourished on admission to the intensive care unit. He is initially alert but unable to wean from the ventilator postoperatively. He is started on parenteral nutritional therapy with 35 kcal/kg/day with 60% as carbohydrates, 30% as lipids, and 10% kcal as protein. His prealbumin slowly improves over the next several days and his glucose levels remain relatively stable (130–190). Over a 10-day period the patient fails to wean from the ventilator and becomes more confused and lethargic. He also gradually develops a worsening picture of cardiogenic shock. For definitive management of this patient's underlying problem, which of the following is most appropriate to be administered?

(A) Thiamine
(B) KPO_4^-
(C) Niacin
(D) Insulin
(E) Lipids

10. A 65-year-old man underwent resection of the distal 150 cm of his small bowel for severe mesenteric ischemia 3 months ago. He has since recovered and is receiving supplemental enteral nutritional support through a gastrostomy tube in addition to eating small amounts of food each day. He now presents with the complaint of worsening fatigue and malaise over the past several weeks. He has noted an improvement in his appetite and denies any increase in bowel habits. On examination, he appears pale but without muscle wasting or other signs of weight loss. His laboratory results: $K^+ \times 4.5$, $Cl^- = 110$, blood urea nitrogen = 14, creatinine = 1.2, $Mg^{2+} = 2.5$, $PO_4^- = 5.0$, and $Ca^{2+} = 8.5$. His hematocrit is 25%, white blood cell count is 5,000, platelets are 150,000, and mean red cell volume is 125. Which of the following would be the most appropriate therapy in the definitive management of this patient's current condition?

(A) Vitamin B_{12} supplementation
(B) Folate supplementation
(C) Iron supplementation
(D) Administration of 2 U packed red blood cells
(E) Essential fatty acid supplementation

Answers and Explanations

1–D. Medium chain triglycerides are absorbed directly by enterocytes and transported to the liver via the portal vein. Unlike long chain triglycerides, medium chain triglycerides do not require bile salts or pancreatic lipase for absorption. Once long chain fatty acids are degraded to and absorbed by the enterocyte, they are then reconverted to triacylglycerols to form chylomicrons that are transported through lymphatic channels and then into the bloodstream. Medium chain triglycerides do not undergo this process and therefore are considered useful in patients with pancreatic insufficiency. Malabsorption of long chain triglycerides may also lead to steatorrhea, which may be prevented with the use of medium chain triglycerides.

2–E. Carbohydrates produce ~4 kcal/g of substrate while lipids produce ~9 kcal/g substrate. Proteins produce ~4 kcal/g of substrate as well. Protein content may be frequently expressed as grams of nitrogen: 6.25 g of protein = 1 g of nitrogen. Therefore 0.2 g/kg/day of nitrogen = 1.25 g/kg/day of protein. Using these values, this patient is receiving approximately [(4 kcal/g × 5 g carbohydrates) + (9 kcal/g × 0.6 g lipids) + (4 kcal/g × 1.25 g protein)] × 70 kg = 2128 kcal/day.

3–D. Alanine produced by the muscle tissue is a major precursor for gluconeogenesis in the liver and therefore is likely to be elevated in the setting of severe stress where glucagon, cortisol, and catecholamines all play a role in stimulating gluconeogenesis. Frequently in this setting patients become hyperglycemic because of a relative inhibition of insulin secretion as well as a peripheral resistance to the effects of insulin. This would be associated with a relatively low insulin/glucose ratio. In severe stress, there is generally a net proteolysis, resulting in a negative nitrogen balance, while the goal of nutritional therapy and recovery is to produce neutral nitrogen balance. Glutamine levels decrease during stress. In addition, with a relatively prolonged stress (postoperative day 3) there is significant utilization of lipids (lipolysis) resulting in a respiratory quotient (RQ) of ~ 0.7.

4–B. This patient's triad of symptoms (dermatitis, diarrhea, and dementia) is characteristic of pellagra associated with niacin deficiency. In humans, despite inadequate intake of niacin, tryptophan can be converted to niacin. However, in patients with carcinoid syndrome, tryptophan may be diverted to synthesis of serotonin, resulting in an increased risk of niacin deficiency. Thus, in this patient, supplementation with vitamins, specifically niacin, may help to relieve his current triad of symptoms. Zinc deficiency is not associated with this triad of symptoms. Although excess serotonin can lead to diarrhea, treatment of serotonin excess with octreotide will not treat the underlying vitamin deficiency, nor will administration of the antidiarrheal agent, loperamide.

5–D. A high-grade small bowel obstruction is a contraindication to the use of enteral nutritional support. Although severe ulceration of the esophagus may be a relative contraindication to placement of a nasoenteric feeding tube, this patient is still an excellent candidate for a gastrostomy tube or a jejunostomy tube for enteral nutritional support. Sepsis is not a contraindication to enteral nutritional support although attention should first be focused on the underlying cause of sepsis before nutritional therapy is initiated. This patient's extensive oropharyngeal resection is not a contraindication to placement of a direct enteral feeding tube such as a gastrostomy tube, which can be placed percutaneously as well as with an open surgical technique in the setting of previous abdominal surgery with significant adhesions.

6–E. This patient is suffering from sequelae of essential fatty acid deficiency. Today, this is generally avoided in patients receiving parenteral nutritional therapy by co-administering lipid emulsions with the carbohydrate and amino acid solutions characteristic of parenteral therapy, although inadvertent failure to administer such lipids may result in essential fatty acid deficiency. Characteristics of such a deficiency include fatigue, dermatitis, ecchymoses, alopecia, anemia, edema, thrombocytopenia, and respiratory distress. This patient's signs and symptoms are not characteristic of niacin deficiency (pellagra), vitamin C deficiency (scurvy), or zinc deficiency. Although a coexisting iron deficiency could contribute to the anemia, administering iron would not address the primary deficiency causing the entire myriad of findings.

7–C. Studies have shown a significant benefit of enteral nutritional therapy in improving overall outcome in patients with severe burn injuries. In addition, this benefit is increased if enteral therapy can be initiated early in the course of therapy for burn injury and even as early as at the time of initial admission. Facial and oropharyngeal burn injury does not preclude the use of enteral nutrition support nor does the risk of aspiration associated with gastric ileus. Generally speaking, although particularly true for burn patients, enteral nutritional support is preferred over parenteral nutritional support when the gastrointestinal tract is functional and available.

8–D. During severe stress such a significant thermal injury, cortisol, glucagon, catecholamines, and sympathetic nervous stimulation all play a role in stimulating glucose production via lipolysis and hepatic gluconeogenesis. To provide substrates for gluconeogenesis, these agents also stimulate net protein catabolism. Glycogen stores within the body are rapidly depleted in the setting of severe injury within 12–24 hours, therefore after this period glycogenolysis is not the major source of glucose production. Patients with burn injuries have a significantly increased requirement for protein intake given the massive proteolysis. This requirement is ~1.5–2.5 g protein/kg/day and protein restriction should not be initiated because of the risk of worsening azotemia. Insulin is a major stimulus for lipogenesis.

9–A. This patient is manifesting symptoms of thiamine deficiency including Wernicke's encephalopathy, and eventual cardiomyopathy (wet beriberi). This may be seen in severely malnourished patients, particularly in alcoholics. Thiamine supplementation in this setting is the most appropriate therapy. The time course is not consistent with acute refeeding syndrome and hypophosphatemia. Additionally, his glucose levels appear to be stable, thus additional insulin would not treat the underlying condition. The clinical manifestations are also not consistent with either a niacin deficiency or an essential fatty acid deficiency.

10–A. This patient has findings characteristic of megaloblastic anemia caused by inadequate supplementation of vitamin B_{12} after extensive resection of the distal small bowel. The worsening fatigue and malaise in association with the significant decrease in the hematocrit and a large mean cell volume are characteristic. Vitamin B_{12} is primarily absorbed in the terminal ileum and resection can result in a B_{12} deficiency. B_{12} is currently not available as an enteral supplement so must be provided by intravenous or intramuscular administration in this setting. Although folate may be associated with a megaloblastic anemia, this would not be associated with resection of the terminal ileum. The clinical picture and laboratory data are also not consistent with iron or essential fatty acid deficiency. Administration of packed red blood cells would acutely help with the anemia but it would not address the underlying condition.

4

Surgical Infections

Traves D. Crabtree

I. Perioperative Wound Infections

A. Operative cases

—are classified by the level of bacterial contamination (Table 4-1).

1. Clean operative cases

—are associated with a wound infection rate of less than 3%.

2. Clean-contaminated cases

—are associated with a wound infection rate of 3% to 10%.

3. Contaminated cases

—are associated with a wound infection rate of 5% to 15%.

4. Dirty cases

—are associated with a wound infection rate as high as 10% to 40% if wounds are closed primarily. These wounds should be left open and allowed to heal by secondary intention.

B. Perioperative antibiotic prophylaxis

—has been shown to **decrease the postoperative wound infection** rate in **clean-contaminated procedures.**

1. Other indications for prophylaxis

a. Some clean cases (e.g., elective inguinal hernia repairs, breast surgery) may also benefit from antibiotic prophylaxis.

b. Antibiotic prophylaxis is generally accepted with procedures that involve insertion of prosthetic material or foreign bodies; clean operations in patients with impaired host defenses; and neurosurgical, cardiac, and ophthalmologic procedures.

c. Other considerations are the patient's **overall health status** and the **length of operation.**

Table 4-1. Classification of Operative Cases Based on Potential Bacterial Contamination

Wound Classification	Viscus Injury	Spillage	Break in Surgical Technique	Trauma	Finding of Infection or Inflammation	Example
Clean	None	None	None	None	No inflammation	Elective inguinal hernia
Clean-contaminated	**Controlled/planned viscus entry**	Minimal	Minimal	None	Emergent clean case, reopen clean case	Elective bowel resection
Contaminated	**Unintended viscus entry**	**Gross GI spillage**	Major	Injury < 4 hours old	Presence of infected urine or bile	Colon injury during cholecystectomy
Dirty	Perforated viscus encountered	**Fecal contamination present**	–	Injury > 4 hours old, foreign body, devitalized tissue	**Purulent material encountered**	Traumatic colon injury

GI = gastrointestinal.

2. **Prophylactic antibiotics**

—should be administered **within 1 hour** before incision. If given more than 24 hours postoperatively, antibiotics have not been shown to provide additional benefit in decreasing infection rates.

a. **A preoperative bowel preparation**

—with nonabsorbable antibiotics and cathartic agents [e.g., polyethylene glycol (GoLYTELY)], in conjunction with antibiotics, may decrease the postoperative wound infection rate in surgery of the lower alimentary tract.

b. **Antibiotic prophylaxis**

—plays a small role in preventing wound infections relative to the role of **adequate surgical débridement** and meticulous attention to **proper surgical technique.**

3. **Contaminated and dirty wounds**

—generally require a course of antibiotic therapy after appropriate débridement and drainage have been performed.

C. The **American Heart Association** has provided recommendations for perioperative antibiotic prophylaxis in patients at risk for **bacterial endocarditis.**

1. **Antibiotic prophylaxis is recommended in patients with**

—prosthetic cardiac valves.

—rheumatic valvular dysfunction.

—most congenital cardiac malformations.

—mitral valve prolapse with regurgitation.

—previous history of bacterial endocarditis.

2. **Antibiotic prophylaxis is not required in patients with**

—previous coronary artery bypass grafting.

—isolated secundum atrial septal defect.

—physiologic/functional heart murmurs.

3. **Prophylaxis for endocarditis in at-risk patients**

—is generally recommended in **procedures with a significant risk for transient bacteremia** (e.g., abdominal surgery, most urologic procedures, many dental procedures).

4. **For general surgical procedures**

—a regimen of **ampicillin** and **gentamicin** is recommended perioperatively.

—Patients with penicillin allergies may receive vancomycin and gentamicin.

D. **Prophylaxis against tetanus** for traumatic injuries depends on the **characteristics of the injury** and the patient's **immunization status.**

1. **Characteristics of tetanus-prone wounds** include

—wounds over 6 hours old.

—injuries more than 1-cm deep.

—irregular skin borders.

—the presence of devitalized tissue or obvious contamination.

—crush, burn, frostbite, and missile injuries.

2. **Tetanus immune globulin**

—is administered only in tetanus-prone wounds in unimmunized patients or if the immunization status is unknown.

3. **Tetanus toxoid**

—is administered depending on the patient's immunization status as outlined in Table 4-2.

II. Skin and Soft Tissue Infections

A. Primary infections of the skin (pyodermas)

—include impetigo, erysipelas, cellulitis, and folliculitis.

1. Most of these infections are caused by ***Staphylococcus*** and ***Streptococcus*** species.
2. Antibiotics alone are often sufficient treatment because the vascular supply to the area of infection remains intact.
3. Specific environments may predispose to primary skin infections with uncommon organisms; for example, *Pseudomonas* species can cause "hot-tub folliculitis."

B. Abscesses

—are infections that contain a **nonvascular central portion** comprised of necrotic debris from leukocytes, bacteria, and tissue components.

1. **Treatment**
   - a. **Drainage** of an abscess is the **definitive** treatment, with antibiotics serving as adjunctive therapy.
   - b. **Antibiotics alone** are **insufficient** treatment because of the poor vascular supply to an abscess.
2. **The organisms within abscesses**

Table 4-2. Schedule for Administration of Tetanus Toxoid in Traumatic Injuries

		Tetanus Immunization History		
Wound Class	**Unknown or < 3 Doses**	**≥ 3 Doses**	**≥ 3 Doses and > 5 Years Since Booster**	**≥ 3 Doses and > 10 Years Since Booster**
Tetanus-prone	Yes	No (yes if wound > 24 hours old)	Yes	Yes
Nontetanus-prone	Yes	No	No	Yes

Adapted from *MMWR* 1990;39:37–41.

—may include one predominant bacteria or multiple bacteria, both aerobic and anaerobic, depending on the original source of bacteria.

a. Soft tissue abscesses above the waist are often associated with ***Staphylococcus* or *Streptococcus* species.**

b. Perirectal and **intra-abdominal abscesses** often contain **mixed aerobic and anaerobic pathogens** originating from fecal or intestinal flora.

C. Bite wounds

—may become infected 15% to 20% of the time.

1. Organisms in human bite wounds

—include ***Staphylococcus*** species, oral anaerobes, *Eikenella* species, and *Haemophilus influenza.*

a. *Eikenella* species cause **permanent joint injury.**

b. Closed-fist injuries should be carefully examined for joint involvement.

c. These closed-fisted wounds should **not be closed** and should be **débrided appropriately.**

d. Appropriate antibiotics and **tetanus prophylaxis** should also be instituted.

2. Organisms in animal bites

—may include **streptococci, staphylococci,** anaerobes, and ***Pasteurella multocida*** (more common in cat bites).

D. Necrotizing soft tissue infections

1. Organisms producing gangrene or necrosis of soft tissue

—most often include ***Streptococcus*** species and then ***Clostridium*** species. Other organisms often cultured from such infections include *Bacteroides, Enterobacter,* and *Enterococcus.*

2. Classic "gas gangrene"

—is **myonecrosis produced by *clostridium* species,** and less frequently by *staphylococcus* and *streptococcus* species.

a. *Clostridium* and *streptococcus* species

—may produce a **rapid fulminant course** with severe toxemia occurring within 24 hours of wound inoculation.

b. Characteristic findings include

—**severe pain.**

—**"dishwater-like" nonpurulent discharge.**

—**early toxemia.**

—wound edema and crepitus.

—nonerythematous skin with bullous lesions.

—late skin necrosis.

c. Treatment

—The **primary** therapy is **early aggressive surgical débridement.**

—Penicillin G provides adequate coverage for these *clostridium* and *streptococcus* species.

—Additional coverage for potential mixed infections may be appropriate (e.g., aminoglycoside).

—Adjunctive hyperbaric oxygen therapy may also be of some benefit.

3. **Fournier's gangrene**

—refers to necrotizing soft tissue infections of the perineal/scrotal region.

a. **Bacteria** often originate from a primary colonic or genitourinary source.

b. **Etiologies** include rectal trauma, perirectal abscesses, pilonidal cysts, posthemorrhoidectomy infections, and various primary and secondary urologic infections.

c. Diabetes is a significant **risk factor** for development of these infections.

d. Infections are polymicrobial and require **aggressive débridement** of the perineum and scrotum with **sparing of the testes.**

E. **Toxic shock syndrome (TSS)**

—is most frequently caused by ***staphylococcus*** species, although ***streptococcus*** species may also produce this syndrome.

1. **Staphylococcal TSS**

—often originates from infections involving **mucous membranes** as well as soft tissue infections.

—may result from colonization of wounds **without overt infection.**

2. **Streptococcal TSS**

—often originates from invasive skin and soft tissue infections.

3. **Characteristics** include

—**rapid onset of fever.**

—**refractory hypotension.**

—**diffuse erythematous desquamating rash.**

—vomiting and diarrhea.

—conjunctival injection.

—strawberry tongue.

—multisystem organ failure.

4. **Treatment**

—involves aggressive **fluid resuscitation** used in conjunction with **antibiotics** and **surgical débridement** when appropriate.

a. Intravenous (IV) administration of **immune globulin against toxic shock syndrome toxin (TSST)** may improve patient outcome.

b. Antistaphylococcal penicillins (e.g., **nafcillin**) are appropriate for staphylococcal-induced TSS.

c. **Penicillin G** in conjunction with **clindamycin** is appropriate antibiotic coverage for streptococcal-induced TSS.

—Clindamycin inhibits protein synthesis and thus may inhibit TSST production.

III. Nosocomial Infections (Table 4-3)

A. Nosocomial pneumonia

—has a mortality rate of 20% to 50%.

1. Risk factors

a. The most important risk factor for the development of nosocomial pneumonia is **mechanical ventilation.**

b. Endotracheal tubes and tracheostomy tubes do not prevent aspiration of oropharyngeal contents even with a cuff inflated.

c. H_2-blocking agents alter gastric pH and allow for bacterial colonization of the stomach, which may increase the risk for pneumonia.

2. **Differential diagnosis** in the critically ill patient includes

—adult respiratory distress syndrome.

—congestive heart failure.

—pulmonary hemorrhage or contusion.

—pulmonary embolus.

—pleural effusion.

—atelectasis.

3. **Diagnostic features** include

—isolation of a predominant organism from sputum or lavage specimens without significant contamination from oral flora.

—characteristic radiographic findings.

—fever.

—productive purulent sputum.

—respiratory compromise.

4. Common pathogens

—include *Pseudomonas aeruginosa, Staphylococcus aureus, Klebsiella, Enterobacter, Escherichia coli, Serratia,* and *Proteus.*

5. Treatment

—involves appropriate **antibiotic therapy** in conjunction with aggressive **management of pulmonary secretions.**

B. Urinary tract infections

—are the most common nosocomial infections.

1. The **greatest risk factor**

—is placement of **urinary catheters.**

2. Common pathogens

—include *E. coli, Pseudomonas, Klebsiella, Staphylococcus epidermidis,* and *Candida albicans.*

3. Treatment

—involves **antibiotic therapy** with meticulous care of indwelling catheters and prompt removal when appropriate.

Table 4-3. Postoperative Nosocomial Infections

Nosocomial Infection	Risk Factors	Signs and Symptoms	Common Pathogens	Diagnosis	Treatment
Pneumonia	**Tracheal intubation**	Purulent sputum, respiratory compromise	***Pseudomonas, Staphylococcus,*** *Klebsiella, Escherichia coli, Serratia, Proteus*	CXR, positive cultures, clinical suspicion	Antibiotics, management of pulmonary secretions
Urinary system infection	Urinary tract catheterization/instrumentation	Urinary frequency, dysuria	*E. coli, Pseudomonas, Klebsiella, Staphylococcus, Epidermidis, Candida albicans*	Pyuria, positive cultures	Antibiotics, prompt removal and meticulous care of indwelling catheters
IV catheter-related infections	**TPN,** Multi-lumen>single lumen, femoral>> subclavian or jugular	Recurrent fever, persistent bacteremia	*Staphylococcus* species, gram-negative rods, *Enterococcus, Candida*	Positive blood cultures, positive catheter tip cultures	Removal of catheter, antibiotics
Sinusitis	Facial fractures, **nasoenteric/ nasotracheal tubes**	Purulent nasal secretions, facial pain	Polymicrobial, gram-negative organisms	Air fluid levels radiographically, positive cultures of sinuses	Removal of foreign bodies, antibiotics
Pseudomembranous colitis	Recent **antibiotic therapy**	Diarrhea, abdominal pain	***Clostridium difficile***	**Cytotoxin** in stool specimen, colonoscopy, *C. difficile* in stool cultures	Oral or IV metronidazole **(Flagyl)**, oral vancomycin

CXR = chest radiograph; IV = intravenous; TPN = total parenteral nutrition.

C. Intravenous catheter-related infections

—are most often caused by ***staphylococcus*** species although **gram-negative bacteria** and ***Candida*** may also be a source.

1. **Relative risk factors** include

—administration of total parenteral nutrition (TPN).

—multilumen catheters (more than single-lumen catheters).

—femoral catheters (more than subclavian or jugular catheters).

2. **Treatment**

—involves prompt removal of the catheter with adjunctive antibiotics.

D. Other potential nosocomial infections in the critically ill patient

1. **Pseudomembranous colitis**

—is caused by an **exotoxin** produced by ***Clostridium difficile.***

—characteristically **presents after a course of antibiotic therapy** secondary to alterations in normal colonic flora.

—can be initiated by **any antibiotic** and can present several weeks after completion of antibiotic therapy.

a. **Signs and symptoms**

—may include watery diarrhea, abdominal pain, and fever.

b. **Diagnosis**

(1) The diagnosis is confirmed by demonstrating the **presence of cytotoxin in stool samples.**

(2) Colonoscopy may also be diagnostic by directly visualizing the characteristic pseudomembranes on the colonic mucosa.

c. **When suspicious of pseudomembranous colitis**

—**prompt diagnosis** is essential for treatment.

d. Adequate **treatment** includes IV or oral **metronidazole therapy** and cessation of inciting antibiotics, if possible.

(1) Oral vancomycin may be used if there is a contraindication to metronidazole therapy or for failure of initial treatment.

(2) **Surgery** is rarely necessary unless complications such as **perforation or toxic megacolon** arise.

2. **Sinusitis**

—accounts for 5% of intensive care unit–acquired infections (see *BRS Surgical Specialties*, Chapter 4 III B).

3. **Other infectious and inflammatory processes** that should be considered in the critically ill postoperative patient include

—deep vein thrombosis.

—thrombophlebitis.

—parotitis.

—perirectal abscess.

—cholecystitis, appendicitis, or other intra-abdominal source.

—pancreatitis.

4. **Fungal infection**

—should be suspected if there are **persistent signs or symptoms of infection** in a critically ill patient despite broad spectrum antibacterial therapy.

IV. Hepatitis B, C, and Human Immunodeficiency Virus (HIV) Exposure in Surgery

A. Hepatitis B virus (HBV)

1. **The risk of transmission**

—to nonimmunized individuals after a needlestick with a **contaminated needle** is 30% overall.

—is 2% if the infected patient is negative for **hepatitis B e antigen (HB_eAg)** and is as high as 40% if the infected patient is HB_eAg-positive.

—is increased with increasing size of the inocula of blood with **hollow needles (e.g., IV catheters),** which pose a greater risk than suture needles.

a. Although rare, transmission with bite wounds and inoculation of mucosal membranes with contaminated blood has been documented.

b. **Bodily fluids,** such as semen, vaginal fluid, and saliva, are also considered potential sources of HBV infection, although their role in occupational transmission is not yet defined.

2. **Immunization for HBV** is now recommended for **newborn children** and **individuals at high risk** for exposure to HBV, including

—health-care and public safety workers.

—hemodialysis patients.

—hemophiliacs.

—homosexual males.

—IV drug abusers.

—household and sexual contacts of HBV carriers.

3. **Administration of the HBV vaccine**

—to **previously vaccinated individuals** after exposure depends on the level of **serum anti-HB_sAg,** as outlined in Table 4-4.

4. **Prophylaxis**

—in **unvaccinated individuals** exposed to HBV (e.g., needlestick) should include **hepatitis B immune globulin (HBIG) and the HBV vaccine** given at **two different sites.** HBIG is considered efficacious if administered within 7 days of exposure.

B. Hepatitis C virus (HCV)

1. **The risk of transmission of HCV**

—in a nonimmunized individual after **percutaneous injury from an infected individual** is 3% to 10%.

Table 4-4. Prophylaxis for Hepatitis B After Exposure to Hepatitis B–Positive Source

	Exposure Source	
Exposed Person	**HBsAg+**	**HBsAg−**
Unvaccinated	HBIG + HB vaccine	HB vaccine
Vaccinated		
Anti-HBs ≥ 10 mIU/mL*	No treatment	No treatment
Anti-HBs < 10 mIU/mL	HBIG + 1 dose HB vaccine	No treatment

Adapted from *MMWR* 1991; 40(RR–13):1–25.
Anti-HBs = serum antibody to hepatitis B surface antigen; HB = hepatitis B; HBIG = hepatitis B immune globulin; HBsAg = serum hepatitis B surface antigen.
*Exposed individuals should be tested for serum anti-HBs antibody titers.

—is low relative to the risk of HBV.

a. Transmission from **contaminated blood** or blood products is the **primary modality of infection.**

b. Blood contamination of mucosal membranes, semen, and vaginal fluid are other plausible sources that have not been reliably confirmed.

2. Currently there are no recommendations for **immunization** against HCV or for postexposure prophylactic therapy, although exposed patients should receive serial serum tests for anti-HCV antibodies after exposure to document seroconversion.

C. **Human immunodeficiency virus (HIV)**

1. **The risk of transmission of HIV**

—after **percutaneous injury from an infected individual** is 0.2% to 0.5%.

—The estimated HIV transmission rate per operation from an HIV-positive patient to the surgeon is 1/130,000.

2. **Chemoprophylaxis**

a. **with an antiretroviral regimen,** including zidovudine (AZT) and lamivudine (3TC) ± a protease inhibitor [i.e., indinavir (IDV)], **decreases the rate of seroconversion** after occupational exposure to HIV.

(1) This ideally should be **administered within 1 to 2 hours** after exposure, although prophylaxis may be considered up to 2 weeks later in high-risk exposures.

(2) Recommendation of postexposure chemoprophylaxis depends on the **exposure risk and the associated morbidity of the antiretroviral regimen.**

(3) Regimens are often individualized based on the source's antiretroviral therapy and the potential for HIV-resistant strains.

b. **after a percutaneous injury** is recommended if exposure involves a **large volume of HIV-positive blood** (i.e., deep large-bore IV injury) or **exposure to blood with a high titer of HIV** [i.e., end-stage acquired immunodeficiency syndrome (AIDS)].

c. should be offered when **blood** or various **bodily fluids** [e.g., semen; vaginal secretions; cerebrospinal fluid (CSF); synovial, pleural, peritoneal, pericardial, and amniotic fluids] are introduced percutaneously or when contact with **mucous membranes** occurs.

d. should be offered with **skin exposure** to these bodily fluids when exposure involves a high titer of HIV, prolonged contact, an extensive area of exposure, or an area with visibly compromised skin integrity.

e. should not be offered when the exposure does not increase the risk of HIV seroconversion.

—For example, there have been no definitively confirmed cases of seroconversion after a solid suture needle injury from an asymptomatic HIV-positive patient.

—This includes exposure to urine, saliva, or feces.

3. Testing of exposed individuals for HIV antibodies

—should be performed at 6 weeks, 12 weeks, and 6 months, with seroconversion typically occurring within 6 to 12 weeks.

Review Test

Directions: Each of the numbered items or incomplete statements in this section is followed by answers or by completions of the statement. Select the ONE lettered answer or completion that is BEST in each case.

Questions 1–4

A 62-year-old man underwent an elective left hemicolectomy with primary anastomosis for Stage II colon adenocarcinoma. Twenty-four hours postoperatively, his temperature was 38.8°C (102°F), his heart rate (HR) was 100 beats/min, and his blood pressure (BP) was 150/90 mm Hg. Breath sounds were diminished in both lung bases, while the rest of the physical examination was unremarkable. Chest radiograph revealed bibasilar atelectasis. Seven days postoperatively, his temperature increased to 39°C (102.2°F), his HR increased to 130 beats/min, and his BP was 90/60 mm Hg. His lungs were clear on physical examination and there was no evidence of wound infection. The patient complained of increasing abdominal bloating and worsening abdominal pain.

1. In regard to this patient's immediate postoperative fever, which of the following is an appropriate statement?

(A) The patient's fever was due to a wound infection
(B) Prophylactic perioperative antibiotics have been shown to prevent the development of nosocomial pneumonia in the postoperative patient
(C) Improved pain control may have indirectly helped to decrease the patient's temperature
(D) All peripheral intravenous catheters should have been immediately removed because of their risk of infection
(E) Pulmonary atelectasis causes fever by bacterial stimulation of inflammatory mediators

2. Which of the following statements is true regarding the use of perioperative prophylactic antibiotics in this patient?

(A) Prophylactic antibiotics should be administered 24 hours before surgery to decrease the rate of wound infection
(B) If no spillage of fecal material occurred, antibiotics are not indicated because it is a clean case
(C) Shaving the evening before surgery decreases the wound infection rate compared with shaving immediately before incision
(D) A preoperative bowel preparation with nonabsorbable antibiotics alone decreases the rate of postoperative infectious complications
(E) The most important intra-operative factor in preventing postoperative wound infections is appropriate dosing of prophylactic antibiotics

3. Which of the following is an appropriate consideration in the diagnosis and treatment of this patient?

(A) This patient probably has an early nosocomial pneumonia
(B) A decrease in this patient's temperature when incentive spirometry is initiated would prove that atelectasis is the source of fever
(C) Antibiotics should be started for treatment of a potential urinary tract infection
(D) An abdominal computed tomography (CT) scan is appropriate to rule out a potential intra-abdominal source of infection
(E) Antifungal therapy should be initiated immediately

4. For wound infections presenting in the early postoperative period (< 48 hours), which of the following statements is true?

(A) *Clostridium* and *streptococcus* species are frequent pathogens
(B) The bacterial contamination leading to wound infection typically occurs in the postoperative period
(C) The rate of wound healing is unaffected by wound infections occurring in the early postoperative period
(D) Débridement of an infected wound should be performed if antibiotic therapy fails
(E) They are generally caused by slow-growing, nonvirulent bacteria

5. A 22-year-old man underwent percutaneous pin fixation of a right ankle fracture as an outpatient. Three days later he presents at the emergency department complaining of vomiting and mild shortness of breath, but denies any pain. The wound is without obvious drainage or erythema. His temperature is 39°C (102.2°F), his heart rate is 140 beats/min, and his blood pressure is 90/40 mm Hg. His chest radiograph is clear and his creatinine is 3.4. Which of the following statements is true regarding this patient?

(A) The causative organism is most likely a clostridial species
(B) An intra-abdominal source of infection is likely
(C) Outpatient antibiotic therapy is indicated
(D) Renal failure is secondary to associated bacteremia
(E) A desquamating erythematous rash is characteristic

6. After a routine right inguinal hernia repair, a 42-year-old man develops erythema over the incision. A wound infection is diagnosed and the patient is discharged to home on 10 days of ciprofloxacin. Three weeks later he returns with complaints of persistent watery diarrhea with a low-grade fever. His temperature is 38.3°C (101°F), his heart rate is 80 beats/min, and his blood pressure is 125/65 mm Hg. Which of the following is the most appropriate next step in the management of this patient?

(A) Intravenous (IV) vancomycin therapy
(B) Colonoscopy
(C) No treatment, because the cause is probably viral
(D) Oral clindamycin

Questions 7–8

A 24-year-old migrant farm worker presents to the emergency department with complaints of pain at the site of a 4-cm laceration on his right leg. The patient states that he was cut by the end of a shovel while working 2 days earlier, but did not seek medical attention at that time because he was able to stop the bleeding. The patient does not recall ever having been immunized for tetanus.

7. Which of the following is the most important initial step in the management of this patient?

(A) Admission to the hospital and administration of intravenous (IV) broad spectrum antibiotics with close observation of the wound
(B) Administration of tetanus toxoid
(C) Oral antibiotics and scheduling of close follow-up as an outpatient
(D) Wound inspection, irrigation, and débridement
(E) Careful closure of the laceration with administration of broad spectrum IV antibiotics

8. Which of the following would be the most appropriate regimen with regard to prophylaxis for tetanus?

(A) Administration of tetanus booster
(B) Administration of a full dose of tetanus toxoid
(C) Administration of tetanus toxoid in the dominant arm and tetanus immune globulin in the nondominant arm
(D) Administration of tetanus toxoid and tetanus immune globulin in the nondominant arm
(E) Administration of tetanus toxoid and tetanus immune globulin in the gluteal region

Directions: Each group of items in this section consists of lettered options followed by a set of numbered items. For each item, select the appropriate lettered option(s) most closely associated with it. Each lettered option may be selected once, more than once, or not at all.

Questions 9–12

(A) *Staphylococcus aureus*
(B) *Clostridium tetani*
(C) *Clostridium difficile*
(D) *Candida albicans*
(E) *Bacteroides fragilis*
(F) *Escherichia coli*
(G) *Pseudomonas aeruginosa*
(H) *Klebsiella pneumoniae*
(I) *Proteus mirabilis*
(J) *Haemophilus influenzae*

Match each scenario with the correct causative organism.

9. A 48-year-old man has been in the intensive care unit for 5 weeks after a severe motor vehicle accident with multiple injuries. He has been on broad spectrum antibiotics for 3½ weeks. He now has persistent fever with associated worsening refractory hypotension. There is no obvious source of infection on physical examination, by abdominal computed tomography (CT), or on chest radiograph. The only new finding is the presence of new retinal lesions on funduscopic examination. (SELECT 1 ORGANISM)

10. A 68-year-old, alcoholic man has been in the hospital for 36 hours after a motor vehicle accident with multiple orthopedic injuries. He develops a fever with painful swelling of his right cheek. There is purulent material noted at the opening of Stensen's duct. There is no other obvious source of infection on physical examination or chest radiograph. (SELECT 1 ORGANISM)

11. A 48-year-old woman has been in the intensive care unit for 3 weeks after repair of a grade III liver laceration and colonic perforation sustained from a motor vehicle accident. She has been ventilator-dependent since admission and has received 2 weeks of broad spectrum antibiotics for a presumed intra-abdominal source of infection. She now has persistent fever with a worsening infiltrate on chest radiograph. Computed tomography (CT) scan reveals no obvious intra-abdominal source of infection and the rest of the physical examination is normal. Sputum cultures reveal gram-negative rods. (SELECT 2 ORGANISMS)

12. A 52-year-old man has been in the intensive care unit for 4 weeks after a surgical débridement for necrotizing pancreatitis. He remains ventilator-dependent and has been on intravenous (IV) antibiotics for aspiration pneumonia. The patient now has a persistent fever without any obvious source of infection on physical examination. His chest radiograph reveals resolution of a right lower lobe infiltrate and CT scan of the abdomen reveals no obvious source of infection. Proctoscopic examination reveals plaque-like lesions on the mucosa of the distal sigmoid colon. (SELECT 1 ORGANISM)

Answers and Explanations

1–C. Fever occurring in the first 48 hours postoperatively without any obvious source of infection after careful evaluation may arise from a pulmonary source of inflammatory mediator stimulation associated with atelectasis. This process is not felt to be bacterial or infectious in nature and can frequently be alleviated by measures that improve the patient's ability to ventilate collapsed alveoli such as incentive spirometry or improved pain control, which may allow for improved respiratory effort. Prophylactic perioperative antibiotics do not decrease the rate of postoperative pneumonia, though they decrease the wound infection rate in selected cases. Although rare, wound infections can occur within the first 24 to 48 hours postoperatively with aggressive strains of *Streptococcus* or *Clostridium*. Inspection of all intravenous (IV) sites is essential in evaluating the postoperative patient with fever; however, immediate removal of all peripheral IV catheters is not warranted.

2–D. For elective surgery on the colon, a preoperative bowel preparation with nonabsorbable antibiotics and cathartic agents decreases the rate of postoperative infectious complications, although prophylactic intravenous (IV) antibiotics may also provide some additional benefit. There is no decrease in infection rates if prophylactic perioperative antibiotics are administered 24 hours preoperatively versus within 1 hour of surgery. In addition, shaving the skin at the incision site the evening before surgery provides no benefit in decreasing wound infection rates and may actually increase the wound infection rate secondary to the induction of microabscess formation. The most important factors in decreasing the postoperative wound infection rate are attention to proper surgical technique and adequate surgical débridement when appropriate. An uncomplicated elective colon resection involves controlled entry into the gastrointestinal tract and is considered a clean-contaminated case.

3–D. Although there are many potential sources of nosocomial infection in the postoperative patient, an intra-abdominal source should always be considered after abdominal surgery. An abdominal computed tomography (CT) scan would be a valuable diagnostic examination in this patient to assess the abdomen for potential sources of infection. Although thorough evaluation for other potential sources of infection is necessary, there is no evidence provided suggesting that the patient has clinically relevant pneumonia, nor is there any evidence of a urinary tract infection at this point. Routine administration of antifungal agents without any evidence of a fungal infection is not indicated.

4–A. Although rare, wound infections occurring within the first 48 hours postoperatively in an otherwise uncomplicated case frequently are caused by fast-growing, virulent strains of *clostridium* or *streptococcus* species. Bacterial introduction into the wound that results in postoperative infection most often occurs intraoperatively rather than postoperatively. Treatment involves adequately débriding devitalized or necrotic tissue and providing adequate drainage of an infected wound, with antibiotics serving as adjuncts in the therapy. Wound infections are a leading cause of wound healing failure. Risk factors for the development of wound infections include the presence of foreign bodies, poor approximation of wound edges, tissue ischemia (i.e., inadequate fluid resuscitation or sutures too tight), and the presence of devitalized tissue, hematomas, or seromas.

5–E. Toxic shock syndrome (TSS) is most often caused by virulent strains of *Staphylococcus* or *Streptococcus* and may frequently produce a rapid fulminant course. A diffuse desquamating erythematous rash, frequently away from the site of injury, is characteristic of TSS and may provide a clue to the diagnosis. The pathogenesis of TSS is related to a toxin called toxic shock syndrome toxin (TSST) produced locally by these bacteria and not necessarily by bacteremia. Although possible, a concomitant intra-abdominal source of infection is unlikely given this scenario. Outpatient management would be inappropriate given his condition and potential for continued rapid deterioration.

6–B. Following a course of antibiotics, one should always be suspicious of the diagnosis of pseudomembranous colitis in a patient with the history given. Although this process could be viral, appropriate diagnostic measures should be taken to rule out pseudomembranous colitis. It is generally appropriate to try to confirm the presence of *Clostridium difficile* cytotoxin in stool specimens, although identifying plaque-like pseudomembranous lesion by colonoscopy would be highly suggestive of such a diagnosis; but this is not routine. Treatment is with oral or intravenous (IV) metronidazole, or nonabsorbable oral vancomycin, although metronidazole is the preferred treatment given the cost considerations and the potential risk of developing vancomycin-resistant *Enterococcus* strains.

7–D. Although intravenous (IV) antibiotics and appropriate tetanus immunization should be administered early in the course of treatment, initial attention should be devoted to inspection, irrigation, and adequate débridement of the injured site. In a dirty wound with exposure to soil contaminants such as this one, closure of the laceration is inappropriate given the high risk of infection. The decision to manage such a patient as an outpatient should be individually based after adequate assessment of the patient and the wound.

8–C. In an unimmunized patient with a tetanusprone wound, a full regimen of both tetanus toxoid and tetanus immune globulin should be administered. When administering the toxoid (antigen) in conjunction with immune globulin (antibody to the antigen) injections should be performed at separate sites to avoid any potential interaction between the antigen and antibody, which could potentially interfere with both the passive and active immunization.

9–D. Definitive diagnostic criteria for disseminated candidal sepsis include endophthalmitis, positive tissue cultures for *Candida,* burn wound invasion, and positive peritoneal cultures in the setting of peritonitis. The presence of *Candida* in blood cultures and in cultures of multiple other sites (three or more sites) is also highly suggestive of the development of candidal sepsis in the critically ill patient. Disseminated candidiasis can often produce a rapid fulminant course with an associated high mortality rate (> 50%). Such infection should be considered in the critically ill patient receiving long-term broad spectrum antibiotics.

10–A. Although parotitis is an uncommon cause of postoperative fever, it should be considered in the differential diagnosis. Dehydration, as may be seen in alcoholic patients, is a risk factor for the development of parotitis with partial obstruction of the parotid duct contributing to the infectious or inflammatory process. The most common organism found in such infections is *Staphylococcus aureus.* Parotitis typically presents with fever, a swollen painful cheek, and purulent exudate from the opening of the parotid duct (Stensen's duct).

11–A, G. Nosocomial pneumonia is a common complication seen in critically ill, hospitalized patients, particularly in patients who require prolonged ventilatory assistance. Diagnostic criteria include productive purulent sputum, radiographic evidence of an infiltrate, positive cultures of sputum or lavage specimens without significant oral contamination, respiratory compromise, and fever. Although many organisms may be identified as the inciting agent, overall, the two most common organisms identified in nosocomial pneumonia are *Pseudomonas aeruginosa* (gram-negative rod) and *Staphylococcus aureus* (gram-positive cocci).

12–C. The diagnosis of pseudomembranous colitis should always be considered as a potential source of infection in any patient receiving long-term antibiotic therapy. Symptomatology may be more subtle in the critically ill patient. Although not routine, the identification of characteristic pseudomembranous lesions on endoscopic examination of the rectosigmoid provides adequate diagnostic criteria for this disease. Confirmation of *Clostridium difficile* cytotoxin in stool specimens may also confirm the diagnosis.

5

Wound Healing and Plastic Surgery

Alan Parungao

I. Wound Healing

A. **Stages or phases of wound healing** (Figure 5-1)

1. **Inflammatory phase** (substrate, lag, or exudative phase)
   —begins immediately after wounding.
   —lasts for 4–6 days in uncomplicated postoperative wound closures (**primary intention** healing).
   a. **Symptoms and signs of inflammation** include
      —redness (rubor).
      —heat (calor).
      —swelling (tumor).
      —pain (dolor).
      —loss of function.
   b. The **two main cells**
      —involved in the inflammatory response are **macrophages** and **polymorphonuclear (PMN) leukocytes.**
      (1) **Macrophages**
         —secrete **basic fibroblastic growth factor (bFGF),** which stimulates fibroblasts and endothelial cells and enhances angiogenesis.
      (2) **PMN leukocytes**
         —are the predominant cells for the **first 48 hours.**
         —release many of the inflammatory mediators and bactericidal oxygen-derived free radicals.
      (3) **Macrophages and PMN leukocytes remove** clots, foreign bodies, and bacteria, which may inhibit wound healing.

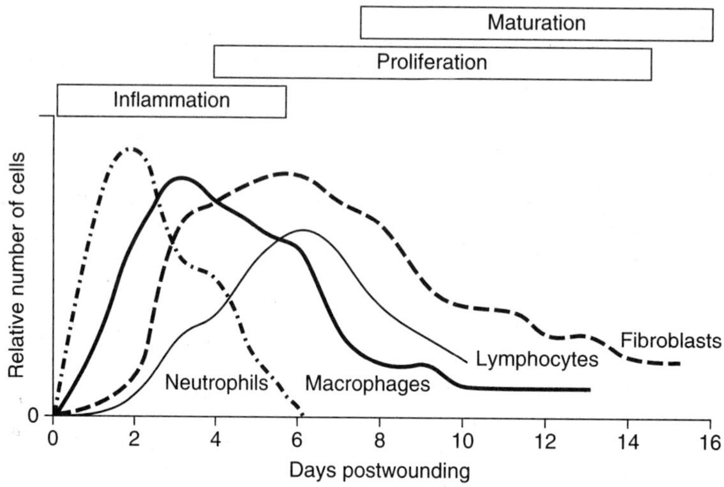

Figure 5-1. The course of the different cells appearing in the wound during the healing process. Macrophages and neutrophils are predominant during inflammation, whereas lymphocytes peak somewhat later and fibroblasts are predominant during the proliferative phase. (Adapted with permission from Wittey MB, Barbul A: General Principles of Wound Healing. In *The Surgical Clinics of North America, "Wound Healing."* Edited by Barbul A. Philadelphia, WB Saunders, 1997, p 512.)

c. **Other factors involved in wound healing** include
   —growth factors (GF) [e.g., platelet-derived GF (PDGF), epidermal GF (EGF), insulin-like GF (IGF), transforming GF (TGF)].
   —interleukin-1.
   —tumor necrosis factor.
   —prostaglandins.
   —collagenase.
   —elastase.

d. **In healing by secondary intention**
   —a contaminated **wound is left open** to prevent wound infection, allowing inflammatory cells to débride the wound.
   —the open full-thickness wound is allowed to close by both **wound contraction and epithelialization.**
   —the inflammatory phase continues until the wound surface is closed by epithelium.
   —In a variation of this technique, called **delayed primary closure,** the skin and subcutaneous tissues are left unopposed and closure is performed after 3–4 days.

2. **Proliferative phase** (collagen or fibroblastic phase)
   —begins only when the wound is covered with epithelium (approximately days 4–42).
   —is characterized by the **production of collagen and glycosaminoglycans** from fibroblasts.

   a. In an incision site, **collagen** production generally begins within **7 days** of wounding and continues for approximately **6 weeks** (Figure 5-2).

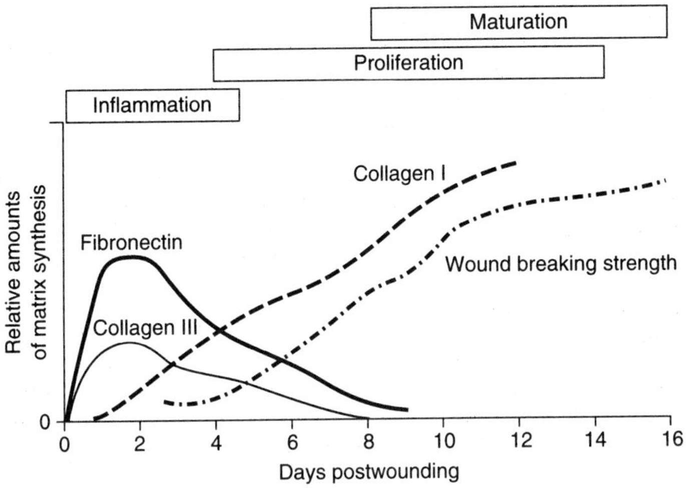

Figure 5-2. The deposition of wound matrix components over time. Although fibronectin and collagen type III constitute the early matrix, collagen type I accumulates later, corresponding to the increase in wound breaking strength. (Adapted with permission from Wittey MB, Barbul A: General Principles of Wound Healing. In *The Surgical Clinics of North America, "Wound Healing."* Edited by Barbul A. Philadelphia, WB Saunders, 1997, p 516.)

b. Hydroxyproline and hydroxylysine are key amino acids in collagen that require specific enzymes for their synthesis.

c. Hydroxylation of these amino acids requires **iron, α-ketoglutarate, and ascorbic acid (vitamin C)** as cofactors.

d. Removal of terminal amino acids from the α chains produces tropocollagen, which aggregates to form collagen fibrils that cross-link with other fibrils.

e. Postoperative wounds achieve **80%–90% of their final strength within 30 days.**

f. Mechanical stresses, such as movement over a joint, affect the quantity, aggregation, and orientation of collagen fibers.

3. **Remodeling phase** (maturation stage)

—begins at 6 weeks and may last as long as 2 years in adults and even longer in children.

—is characterized by the maturation of collagen by cross-linking and continued turnover.

a. This **cross-linking** is primarily responsible for the wound's tensile strength.

b. There is generally **little net collagen production** after day 42.

c. **Maturation** leads to flattening of scar.

B. Wound contraction

1. **Open wounds heal** by a bimodal process of **epithelial migration and contraction of the wound edges.**

2. The **main cell** responsible for wound contraction is the **myofibroblast,** which is a specialized fibroblast with contractile properties.

3. **Collagen formation** is **not essential** for wound contraction.

C. Factors impeding wound healing (Table 5-1)

1. Local factors affecting wound closure

a. **Hematoma formation** provides a medium for bacterial proliferation and inhibits foreign body removal.

b. **Foreign bodies,** including sutures, decrease the number of bacteria required to cause a wound infection.

c. Impaired **local host defenses** also inhibit healing.

(1) **Without impaired host defenses** or the presence of hematomas or foreign bodies, a wound can withstand a level up to **10^5 organisms per gram of tissue** and still heal successfully.

(2) An exception is wounds contaminated with β-hemolytic streptococci, which can cause a wound infection if present in significantly lower numbers.

d. **Oxygen deprivation**

(1) **Tissue hypoxia** is the **most common cause** of poor wound healing.

(2) Oxygen is important in cell migration and multiplication, and protein and collagen synthesis.

(3) The oxygen gradient determines the rate of angiogenesis.

(4) Conditions that lower oxygen delivery to tissues include hypotension, hypovolemia, anemia, lung disease, low inspired oxygen concentrations, hypothermia, alkalosis, and edema.

2. Systemic factors affecting wound closure

a. **Cytotoxic drugs**

—such as 5-fluorouracil, methotrexate, and cyclophosphamide impair wound healing by suppressing collagen synthesis and fibroblast replication.

b. **Chronic glucocorticoid therapy**

(1) **Glucocorticoids**

—can prevent macrophages from migrating into the wound.

(2) **The inflammatory response** is decreased.

—There is a delay in angiogenesis, fibroblast proliferation, and synthesis of collagen and proteoglycan.

Table 5-1. Local and Systemic Factors that May Impair Wound Healing

Local Factors	Systemic Factors
Infection	Malnutrition
Ischemia	Cancer
Cigarette smoking	Diabetes mellitus
Radiation	Uremia
Previous trauma	Alcoholism
Venous insufficiency	Chemotherapeutic agents
Local toxins (e.g., spider venom)	Jaundice
Mechanical stress	Old age
Blood flow	Chronic steroid therapy
Bacterial contamination	

(3) **Supplemental vitamin A**

—may counteract the deleterious effects of steroids.

—increases the fibroblast receptor for EGF and increases fibroblast multiplication.

—stabilizes the lysosomal membrane, opposing the effect of glucocorticoids.

c. **Diabetes mellitus**

—is associated with inhibition of the early inflammatory response and proliferation of fibroblasts and endothelial cells.

(1) **Hyperglycemia** interferes with the cellular transport of ascorbic acid into fibroblasts and leukocytes and inhibits leukocyte chemotaxis.

(2) **Other indirect effects** that may contribute to poor wound healing include dehydration, metabolic acidosis, and inadequate tissue perfusion.

D. **Excessive wound healing: hypertrophic scars and keloids** (Table 5-2)

E. **Squamous cell carcinoma**

1. **Some wounds may rarely develop** a focus of **squamous cell carcinoma** years after the original injury.
2. These lesions characteristically present as a **persistent nonhealing ulcer** at the site of previous injury, and are frequently referred to as **Marjolin ulcers.**
3. Appropriate **management** of suspicious lesions involves prompt **biopsy** with subsequent **resection** of cancerous lesions.

II. Skin Grafts and Tissue Flaps

A. **Classification of skin grafts by thickness** (Figure 5-3)

1. **Split-thickness skin grafts** include the epidermis and part of the dermis.

a. The **dermal skin appendages** within these grafts (e.g., sweat glands, hair follicles, and sebaceous glands) **contribute to epithelialization.**

b. **Thinner grafts** are associated with a higher percentage of graft survival.

—Thicker grafts are associated with less wound contraction.

c. **Advantages** include

—large supply of donor areas.

—ease of harvesting.

—availability of donor site for reuse in 10–14 days.

—coverage of large surface areas.

—ability to be stored for later use.

d. **Disadvantages** include

—cosmetic inferiority to full-thickness skin grafts.

Table 5-2. Characteristics of Hypertrophic Scars and Keloids

	Hypertrophic Scars	Keloids
Causes	Increased degree and time of inflammation (e.g., healing by secondary intention), **unnecessary tension** that produces uncontrolled would contraction	Pre-disposition to excessive scar formation.
Clinical appearance	**Collagen mass remains within the original bounds of the wound**	Collagen mass extends **beyond the original bounds of the wound,** lesion is raised and firm, overlying skin is often darker than normal surrounding skin
Common location	Anywhere	Sternum, mandible, deltoid (rarely occurs distal to wrist or knee)
Natural history	Usually **regresses with time**	**Does not regress**
Microscopic	Histologically similar to keloids; collagen tends to whorl about clusters of macrophages, fibroblasts and vessels; perivascular necrosis	Thick, homogenous bands of collagen; paucity of cellular elements; perivascular necrosis; density of fibroblasts and collagen similar to hypertrophic scars
Treatment	Z-plasty to change direction of scar, direct pressure, intralesional steroids (Surgical treatment is possible because the healing mechanisms are normal.)	Intralesional steroids (i.e., triamcinolone every 3–4 weeks) followed by excision, excision followed by radiation therapy (alternative), experimental pharmacologic manipulations [e.g., penicillamine, colchine, vitamin A (as retinoic acid), interferons α and γ]

—decreased durability.

—hyperpigmentation.

—increased secondary contracture.

2. **Full-thickness skin grafts** are comprised of the epidermis and the **full thickness of dermis** without subcutaneous fat.
   a. **The greater the proportion of dermis** the **less contraction** that occurs during healing.
      —This provides better coverage, but is less likely to survive than a split-thickness skin graft because the greater thickness leads to slower revascularization.
   b. These grafts are **frequently used** on the
      —**face** because they provide a better color match than split-thickness grafts.
      —**finger** to decrease contracture formation.
   c. **Advantages** include
      —cosmetic superiority to split-thickness skin grafts.
      —decreased secondary contractures.
      —increased durability.

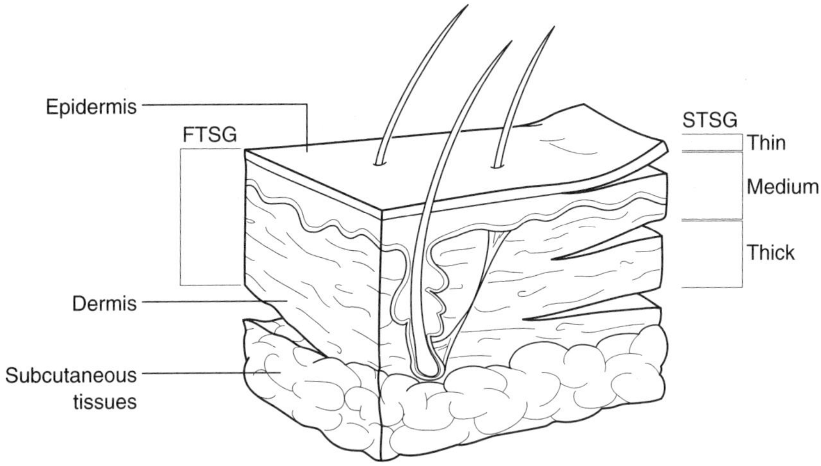

Figure 5-3. A split-thickness skin graft (STSG) includes epidermis and a portion of the dermis. Because dermis is left behind, the donor site heals by epithelialization. A full-thickness skin graft (FTSG) includes the epidermis and all layers of the dermis. Because no dermis is left behind, the donor wound must be closed primarily. (Adapted with permission from Marks MW, Marks C: Grafts and Implants. In *Fundamentals of Plastic Surgery,* 1st ed. Edited by Marks MW, Marks C. Philadelphia, WB Saunders, 1997, p 67.)

d. The main **disadvantage**

—is the **limited number of donor sites.**

B. Skin graft survival

1. Initially, both types of grafts survive

—via **diffusion** of nutrients from the recipient bed, a process called **plasma imbibition.**

2. Three to five days after graft placement

—revascularization occurs by ingrowth of vessels from the recipient site.

3. Common reasons for graft loss include

—**hematoma or seroma** formation under the graft (**most common**); meshing the skin graft allows for seroma drainage.

—shearing forces between the graft and recipient site (e.g., poor immobilization of an extremity).

—poorly vascularized recipient site (e.g., bone).

—infection.

4. Poorly vascularized beds that generally are not good recipient sites for skin grafts include

—bare **tendons.**

—**cortical bone** without periosteum.

—**irradiated wounds.**

—**infected wounds.**

C. Flaps

—consist of tissues transferred from their bed to an adjacent or distal area while retaining a **functioning vascular attachment** or pedicle.

1. **Flaps classified by surgical technique**
   a. In **pedicled flaps,** the arterial and venous vessels remain in their native bed.
   b. In **free flaps,** the arterial and venous vessels are anastomosed by microvascular techniques to recipient vessels.
2. **Skin flaps**
   —include random pattern, axial pattern, and island flaps.
   a. **Random pattern flaps lack specific vessels** but are based on a random blood supply from the intradermal and subdermal plexus, which **limits the length of these flaps.**
      (1) **Rotation flaps** are semicircular flaps of skin and subcutaneous tissue that rotate about a pivot point (Figure 5-4).
      (2) **Transposition flaps** are rectangular or square flaps of skin and subcutaneous tissue that transpose around a pivot point into an adjacent wound such as Z-plasty (Figure 5-5).
      (3) **Advancement flaps depend on stretching** of the skin in a straight line to fill a wound or defect.
   b. **An axial pattern flap** is a single-pedicled flap with a defined arteriovenous system running along its long axis.
   c. **Island flaps** are dissected so that the flap is attached only by axial vessels.
      (1) This improves flap mobility, thus permitting rotation through an arc of 180° or greater.
      (2) A neurovascular island flap includes a nerve within the pedicle, thereby permitting the skin to retain sensation.
3. **Muscle and musculocutaneous flaps**
   a. A muscle may be **detached from its origin** and insertion sites and transposed on its vascular pedicle to an adjacent area.
      —Alternatively, the vascular pedicle may be detached at its origin and reattached by microvascular techniques.
   b. **Muscle flaps provide**
      —**additional blood supply** to the recipient area.
   c. **Muscle can obliterate large cavities**
      —and aid in combating low-grade infections.

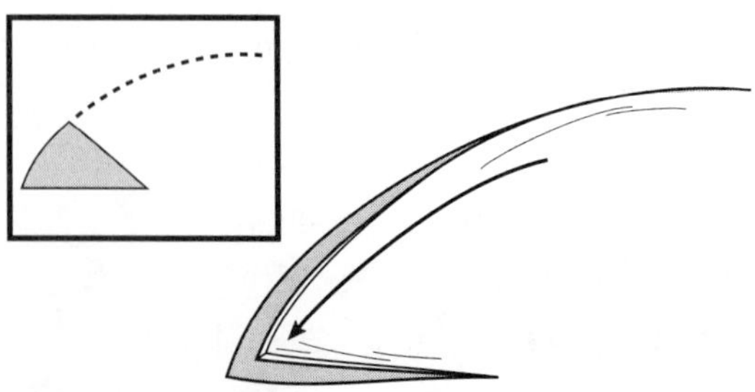

Figure 5-4. A rotation flap. A semicircular flap of skin and subcutaneous tissue is rotated about a pivot point into the defect. (Adapted with permission from Marks MW, Marks C: Grafts and Implants. In *Fundamentals of Plastic Surgery,* 1st ed. Edited by Marks MW, Marks C. Philadelphia, WB Saunders, 1997, p 84.)

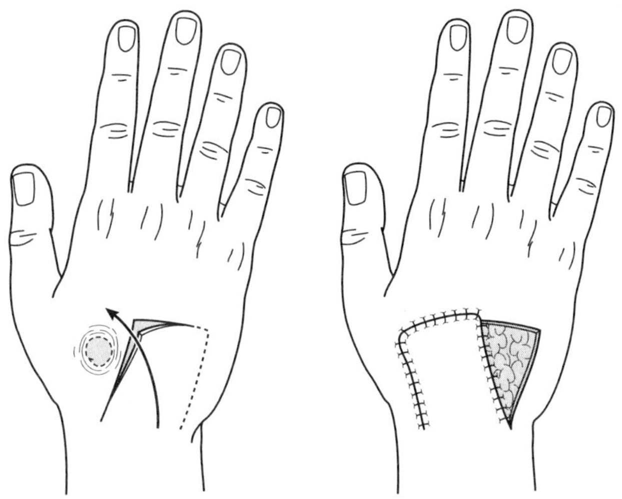

Figure 5-5. A transposition flap. The flap is elevated and transposed into an adjacent defect. The donor defect is either closed primarily or grafted. (Adapted with permission from Marks MW, Marks C: Grafts and Implants. In *Fundamentals of Plastic Surgery,* 1st ed. Edited by Marks MW, Marks C. Philadelphia, WB Saunders, 1997, p 85.)

d. The **exposed surface of muscle** provides
   —an excellent recipient area for **split-thickness skin graft** if skin is not transposed with the muscle unit.

e. **Commonly used muscle flaps** include
   —temporalis or trapezius muscle flaps for **head and neck defects.**
   —pectoralis major, latissimus dorsi, rectus abdominis, or gluteus maximus flaps for **defects of the trunk.**
   —tensor fascia lata, gracilis, rectus femoris, gastrocnemius, or soleus muscle flaps for **defects of the lower extremity.**

4. **Fasciocutaneous flaps**
   —are **well vascularized and easy to manipulate.**
   —avoid the need for sacrifice of a muscle.

III. Hand Surgery

A. Anatomic considerations

1. **Compromise of the skin's surface area** or **elasticity**
   —will **inhibit range of motion** and **constrict circulation.**

2. **Fascia anchors palmar skin to bone**
   —to make pinch and grip stable.

   a. In the form of **sheaths** and **pulleys** fascia holds tendons in the concave portions of arched joints.

   b. **Fascial compartments** provide an avenue for **dissemination of infection.**

   c. **Across the wrist** the dense carpal ligament forms a roof over the bony carpal canal (**carpal tunnel**).

—All **eight finger flexors** as well as the **flexor pollicis longus** and **median nerve** pass through this canal.

3. The **four joints of each finger** include
   —distal interphalangeal (DIP).
   —proximal interphalangeal (PIP).
   —metacarpophalangeal (MCP).
   —metacarpocarpal (MCC).

4. **Flexor tendons and extensor tendons**
   —control motor function of the hand.
   a. **Flexor digitorum superficialis**
      —inserts on the base of each **middle** phalanx.
   b. **Flexor digitorum profundus**
      —inserts on the base of each **distal** phalanx.
   c. **Long extensor tendons**
      —insert at the base of the **middle** phalanx.
   d. **Lateral bands**
      —originating from the lumbricals and interossei travel on each side of the finger and insert on the distal phalanx to act as MCP flexors and IP extensors.
   e. **No Man's Land** (Figure 5-6)
      —is the zone from the middle of the palm to just distal to the PIP joint.
      —is where the superficialis and profundus tendons lie ensheathed together.
      —is where **recovery of function is difficult after injury.**

5. **The nerves most important to hand function**

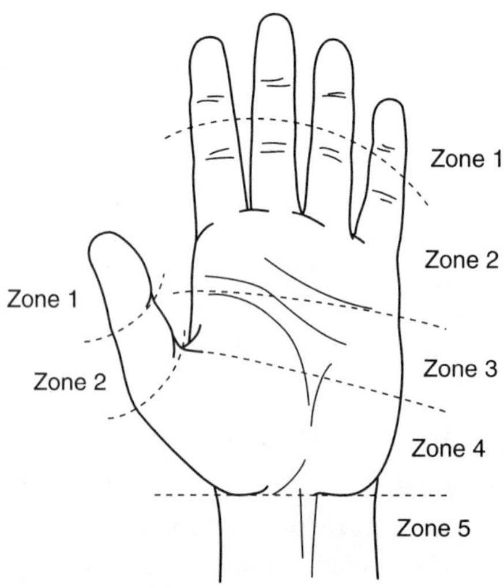

Figure 5-6. Flexor tendon zones of the hand. These zones are defined by their relevance to flexor tendon injuries. Tendon injuries that occur in Zone 2 (No Man's Land) are generally associated with poor recovery of function. (Adapted with permission from Winograd J: Plastic Surgery. In *Advanced Surgical Recall,* 1st ed. Edited by Blackbourne LH, Fleischer KJ. Baltimore, Williams & Wilkins. 1997, p 1028.)

—are the **musculocutaneous, radial, ulnar, and median nerves.**

a. Together, the **musculocutaneous and radial nerve** control forearm supination.

b. The **radial** nerve innervates the extensor muscles.

c. The **ulnar** nerve innervates 15 of the 20 intrinsic muscles.

d. The **median** nerve innervates most of the long flexors, the pronators of the forearm, and the thenar muscles.

e. Figure 5-7 demonstrates the sensory distribution of the ulnar, radial, and median nerves.

B. Hand infections

1. Paronychia

—is an infection at the radial or ulnar side of the **nail.**

a. Tissue tension that forms about the rigid nail causes **exquisite pain.**

b. Early **treatment** before abscess formation involves water-soaked or zinc oxide dressings, elevation, immobilization, and antibiotics.

c. If purulent material forms under the nail, the nail should be removed for adequate drainage.

2. Felon

—is an infection of the **volar distal fat pad of the finger.**

—The abscess is drained by a **longitudinally oriented incision** over the central portion of the fat pad.

3. Tenosynovitis

—is an infection of the synovial **tendon sheaths.**

a. Kanavel's four signs of tenosynovitis include

—**flexion** of the affected finger.

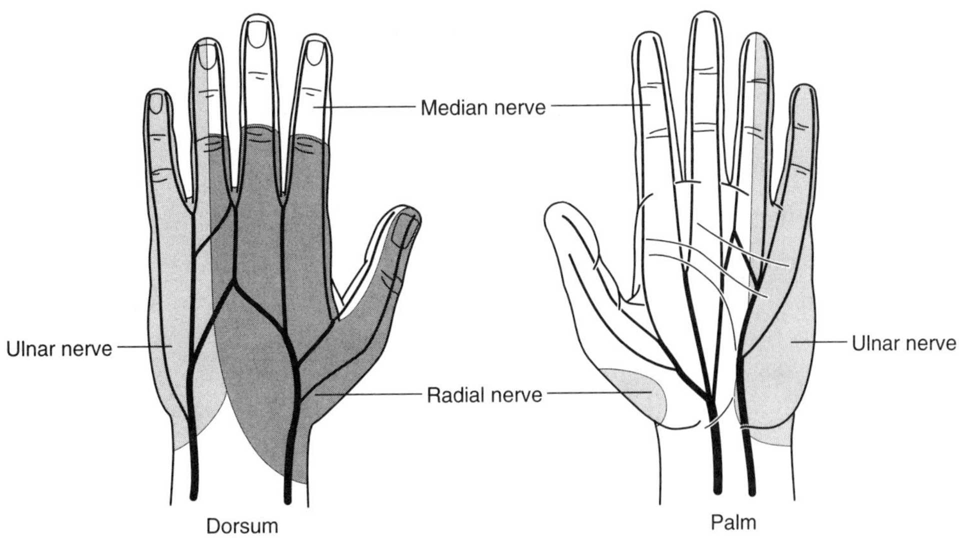

Figure 5-7. Sensory innervation of the hand. (Adapted with permission from Winograd J: Plastic Surgery. In *Advanced Surgical Recall,* 1st ed. Edited by Blackbourne LH, Fleischer KJ. Baltimore, Williams & Wilkins. 1997, p 1016.)

—**swelling.**

—**pain with passive extension.**

—**tenderness** over the **flexor tendon sheath.**

b. **Treatment** is by incision, drainage, and irrigation of the tendon sheath.

4. **Human bites to the hand**

—frequently become infected (see Chapter 4 II C).

—should be treated by aggressive débridement and broad spectrum antibiotics.

—The wound should be left **unsutured.**

C. **Fractures**

1. **Metacarpal fractures**

—are usually transversely oriented and **tend to rotate.**

a. **Rotation of a finger**

—causes it to cross over an adjacent finger during flexion.

—interferes with grasping and making a fist.

b. **Unstable fractures**

—are those that **tend to redisplace.**

—Treatment involves either **percutaneous pinning or open reduction with internal fixation.**

c. **A boxer's fracture**

—is a transverse fracture of the distal **fourth or fifth metacarpal** with palmar displacement of the metacarpal head.

—can usually be reduced with traction and application of dorsal pressure on the distal fragment.

—requires percutaneous pinning, if unstable.

2. **Proximal and middle phalangeal fractures**

—also tend to rotate.

—require percutaneous pinning or fixation.

3. **Nondisplaced distal phalangeal fractures**

—may be treated by splinting at the DIP joint for 2–3 weeks.

D. **Noninfectious inflammatory disorders of the hand**

1. **Trigger finger** is a stenosing flexor tenosynovitis of the proximal digital pulley.

a. Pain is felt over the DIP joint and the digit may be locked in flexion.

b. The patient may notice a painful "click" as the finger goes into extension.

—This occurs as the bulge in the tendon passes through the tight pulley.

2. **de Quervain tenosynovitis** involves the pulley over the radial styloid.

a. This pulley houses the abductor pollicis longus and extensor pollicis brevis.

b. A characteristic finding includes local tenderness and pain with active or passive stretching of these tendons (**Finklestein's test**).

3. Carpal tunnel syndrome is caused by compression of the **median nerve** as it passes under the volar carpal ligament.

a. Patients experience **sleep disturbance** by the aching and numbness over the distribution of the nerve (most often the **long and ring fingers**).

b. Severe constriction causes **paralysis** of the abductor pollicis brevis.

—This can manifest itself as atrophy of the thenar eminence.

4. Ulnar nerve compression may occur in three places:

—Behind the **medial epicondyle (cubital tunnel).**

—Between the heads of the **flexor carpi ulnaris.**

—**Guyon's canal** from the pisiform bone to the hook of the hamate (this canal contains both the ulnar artery and nerve).

5. Dupuytren contracture is a fibrous contraction of the palmar fascia of unknown etiology.

a. Risk factors include **Celtic** origin, **epilepsy, diabetes, alcoholism,** and a **family history** of the disease.

b. On physical **examination,** patients may have **nodules or cordlike bands** in their palms that restrict their ability to completely extend the fingers.

c. Treatment is by **partial fasciectomy,** although recurrence is common.

E. Tumors of the hand (Table 5-3)

1. A **ganglion**

Table 5-3. Tumors of the Hand

Tumor	Pathology	Clinical Presentation	Treatment
Ganglion*	Protrusion of synovium filled with synovial fluid	Most commonly found on the wrist (radiodorsal or radiovolar)	Asymptomatic: none Symptomatic: excision
Inclusion cyst	Subcutaneous mass containing a nidus of epithelial cells	Associated with penetrating trauma	Excision
Xanthoma (giant cell tumor)	Yellow, nodule-like tumor containing connective tissue histiocytes	May be cystic, solid, or multilocular; often hard and painless	Excision
Enchondroma	Lobules of hyaline cartilage with areas of calcification	Frequently presents as a pathologic fracture	Curette and bone grafting
Glomus	Comprised of blood vessels and unmyelinated nerves	Found in pad of finger and under nail, associated with cold sensitivity	Excision

*Ganglion tumors are the most common tumor of the hand.

—is a protrusion of synovium filled with **synovial fluid.**

—typically appears insidiously, although sudden forceful bending of a joint may be associated with an acute presentation.

—is most commonly located on the **radiodorsal or radiovolar area of the wrist.**

a. A **mucous cyst** is a **DIP ganglion** that may deform the nail.

b. Asymptomatic ganglia generally do not require treatment, while symptomatic cysts require surgical excision.

2. **An inclusion cyst**

—forms when viable **epidermal cells** are found deep in the dermis, in subcutaneous fat, or in bone (frequently induced by **traumatic injury**).

a. With growth of these cells, keratinized cells accumulate into a ball or cyst.

b. These lesions can be removed surgically.

3. **Xanthoma (i.e., giant cell tumor)**

—is an insidiously growing, benign, often multinodular tumor that arises from the fibrous flexor sheath, ligaments, or fascia.

—is usually **hard and painless.**

4. **Enchondromas**

—are benign tumors that constitute 90% of bone tumors of the hand.

—The classic finding is **calcific stippling** of the lytic bone defect, which is commonly seen in the proximal phalanges and distal metacarpals.

5. **Glomus tumors**

—are comprised of blood vessels and unmyelinated nerves of a **heat-regulating arteriovenous shunt.**

a. Although most patients will have no symptoms, lesions under the fingernail may be associated with severe pain.

b. Treatment is by total excision.

F. **Compartment syndromes of the upper extremity**

1. This syndrome **develops** when a compartment of tissue (e.g., muscle) bounded by noncompliant structures (e.g., fascia, bone) develops a significant increase in pressure.

—The most **common cause** of compartment syndrome is **trauma.**

a. Increased pressure leads to **inhibition of venous outflow** with a subsequent decrease in arterial inflow, resulting in **tissue ischemia.**

b. Compartment **pressures greater than 30–40 mm Hg** significantly inhibit muscle perfusion.

c. **Volkmann ischemia** is **irreversible** muscle necrosis that may occur within **2 hours** of onset of injury.

d. Nerve compression results in paresthesia and hypoesthesia.

e. Flow through major vessels is generally maintained, thus **distal pulses may remain palpable, even after irreversible muscle necrosis.**

2. The **most common site** of compartment syndrome in the upper extremity is in the **anterior forearm compartment.**
   a. **Signs and symptoms** occur in the following order
      —**pain** out of proportion to the injury.
      —**weakness** of the compartment muscles.
      —increased **tenseness** of the compartment.
      —**hypoesthesia** of nerves passing through the compartment.
   b. Compartment syndrome may **present**
      —as flexion of the digits with resistance to passive extension.
   c. The **diagnosis**
      —**is clinical,** based on a high index of suspicion from the history of a predisposing trauma or medical condition and progressive signs of muscle and nerve ischemia.
      —**can be confirmed** by compartment pressure measurements that are **above 30 mm Hg.**
3. **Prompt surgical decompression by adequate fasciotomy** is the only treatment for the early stage of compartment syndromes.
   a. The important features of the incision used are adequate exposure, maintenance of skin coverage of the median nerve at the wrist, and avoidance of longitudinal cuts across the wrist and elbow skin creases.
   b. Judicious débridement of necrotic muscle should be performed.

Review Test

Directions: Each of the numbered items or incomplete statements in this section is followed by answers or by completions of the statement. Select the ONE lettered answer or completion that is BEST in each case.

1. Which of the following characteristics of keloids most appropriately differentiates a keloid from a hypertrophic scar?

(A) Decreased fibroblast density
(B) Increased fibroblast density
(C) Increased collagen density
(D) Increased perivascular sclerosis
(E) Growth beyond the incision site

2. Which of the following is a mechanism of keloid formation?

(A) Altered ratio of collagen production and collagenase activity
(B) Excessive fibroblast proliferation
(C) Excessive collagenase synthesis
(D) Excessive collagen cross-linking
(E) Prolonged acute inflammation

3. A 16-year-old girl sustains a needle prick to the left index finger over the distal palmar surface. Initially, she notices little discomfort. However, 3 days after the injury she develops intense pain in the distal phalanx that wakes her up at night. Regarding this situation, which of the following is the most appropriate statement?

(A) She has an acute paronychial infection
(B) Drainage is accomplished via an incision over the most tender region
(C) Incision through the volar surface of the finger often results in a tender scar
(D) Cultures of the finger will most likely produce a gram-negative rod
(E) Late sequelae of this type of infection seldom involve the bone

4. A 62-year-old woman has had a clicking sensation of her thumb for 4 months. On examination, she has tenderness and a palpable nodule at the level of the proximal interphalangeal joint. The thumb exhibits full active and passive range of motion, but active extension results in a clicking noise. Which of the following is the most appropriate initial step in the management of this patient?

(A) Physical therapy
(B) Splinting of the thumb
(C) Oral administration of an anti-inflammatory agent
(D) Injection of a corticosteroid into the flexor tendon sheath
(E) Surgical release of the A1 annular pulley

Questions 5–6

A 16-year-old boy presents to the office immediately after a cut injury to the palm of his right hand. The cut was caused by a clean razor blade. Physical examination reveals a 2-cm laceration at the base of the long finger. The patient is able to flex the metacarpophalangeal (MCP) joint but he cannot flex either interphalangeal joint in that finger.

5. Which of the following is the most likely diagnosis?

(A) Lacerated flexor digitorum profundus tendon
(B) Lacerated flexor digitorum superficialis tendon
(C) Combined laceration of the superficialis and profundus tendon
(D) Laceration of the intrinsic muscle to the long finger
(E) Transection of the radial nerve

6. Which of the following is the most appropriate treatment plan for this patient?

(A) Immediate tendon repair
(B) Regional anesthesia, extension of the skin wound, and exploration to confirm the diagnosis
(C) Careful cleansing of the wound, placement of the appropriate dressing, and hand immobilization before definitive primary surgical repair
(D) Cleansing of the wound, primary skin closure, hand immobilization, and delayed repair using tendon graft
(E) Observation only

Questions 7–9

A 45-year-old man suffers a 45% total body surface area (TBSA, partial and full-thickness) burn to the neck, face, trunk, and lower extremities sustained in an industrial explosion. Other injuries include a severe LeFort II maxillary fracture, a pulmonary contusion with rib fractures, and a crush injury to the right arm and hand. The patient is unresponsive with labored respirations and his current blood pressure is 70/40 mm Hg.

7. Which of the following should be the primary concern in the emergency room?

(A) The facial fractures
(B) The 45% TBSA burns
(C) Endotracheal intubation
(D) The crush injury to the right upper extremity
(E) Splinting of the chest for the rib fractures

8. The patient is appropriately resuscitated and further work-up reveals no additional thoracic or intra-abdominal injuries. Thirty-six hours after the injury, his blood pressure is 130/85 mm Hg and urine output is maintained at 30 mL/hour. The patient is also awake and alert. Physical examination of his right arm reveals it to be tense and painful. Pulses in the extremity are noted by Doppler examination. Which of the following is the most appropriate next step in the management of this patient?

(A) High-dose corticosteroids
(B) Arm evaluation, analgesics, and close observation
(C) Fasciotomies
(D) Compressive dressings
(E) Burn excision and grafting

9. Three days after the initial injury, the patient's wounds are débrided in the operating room. Coverage of the burns to his thorax, abdomen, and lower extremities is best accomplished via which of the following?

(A) Local (random pattern) skin flaps
(B) Free flaps using microvascular transfer
(C) Full-thickness skin grafts
(D) Split-thickness skin grafts
(E) Myocutaneous flaps

10. Which of the following statements is correct regarding wound healing and persistent local tissue hypoxia?

(A) Fibroblasts are stimulated by low oxygen tension
(B) High lactate levels inhibit macrophage production of angiogenesis factor
(C) Low oxygen tension is the most common cause of poor wound healing
(D) Collagen synthesis is stimulated by hypoxia
(E) Wound healing is not affected by alterations in tissue oxygen tension

11. During the first 4 days after an injury, which of the following cells are most critical to wound healing?

(A) Fibroblast
(B) Lymphocyte
(C) Myofibroblast
(D) Platelet
(E) Macrophage

12. A 45-year-old, obese man develops a wound infection on postoperative day 10. The patient undergoes wound débridement, followed by dressing changes to the open wound and systemic antibiotics. Allowing this wound to heal by wound contraction and epithelialization (i.e., secondary intention) means that the wound will spend a prolonged period of time in which of the following phases?

(A) Inflammatory
(B) Proliferative
(C) Fibroblastic
(D) Remodeling
(E) Maturation

13. Which of the following is the most appropriate option for closing a large wound once the wound appears "clean"?

(A) Split-thickness skin graft
(B) Full-thickness skin graft
(C) Local skin flap
(D) Myocutaneous flap
(E) Cadaveric skin grafting

Directions: Each of the numbered items or incomplete statements in this section is negatively phrased, as indicated by a capitalized word such as NOT, LEAST, or EXCEPT. Select the ONE lettered answer or completion that is BEST in each case.

14. A 65-year-old man with a past medical history of chronic obstructive pulmonary disease (COPD), diabetes mellitus, and peripheral vascular disease undergoes an uncomplicated three-vessel coronary artery bypass grafting (CABG) using both internal mammary arteries. His sternal wound is closed primarily using sternal wires and buried subcuticular sutures using absorbable, synthetic suture. Eight days postoperatively, the patient develops a fever, and on examination there is crepitance in the sternal wound. Factors predisposing the patient to a sternal wound infection include all of the following EXCEPT

(A) Male gender
(B) COPD
(C) Diabetes mellitus
(D) Peripheral vascular disease
(E) Use of both internal mammary arteries versus using only one

Answers and Explanations

1–E. Unlike hypertrophic scars, keloids typically overgrow the boundaries of the initial incision site. This differentiation is generally made by clinical examination. Light microscopy alone cannot be used to make this differentiation because there are no differences in the architecture or quantity of collagen or the number of fibroblasts. Perivascular sclerosis also occurs in both disorders. Although the specific biochemical cause of abnormal scar production has not been identified, increased collagen production and decreased collagen lysis have been demonstrated.

2–A. Studies of the origin of keloids and hypertrophic scars suggest that both excessive collagen production and decreased collagenase activity may be responsible for abnormal collagen formation. Excessive cross-linking and prolonged inflammation are not thought to be primary mechanisms. Although collagen production is increased in hypertrophic scars and keloids, it does not result from an excessive number of fibroblasts in the wound or from specific abnormal types of fibroblasts.

3–B. This patient has a felon, not a paronychial infection. Untreated, the infection may progress to involve the distal phalanx. The most likely organisms are gram-positive cocci. The scar on the volar surface may be tender initially, but no more so than a scar elsewhere on the hand. Incision and drainage is indicated in this situation, with the incision placed directly over the point of maximal tenderness.

4–D. This patient has stenosing flexor tenosynovitis of the thumb (trigger thumb). When she flexes or extends her thumb, triggering occurs. Primary, or idiopathic, trigger finger is common, and middle-aged women are most frequently affected. Secondary causes include gout, rheumatoid arthritis, diabetes mellitus, and other diseases that cause connective tissue changes. The most appropriate initial treatment is to inject corticosteroid into the flexor tendon sheath. Splinting and corticosteroid injection are equally effective in treating trigger finger, but corticosteroid injection has been shown to be more successful when the thumb is affected. Surgical release of the A1 annular pulley is indicated when corticosteroid injection fails or if the digit is locked. Physical therapy has no effect on the nodule causing the triggering. Anti-inflammatory agents are not likely to be successful as the sole treatment of this disease.

5–C. Flexion of the metacarpophalangeal (MCP) joint is accomplished via intrinsic muscles of the hand. This may be preserved even when the extrinsic flexion mechanism is disrupted. The goal of flexor tendon repair is to restore interphalangeal joint flexion. The flexor digitorum superficialis inserts on the base of each middle phalanx and causes proximal interphalangeal (PIP) flexion. The flexor digitorum profundus inserts on the base of each distal phalanx and is responsible for distal interphalangeal (DIP) flexion. Laceration of the intrinsic muscle to the long finger would not explain the patient's inability to flex the PIP and DIP joints. The radial nerve is responsible for the extensors, not flexors, of the hand.

6–C. The goal of flexor tendon repair is to restore interphalangeal joint flexion. Proper wound cleansing, dressing, immobilization, and prophylactic antibiotics allow delay of primary repair if a hand surgeon is not immediately available. With this cut, primary repair of the tendon is the most appropriate operative technique without the need for tendon grafts. Delayed repair (2–6 days after injury) is indicated when the degree of wound contamination is uncertain or if the initial treatment has been delayed beyond several hours. Grossly contaminated wounds, those with significant tendon disruption, or wounds with significant associated injuries to the soft tissue, bone, nerve, or blood vessels are treated by secondary repair in 3–6 weeks, after the wound has healed and edema and callus formation subside.

7–C. Trauma evaluations are generally approached in the same systematic manner to avoid missing life-threatening injuries. The ABCs (airway, breathing, circulation) of trauma is a useful mnemonic for the sequential approach to potential life-threatening injuries during a trauma evaluation. While the crush injury and burns may be quite disfiguring and obvious, in patients with respiratory distress initial attention should be directed toward providing an adequate airway, typically via endotracheal intubation. Facial fractures can also be dealt with once the life-threatening injuries are controlled.

8–C. The patient is developing a compartment syndrome secondary to his crush injuries. Immediate treatment includes fasciotomies to prevent irreversible muscle necrosis and nerve damage. There is no role for corticosteroids in the treatment of his compartment syndrome. Arm elevation may be a temporizing measure before fasciotomy but is not adequate for definitive treatment. Compressive dressings may mask his findings and irreversible necrosis can ensue. Pulses may be present even during the late stages of compartment syndrome. Although burn excision and grafting are important, initial attention to release of compartment pressure with fasciotomy is essential.

9–D. This patient has a large amount of surface area that requires coverage. This is best accomplished using meshed split-thickness skin grafts, which are harvested at a thickness of 12–15 one-thousandths of an inch. Skin and myocutaneous flaps will not adequately cover his wounds, and the donor site morbidity precludes their use. Similarly, full-thickness skin grafts require the donor sites to be covered with skin grafts and this too limits their use. In this patient, split-thickness skin grafts will accomplish the coverage needed while minimizing donor site morbidity.

10–C. Oxygen deficiency of the tissues is the most common cause of poor wound healing. Proper tissue oxygenation requires sufficient inspired PO_2, transfer of oxygen to hemoglobin, ample hemoglobin for transport, and adequate vascularity of the tissues. Most healing problems associated with diabetes mellitus, irradiation, small vessel atherosclerosis, and chronic infection are a result of a faulty oxygen delivery system. Transiently low wound tissue oxygen levels stimulates cell migration, growth factor release, and collagenase production. Similarly, high lactate levels stimulate the macrophage to produce angiogenesis factors. Fibroblasts are oxygen sensitive and are inhibited by low tissue oxygen tension. Collagen synthesis is also inhibited by low tissue oxygen.

11–E. Macrophages play a critical role in the inflammatory phase of wound healing and in the modulation of collagen production. These cells affect wound healing through multiple secretory factors and receptors. Studies of the role of macrophages have shown a marked inhibition in the process of wound débridement and collagen production with administration of antimacrophage serum early in wound healing. Although lymphocytes also modulate wound healing by secreting interleukin-2, transforming growth factor-β, and other lymphokines, these substances do not appear until inflammation has resolved, approximately 3 days after injury.

12–A. In healing by secondary intention, the inflammatory phase continues until the wound surface is closed by epithelium. In this case, coverage with epithelium may not be complete for several weeks to months, depending on the size of the defect. When a wound is closed primarily, the inflammatory phase usually lasts from 4–6 days. The rest of the phases listed should proceed normally once the wound has closed by contraction and epithelialization.

13–D. The choice for coverage depends on the wound's size and depth. Because bone will probably be débrided before definitive closure, the resulting defect will have a significant amount of dead space. A myocutaneous flap provides excellent coverage and obliterates the dead space. In addition, the added vascularity of the transposed muscle will aid in fighting infection by allowing the egress of inflammatory cells. Skin grafts and a local skin flap will not provide the bulk needed to close the dead space. Cadaveric skin grafts serve as a temporary biologic dressing before definitive closure; they are not appropriate for long-term use.

14–A. Tissue hypoxia is the most common cause of poor wound healing. Conditions that lower oxygen delivery to tissues include lung disease, cigarette smoking, hypovolemia, anemia, hypotension, and low concentrations of inspired oxygen. Peripheral vascular disease is associated with tissue hypoxia and poor wound healing. Diabetes mellitus has multiple effects on different aspects of wound healing and predisposes this patient to wound infection. For example, diabetes is associated with an inhibition of the early inflammatory response and proliferation of fibroblasts and endothelial cells. The use of bilateral internal mammary arteries for revascularization procedures (e.g., CABG) has recently been demonstrated as being associated with an increased risk of postoperative sternal wound infection, verus using only a single internal mammary artery while maintaining adequate perfusion of the area by the remaining mammary artery. While old age may lead to impaired wound healing, being male does not.

6

Immunology and Transplantation

Shawn J. Pelletier

I. Immunology

A. Types of immunity

1. **Characteristics**

   —of innate (natural) and acquired immunity are outlined in **Table 6-1.**

2. **Cellular immunity** is predominantly mediated by **T lymphocytes.** Major groups include

   —helper T cells (CD4+).

   —cytotoxic/suppressor T cells (CD8+).

   a. **Cytokines**

      —that mediate lymphocyte function are described in **Table 6–2.**

   b. The **major functions** of the **cellular immune response** include

      —regulation of antibody response.

      —host defense against intracellular bacteria (e.g., *Mycobacterium tuberculosis*).

      —host defense against viruses, fungi, and parasites.

      —acute and chronic graft rejection.

      —tumor rejection.

3. **Humoral immunity**

   —is predominantly mediated by **B lymphocytes and plasma cells.**

   a. The **major function**

      —is production of **antibodies.**

   b. The **antibody response to infection** is important in

      —opsonization of bacteria.

Table 6-1. Types of Immunity

Immunity	Characteristics	Examples
Natural	Nonspecific, innate, not acquired through contact with an antigen	Skin and mucous membranes, natural killer cells, phagocytosis, complement cascade
Acquired	Specific, occurs after exposure to an antigen, may be active or passive	
	Active: Production of antibodies or specific lymphoid cell response after contact with foreign antigen, long-term slow onset	Tetanus toxoid, resistance to mumps after receiving vaccine
	Passive: Resistance based on antibodies preformed in another host, rapid availability, short half-life	Antitetanus immunoglobulin

Table 6-2. Characteristics of Cytokines

Cytokine	Predominant Source	Effect
IL-1	Macrophages	Activates T cells, B cells, neutrophils, epithelial cells, fibroblasts
IL-2	Helper T cells	Stimulates helper and cytotoxic T cells, synergistic with IL-4 to stimulate B cells
IL-4	Helper T cells	Promotes growth and differentiation of B cells, enhances synthesis of IgE, increases MHC II induction on B cells
IL-6	Predominantly macrophages, monocytes, T cells	Stimulates fibroblast and B cell proliferation, and acute phase protein synthesis by the liver*
IL-10	Helper T cells, macrophages	Increases MHC II on B cells, inhibits T helper response, decreases cytokine release from macrophages
IFN-γ	Helper T cells, cytotoxic lymphocytes	Differentiation of B cells to IgG, kills T cells, increases MHC I and II on macrophages and other cells, antiviral
TNF-α	Predominantly macrophages, monocytes	Activates macrophages and induces NO production, mobilizes neutrophils, pyrogenic, activates B and T lymphocytes

*Acute phase proteins include ceruloplasmin, C3 complement, α_1-antitrypsin, fibrinogen, C-reactive protein, and amyloid-A-protein.
IL = interleukin; Ig = immunoglobulin; MHC = major histocompatibility complex; IFN = interferon; NO = nitric oxide.

—neutralization of toxins and viruses.

—allergy (i.e., hay fever).

—pathogenesis of autoimmune disorders and hyperacute rejection.

B. Major histocompatibility complex (MHC) and transplantation (Table 6-3).

Table 6-3. Major Histocompatability Complex (MHC)

MHC Class	Genomic loci	Cells Expressing Specific MHC	Immunologic Significance
Class I	HLA-A, HLA-B, HLA-C	Nearly universal to all nucleated cells	Associated with cytotoxic or T cell function (CD8) response to antigen
Class II	HLA-DP, HLA-DQ, **HLA-DR**	Macrophage, B cells, dendritic cells of the spleen, and Langerhans' cells of skin	Associated with T helper function (CD4)

HLA = human leukocyte antigen.

1. The **MHC**

—is located on chromosome 6.

—encodes the genes for **human leukocyte antigens (HLA).**

a. **HLA proteins**

—are **alloantigens** (i.e., they differ among members of the same species).

b. **Each person has 2 haplotypes,** or 2 sets of these genes, maternal and paternal.

—The proteins encoded by both the maternal and paternal chromosomes are expressed (**codominance**).

c. **Class I and II antigens**

—are detected in the laboratory either by

(1) A **serologic test** that reacts lymphocytes with known specific antibodies and complement to determine cell lysis.

(2) **Polymerase chain reaction** (PCR) analysis.

d. The **haplotypes of class I and II antigens**

—are usually determined for both the donor and recipient before kidney transplantation.

(1) The **main loci** include

—**HLA-A.**

—**HLA-B.**

—**HLA-DR.**

—A **heterozygous** individual will have **6 antigens (2 of each).**

(2) A **higher frequency of matching**

—of these antigens between the recipient and the donor may be associated with a **lower rate of graft rejection** for some organs.

e. **Attempting to match antigens**

—may offer significant advantage, particularly for kidney and pancreas transplantation.

(1) A small advantage is probably offered for heart transplantation by HLA matching.

(2) HLA matching is less important for liver transplantation.

f. **In addition to these major antigens**

—there are **minor antigens** coded for by genes other than the MHC.

g. Compatibility between blood type

—(i.e., A, B, and O) encoded for by genes other than the MHC is also required for successful transplantation.

—Liver transplantation can be performed across blood type barriers.

C. Clinical syndromes of the immune response

1. Hypersensitivity reactions

—are listed in **Table 6-4.**

2. Hyperacute rejection

—is the response to **preformed antibodies** that bind to the allograft at the time of implantation.

—results in the destruction of the graft in **minutes to hours.**

a. This typically occurs in the presence of

—ABO incompatibility.

—high titer of anti-donor class I HLA antibodies.

b. Liver allografts

—are relatively resistant to hyperacute rejection.

c. A panel reactive antibody (PRA) test

—can be performed by adding recipient serum to a panel of cells with known HLA to determine the percent of cells that react with the recipient serum.

Table 6-4. Four Main Types of Hypersensitivity Reactions

Type	Description	Mechanism	Examples
I	**Anaphylactic**	Antigen induces IgE production and release of mast and basophil granules containing histamine, serotonin, prostaglandins	Hay fever, asthma, urticaria
II	**Cytotoxic**	IgG or IgM binds to antigen on cell membrane and activates complement	ABO transfusion reaction, Goodpasture's syndrome, rheumatic fever
III	**Immune-Complex**	Antigen and antibody form complexes that deposit in organs and may activate complement	Arthus reaction, serum sickness, poststreptococcal glomerulonephritis
IV	**Delayed**	CD4 T lymphocytes form mononuclear infiltrate within hours to days after exposure to antigen	Tuberculin skin test (PPD), contact hypersensitivity

Ig = immunoglobulin.

(1) A **normal individual**

—will not have anti-HLA antibodies (i.e., PRA = 0%–5%).

(2) An **elevated PRA**

—may be due to previous blood transfusions, transplantation, pregnancy, or autoimmune disorder.

—suggests an increased likelihood of a positive crossmatch.

d. Crossmatching

—is used to prevent hyperacute rejection by determining if a recipient has preformed antibodies to donor lymphocyte surface antigens.

e. Hyperacute rejection

—is a major barrier to transplantation from other species (i.e., xenotransplantation).

3. Acute rejection

—usually occurs days to weeks after transplantation but may occur at any time after transplantation.

a. Acute rejection is initiated

—by **T cell dependent immunity.**

b. Most current immunosuppressive regimens

—are directed toward preventing acute rejection with inhibition of T cell immunity.

4. Chronic rejection

—occurs months to years after transplantation.

a. Chronic rejection is characterized by

—the loss of normal histologic structure.

—fibrosis.

—atherosclerosis.

b. Factors contributing to **chronic rejection** include

—**repeated bouts of acute rejection.**

—drug toxicity.

—recurrent infections.

—ischemic damage at the time of harvest or transplant.

—use of older or suboptimal organs.

—noncompliance with immunosuppression.

c. Prevention of chronic rejection

—requires specific attention to these causes.

II. Immunosuppression

A. The current clinical use of immunosuppressive agents

—depends on the organ transplanted.

—frequently varies by institution.

B. General principles of immunosuppression

1. Induction therapy

—involves administering high doses of immunosuppression (usually antibody therapy) at the time of transplantation to prevent rejection.

2. **Maintenance therapy**

—involves administering lower, less toxic doses of immunosuppressive agents following high-dose induction therapy.

C. **Characteristics of the various agents**

—used are outlined in **Table 6-5.**

D. **Complications of immunosuppressive therapy**

—are also outlined in Table 6-5.

1. **Immunosuppressed individuals**

—are more **susceptible to infection** by typical bacterial pathogens and also by unusual organisms.

a. The **common pathogens**

—and timing of infection are demonstrated in **Figure 6-1.**

b. **Chronic suppression**

—of the immune system can also lead to **malignancy.**

(1) **Squamous cell carcinoma**

—is the most common.

—is generally not aggressive.

—can be treated by local excision.

(2) **Post-transplant lymphoproliferative disease (PTLD)**

—is the next most common.

—may be related to malignant transformation by **Epstein-Barr virus.**

—Treatment includes the reduction or withdrawal of immunosuppression.

—Conventional chemotherapy and radiation therapy are used for aggressive tumors.

(3) **Other malignancies include**

—**Kaposi's sarcoma** and **cervical carcinoma** related to papilloma virus.

(4) The incidence of more **common neoplasms**

—(i.e., breast, lung, and colon) may be slightly **increased** in the transplant population.

III. Classification of Organ Transplants

A. **An autograft**

—is the transfer of an individual's own tissue from one site to another.

—is not associated with a specific immune response against the tissue.

B. **An isograft** (syngeneic graft)

—is transplantation between identical twins.

Table 6-5. Clinical Immunosuppressive Agents

Drug	Mechanism of Action	Clinical Use	Side Effects
Glucocorticoids	Hormone receptor-steroid complex binds to DNA, alters transcription and translation, affects T cells and macrophages	Key component of maintenance therapy, treatment for rejection	Cushingoid features, hypertension, weight gain, hyperglycemia/glucose intolerance, osteoporosis poor wound healing, pancreatitis, peptic ulcer, psychosis
Azathioprine	Inhibits purine synthesis, blocks RNA/DNA synthesis; affects T cells > B cells	Maintenance therapy: allows lower doses of glucocorticoids and cyclosporine	Leukopenia, thrombocytopenia, hepatitis, pancreatitis, dermatitis, alopecia, infections
Mycophenolate mofetil	Inhibits inosine monophosphate dehydrogenase, blocks DNA synthesis; more specific for lymphocytes	Decreases incidence of rejection versus azathioprine in renal transplantation	GI symptoms (e.g., nausea, diarrhea, cramping), leukopenia, anemia, infections
Cyclosporine	Binds to cyclophilin (an isomerase enzyme); decreases IL-2 and other cytokine release from T cells	Induction therapy and maintenance	Nephrotoxicity, hypertension, hyperkalemia, hyperuricemia, gout, gingival hypertrophy, hirsutism, tremors, seizures, hyperglycemia, hemolytic uremic syndrome
Tacrolimus (FK506)	Binds to FK binding proteins, effects similar to cyclosporine	Induction and maintenance therapy, "rescue" of grafts failing on cyclosporine	Nephrotoxicity, neurotoxicity, diabetes
Antithymocyte globulin (ATG)	Polyclonal antibodies directed against T cell receptors (CD2, CD3, CD4, CD8) as well as B cells, monocytes, and granulocytes	Induction therapy, treatment of steroid resistance, recurrent, or severe rejection	Fever, chills, nausea, vomiting, leukopenia, thrombocytopenia, myalgia/arthralgia, diarrhea, headache, rash, pruritis, urticaria, phlebitis
OKT3	Murine monoclonal antibody directed against the CD3 complex on T cells	Induction therapy, treatment of steroid resistant, recurrent, or severe rejection	Cytokine release syndrome, fever, chills, dyspnea, wheezing, pulmonary edema, tachycardia, hypotension, anaphylaxis

GI = gastrointestinal; IL = interleukin.

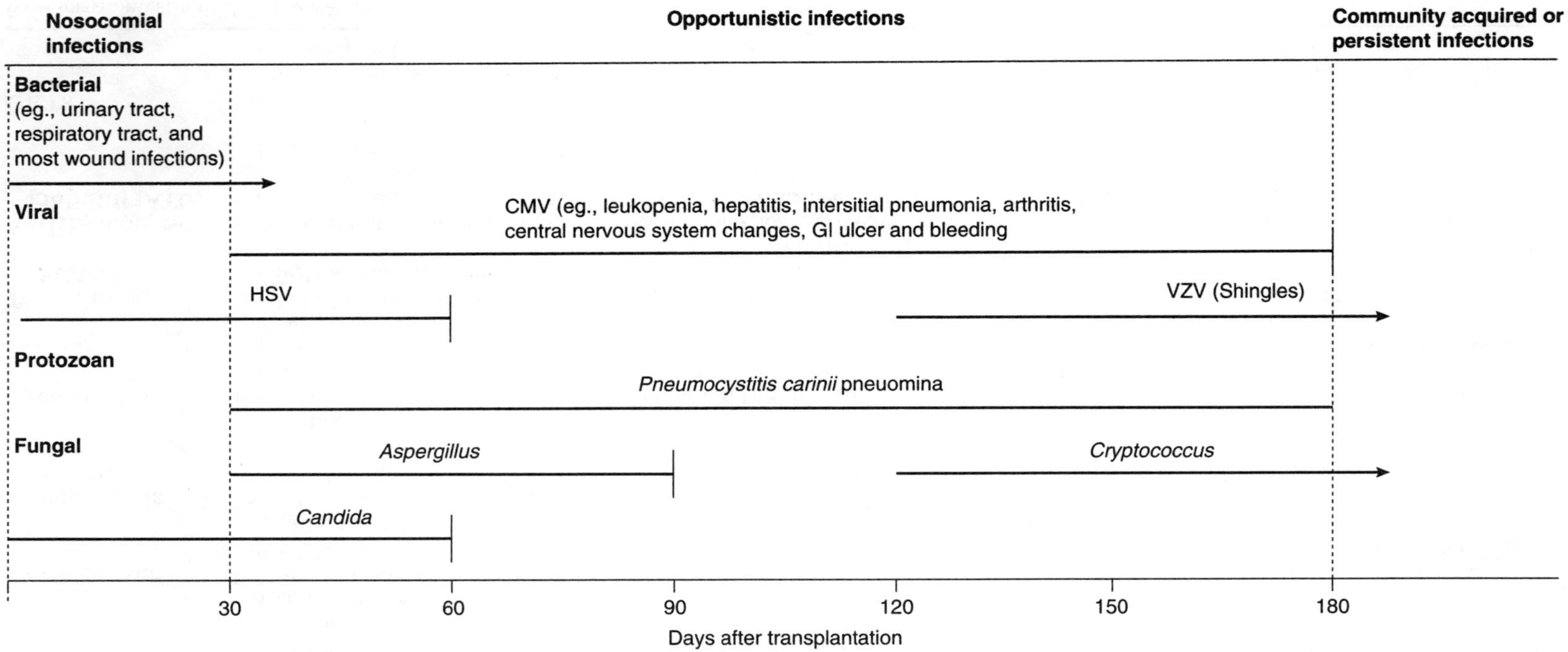

Figure 6-1. Major pathogens and usual timing for infections after organ transplantation. (Adapted with permission from Rubin RH, Wolfson JS, Cosimi AB, Tolkoff-Rubin NE: Infection in renal transplant recipients. *Am J Med* 1981;70:406.) CMV = cytomegalovirus; GI = gastrointestinal; HSV = herpes simplex virus; VZV = varicella-zoster virus.

—is accepted without immunosuppression (e.g., the first successful kidney transplant).

C. An allograft (homograft)

—is a graft between genetically different members of the same species (i.e., from one human to another).

D. A xenograft (heterograft)

—is a graft transplanted between 2 species (e.g., a baboon heart to a human recipient).

—These result in **hyperacute rejection** in an immunocompetent host.

—Xenograft transplantation is currently undergoing experimental evaluation for clinical application.

IV. Kidney Transplantation

A. Donors for kidney transplants

—come from **3 sources:** cadaver, living related, and living unrelated donors.

1. **All donors,** both living and cadaveric, should
   —have good renal function.
   —be free of systemic infection or cancer (except for a primary brain tumor).
   —be screened for human immunodeficiency virus (HIV) and hepatitis.
2. **Renal recipients**
   a. **About 30% have a living relative suitable for donation.**
   b. **The relative must be**
      —ABO compatible.
      —in good medical and psychological condition.
      —of legal age.
      —willing to donate.
3. **Living donors**
   —have a low risk of complications.
   a. The **remaining kidney hypertrophies**
      —and provides up to 80% of the original renal function after several months.
   b. The **most common complication**
      —is **wound infection** (~1%).
   c. The **most common cause of death**
      —(~1 in 5000) is pulmonary embolus.
   d. Laparoscopic donor nephrectomy can now be safely performed.
4. **Donor evaluation**
   a. Before donation, **donors should be evaluated** with
      —history and physical.
      —chest radiograph.

—electrocardiogram (ECG).
—urinalysis.
—complete blood count.
—blood urea nitrogen (BUN).
—creatinine (Cr).

b. **Suitable donors** should then be evaluated with
—an **arteriogram.**
—**spiral computed tomography (CT) scan, or magnetic resonance imaging (MRI).**
(1) Organs with multiple renal arteries will require anastomosis of the small accessory arteries.
(2) Small accessory renal veins may be ligated.

5. The **need for cadaver donors**
—**far outweighs the supply.**

a. **Brain death** must be established
—before removal of organs.
(1) **Clinical criteria for brain death**
—are the absence of spontaneous respiration, cranial reflexes, and response to stimuli.
—A known cause for the condition must exist over a period of time, and must be irreversible.
(2) **Confirmatory findings include**
—absence of cerebral blood flow.
—an isoelectric electroencephalogram.
—sustained apnea in the presence of an elevated CO_2.

b. **Organs are removed**
—before or shortly after cardiac arrest.

c. **Solutions used to preserve the organs**
—after harvest and before transplantation include **Euro-Collins** or **University of Wisconsin** (UW) solution.
(1) These contain large sugars not absorbed by cells creating an osmotic gradient that prevents swelling of cells.
(2) Antioxidants, electrolytes, and nutrients are also present.

d. **The kidney**
—should then be transplanted within **30 hours** to prevent a high rate of **acute tubular necrosis.**
—may also be preserved for 3 days with continuous **pulsatile perfusion.**

B. **Disease states**
—leading to the need for **renal transplantation** are listed in **Table 6-6.**

1. **Most patients**
—will require **hemodialysis** or **peritoneal dialysis** while awaiting the availability of a suitable organ.

2. **Recipients receiving an organ from a living donor**

Table 6-6. Causes of End-Stage Organ Disease Leading to Transplantation*

Kidney	Liver	Pancreas	Heart	Heart–Lung	Lung
Diabetes mellitus (30%) Glomerulonephritis (25%) Hypertension Polycystic kidney disease Reflux pyelonephritis Goodpasture's syndrome Congenital renal hypoplasia Renal cortical necrosis Alport's syndrome Systemic lupus erythematosus	Hepatitis C (30%) Alcoholic cirrhosis (25%) Hepatitis B Autoimmune hepatitis Cryptogenic hepatitis Primary biliary cirrhosis Primary sclerosing cholangitis Fulminant hepatic failure Malignant neoplasms Biliary atresia Budd-Chiari syndrome Wilson's disease Hemochromatosis α_1-antitrypsin deficiency	Insulin-dependent diabetes mellitus	Ischemic cardiomyopathy (40%) Idiopathic cardiomyopathy (35%) Congenital cardiomyopathy Familial cardiomyopathy	Primary pulmonary hypertension Fibrotic lung disease Cor pulmonale Cystic fibrosis Congenital heart disease with Eisenmenger's syndrome α_1-Antitrypsin deficiency	Chronic obstructive pulmonary disease (30%) Idiopathic pulmonary fibrosis (17%) α_1-Antitrypsin deficiency Cystic fibrosis Primary pulmonary hypertension Sarcoidosis Idiopathic bronchiectasis Lymphangiomyomatosis Pulmonary fibrosis from previous chemotherapy or radiation therapy

*Percent given in parentheses for more common indications.

—may be transplanted before the need for dialysis.

C. Few absolute contraindications exist

—for kidney transplantation recipients.

—Children younger than 1 year old and adults older than 70 have received transplants.

1. Absolute contraindications include

—active malignancy.

—septicemia.

—severe cardiopulmonary debilitation.

2. Five-year survival and **quality of life are improved** in renal transplant recipients compared to those on hemodialysis.

—Five-year survival of a diabetic patient on dialysis is ~40%.

D. Surgical procedure

1. The **renal graft**

—is commonly **placed in the iliac fossa** via an oblique, lower abdominal incision (heterotopic).

2. The **donor renal artery**

—and vein are anastomosed to the recipient's iliac artery and vein, respectively.

3. Continuity of the urinary tract

—is often reestablished by ureteroneocytostomy (donor ureter to recipient bladder).

—A **Foley catheter** is used for **several days** postoperatively to decompress the bladder and protect the anastomosis.

4. Bilateral nephrectomies

—are rarely required.

5. **Indications for bilateral nephrectomies** include

—polycystic kidney disease with recurrent infections.

—recurrent hematuria requiring multiple transfusions.

—refractory, severe hypertension.

E. Complications

1. Vascular complications

—occur in less than 1% of recipients.

a. Renal artery stenosis

—may result in **severe hypertension** and be secondary to rejection.

b. Renal vein thrombosis

—or iliofemoral thrombosis may be treated with anticoagulation or urokinase.

2. **Urine extravasation** may occur because of

—ureteroneocystostomy leakage.

—ureteral necrosis.

—ureteral obstruction.

—Surgical intervention is often required.

3. A lymphocele

—may occur from leakage of nearby lymphatics in the iliac fossa.

a. Lymphoceles may become infected or large enough to obstruct the ureter or renal vasculature.

b. These frequently need to be drained surgically.

4. Recipients may experience complications

—of immunosuppression (see II D) including **cyclosporine-induced or tacrolimus-induced nephrotoxicity.**

5. Acute cellular rejection

—usually occurs within the first 3 months but may occur sooner or years later.

a. Diagnosis

—is made by multiple findings.

(1) Signs and symptoms may include

—fever.

—malaise.

—oliguria.

—hypertension.

—tenderness over the graft.

(2) Laboratory evaluation

—of blood and urine usually reveal a rising BUN and serum Cr.

(3) A renal ultrasound

—may be useful in ruling out obstruction of the ureter and for assessing blood flow to the kidney.

(4) A radioisotope perfusion scan may be useful to evaluate

—renal blood flow.

—tubular function.

—the patency of the ureter.

(5) Percutaneous kidney biopsy

—is frequently used to evaluate patients with suspected rejection.

b. The **differential diagnosis** includes

—infection

—acute tubular necrosis from preservation injury or ischemia.

—cyclosporine nephrotoxicity.

—urinary obstruction or extravasation.

—return of original disease.

—chronic rejection.

c. Treatment to prevent loss of allograft

—includes the prompt administration of antirejection therapy [e.g., high-dose steroids, OKT3, or antithymocyte globulin (ATG)].

V. Liver Transplantation

A. A suitable liver donor

—is usually a brain-dead, heart-beating donor.

1. Preferably, donors

—are hemodynamically stable.

—have acceptable liver function tests.

—have serum Na^+ less than 170.

2. Features that predict poor graft function include

—steatosis in over 30% of hepatocytes.

—**cold preservation time over 18 hours.**

—increasing donor age.

3. Reduced-size grafting

—(i.e., transplantation of the left lobe or left lateral segment only) can be used to transplant an adult liver to an adult or pediatric recipient.

—Success of reduced-size grafting has led to **living-related liver transplantation** at some centers.

B. Causes of end-stage liver disease

—leading to liver transplantation are listed in **Table 6-6.**

1. Transplantation is indicated

—when the chance of a life-threatening complication occurring over a 1–2 year period is estimated to be greater than 50%.

2. Contraindications to transplantation in a recipient include

—extrahepatic malignancy.

—septicemia.

—severe cardiopulmonary disease.

—active substance abuse (e.g., alcohol).

C. Surgical implantation of the liver

—includes the associated factors below.

1. Hemodynamic instability

—may occur during clamping of the inferior vena cava (IVC).

—may be avoided by using **venovenous bypass.**

2. Revascularization of the allograft

—is commonly performed by anastomosis of the donor suprahepatic-IVC, infrahepatic-IVC, portal vein, and hepatic artery to corresponding structures in the recipient.

3. Biliary tract continuity

—is commonly performed by **choledochocholedochostomy** (anastomosis of donor to recipient bile duct) or choledochoenterostomy.

D. Post-transplant complications

1. Technical complications include

—bleeding.

—hepatic artery thrombosis.

—portal vein thrombosis.

—biliary stenosis and leaks.

—intra-abdominal infection.

—**Primary nonfunction** immediately after implantation requires retransplantation within 5–7 days.

2. Complications

—of infection and immunosuppression may also occur (see II D and Table 6-5).

3. Acute allograft rejection

—occurs in ~50% of liver recipients.

—is most common within the first 4 weeks after transplantation.

a. Symptoms

—are nonspecific and include fever and general malaise.

b. Liver function tests

—are usually elevated.

c. Evaluation includes

—**Doppler ultrasound** to assess hepatic blood flow.

d. Percutaneous liver biopsy

—is frequently performed.

e. The **differential diagnosis includes**

—the technical complications listed in Section V D 1 and drug toxicity.

E. Survival

—Overall 1-year survival is ~80%−85%.

VI. Pancreas Transplantation

A. A **pancreas is typically procured from** someone who

—is a heart-beating donor.

—is 3–55 years old.

—does not have acute pancreatitis or pancreatic injury.

—does not have a history of diabetes.

1. Organs are preserved safely

—**for 20–30 hours** using UW solution and hypothermia.

2. Living related segmental grafts

—have been transplanted.

B. The **indication for pancreatic transplantation**

—although controversial, includes Type I **insulin-dependent diabetes mellitus.**

1. If possible, transplantation should be performed **before the development of end-stage complications.**
   a. **These complications include**
      —blindness caused by retinopathy.
      —disabling neuropathy.
      —extensive vascular disease.
      —end-stage nephropathy.
   b. These are **not,** however, **contraindications** to transplantation.
2. **In patients with renal failure, transplantation**
   —can occur prior to, at the same time as, or after kidney transplantation.
3. **Contraindications to transplantation are**
   —similar to those for kidney transplantation (see IV C).

C. **Multiple techniques exist**

—for the recipient transplant operation.

1. The **arterial blood supply is reconstructed**
   —using the donor celiac axis or donor iliac artery.
2. **Pancreatic exocrine drainage**
   —via donor duodenum can be established enterically or into the bladder (**Figure 6-2**).
   a. **Measuring urinary amylase**
      —after a bladder anastomosis allows for early detection of rejection.
   b. A **bladder anastomosis** is associated with metabolic acidosis from
      —HCO_3^- loss in the urine.
      —hematuria.
      —urethral strictures.
      —frequent urinary tract infections.
      —reflux pancreatitis.

D. **Complications may include**

—pancreatic thrombosis.

—peripancreatic fluid collections.

—adult respiratory distress syndrome.

—bleeding.

—pancreatic fistula formation.

E. **Monitoring for rejection**

—can be difficult.

1. **Hypoglycemia**
   —may occur after **irreversible** rejection occurs.

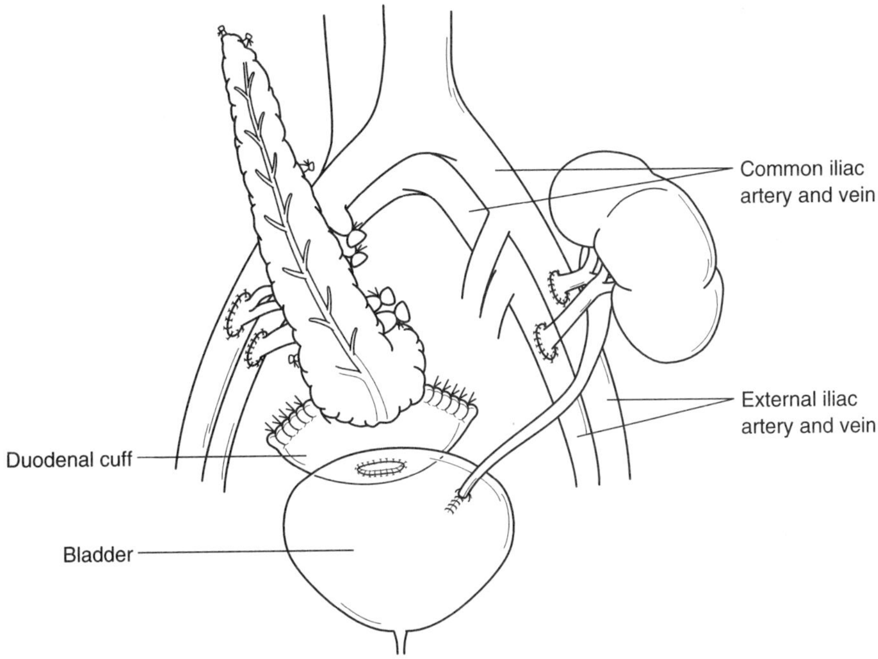

Figure 6-2. Vascular and bladder anastomoses in a kidney and pancreas transplantation. (Adapted with permission from Sollinger SW, Knechtle SJ: Pancreas Transplantation. In: *Textbook of Surgery: The Biological Basis of Modern Surgical Practice,* 15th ed. Edited by David C. Sabiston, Jr. Philadelphia, WB Saunders, 1996, p 474.)

2. Rejection of a renal allograft

—**usually occurs before pancreatic rejection.**

—can be useful if both were transplanted simultaneously.

3. Urinary amylase monitoring

—is useful if a bladder anastomosis was performed.

F. Survival

—Overall 1-year survival is ~90%.

VII. Heart Transplantation

A. Characteristics of suitable brain-dead **cardiac donors** generally include

—being younger than 60 years old.

—no history of cardiac disease.

—normal ECG and echocardiogram.

—ABO compatibility.

—donor within 20%–50% of recipient size.

—minimal vasopressor support.

B. Allografts can be **preserved** with

—cardioplegia and hypothermia **for 4 hours.**

C. **Recipients usually have** Class IV heart failure

—[New York Heart Association (NYHA) classification] with less than 1 year expected survival.

1. **Common causes of heart failure**

   —that require transplantation are listed in **Table 6-6.**

2. **Recipients must have cardiac disease**

   —not amenable to conventional medical or surgical therapy.

3. **Pulmonary hypertension** in the recipient is associated with

   —**increased perioperative morbidity and mortality.**

   —an increased risk of **graft failure.**

4. **Recipients should also be HIV-negative**

   —and free of malignancy or active infection.

D. **Donor and recipient operations**

—are done in concert because of a relatively short cold preservation time.

1. The **recipient heart**

   —is excised, leaving portions of the right and left atria.

2. The **donor right and left atria**

   —are trimmed appropriately and then anastomosed to the corresponding donor atria.

3. The **aortic and pulmonary anastomoses**

   —are then performed.

4. The **heart rate**

   —is initially supported by isoproterenol or atrial pacing because the graft is denervated.

E. **Post-transplant complications include**

—immunosuppression toxicity.

—infection, including mediastinitis and sternal wound infection.

—**accelerated allograft coronary artery disease.**

F. **Diagnosis**

—**of cardiac rejection can be difficult.**

1. **Clinical signs** include the new onset of

   —cardiac arrhythmia.

   —fever.

   —malaise.

   —hypotension.

   —shortness of breath.

2. **Echocardiography**

   —is frequently used to characterize a poor functioning heart secondary to rejection.

3. Routine endomyocardial biopsies

—remain the mainstay of diagnosis.

G. Survival

—Overall 1-year survival is ~80%–90%.

VIII. Combined Heart–Lung Transplantation

A. For combined heart–lung transplantation

—a **close size match** is necessary, with the donor being either smaller or the same size as the recipient.

1. The **donor lungs** should
   - **a.** demonstrate **adequate gas exchange** with
     - —the PO_2 higher than 400 mm Hg on 100% O_2.
     - —normal compliance demonstrated by peak airway pressures of less than 30 mm Hg with normal tidal volumes.
   - **b.** They should also be
     - —absent of purulent secretions.
     - —clear on chest radiograph.
2. The donor **heart and lungs are removed**

   —**en bloc** and can be **preserved for 4 hours.**

B. Indications for heart–lung transplantation

—are listed in **Table 6-6.**

—General indications include end-stage disease in both organs or end-stage disease in one organ with poor function in the other, prohibiting single organ transplantation.

C. The **surgical procedure involves**

—transplantation of the heart and lungs en bloc by anastomosis of the trachea, right atrium, and aorta.

D. Post-transplant complications include

—those related to infections and immunosuppression.

—those seen with heart or lung transplant individually (see VII E).

1. **Most recipients experience**

   —an **episode of rejection within the first 2 weeks.**
   - **a. Rejection in the heart**

     —does not necessarily correspond to that seen in the **lung,** which **is more common.**
   - **b. Routine endomyocardial biopsies**

     —should be obtained.
   - **c.** Rejection of a **lung allograft is diagnosed on clinical parameters** including

—decreased oxygenation.

—infiltrate on chest film.

—fever and general malaise.

—characteristic histologic findings of rejection on **transbronchial lung biopsy.**

d. **Bronchiolitis obliterans**

—may represent a form of chronic rejection in the lung.

—occurs in ~50% of recipients.

—begins to appear several months after transplantation.

(1) **Patients develop** shortness of breath and have a decreased forced expiratory flow $(FEF)_{25\%-75\%}$.

(2) **Treatment** primarily involves increased immunosuppression, but is generally **not very effective.**

2. **Strictures and breakdown of bronchial anastomoses**

—may occur and usually represent the presence of ischemia.

IX. Lung Transplantation

A. Criteria for potential donors

—are similar to those described for cardiopulmonary transplantation (see VIII A 1).

B. Eligible lung transplant recipients are those with

—end-stage lung disease.

—a life expectancy of 1–2 years.

1. **Common causes of lung disease**

—requiring transplantation are listed in **Table 6-6.**

2. **Contraindications to transplantation** include

—uncontrolled sepsis.

—active malignancy.

—continued smoking.

C. The surgical procedure

—may involve a **single or bilateral lung transplantation.**

—Potential recipients with cystic fibrosis or other septic lung disease usually undergo bilateral lung transplantation.

D. Post-transplant complications

—are similar to those described for the lung under heart–lung transplantation (see VIII D).

E. Survival

—Overall 1-year survival for **single lung transplantation** is ~65%.

—Overall 1-year survival for **bilateral lung transplantation** is ~70%.

Review Test

Directions: Each of the numbered items or incomplete statements in this section is followed by answers or by completions of the statement. Select the ONE lettered answer or completion that is BEST in each case.

1. A 47-year-old man with a history of alcoholic liver disease (his last drink was over 3 years ago) is admitted to the intensive care unit because of variceal bleeding. During evaluation for blood transfusions, he is found to have blood type A^+. During the first 7 days in the ICU, he develops ascites refractory to medical therapy, encephalopathy, and hepatorenal syndrome. Because he is not expected to survive more than another week, he is listed for liver transplantation. Which of the following is the most appropriate donor organ for this patient?

(A) The left hepatic lobe from his 17-year-old son
(B) A liver from a brain-dead 38-year-old man with human immunodeficiency virus (HIV)
(C) A liver from a brain-dead 38-year-old man with hepatitis C
(D) A pig liver
(E) A liver from a donor with blood type O^+

2. A 27-year-old woman develops oliguria 10 days after an uncomplicated kidney transplant. Evaluation includes a kidney biopsy that demonstrates a lymphocytic infiltrate in the tubular interstitium. Because she does not respond to steroid boluses over several days, a repeat biopsy is performed. OKT3 therapy is started for steroid resistant rejection. That afternoon, the patient develops severe rigors, a temperature of 39.3°C, a blood pressure of 89/64 mm Hg, and shortness of breath. Which one of the following is the most likely explanation for these findings?

(A) Fluid overload due to renal insufficiency
(B) Treatment with OKT3
(C) Cytomegalovirus viremia
(D) Renal graft rejection
(E) *Pneumocystis carinii* pneumonia

3. During cardiac transplantation, a recipient requires multiple blood transfusions from blood loss during surgery. During the operation, the patient develops sudden hypotension, bleeding from intravenous sites and wound edges, along with severe tachycardia. Which of the following is the most likely cause of these findings?

(A) Type I immediate hypersensitivity
(B) Type II cytotoxic hypersensitivity
(C) Previous aspirin therapy
(D) Type IV delayed hypersensitivity
(E) Previous warfarin therapy

4. After an uncomplicated renal transplantation, a patient inadvertently removes his Foley catheter on the first postoperative day. Why should the Foley catheter be reinserted?

(A) Hourly urine output monitoring is necessary.
(B) Foley catheters decrease the risk of urinary tract infections (UTI).
(C) Foley catheters decompress the bladder.
(D) Urethral strictures occur more commonly after kidney transplantation.
(E) Use of Foley catheters prevents acute rejection.

5. A 49-year-old woman develops markedly increased liver enzymes on the ninth postoperative day after liver transplantation for hepatitis C. Further evaluation includes a Doppler ultrasound demonstrating adequate hepatic blood flow, and liver biopsy demonstrating endothelialitis and bile duct damage. Which of the following therapies is most likely to be effective?

(A) Interferon therapy for recurrent hepatitis C
(B) Steroid bolus therapy for rejection
(C) Reoperation for portal vein thrombosis
(D) Reoperation for bile duct stricture
(E) Observation with repeat biopsy in 1 week

6. A 59-year-old man with chronic renal insufficiency presents for repeat kidney transplantation after loss of a previous graft. After the arterial and venous anastomosis are complete, the vascular clamps are removed and excellent perfusion of the kidney is observed. Thirty minutes later, the kidney is noted to have a bluish discoloration, loss of perfusion, and lack of urine production. Which of the following statements is true regarding this patient?

(A) This is due to class II HLA antibodies.
(B) A similar reaction is the major barrier to xenotransplantation.
(C) This reaction cannot be avoided.
(D) This reaction does not occur in cardiac recipients.
(E) Emergent treatment with OKT3 is indicated.

7. An 18-year-old woman with cystic fibrosis underwent bilateral lung transplantation 15 months ago. She now presents with a dry cough, and dyspnea refractory to bronchodilators. She has been observed to have a serial decline in her forced expiratory volume (FEV) over the past 3 months. Transbronchial lung biopsy is consistent with obliterative bronchiolitis (OB). Which of the following statements is true?

(A) No satisfactory treatment for reversal of this condition currently exists.
(B) The fibrosis can be reversed with increased immunosuppression.
(C) Most patients stop progressing with adequate therapy.
(D) OB occurs in less than 5% of all lung transplants.
(E) OB is a manifestation of acute rejection.

Directions: Each set of matching questions in this section consists of a list of four to twenty-six lettered options followed by several numbered items. For each numbered item, select the appropriate lettered option(s). Each lettered option may be selected once, more than once, or not at all.

Questions 8–10

(A) Cyclosporine
(B) Mycophenolate mofetil
(C) OKT3
(D) Cyclophosphamide
(E) Antithymocyte globulin (ATG)
(F) Azathioprine
(G) Tacrolimus
(H) Glucocorticoids

Match each immunologic drug with the most likely associated description.

8. A 49-year-old man with steroid resistant rejection of a renal allograft develops high fever, tachycardia, and shortness of breath 30 minutes after administration of this medication. (SELECT 1 DRUG)

9. Patients receiving this agent specifically have significantly decreased production of interleukin (IL)-2. (SELECT 2 DRUGS)

10. When used in transplant recipients, this agent specifically binds to multiple cell surface receptors on the T cell. (SELECT 1 DRUG)

Answers and Explanations

1–E. The patient described has acute or chronic hepatic failure and is not expected to live beyond 7 days. He is, therefore, a United Network for Organ Sharing (UNOS) status IIA and requires urgent liver transplantation. Although not ideal, living related liver donation is acceptable, however, the donor should be 18 years or older. Transplantation from donors with hepatitis C has a high rate of occurrence of these viral infections in the recipient. Xenotransplantation is experimental at this time. Liver transplantation can be performed across blood type barriers (e.g., B donor, O recipient) but this is associated with a decreased survival. A donor with blood type O, however, is an appropriate donor for liver transplantation.

2–B. Cytokine release syndrome from treatment with OKT3 is the most likely explanation for the findings described. The binding of OKT3 to CD3 antigens on T cells leads to the release of cytokines, resulting in symptoms similar to this patient's. Cytokine release syndrome is associated most commonly with the first dose. Pretreating with diphenhydramine, acetaminophen, steroids, and narcotics can reduce the symptoms. Fluid overload is not commonly associated with fevers and rigors. Cytomegalovirus and *Pneumocystis carinii* pneumonia do not commonly occur within the first month after transplantation. Allograft rejection itself is associated with fever but would be less likely to explain the other symptoms.

3–B. Blood transfusion reaction—a type II cytotoxic hypersensitivity—commonly is associated with hypotension, tachycardia, and diffuse bleeding in an anesthetized patient. This reaction occurs when preformed antibodies to transfused red blood cell antigens are present in the recipient, leading to complement mediated lysis. Type I reactions are mediated by immunoglobulin (Ig)E to allergen, leading to mast cell or basophil degranulation. Previous aspirin or warfarin therapy would likely be associated with persistent bleeding throughout the operation and would not lead to sudden hypotension. Type IV sensitivity occurs 48–72 hours after exposure to antigen and is associated with sensitized helper T cells.

4–C. After ureteroneocystostomy, decompression of the bladder for several days using a Foley catheter allows healing of the anastomosis. Urine output monitoring aids in detection of renal hypoperfusion and graft rejection but can be accurately measured in this setting without the use of a Foley catheter. Foley catheters are associated with an increased rate of urinary tract infections. Overdistension of the bladder can lead to breakdown of the anastomosis of the ureter to the bladder. Although ureter strictures are not uncommon after renal transplantation, urethral strictures are rare. Foley catheters do not prevent rejection.

5–B. The pathologic findings and time course described are consistent with acute cellular rejection. More than half of liver transplant recipients will develop acute rejection, most within the first 4 weeks. Initial therapy often includes steroid boluses. Hepatitis C, like many other indications for transplantation, may recur 3–6 months after transplantation. Adequate hepatic blood flow on Doppler ultrasound decreases the likelihood of portal vein thrombosis. Bile duct strictures are often associated with jaundice and characteristic pathologic findings. Observation alone may lead to graft loss due to rejection.

6–B. The development of a bluish discoloration, and loss of perfusion and function within minutes to hours after revascularization is rare, but often due to hyperacute rejection. Hyperacute rejection occurs when preformed recipient antibodies act against class I donor antigens. Humans have preformed antibodies to animal antigens, making hyperacute rejection the major barrier to xenotransplantation. This reaction can almost always be avoided by performing a crossmatch. This assay is performed by adding donor serum to recipient lymphocytes in the presence of complement. If preformed antibodies are in the donor serum, cell lysis will occur. Although liver allografts are relatively resistant to hyperacute rejection, heart, pancreas, lung, and kidney are susceptible. Hyperacute rejection is refractory to therapy and almost always results in loss of the graft. OKT3 is indicated in the setting of acute rejection but has less of a role in hyperacute rejection.

7–A. Obliterative bronchiolitis (OB) has become recognized as the main impediment to long-term survival after lung transplantation. At present, no satisfactory therapy can reverse the fibrosis once it occurs. Although current treatment often involves increased immunosuppression, most patients continue to have progression of disease. OB occurs in ~50% of lung transplant recipients and is believed to be a manifestation of chronic rejection.

8–C. OKT3 is a monoclonal antibody directed against the CD3 complex commonly used for induction therapy and treatment of steroid resistant rejection. Binding of OKT3 to the CD3 complex induces the release of multiple cytokines, and is associated with fever, chills, wheezing, pulmonary edema, tachycardia, hypotension, and rarely, death. This occurs most commonly within 30 minutes to 4 hours after the first dose and usually subsides with subsequent doses.

9–A and G. Cyclosporine and tacrolimus both function by decreasing the release of interleukin (IL)-2. Cyclosporine is useful for induction and maintenance therapy but has no benefit in treating rejection. In contrast, tacrolimus can be used for resistant rejection and "rescue therapy" of grafts failing on cyclosporine.

10–E. Antithymocyte globulin (ATG) and antilymphocyte globulin are polyclonal antibodies directed against T cell antigens including CD2, CD3, CD4, and CD8, as well as B cell, platelet, monocyte, and granulocyte antigens. OKT3 is a monoclonal antibody directed against the CD3 antigen of T cells. These three agents are used for induction therapy as well as treatment of resistant or severe rejection.

7

Fluids, Electrolytes, and Critical Care

James F. Calland

I. Fluids

A. Water

1. Estimation of total body water

—is based on the **"rule of thirds."**

a. **Total body water** equals two thirds of total body weight.

b. **Intracellular water** is approximately two thirds of total body water.

c. **Extracellular water** is approximately one third of total body water.

(1) One third of extracellular water is intravascular.

(2) Two thirds of extracellular water is interstitial.

d. **Third space fluids** collect outside of the functional or "exchangeable" extracellular space (e.g., pleural effusions, ascites).

(1) Large amounts of fluid may be unavailable to the circulation in third spaces.

(2) The **abdominal peritoneum** can hold up to 18 L of third space fluids in the presence of an inflammatory process (e.g., peritonitis, postoperatively).

e. **Circulating blood volume** is 7% of body weight in adults.

2. Alterations in water balance

—are common in surgical patients.

a. **Hypovolemia**

(1) **Causes of hypovolemia**

—include **hemorrhage, gastrointestinal losses** [e.g., diarrhea, fistula, nasogastric (NG) tube drainage], **third space losses,** insensible losses, and inadequate intake.

(2) **Early signs**

—include decreased urine output, thirst, and poor skin turgor.

(3) **Late signs**

—include tachycardia, confusion, and alterations in body temperature.

(4) **Laboratory values**

—may include an elevated blood urea nitrogen (BUN), BUN/creatinine (Cr) > 20, high urine specific gravity (> 1.020), osmolarity (> 500 mOsm/L), and low urine Na^+.

b. **Hypervolemia**

(1) **Causes of hypervolemia**

—include heart, renal, and liver failure and depleted serum albumin.

(2) **Characteristics**

—include peripheral edema, dyspnea, pulmonary edema, and jugular venous distention.

—**Excessive intravenous (IV) fluid administration or excess salt intake** can exacerbate these conditions.

(3) **Measuring daily weight changes**

—is an accurate method for monitoring potential hypervolemia.

B. IV fluids

1. **Crystalloid versus colloid solutions**

a. **Crystalloid solutions** use ions in the form of salts (e.g., NaCl) as osmotically active particles (Table 7-1).

b. **Colloid solutions** use proteins, polysaccharides, and other macromolecules as osmotically active particles.

(1) **Hetastarch**

—is a synthetic solution containing polysaccharides.

(2) **Albumin solutions (5% or 25%)**

—are made from human plasma.

—are commonly used in the management of hypoalbuminemia and hypovolemia despite a lack of evidence supporting their use versus crystalloid.

—Use of albumin solutions is also questioned because of their high cost and short half-life (< 24 hours).

(3) **Fresh frozen plasma (FFP)**

Table 7-1. Electrolyte Concentration of Common Intravenous (IV) Solutions

IV Solutions	Na^+*	Cl^-*	HCO_3^-*	K^+*	Ca^{2+}*	Glucose (g/L)
0.9% NaCl (normal saline)	154	154	—	—	—	—
0.45% NaCl (½ normal saline)	77	77	—	—	—	—
Lactated Ringer's	130	109	28†	4	2.7	—
5% dextrose in H_2O	—	—	—	—	—	50
3% NaCl (hypertonic saline)	513	513	—	—	—	—

*These electrolytes are measured in mEq/L.
†Lactate in solution is metabolized in HCO_3^-.

—from human donors is a colloid solution frequently used for **repletion of clotting factors** during resuscitation.

c. The use of colloid solutions for volume resuscitation has not been shown to provide additional benefit versus crystalloid solutions.

2. Maintenance fluids

—provide the minimal requirements for daily water and electrolyte balance.

a. Obligatory urine production necessary for excretion of the daily solute load varies by a patient's age and size (500–1000 mL/24 hr for a 70-kg patient).

b. Insensible losses account for about 500 mL/day for an average 70-kg patient.

(1) Evaporative skin losses

—During fever, patients lose an extra 500 mL for each degree C above 37.

(2) Respiratory losses are increased in patients with tachypnea or a tracheostomy.

—Humidified oxygen reduces these losses.

(3) Losses in stool account for 250 mL/day in normal patients.

c. Estimations for maintenance IV fluids

(1) For the first 10 kg of body weight

—give 100 mL/kg divided over 24 hours.

(2) For the second 10 kg of body weight

—administer 50 mL/kg.

(3) All weight thereafter requires 20 mL/kg divided over 24 hours.

(4) Alternatively, the "4–2–1 rule" uses

—4 mL/kg/hr for the first 10 kg

—2 mL/kg/hr for the second 10 kg

—1 mL/kg/hr for the remaining weight.

3. Maintenance electrolyte replacement

—also depends on body weight.

a. Na^+ requirements are highly variable.

—Administration of 1–2 mEq/kg/24 hr is generally sufficient.

b. K^+ average 0.5–1.0 mEq/kg/day with care to avoid hyperkalemia.

4. Replacement of additional fluid losses

—should approximate in volume and electrolyte concentration the fluid that is being lost (Table 7-2).

a. Blood losses

—should be replaced 1:3 with normal saline or lactated Ringer's solution because of redistribution of crystalloid solutions into the extravascular space.

b. NG tube losses

—are most appropriately replaced with K^+ in excess of that found in the NG tube aspirate.

(1) K^+ and H^+ losses from NG tube drainage can result in **metabolic alkalosis** with paradoxic aciduria.

Table 7-2. Composition of Gastrointestinal Secretions

Source	Volume (mL/24 hr)	Na^+ (mEq/L)	K^+ (mEq/L)	HCO_3^- (mEq/L)
Stomach	1000–2000	60–100	10–20	—
Small intestine	2000–4000	120–140	5–10	30–40
Pancreas	300–800	135–145	5–10	95–120
Bile	300–600	135–145	5–10	30–40

(2) **Paradoxic aciduria** results from an aldosterone-mediated compensatory renal loss of H^+ in an effort to resorb K^+ in the distal tubules.

c. **Diarrhea losses**

—should be replaced with HCO_3- and K^+-rich fluids if necessary.

d. **Before replacing fluid losses**

—assess the patient's respiratory status, cardiac status, and overall fluid balance.

C. Blood products

1. Transfusion of blood

—is used in patients when a critical **reduction in red blood cell (RBC) mass results in tissue ischemia** (e.g., severe hemorrhage or anemia).

a. **Hematocrit (Hct) levels**

—Specific indications vary greatly depending on the patient's overall condition; however, a Hct < 30 [hemoglobin (Hgb) < 10] is a relative indication for transfusion.

b. **A type and cross-match of the recipient's blood** should be attempted before transfusion.

(1) **Blood typing**

—identifies the patient's specific **ABO and Rh antigen** types (5–10 minutes).

(2) **A "screen"**

—tests the **recipient's serum for antibodies** to antigens other than ABO (45 minutes).

(3) **A cross-match**

—tests the **compatibility** of the donor's RBCs and the recipient's serum (45–60 minutes).

c. **Whole blood** is sometimes used in severe hemorrhage.

—Transfusion of concentrated **packed red blood cells (PRBCs)** is generally preferred.

(1) Stored blood is often **deficient** in **platelets, factor V, factor VIII,** and **calcium.**

(2) Administration of 1 unit of PRBCs usually results in a 3–4-point increase in the Hct.

d. **In an emergency,** transfusion of **type-specific blood** or **O^- blood (universal donor)** may be required.

e. **For elective surgery,** patients may donate their own blood before surgery should it be needed for transfusion.

2. **FFP (human)**

—is used primarily as a replacement for depleted clotting factors, and is sometimes used as a volume expander.

3. **Cryoprecipitate**

—is used for replacement of von Willebrand factor, factor VIII, and fibrinogen.

4. **Other blood components**

—such as **factor VIII concentrate** and **factor IX concentrate** are used to correct specific coagulation defects (see Chapter 2).

5. **Complications of transfusion**

—are outlined in Table 7-3.

a. **A febrile response**

—may frequently result due to a reaction between the recipient's cells and the donor's leukocytes.

(1) This may be prevented by administration of **leukocyte-depleted blood.**

(2) Treatment generally consists of antipyretic therapy.

b. **Anaphylaxis**

—may occur with itching, rash, dyspnea, and even shock.

(1) **Mild symptoms** may be treated with antihistamines and observation.

Table 7-3. Complications of Transfusion of Blood Products

Reaction	Cause	Characteristics	Treatment
Hemolytic	ABO incompatibility (often due to clerical error)	Fever, chills, back pain, abdominal pain, shock, spontaneous bleeding, hemoglobinuria	Stop transfusion, IV fluids, mannitol
Febrile	Reaction with donor leukocytes	Fever, chills	Antipyretics, leukocyte-depleted PRBCs
Anaphylactic	Recipient antibodies against donor serum proteins	Itching, urticaria, broncospasm	Severe: stop transfusion, antihistamines, epinephrine, steroids
Viral transmission	Hepatitis C (< 1/30,000); HIV (< 1/300,000)	Hepatitis, cirrhosis, AIDS	Prevention, pharmacotherapy (see Chapter 4)
Fluid overload	Rapid administration of blood products (especially in the elderly)	Dyspnea, pulmonary edema	Diuretics, slow rate of administration
Bacterial contamination	Introduction of skin flora (*Staphylococcus* and *Streptococcus* sp.)	Bacteremia, sepsis	Treat infection (i.e., with antibiotics)

HIV = human immunodeficiency virus; IV = intravenous; PRBCs = packed red blood cells.

(2) **Advanced symptoms** require immediate **cessation of transfusion,** proper airway control, fluid resuscitation, bronchodilators, and steroids.

c. **ABO incompatibility**

—Although rare, it is a life-threatening condition.

(1) **Characteristics**

—include fever, chills, back pain, abdominal pain, shock, spontaneous bleeding, hemoglobinuria, and oliguria.

(2) **Intraoperative excessive bleeding**

—may be an early sign of a severe reaction.

(3) **Renal failure**

—is a frequent complication.

(4) **Treatment** involves

—immediate **cessation of the transfusion.**

—aggressive **fluid resuscitation.**

—administration of mannitol.

II. Shock

—is defined as **inadequate perfusion of vital tissues.**

A. **Hypovolemic shock** is the result of inadequate circulating blood volume.

1. **Causes**

—include hemorrhage, gastrointestinal losses, dehydration, and burn injury.

2. **Early signs**

—include tachycardia, diaphoresis, and apprehension.

—More progressive shock may be associated with orthostatic hypotension, thirst, and oliguria.

3. **Late signs**

—include decreased mental status, agitation, and tachypnea.

4. **Physiologic signs**

—include high systemic vascular resistance (SVR), low central venous pressure (CVP), and decreased cardiac output.

5. **Management** involves

—**treatment of the underlying cause** of fluid loss.

—**aggressive resuscitation** with fluid administration.

a. **Continuous monitoring** of vital signs, CVP, and urine output are useful for measuring adequacy of resuscitation.

b. **During the initial resuscitation,** hypovolemic patients generally respond to **rapid infusion** of 2 L of fluid with some clinical improvement.

c. **Failure to respond** to this initial bolus may be a marker of severe ongoing blood loss, requiring early **transfusion,** early operative intervention, or both.

B. Septic shock results from the systemic effects of infection (e.g., abscess, pneumonia).

1. Potential mediators

—include bacterial products such as **lipopolysaccharide** and inflammatory mediators such as **interleukin-1** and **tumor-necrosis factor-α.**

2. Manifestations

—include confusion, fever, flushed skin, tachycardia, and hypotension.

3. Unlike hypovolemic shock, septic shock is associated with

—a **decrease in SVR.**

—an increase in cardiac output.

—low central venous pressure.

4. Management involves

—effective treatment of the underlying infectious source.

—administration of antibiotics.

—volume resuscitation.

C. Cardiogenic shock is defined as an **inability of the heart to meet the perfusion needs** of vital tissues and may be due to intrinsic or extrinsic causes.

1. Intrinsic causes

—include **ischemic heart disease** (e.g., infarction), valvular heart disease, arrhythmias, and myocardial contusion.

2. Extrinsic causes

—include cardiac tamponade and tension pneumothorax.

3. Manifestations

—include cool, diaphoretic skin; jugular venous distention; peripheral edema; and anxiety.

4. High adrenergic tone

—results in an elevated SVR, high CVP, and low cardiac output.

5. Management involves

—**optimizing preload** (left-ventricular filling pressure).

—pharmacologic **inotropic** (contractility) **support.**

—**afterload reduction.**

a. Preload

—is measured indirectly by CVP monitoring or by Swan-Ganz catheterization.

(1) If preload is low, administer fluids.

(2) If preload is high, diuresis may be necessary.

b. Inotropic support

—involves the use of pharmacologic agents (e.g., dobutamine, milrinone) that increase contractility and cardiac output.

c. Afterload reduction

—is most commonly achieved with pharmacologic agents such as hydralazine, nitroglycerin, and nitric oxide.

d. **Cardiac tamponade** and **tension pneumothorax** require **immediate decompression** of the pericardial or pleural space, respectively.

D. **Neurogenic shock** results from injury to the brain or spinal cord, anaphylaxis, or fainting (**psychogenic shock**).

1. **In surgical patients,** neurogenic shock generally presents as **hypotension** in the setting of paralysis or **spinal cord injury.**

a. **An aggressive search for other causes of hypotension** (e.g., hemorrhage) should be performed before a diagnosis of neurogenic shock is made.

b. **Patients are normovolemic** but lack vascular tone resulting in decreased CVP, tachycardia, and **low SVR.**

2. **Management** involves

—optimizing preload.

—increasing afterload with phenylephrine or norepinephrine.

—treating neurologic dysfunction.

III. Electrolytes

A. **Disorders of Na^+ balance**

1. **Hyponatremia** is defined as a serum $Na^+ < 130$ mEq/L.

—Hyponatremia can occur when total body Na^+ is normal, elevated, or depleted.

—Hyponatremia occurring when serum osmolality is **normal** (280–295 mOsm/kg) suggests that total body Na^+ is normal or elevated (**pseudohyponatremia**).

a. **Causes of pseudohyponatremia**

—may include hyperglycemia, uremia, or hyperlipidemia.

b. **Symptoms**

—may include irritability, hyperactive deep tendon reflexes, and **seizures** when serum Na^+ is **< 120 mEq/L.**

c. **The etiology and management of hyponatremia**

—depends on the volume status of the patient (hypovolemic, euvolemic, hypervolemic) as outlined in Table 7-4.

d. **Symptomatic hyponatremia**

—should be corrected at a rate no greater than 0.5–2.0 mEq/hr because of the risk of **central pontine myelinosis.**

—Correction with **normal saline** is appropriate although hypertonic saline may be used on rare occasions.

2. **Hypernatremia** is defined as a serum $Na^+ > 145$ mEq/L.

a. **Causes**

—include inadequate free water replacement (most common), IV ad-

Table 7-4. Characteristics of Hyponatremia

Imbalance	Causes	Management
Hyponatremia with euvolemia	Excess ADH (e.g., postoperatively, SIADH), psychogenic polydipsia, excessive infusion of hypotonic fluids, escess hyperosmotic solute in the blood (pseudo-hypernatremia)	Restrict intake of hypotonic fluids (free water restriction)
Hyponatremia with hypervolemia	Congestive heart failure, renal failure, liver failure, ascites, excessive fluid resuscitation	Fluid restriction
Hyponatremia with hypovolemia	Inadequate volume resuscitation with hypotonic fluids, hypovolemia with excessive ADH secretion (e.g., postoperatively, closed head injury)	Oral salts, resuscitation with normal saline (0.9%)

ADH = antidiuretic hormone; SIADH = syndrome of inappropriate antidiuretic hormone.

ministration of saline solutions, and excess free water loss (e.g., in diabetes insipidus).

b. Characteristics

—are those of **dehydration.**

—include orthostatic hypotension, poor skin turgor, dry mucous membranes, and lethargy.

c. Treatment

—is based on the underlying defect.

(1) Stop ongoing administration of Na^+-rich fluids and administer free water according to the free water deficit.

(2) Desmopressin (DDAVP) may be administered in the setting of diabetes insipidus.

B. Disorders of K^+ balance (Table 7-5)

1. Hypokalemia is generally defined as a serum $K^+ < 3$ mEq/L.

a. Potential causes in surgery patients include

—**gastrointestinal losses** (e.g., diarrhea, fistula, NG tube losses).

—**renal losses** (e.g., diuretics, hypomagnesemia, hyperaldosteronemia).

—**inadequate intake** (e.g., inadequate K^+ in postoperative fluids).

—**third space losses** (e.g., peritonitis, small bowel obstruction).

—**intracellular shift of K^+** (e.g., insulin overdose, severe metabolic alkalosis).

b. Signs and symptoms

—include muscle weakness, paresthesias, paralytic ileus, and arrhythmias (e.g., ventricular fibrillation).

c. Characteristic electrocardiogram (ECG) changes

—include T wave flattening, U waves, ST depression, and PR and QT widening.

d. Treatment involves

Table 7-5. Disorders of Potassium Balance

Disorder	Causes	Characteristics	ECG Findings	Management
Hypokalemia (< 3 mEq/L)	Diuretics, GI losses (e.g., diarrhea, NG tube, fistulae), severe metabolic alkalosis, hypomag-nesemia, hyperal-dosteronemia	Muscle weakness, ileus, arrhythmias (e.g., ventricular fibrillation), hypotension, digitalis toxicity	Flat T waves, U waves, ST depression, PR and QT widening	IV or oral replacement with K^+ solutions (e.g., KCl, KPO_4)
Hyperkalemia (> 6 mEq/L)	Renal failure, excess administra-tion, cell death and intracellular release of K^+ (e.g., crush injuries, reperfusion of ischemic tissue)	Paresthesias, severe muscle weakness, cardiac irritability and arrhythmias	Peaked T waves, flat P waves, QRS prolongation, deep S waves, sine wave appearance of QRS complex	**Mild:** saline, kayexalate glucose, insulin, HCO_3^- **Severe (ectopy):** emergent IV Ca^{2+}, hemodialysis, in addition to treatment measures for mild hyperkalemia

ECG = electrocardiogram; GI = gastrointestinal; IV = intravenous; NG = nasogastric.

—oral or IV replacement with **K^+ salts** (e.g., KCl).

2. **Hyperkalemia** is generally defined as a serum $K^+ > 6$ mEq/L.
   a. **Potential causes** include
      —**renal failure.**
      —**unchecked K^+** administration.
      —**drugs** (e.g., K^+ penicillin, digitalis, succinylcholine).
      —**tissue necrosis** with cellular release (e.g., **crush injuries,** compartment syndrome, major burns, rewarming after hypothermia).
      —**adrenal insufficiency** (e.g., low aldosterone state).
      —**inappropriately obtained blood sample** (e.g., hemolysis of sample).
   b. **Signs and symptoms**
      —include paresthesias, severe muscle weakness, and arrhythmias, including ventricular fibrillation.
   c. **ECG changes**
      —include peaked T waves, flattened P waves, prolonged QRS complex, and disappearance of the QRS complex into a sine wave.
   d. **Treatment**
      (1) **Hemodialysis** is the most effective treatment of hyperkalemia.
      (2) **Sodium polystyrene sulfonate (Kayexalate)** given orally or rectally prevents resorption of K^+ in the stool.
      (3) **Insulin (+ glucose) and HCO_3^-** cause an intracellular shift of K^+.
      (4) **IV calcium gluconate or $CaCl_2$** should be given in cases of **severe** hyperkalemia (i.e., marked ECG changes, arrhythmias, $K^+ > 7.5$ mEq/L).
         —Without lowering K^+, **Ca^+** protects against hyperkalemia by **decreasing the excitability** of the myocardium.
      (5) With **severe hyperkalemia,** all of these therapies should be initiated [see III B 2 d (1)–(4)].

C. **Disorders of Ca^{2+} balance**

1. **Hypocalcemia** (Table 7-6) is defined as a serum $Ca^{2+} < 8$ mg/dL or an ionized $Ca^{2+} < 2.5$ mEq/L.
   a. **Serum Ca^{2+} values are falsely elevated** in hypoalbuminemic states.
      —True calcium = observed calcium − (3.5 − serum albumin) × 0.8.
   b. Significant **risk factors** for hypocalcemia include
      —**elective parathyroidectomy.**
      —inadvertent parathyroidectomy during thyroid surgery.
   c. **Signs and symptoms**
      —include muscle cramps, perioral tingling, spasm, seizures, and laryngeal stridor.
   d. **ECG changes**
      —include prolonged PR interval.
   e. **Treatment** involves

Table 7-6. Characteristics of Hypocalcemia

Causes	Characteristics	Treatment
Vitamin D deficiency Chronic renal failure Inadequate intake Postparathyroidectomy Excessive administration of Ca^{2+} (poor fluids) Massive transfusion (i.e., citrate binding of Ca^{2+})	Muscle cramps Perioral tingling Paresthesias Hyperactive deep tendon reflexes Laryngeal stridor Seizures Carpopedal spasm (Trousseau's sign) Facial twitching with palpation (Chvostek's sign)	**Mild to moderate:** Vitamin D and oral Ca^{2+} replacement **Severe: IV** replacement with calcium gluconate

IV = intravenous.

—oral or IV Ca^{2+} replacement.

—vitamin D replacement.

—IV calcium gluconate for severe hypocalcemia.

2. **Hypercalcemia** is defined as a serum $Ca^{2+} > 10.5$ mg/dL or an ionized $Ca^{2+} > 4.5$ mEq/L.

   a. **Most frequent causes in surgery**

   —include **hyperparathyroidism** and malignant metastases to bone.

   b. **Signs and symptoms**

   —include weakness, nausea, vomiting, abdominal and musculoskeletal pain, nephrolithiasis, and neuropsychiatric symptoms.

   c. **ECG changes**

   —include short QT interval and prolonged PR interval.

   d. **Initial treatment** involves

   —**restriction of Ca^{2+} intake.**

   —**rehydration** with crystalloid.

   e. **Other therapies** include

   —**furosemide,** which may also be used to promote urinary Ca^{2+} excretion.

   —steroids.

   —phosphate.

   —biphosphonates (e.g., etidronate).

   —calcitonin.

   —mithramycin.

   —**surgical resection of the parathyroids** (see Chapter 19).

D. Disorders of Mg^{2+} balance (Table 7-7)

1. **Hypomagnesemia** is defined as $Mg^{2+} < 1.5$ mEq/L

Table 7-7. Characteristics of Magnesium Disorders

Disorders	Causes	Characteristics	Treatment
Hypomagnesemia	Inadequate intake, malabsorption, medications (cyclosporine, tacrolimus, amphotericin)	Anorexia, nausea, vomiting, weakness, increased deep tendon reflexes, asterixis/ tremor, hypokalemia, ECG changes (torsades de pointes)	Oral salts or IV replacement with magnesium solutions ($MgSo_4$), potassium replacement
Hypermagnesemia	Excessive administration (i.e., to treat eclampsia), renal failure, adrenal insufficiency	Sedation/obtundation, decreased deep tendon reflexes, weakness, bradycardia/hypotension, respiratory paralysis	IV calcium salts

ECG = electrocardiogram; IV = intravenous.

and is common in surgical patients secondary to inadequate provision of Mg^{2+} postoperatively.

a. **Presentation** is similar to that of hypocalcemia.
   —Severe refractory arrhythmias (e.g., **torsade de pointes**) may occur.

b. **Treatment** involves
   —oral or IV replacement with Mg^{2+} salts.

2. **Hypermagnesemia** is defined as $Mg^{2+} > 4$ mEq/L and is frequently caused by renal failure.

   a. **Symptoms of hypermagnesemia**
      —rarely occur with $Mg^{2+} < 8$ mEq/L.
      —may include weakness, fatigue, somnolence, bradycardia, hypotension, and respiratory paralysis.

   b. **Treatment** involves
      —**hydration.**
      —administration of **Ca^{2+} salts.**
      —hemodialysis to remove Mg^{2+} from the serum (rare).

IV. Acid–Base Disorders

A. Primary and compensatory mechanisms of acid–base disorders (Table 7-8)

B. Acidosis

1. **Respiratory acidosis**
   —is caused by alveolar hypoventilation.
   —is compensated by retention of HCO_3^- in the proximal tubules of the kidneys.

   a. **Criteria for diagnosis**
      —is **hypercarbia** in the setting of acidosis.

Table 7-8. Primary and Compensatory Mechanisms of Acid–Base Disorders

Abnormality	Primary Change	Compensatory Change
Metabolic acidosis	↓[HCO_3^-]	↓$PaCO_2$: 1.2 mm Hg ↓ in $PaCO_2$ for every 1 mEq/L ↓ in [HCO_3^-]
Metabolic alkalosis	↑[HCO_3^-]	↑$PaCO_2$: 0.7 mm Hg ↑ in $PaCO_2$ for every 1 mEq/L ↑ in [HCO_3^-↑]
Respiratory acidosis	↑$PaCO_2$	↑HCO_3^- Acute: 1 mEq/L ↑ in [HCO_3^-] for every 10 mm Hg ↑ in $PaCO_2$ Chronic: 3.5 mEq/L ↑ in [HCO_3^-] for every 10 mm Hg ↑ in $PaCO_2$
Respiratory alkalosis	↓$PaCO_2$	↓HCO_3^- Acute: 2 mEq/L ↓ in [HCO_3^-] for every 10 mm Hg ↓ in $PaCO_2$ Chronic: 4 mEq/L ↓ in [HCO_3^-] for every 10 mm Hg ↓ in $PaCO_2$.

b. **Acute respiratory acidosis is often caused by** suppression of respiratory drive either by drugs or injuries to the central nervous system or chest.

c. **Treatment of acute respiratory acidosis** includes

—correcting the underlying disorder.

—**increasing ventilation.**

(1) Ventilated patients unable to compensate by increasing their ventilation may benefit from increases in the ventilatory rate or tidal volume.

(2) For acute rises in $PaCO_2$ of 10 mm Hg, there is a decrease in pH of 0.08.

d. **Chronic respiratory acidosis**

—is often found in patients with chronic obstructive pulmonary disease (COPD), pneumonia, and pulmonary defects such as shunting.

(1) **These patients**

—frequently have a high baseline PCO_2.

—may decompensate rapidly under stress (e.g., infection, surgery).

(2) **Management** involves

—treating the underlying disorder.

—appropriate ventilatory support if acute decompensation occurs.

2. **Metabolic acidosis**

a. **Causes of metabolic acidosis** (Table 7-9)

—are differentiated based on the presence or absence of an **anion gap.**

(1) Anion gap = $Na^+ - (Cl^- + HCO_3^-)$; normal range = 5–12.

(2) An **elevated** anion gap indicates

—the loss of HCO_3^-.

—replacement with an unmeasured base (e.g., lactate, α-ketoglutarate).

—In surgery patients, the most common cause of metabolic acidosis is poor tissue perfusion from **hypovolemia or inadequate cardiac output.**

b. Treatment (see Table 7-9)

c. Hyperventilation with subsequent respiratory alkalosis is a **compensatory mechanism** for metabolic acidosis.

C. Alkalosis

1. Respiratory alkalosis results from elevated alveolar minute ventilation (hyperventilation).

a. Causes may include

—anxiety-pain or apprehension associated with a procedure.

—fever.

—iatrogenic-tidal volume or respiratory rate set too high on the ventilator.

(1) Hypoxia-hyperventilation may be an early sign of pulmonary embolus.

(2) Liver failure-high ammonia levels can stimulate ventilation.

b. Respiratory alkalosis can cause

—hypokalemia, hypocalcemia, hypomagnesemia, decreased O_2 release from Hgb, and cerebral hypoperfusion secondary to vasoconstriction.

c. Treatment

—focuses on identification and treatment of the underlying cause.

Table 7-9. Treatment of Common Causes of Metabolic Acidosis

Classification	Causes	Treatment
High anion gap (>12)	Lactic acidosis (e.g., shock)	Volume resuscitation, optimize cardiac output
	Diabetic ketoacidosis	Hydration, insulin, electrolyte replacement
	Uremia (renal failure)	Hemodialysis, $NaHCO_3$, electrolyte replacement
	Ingestions:	
	Alcohol	Glucose administration (starvation-like state)
	Methanol	Ethanol, hemodialysis, IV folate
	Ethylene glycol	Ethanol, hemodialysis
	Salicylates	Hemodialysis, alkalinize urine
	Paraformaldehyde	Water, milk, ammonium salts, $NaHCO_3$, dialysis
Normal anion gap (hyperchloremic) (5–12)	GI losses (e.g., diarrhea, fistulae)	Appropriate volume and electrolyte replacement
	Renal tubular acidosis	
	Carbonic anhydrase inhibitors (e.g., acetazolamide)	Discontinue medication
	Excessive Cl^- administration (i.e., TPN solutions)	Adjustment of fluid electrolyte concentrations

GI = gastrointestinal; IV = intravenous; TPN = total parenteral nutrition.

2. **Metabolic alkalosis** is generally caused by depletion of acids associated with fluid losses.

—Excessive administration of citrate found in transfused blood may be converted to HCO_3^-, which causes metabolic alkalosis, although this occurs infrequently.

a. **Causes**

—include gastrointestinal losses (e.g., **prolonged NG suctioning**), diuretic therapy, hyperaldosteronism, and corticosteroid excess (e.g., iatrogenic, Cushing's syndrome).

b. **Treatment** involves

—replacement of fluid losses.

—correction of the underlying cause.

V. Principles of Critical Care

A. **The initial assessment of critically ill patients** focuses on their pulmonary, cardiovascular, and neurologic condition.

—Airway, breathing, and circulation (ABCs) are the primary focus of the initial assessment.

1. **Pulmonary assessment evaluates**

—the ***A*irway,** or work of breathing.

—the adequacy of oxygenation and ventilation (***B*reathing**).

a. **The initial pulmonary assessment includes**

—evaluation of the patient's general appearance.

—auscultatory examination.

—chest radiograph.

—arterial blood gases.

b. General indications for **intubation** include

—**impending respiratory failure.**

—**inability to protect the airway** (i.e., risk of aspiration in obtunded patient).

—**hypoventilation (PCO_2 > 70 mm Hg).**

—**hypoxemia (PO_2 < 50 mm Hg).**

—extreme respiratory fatigue.

c. Potential **causes** of **respiratory failure**

—include pneumonia, acute respiratory distress syndrome, sepsis, congestive heart failure, aspiration, lung and chest trauma (e.g., contusion, multiple rib fractures), pulmonary embolus, and neurologic injury (e.g., trauma, pharmacologic).

d. **Acute respiratory distress syndrome**

—is a syndrome of diffuse respiratory failure seen frequently in critically ill patients.

—may be associated with sepsis, severe infection, shock, severe trauma or burn injury, aspiration, inhalation injury, and pancreatitis.

—Treatment involves mechanical ventilation when necessary and treatment of the underlying illness.

e. **Summary of common ventilator settings** (Table 7-10)

2. **Cardiovascular assessment (Circulation)**

—evaluates volume status, vascular tone, and myocardial function.

a. **Useful initial tests**

—include evaluation of vital signs, heart rhythm, chest radiograph, weight, and urine output.

b. **Hemodynamically unstable patients** (e.g., patients with hypotension)

—may benefit from invasive monitoring when the cause is unclear (i.e., hypovolemia versus heart failure).

(1) **A pulmonary artery catheter (Swan-Ganz)**

—allows for indirect measurement of **cardiac output and SVR.**

(2) **The pulmonary arterial wedge pressure (PAWP)**

Table 7-10. Common Ventilator Settings

Ventilator Mode	Mechanism	Clinical Utility
SIMV	Provides a minimum number of breaths/min at a set tidal volume. Synchronized with patient breaths, if present. Work of spontaneous breaths done by patient.	Useful in most settings, especially ventilator weaning.
ACMV	Provides a minimum number of breaths/min. Allows for complete mechanical control of the pressure and/or volume of each breath delivered.	Frequently used in patients with altered lung compliance.
Pressure control	Type of ACMV. Delivers variable tidal volume with each breath at a preset pressure to protect the lungs from barotrauma (pneumothorax).	Used in the setting of decreased lung compliance (i.e., large ↑ in pressure resulting from small ↑ in volume).
PS	Provides positive pressure during voluntary inspiration to improve tidal volume with each breath the patient takes.	Especially useful for patients weaning from the ventilator.
CPAP	Supplies a continuous airway pressure that traps gas in the lungs and increases expiratory reserve volume and functional residual capacity.	Often used during ventilator weaning.
PEEP	Provides positive pressure during expiration to prevent airway collapse. "Physiologic PEEP" normally caused by partially closed glottis with expiration about 5 cm H_2O.	Can be used with most ventilator settings. ↑ PEEP may improve oxygenation.

ACMV = assist controlled mechanical ventilation; CPAP = continuous positive airway pressure; PEEP = positive end-expiratory pressure; PS = pressure support; SIMV = synchronized intermittent mandatory ventilation.

—is an indirect measure of left ventricular end-diastolic pressure.

—is useful for optimizing preload and cardiac function.

(3) Complications of pulmonary artery catheters

—may include infection, arrhythmia, pneumothorax, and pulmonary artery or cardiac rupture.

c. **Hypovolemia** is a frequent cause of cardiovascular instability.

—Treatment involves adequate **volume resuscitation.**

d. **Pharmacologic agents**

—may be used to optimize cardiac output, SVR, and ultimately **tissue perfusion** (BP = CO × SVR).

(1) Inotropic drugs

—include dopamine, dobutamine, and epinephrine.

(2) Vasoconstrictors

—include norepinephrine and phenylephrine.

(3) Vasodilators

—include hydralazine, nitrates, nitric oxide, and angiotensin-converting enzyme (ACE) inhibitors.

3. **Neurologic assessment**

—is an essential part of the initial evaluation of the critically ill patient.

a. **The Glasgow Coma Scale (GCS)**

—helps to standardize the patient's response in three basic neurologic categories:

(1) Verbalization

(2) Motor response

(3) Eye opening

b. **Standard tests**

—are also useful for evaluating mentation, strength, and sensory function.

c. **Useful tests for patients with known or suspected brain injury**

—include computed tomography (CT) scans, electroencephalogram (EEG), and intracranial pressure monitoring (see *BRS Surgical Specialties,* Chapter 7).

4. **Further assessment**

—should include evaluation for potential infection and abnormalities of other organ systems (e.g., renal, hepatic, gastrointestinal, skin).

5. **The patient's immune reaction to stresses** (i.e. trauma, surgery, infection)

—may also cause physiologic abnormalities.

a. **The systemic inflammatory response syndrome (SIRS) is characterized by**

—temperature > 38°C or < 36°C.

—heart rate > 90 beats/minute.

—respiratory rate > 20 breaths/minute or $PaCO_2 < 32$ mm Hg.

—white blood cell count > 12,000 or < 4000 cells/mm^3.

b. **Sepsis** may be used to describe **SIRS as a result of infection.**

c. **Septic shock** is refractory hypotension resulting from sepsis.

d. **Multiple system organ failure**

—is a late manifestation of SIRS associated with a very **high mortality.**

(1) **Severe failure**

—of the respiratory, cardiovascular, renal, and hepatic systems may be present.

(2) **Causes**

—may include infection, severe trauma, and massive burn injuries.

Review Test

Directions: Each of the numbered items or incomplete statements in this section is followed by answers or by completions of the statement. Select the ONE lettered answer or completion that is BEST in each case.

1. A 5-year-old, 25-kg boy is now postoperative day 1 from an open appendectomy for nonperforated appendicitis. He is still experiencing some nausea and has minimal bowel sounds upon physical examination. The patient is afebrile and is otherwise healthy. Which of the following electrolyte solutions and rate of administration would be most appropriate for providing maintenance postoperative hydration in this patient?

(A) 5% dextrose in $\frac{3}{4}$ normal saline at 65 mL/hr
(B) 5% dextrose in normal saline at 85 mL/hr
(C) Normal saline (0.9%) at 65 mL/hr
(D) 5% dextrose in $\frac{1}{4}$ normal saline at 85 mL/hr
(E) 5% dextrose in $\frac{1}{4}$ normal saline at 65 mL/hr

2. A 64-year-old man undergoes upper endoscopy for chronic gastrointestinal bleeding that reveals mild gastritis but no evidence of ulceration or active bleeding. Rectal examination is heme-positive but without gross blood. Immediately after starting a blood transfusion for symptomatic anemia, the patient becomes confused. His blood pressure is 70/30 mm Hg, his heart rate is 145 beats/min, and his temperature is 39°C (102.2°F). Which of the following is the most appropriate next step in the management of this patient?

(A) Slow the rate of infusion of blood and give diphenhydramine
(B) Discontinue blood transfusion and give intravenous (IV) antibiotics
(C) Increase rate of infusion of blood and perform immediate upper endoscopy
(D) Discontinue blood transfusion and administer a bolus of crystalloid solution
(E) Discontinue blood transfusion and administer calcium gluconate intravenously

3. A 53-year-old woman is undergoing an elective sigmoid resection for recurrent diverticulitis. Intraoperatively, the patient requires transfusion of 2 units of packed red blood cells (PRBCs) for significant blood loss early in the case. After starting the transfusion, the anesthesiologist notes that the patient's blood pressure is now 70/40 mm Hg, having dropped from 120/80 mm Hg. There is no intra-abdominal bleeding noted, however her urine has suddenly become very dark. Electrocardiogram (ECG) reveals sinus tachycardia without evidence of myocardial ischemia. Which of the following is the most frequent cause of this patient's current condition?

(A) Primary bacterial contamination of donor blood
(B) Clerical errors in matching donor blood to recipient
(C) Inadequate screening of donor blood for leukocytes
(D) Recipient antibody formation to minor antigens on donor blood cells
(E) Binding of serum calcium by citrate present in donor blood

4. A 19-year-old man sustains orthopedic injuries after a motor vehicle accident. During evaluation and treatment, he receives 4 units of packed red blood cells (PRBCs) for significant blood loss. His family asks about the risk of his contracting human immunodeficiency virus (HIV) from blood transfusion. Which of the following is the approximate risk of transmission of HIV from each unit of PRBCs?

(A) 1/300
(B) 1/3000
(C) 1/50,000
(D) 1/300,000
(E) 1/1,000,000

5. A 62-year-old, 90-kg woman undergoes exploratory laparotomy and resection of an obstructing sigmoid colon cancer. Postoperatively, the patient is transferred to the surgical floor where she receives normal saline at 100 mL/hr. The next morning she is tachycardic with a heart rate of 120 beats/min and a blood pressure of 95/60 mm Hg. Her urine output is diminished to 20 mL/hr. Her physical examination is remarkable for a distended abdomen without bowel sounds and with mild tenderness. Her hematocrit is now 36% (it was 33% the night before). Abdominal radiograph shows a gasless abdomen, and a chest radiograph is read as "normal." Which of the following is the most likely source for her hypotension in the intensive care unit the day after surgery?

(A) Renewed bleeding within the abdominal cavity
(B) Gastrointestinal bleeding from stress ulceration
(C) Acute gastric dilation with a vasovagal response
(D) Third space losses within the peritoneum
(E) Septic shock from gram-negative organisms

6. A 26-year-old man sustains multiple injuries in a motor vehicle accident, including multiple rib fractures, a pulmonary contusion, pelvic fracture, and a left femur fracture. On hospital day 2 the patient is on the ventilator in synchronized intermittent mandatory ventilation (SIMV) mode set at a rate of 14. FIO_2 is 50%, tidal volume is set at 800 ml, and positive end-expiratory pressure (PEEP) is 2 cm H_2O. An arterial blood gas reveals a pH of 7.38, $PaCO_2$ of 38 mm Hg, PaO_2 of 60 mm Hg, and a HCO_3^- of 22 mEq/L. Which of the following ventilatory changes would be most appropriate for improving this patient's oxygenation?

(A) Increase the PEEP from 2 to 8 cm H_20
(B) Increase the respiratory rate from 14/min to 18/min
(C) Increase the tidal volume from 800 ml to 1000 ml
(D) Increase the FIO_2 to 75%
(E) Change from SIMV mode to pressure-control mode

7. A 32-year-old man sustained a left femur fracture after a steel beam fell on his legs and trapped him underneath. It was approximately 2 hours before coworkers were able to locate him and remove the beam. On admission, the patient received 2 units of packed red blood cells (PRBCs) for hypotension and had significant blood loss from the femur fracture. On hospital day 2, the patient is noted to have frequent runs of ectopy on the electrocardiogram (ECG) monitor. Widened QRS complexes are also noted. His urine is dark red, but microscopic examination of the urine reveals no red blood cells (RBCs). Which of the following events is most likely responsible for this patient's current findings?

(A) Hemolysis secondary to the blood transfusion
(B) Acute tubular necrosis secondary to hypovolemia
(C) An unrecognized kidney laceration
(D) Fat embolus syndrome
(E) Rhabdomyolysis

8. A 65-year-old man with non–insulin-dependent diabetes mellitus (NIDDM) is postoperative day 2 after undergoing an elective colon resection for adenocarcinoma. The patient is poorly responsive. On examination, the patient is obtunded, his pupils are pinpoint, his heart rate is 130 beats/min, and his blood pressure is 70/50 mm Hg. A patient care assistant states that the patient was awake 1 hour before, but somewhat confused. Arterial blood gas reveals a pH of 7.29, $PaCO_2$ of 75 mm Hg, PaO_2 of 70 mm Hg, and a HCO_3^+ of 23 mEq/L. Which of the following is the most appropriate initial step in the management of this patient?

(A) Administer an insulin bolus immediately
(B) Obtain a chest radiograph immediately
(C) Administer naloxone and control the airway
(D) Administer sodium bicarbonate
(E) Obtain a ventilation-perfusion (V/Q) scan to rule out pulmonary embolus

9. A 55-year-old woman underwent a Whipple procedure for pancreatic adenocarcinoma. Postoperatively, she develops a pancreaticocutaneous fistula, which drains approximately 400 mL/day. On evaluation, the patient is noted to be tachycardic with a heart rate of 115 beats/min and a blood pressure of 100/80 mm Hg. Her skin is noted to be dry, and her urine output has decreased significantly over the past 2–3 days. Labs reveal a Na^+ of 140 mEq/L, Cl^- of 120 mEq/L, and HCO_3^- of 15 mEq/L. To resuscitate this patient, which of the following is the most appropriate fluid?

(A) 5% dextrose in normal saline (0.9%)
(B) 5% dextrose in ½ normal saline (0.45%)
(C) 5% albumin solution
(D) Lactated Ringer's solution
(E) 5% dextrose in water + insulin bolus

Directions: Each set of matching questions in this section consists of a list of four to twenty-six lettered options followed by several numbered items. For each numbered item, select the appropriate lettered option(s). Each lettered option may be selected once, more than once, or not at all.

Questions 10–16

(A) Cardiogenic shock due to extrinsic causes
(B) Cardiogenic shock due to intrinsic causes
(C) Hypovolemic shock secondary to blood loss
(D) Hypovolemic shock secondary to third space losses
(E) Hypovolemic shock secondary to insensible losses
(F) Septic shock
(G) Neurogenic shock

For each patient description, select the associated type(s) of shock.

10. A 65-year-old, otherwise healthy man underwent laparoscopic cholecystectomy 3 weeks ago for acute cholecystitis and cholelithiasis. Now he presents with fever, chills, and right upper quadrant (RUQ) pain, and a new onset of confusion, according to his wife. He is tachycardic (130 beats/min), he appears flushed, and his skin is warm. (SELECT 1 TYPE OF SHOCK)

11. A 19-year-old man presents to the emergency department by ambulance with a stab wound adjacent to the left nipple region. His blood pressure is 50/30 mm Hg and he is unresponsive. (SELECT 2 TYPES OF SHOCK)

12. A 23-year-old medical student suddenly becomes faint and dizzy while observing a right inguinal hernia repair in the operating room. The student collapses and during evaluation is noted to have a blood pressure of 85/50 mm Hg. (SELECT 1 TYPE OF SHOCK)

13. A 42-year-old, obese woman presents with a 2–3 day history of persistent nausea and vomiting. Her blood pressure is 80/50 mm Hg with a heart rate of 140 beats/min. She is noted to have an unreducible umbilical hernia on examination. Abdominal radiograph reveals a high-grade small bowel obstruction. During operative repair of the incarcerated hernia, there is no evidence of strangulation. (SELECT 1 TYPE OF SHOCK)

14. A 25-year-old man is admitted to the neurosurgery intensive care unit after a motor vehicle accident. On admission the patient is noted to have a blood pressure of 120/80 mm Hg with a heart rate of 105 beats/min. Upon evaluation he is found to have a complete spinal cord injury at the sixth cervical vertebrae, as well as a bruise on his abdomen in the distribution of his seatbelt and a bruise on his chest from hitting the steering wheel. Six hours after admission the patient's blood pressure gradually falls to 60/40 mm Hg and the patient becomes unresponsive. (SELECT 4 TYPES OF SHOCK)

15. A 35-year-old man sustains a 50% full-thickness burn injury to his torso and lower extremities during a house fire. Over the next 2 days, the patient develops a worsening paralytic ileus and a gradual decrease in his blood pressure to 80/60 mm Hg despite following the Parkland formula for determining the amount of fluid to give after a burn injury. (SELECT 2 TYPES OF SHOCK)

16. During placement of a triple lumen catheter in a 72-year-old woman, the patient suddenly becomes hypotensive with a blood pressure of 60/30 mm Hg during advancement of the guidewire. (SELECT 3 TYPES OF SHOCK)

Answers and Explanations

1–E. The standard formulas for determining the rate of administration of maintenance fluids are as follows:

$$[(100 \text{ mL/kg} \times 10 \text{ kg}) + (50 \text{ mL/kg} \times 10 \text{ kg}) + (20 \text{ mL/kg} \times 5 \text{ kg})]/24 \text{ hr}$$

or

$$(4 \text{ mL/kg/hr} \times 10 \text{ kg}) + (2 \text{ mL/kg/hr} \times 10 \text{ kg}) + (1 \text{ mL/kg/hr} \times 5 \text{ kg})$$

Using these formulas, a 25-kg patient would require a rate of approximately 65 mL/hr over 24 hours. In addition, ¼ normal saline (38.5 mEq/L of Na^+) would most appropriately provide the daily maintenance sodium requirements of 1–2 mEq/kg/day (25–50 mEq/day) in this patient, whereas administration of normal saline (145 mEq/L Na^+) would give well in excess of normal daily maintenance requirements. It is important to remember, however, that these formulas serve only as guidelines. Clinical assessment of the patient's condition and fluid status are the most important components of determining the rate and type of fluid administered.

2–D. This patient is showing signs of rapid clinical deterioration secondary to ABO incompatibility. In this setting, immediate steps include discontinuing the transfusion and administering crystalloid solution. These steps, in association with appropriate management of the respiratory system [airway, breathing, and circulation (ABCs)], are crucial in the treatment of these patients. Administration of antibiotics or calcium gluconate would not treat the primary origin of the problem, nor would they provide significant benefit in the volume resuscitation of a hemodynamically unstable patient in this situation. Although one should always be concerned about acute massive gastrointestinal bleeding in patients that deteriorate so rapidly, the absence of significant pathology on recent endoscopy and the temporal relationship to the blood transfusion make a transfusion reaction more likely, thus negating the need for immediate upper endoscopy at this point in the evaluation.

3–B. This patient is having a severe transfusion reaction secondary to ABO incompatibility. The cardiovascular instability and hemoglobinuria are temporally related to transfusion without other obvious causes for the clinical scenario. The most common cause of a transfusion reaction occurring secondary to ABO incompatibility is a clerical error in matching the appropriate donor blood to the recipient. Although this occurs rarely, it can result from errors in the blood bank or with the medical personnel administering the blood. Thus, great care should be taken to assure appropriate matching occurs at all levels. Recipient antibody formation to antigens other than ABO system may rarely cause mild immune reactions, although this occurs infrequently. Binding of serum calcium and primary bacterial contamination of donor blood is rare. Screening of donor blood for leukocytes is not routinely performed or required.

4–D. Although viral transmission with blood transfusion is rare, it can still occur and must be considered when transfusions are performed. The reported risk of transmission of human immunodeficiency virus (HIV) per unit of blood transfused is estimated to be approximately 1/300,000. Donated blood is routinely screened for HIV contamination; however, despite an excellent sensitivity of these tests, they do not identify absolutely all HIV-contaminated blood samples.

5–D. The most likely cause of volume loss and hypotension in this patient is inadequate provision of fluid in the setting of significant third space losses after major intra-abdominal surgery. The peritoneum and the intestinal lumen can accommodate a large amount (approximately 18 L) of third space fluid, which can occur in the setting of intra-abdominal infections, intestinal obstruction, and even postoperatively. The increase in the hematocrit may be secondary to volume loss (i.e., plasma loss) with hemoconcentration of the red blood cells (RBCs). This also makes massive bleeding unlikely in this setting. Acute gastric dilation can result in hypotension, although this would have been noted on the abdominal radiograph. Septic shock occurring this early in the postoperative course for elective surgery is unlikely unless perforation has occurred. However, perforation is frequently associated with other signs and symptoms, such as peritoneal signs (e.g., guarding, rebound pain) and identification of free peritoneal air on radiograph evaluation.

6–A. The most appropriate measure to manage this patient's hypoxia is to increase the positive end-expiratory pressure (PEEP) from 2 cm H_2O to 8 cm H_2O. This helps to improve ventilation of collapsed alveoli and the ventilation/perfusion mismatch resulting from this collapse. Increasing the FIO_2 would also help to improve oxygenation but is also associated with other complications if used chronically (e.g., direct pulmonary toxicity). Excessive PEEP may also be associated with complications such as pneumothorax, although this rarely occurs with low levels of PEEP (i.e., 2 cm H_2O to 8 cm H_2O). Increasing the respiratory rate and increasing the tidal volume would improve ventilation (i.e., $PaCO_2$) but would not specifically address the issue of oxygenation. Altering the mode of ventilation is not necessary in this situation because simpler measures are available to address the hypoxia.

7–E. The most likely cause of the findings in this patient is hyperkalemia associated with rhabdomyolysis. Extensive necrosis of muscle tissue can occur after crush injuries without visible signs of necrosis noted at the level of the skin. Necrosis of muscle cells with subsequent lysis can lead to release of large amounts of K^+ from the cytoplasm of these cells, resulting in the widened QRS complex and ectopy seen on the ECG. Hemolysis related to blood transfusion would generally not result in severe hyperkalemia unless it was associated with ABO incompatibility, which occurs within minutes to hours of transfusion. Acute tubular necrosis may occur after periods of hypovolemia and may lead to renal failure and hyperkalemia; however, this generally does not present acutely, as in this patient. Unilateral kidney injuries can occur in the absence of hematuria, although in an otherwise healthy individual this would not affect renal function. Hyperkalemia is not a typical characteristic of fat embolus syndrome.

8–C. This patient has a severe acute respiratory acidosis with a pH of 7.29 and a $PaCO_2$ of 75 mm Hg with minimal compensatory changes in HCO_3^- levels. In a postoperative patient with acute respiratory acidosis and pinpoint pupils, one should be concerned about overdose with narcotic analgesics. Initial treatment of this patient should involve appropriate management of the airway, with intubation if necessary, and administration of naloxone, an antagonist to narcotic analgesics. Hyperglycemia in a patient with non-insulin-dependent diabetes mellitus (NIDDM) is unlikely to present with a severe respiratory acidosis, as opposed to metabolic acidosis and so the insulin bolus is not useful. $NaHCO_3$ does not treat the primary cause of acidosis in this situation and would not be indicated. A chest radiograph may play a role in the evaluation of this patient, but not in the immediate management of acute severe respiratory acidosis. Acute pulmonary embolus is unlikely to be associated with an isolated respiratory acidosis; however, if it is suspected, appropriate diagnostic evaluation and treatment should be initiated after initial resuscitative measures are taken.

9–D. Pancreatic fistulae are frequently associated with a significant loss of HCO_3^-, leading to a metabolic acidosis. This patient's low HCO_3^- level in the absence of a significant anion gap $\{Na^+ (140)–[Cl^- (120) + HCO_3^-(15)] = 5\}$ in the setting of a pancreatic fistula and dehydration suggests a significant loss of fluid and HCO_3^- from this source. Appropriate resuscitation with a crystalloid solution that resembles the fluid being lost is necessary. Lactated Ringer's solution contains 28 mEq/L of lactate, which is quickly metabolized to HCO_3^- by the liver. Other saline and albumin solutions do not contain HCO_3^- and, although they are appropriate solutions in most situations, would not be the best choice for this patient. Insulin should be given when one expects severe hyperglycemia as the primary problem, although the acidosis associated with severe hyperglycemia is generally associated with a large anion gap (> 12).

10–F. Septic shock is associated with severe peripheral vasodilation with increased cardiac output. This leads to flushing and warm skin to palpation, in contrast to hypovolemic shock, which results in peripheral vasoconstriction. Other signs and symptoms are related to the primary infection, such as fever, chills, and leukocytosis. This patient is experiencing symptoms suggestive of cholangitis or a peritoneal infection related to the recent surgery.

11–A, C. Hypovolemia secondary to blood loss is an obvious cause of shock after a stab wound to the chest either from injury to major blood vessels or direct injury to the heart. However, this injury can also result in cardiogenic shock due to extrinsic causes such as cardiac tamponade from injury to the pericardium and tension pneumothorax from lung injury. Theoretically, direct injury to a major coronary vessel can result in a myocardial infarction, even in a young patient. However, consideration of the previous potential causes of shock should be considered first and foremost.

12–G. This is a classic vasovagal response resulting in acute transient peripheral dilation with subsequent hypotension and syncope. This response is a form of neurogenic shock, although different from the typical description of patients with a spinal injury.

13–D. This patient's hypotension is secondary to hypovolemia from third space losses as well as dehydration from frank gastrointestinal losses associated with vomiting. Several liters of fluid can be sequestered ("third spaced") in the intestine when bowel obstruction occurs. If this fluid is not replaced or is combined with other losses from the gastrointestinal tract, it can result in hypotension and even hypovolemic shock.

14–A, B, C, G. Although the spinal injury can result in neurogenic shock in this patient, one must consider several causes of shock, particularly in a patient with traumatic injuries sustained from blunt trauma. The bruise on the abdomen can be a harbinger of intra-abdominal injuries (e.g., splenic or liver trauma), which can result in immediate or delayed hypovolemic shock secondary to blood loss. Blunt trauma to the chest can result in a myocardial contusion, which can infrequently result in impaired cardiac function and intrinsic cardiogenic shock. Blunt chest trauma can also result in a tension pneumothorax or cardiac tamponade (extrinsic cardiogenic shock) by various mechanisms.

15–D, E. Burn injuries can be associated with large amounts of insensible fluid losses from evaporation of fluid directly from the exposed wounds. These patients require large amounts of fluid for maintenance and resuscitation because of these losses. In addition, this patient's paralytic ileus can result in significant third spacing of fluid, also contributing to hypovolemia.

16–A, B, C. Placement of any central venous catheter can cause multiple injuries, resulting in hypotension and shock. Lung injury with tension pneumothorax can result from such placement. In addition, advancement of the guidewire or the catheter itself can perforate the major blood vessels involved and the myocardium, resulting in severe blood loss or cardiac tamponade (extrinsic cardiogenic shock). Advancement of catheters or guidewires through the heart can also incite various arrhythmias, resulting in cardiac failure and intrinsic cardiogenic shock.

II

General Surgery

8

Trauma and Burns

Jeffrey A. Claridge

I. Introduction

A. Trauma

—is a **leading cause of death** in the **first four decades** of life.

B. Head injury

—is the most common cause of immediate death in trauma.

C. Nearly 150,000 trauma deaths

—occur **annually** in the United States.

D. Primary survey and resuscitation of the trauma patient

1. There are **5 steps** of the primary survey (the ABC's)
   - —**A**irway.
   - —**B**reathing.
   - —**C**irculation.
   - —**D**isability.
   - —**E**xposure.
2. The **objectives of the primary survey** are
   - —to **identify immediately life-threatening conditions.**
   - —to initiate resuscitation.
3. **Life-threatening problems**
   - —discovered during the primary survey are treated before proceeding to each consecutive step.

E. Secondary survey (see IV)

F. Definitive care (see V)

II. The Primary Survey

A. Airway and cervical spine (C-spine) control

1. Assessing the airway

a. If the person can speak

—this is generally a sign that the airway is patent.

b. The **tongue**

—is the most common cause of **upper airway obstruction,** particularly in an unconscious patient.

c. If the airway is **not adequately open, immediate sequential steps** may include

—chin lift and/or the jaw thrust maneuver.

—placement of an oral or nasal airway.

—endotracheal intubation.

2. When endotracheal intubation cannot be performed (i.e., severe facial trauma) a **cricothyroidotomy** can be quickly done.

—An incision is made directly through the skin and cricothyroid membrane and a small tube placed through the incised membrane (**Figure 8-1**).

3. C-spine immobilization should be maintained at all times (e.g., neck collar).

—Complete evaluation of the cervical, thoracic, and lumbar spines after trauma is discussed in *BRS Surgical Specialties,* Chapter 7.

B. Breathing

1. Establishing airway patency

a. Once airway is open, the **next step is** to assess for **air movement.**

b. Clinical signs that should initially be evaluated include

—symmetric chest movement.

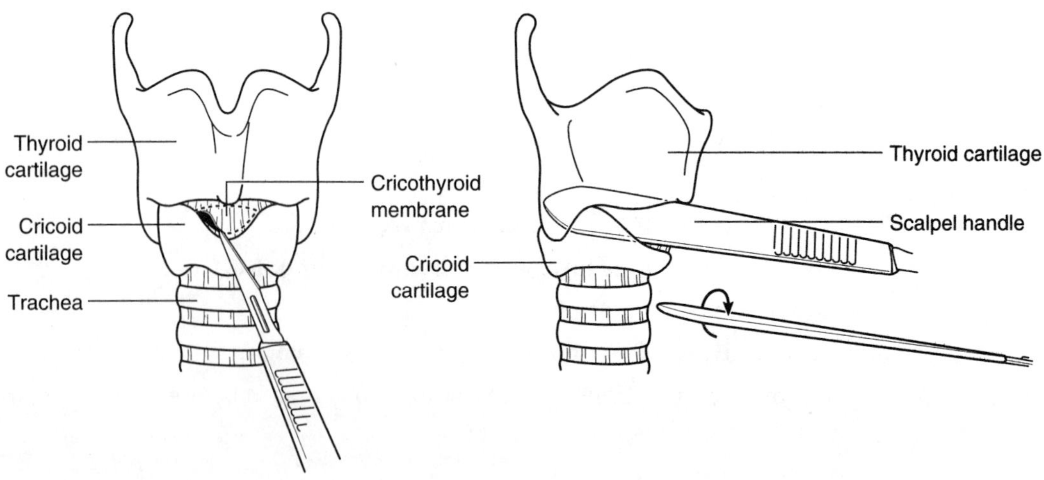

Figure 8-1. Cricothyroidotomy. (*A*) Front view. (*B*) Side view; scalpel is inserted and turned counterclockwise. (Adapted with permission from Lawrence PF: *Essentials of General Surgery,* 2nd ed. Baltimore, Williams & Wilkins, 1992, p 151.)

—cyanosis.

—open chest wounds.

—jugular venous distention (JVD).

—respiratory rate.

—use of accessory muscles of respiration (e.g., sternocleidomastoid).

2. During **auscultation** one should assess for

—bilateral breath sounds.

—wheezing.

—stridor.

3. **Palpation** should be performed to assess for

—tracheal position (a **deviated trachea may indicate a tension pneumothorax**).

—gross deformities.

—subcutaneous emphysema.

—flail segments.

C. Circulation

1. **Evaluate**

—peripheral pulses.

—heart rate.

—blood pressure.

—mental status.

—the appearance of the skin.

a. A **palpable radial pulse**

—suggests that the **systolic pressure ≥ 80 mm Hg.**

b. **Femoral and carotid plus**

—can be felt down to a systolic pressure of 60.

c. **Tachycardia**

—is generally the most sensitive indicator of hypovolemia.

d. A **fall in blood pressure**

—is a **late manifestation** of hypovolemia.

e. **Hypovolemia**

—can cause mental status changes varying from increased **agitation to unconsciousness.**

f. The **skin** in a patient with **hypovolemic shock**

—often feels cold and clammy with **slow capillary refill** (normal is less than 2 seconds).

2. **Aggressive fluid resuscitation**

—should be initiated at this time.

a. **In adults**

—an initial 2 L bolus of crystalloid (e.g., lactated Ringer's) should be given through two large-bore intravenous (IV) lines (i.e., 14–16 gauge).

b. **In children**

—an appropriate initial bolus is 20 mL/kg.

c. A **type and crossmatch**

—should be performed immediately, although Type O negative (O−; universal donor) blood should also be immediately available.

d. **Transfusion with packed red blood cells** is necessary in the case of obvious vigorous hemorrhage or in cases where hematocrit falls below 25 mg/dL with ongoing bleeding.

D. **Disability** (gross, rapid neurologic evaluation)

1. A **rapid assessment** should be performed of

—**mental status.**

—**gross motor function.**

—**gross sensory function.**

2. The **AVPU mnemonic**

—is a quick method to describe the patient's level of consciousness.

—**A** = <u>A</u>lert.

—**V** = responds to <u>V</u>ocal stimuli.

—**P** = responds to <u>P</u>ainful stimuli.

—**U** = <u>U</u>nresponsive.

3. **The Glasgow Coma scale (GCS)**

—is essential for quantitative assessment of the patient's neurologic status (see *BRS Surgical Specialties,* Chapter 7).

4. **Asymmetry in pupillary size and reactivity**

—suggests the presence of an intracranial injury.

5. The **main disabilities discovered** during this phase include

—head injury.

—altered level of consciousness secondary to ethanol or other drugs (diagnosis of exclusion).

E. **Exposure/environmental control**

1. **Remove the patient's clothes**

—to facilitate a thorough examination.

2. **Examine the entire body surface**

—including log-rolling the patient to view the back and buttocks for potential injuries.

3. **Maintain normothermia**

—with warm IV fluids, loose application of warm blankets, and a warm environment.

4. **Consider tetanus immunization**

—and **antibiotic administration,** if necessary.

5. **Perform initial chest and pelvic radiographs.**

III. Initial Management of Life-Threatening Conditions

A. Airway obstruction (see II A 1)

B. Pneumothorax

—is air in the pleural space, causing collapse of the lung, frequently caused by lung parenchymal injury secondary to fractured ribs.

1. A tension pneumothorax

—is air in the pleural space at higher than or equal to atmospheric pressure.

—causes compression of adjacent structures (e.g,. superior vena cava) (**Figure 8-2**).

a. The **diagnosis** should be based on a **combination of clinical findings** including

—dyspnea.

—**jugular venous distension (JVD).**

—tachypnea.

—anxiety.

—pleuritic chest pain.

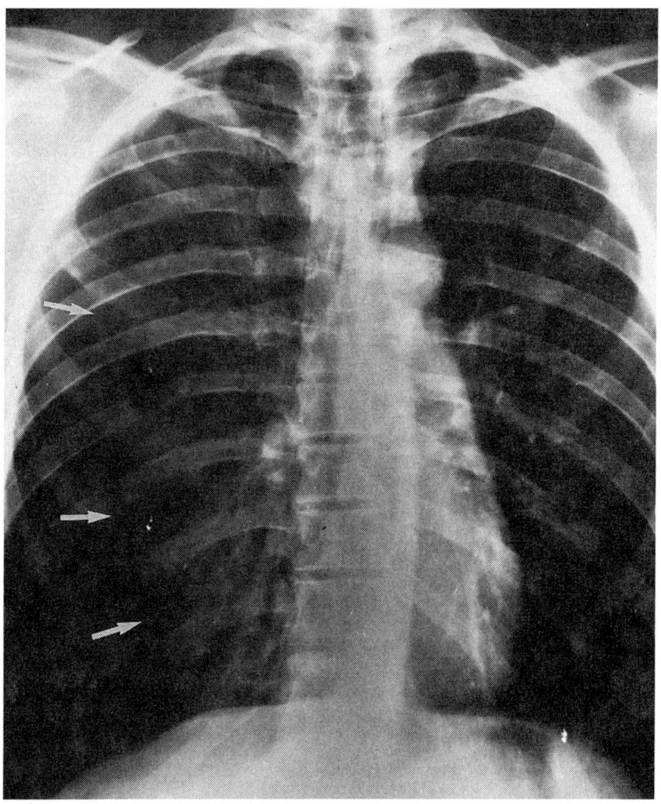

Figure 8-2. Tension pneumothorax. The arrows identify the edge of the collapsed lung and the displacement of the mediastinum toward the left. Note the slight shift of the trachea toward the left. (Reprinted with permission from Daffner RH: *Clinical Radiology: The Essentials,* 2nd ed. Baltimore, Williams & Wilkins, 1999, p 153.)

—**unilateral, decreased or absent breath sounds.**

—**tracheal shift** away from the affected side.

—hyperresonance on the affected side.

b. **Hypotension may result**

—secondary to decreased venous return to the heart.

c. **Treatment** involves

—immediate decompression by chest tube placement or by **needle thoracostomy** if no experienced personnel are present.

d. A **chest tube thoracostomy**

—should then be performed (**Figure 8-3**).

2. An **open pneumothorax**

—("sucking chest wound") is diagnosed by inspection.

a. **Air moves through the chest wall defect**

—during breathing, thereby inhibiting lung expansion and normal respiration.

b. **Treatment involves**

—**insertion of a chest tube.**

—**placement of an occlusive dressing** over the open wound.

—intubation with positive pressure ventilation, if needed.

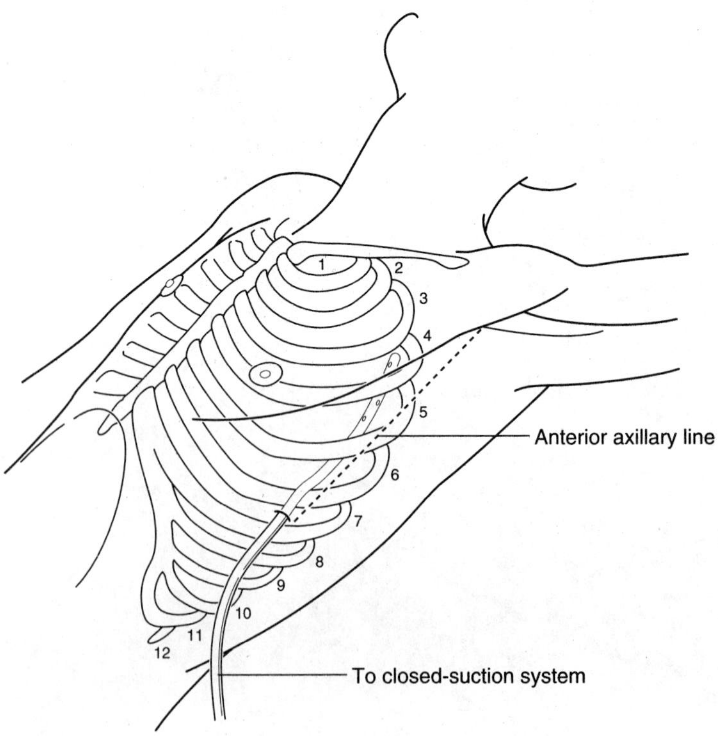

Figure 8-3. Chest tube thoracostomy (chest tube placement). (Adapted with permission from Donovan AJ: *Trauma Surgery: Techniques in Thoracic, Abdominal, and Vascular Surgery.* St. Louis, Mosby, 1994, p 59.)

C. Flail chest

—is caused by the multiple fractures of **4 or more ribs.**

1. **Normal respiration**

   —causes **paradoxical motion** of the affected chest wall.

   —The flail segment moves in with inspiration.

2. **Treatment**

   a. Treatment involves providing adequate pain control (e.g., epidural).

   b. In the presence of respiratory failure, endotracheal intubation and **positive pressure ventilation** are essential.

D. Massive hemothorax

1. This is a **clinical diagnosis characterized by**

   —**hypotension.**

   —**unilateral decreased or absent breath sounds.**

   —dullness to percussion on the affected side.

2. **Chest radiographs**

   —may reveal blood on the affected side.

3. **Treatment**

   —involves fluid resuscitation and **chest tube placement.**

   a. **Removal of the blood**

      —will allow apposition of the pleura, sealing the defect and slowing the bleeding.

   b. If **bleeding continues**

      —at **more than 200 mL per hour,** surgical exploration should be performed to identify the source of bleeding.

E. Cardiac tamponade

—is caused by bleeding into the pericardial sac, resulting in inhibition of cardiac function.

1. Tamponade is **diagnosed clinically** by

   —the presence of **decreased heart sounds.**

   —**JVD.**

   —**hypotension.**

   —These three make up **Beck's triad.**

2. **Initial treatment** involves decompression and fluid resuscitation.

   —If suspected, the pericardial sac is formally explored and a "pericardial window" is placed surgically to allow for decompression.

IV. Secondary Survey

A. To reevaluate the patient during the secondary survey

—perform a **thorough examination from the head to the feet.**

1. **Key elements**

   —to look for are listed in **Table 8-1.**

2. To rely on the **abdominal examination** the patient must be

   —alert and oriented.

   —**without** evidence of **head or spinal cord injury, or drug or alcohol intoxication.**

3. An **abbreviated history**

   —should be taken **(Table 8-2)**.

4. **During the secondary survey**

Table 8-1. Key Elements of the Secondary Survey

Head	Examine for lacerations, contusions, burns, or fractures Reevaluate pupils Reevaluate level of consciousness Evaluate the eye for hemorrhage, penetrating injury, acuity, and hyphema Inspect the ear for **hemotypanum** (associated with basilar skull fractures) Look for evidence of CSF leak from ears (otorrhea) or nose (rhinorrhea) Examine the mouth for dental injuries, fractures, and lacerations **N/G tube placement,** OG tube placement if one suspects maxillofacial injury
Neck	**Maintain C-spine immobilization** (cervical collar) Assess for subcutaneous emphysema Examine **tracheal position** (tension hemo- or pneumothorax associated with tracheal deviation away from side of injury) Palpate the spine for tenderness, swelling, or bony deformity
Chest	Reevaluate the chest as was done in the primary survey Obtain **chest radiograph**
Abdomen	Examine and evaluate for evidence of blunt and penetrating injury Percuss and palpate the abdomen for evidence of rebound and/or guarding Obtain **pelvic radiograph** if indicated
Musculoskeletal	Evaluate for gross evidence of injury Assess for **distal pulses** Palpate for evidence of fracture: crepitation, tenderness, and swelling Obtain necessary films Remember to log-roll the patient and evaluate the back
Perineum	Examine for contusions, hematomas, lacerations, blood at the urethral meatus
Rectum	**Evaluate sphincter tone** (loss of tone associated with severe neurologic injury such as spinal cord injury) Feel for gross bony fragments Palpate the prostate position **Evaluate for blood**
Vagina	Evaluate for blood or lacerations in the vault
Neurologic	Reevaluate the pupils and level of consciousness Examine for extremities for motor and sensory responses Determine the **GCS score**

CSF = cerebrospinal fluid; N/G = nasogastric; OG = orogastric; C-spine = cervical spine; GCS = Glasgow coma scale.

Table 8-2. Brief History During Trauma Evaluation

AMPLE History	Specific Issues
A: Allergies	Medications and IV contrast
M: Medications	Antihypertensives, coumarin (Coumadin), insulin, etc.
P: Past illnesses	Surgeries, chronic illness, heart or respiratory problems
L: Last meal	When they last ate (assessing aspiration risk)
E: Events or Environment related to injury	Mechanism of injury, need to know if other people were involved

IV = intravenous.

—it is important to continually reevaluate the ABC's, looking for any potential changes.

5. It is **also essential to place a Foley catheter**

—to monitor fluid status.

a. **Contraindications to Foley placement** include

—**blood at the urethral meatus.**

—high riding or **"boggy" prostate** in a male.

—severe pelvic fracture.

—obvious perineal injury.

b. If a **urethral injury is suspected**

—a **retrograde urethrogram (RUG)** should be performed (see *BRS Surgical Specialties,* Chapter 6).

B. Laboratory tests

—frequently obtained during the trauma evaluation are listed in **Table 8-3.**

V. Management of Other Specific Injuries

A. Penetrating neck trauma (see *BRS Surgical Specialties,* Chapter 4).

1. The **neck is anatomically divided**

—into **3 zones (Figure 8-4).**

a. **Zone I**

—extends from the **clavicle to the cricoid cartilage.**

b. **Zone II**

Table 8-3. Commonly Obtained Laboratory Tests During Trauma Evaluation

Complete blood count (CBC)
Serum chemistries
Arterial blood gas (ABG)
Prothrombin time (PT) and partial thromboplastin time (PTT)
Ethyl alcohol (EtOH) level
Urine toxicology screen
Lactic acid
Amylase
β-human chorionic gonadotropin (HCG) for females of childbearing age
Type and cross

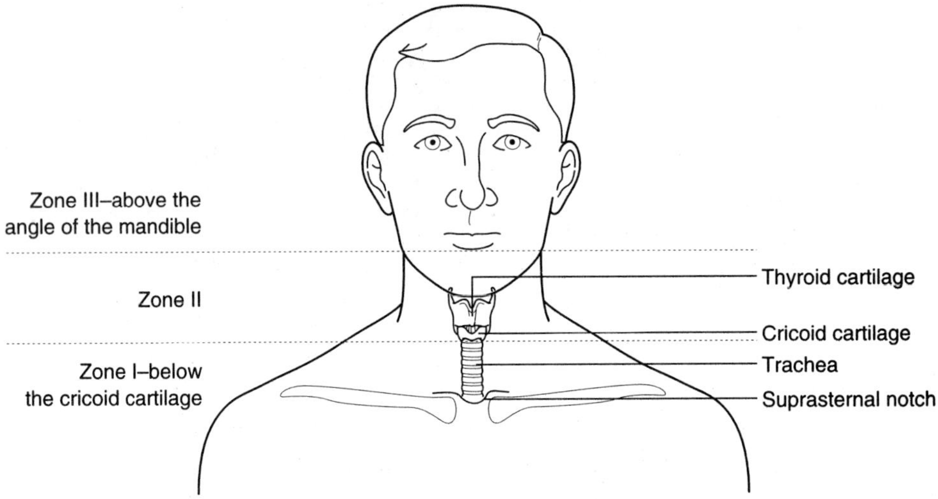

Figure 8-4. Zones of the neck. (Adapted with permission from Lawrence PF: *Essentials of General Surgery,* 2nd ed. Baltimore, Williams & Wilkins, 1992, p 156.)

—extends from the **cricoid cartilage to the angle of the mandible.**

c. **Zone III**

—extends from the **angle of the mandible to the base of the skull.**

2. **Patients**

—**with symptoms,** hemodynamic instability, or signs of underlying injury (e.g., expanding or pulsatile hematoma) require immediate **surgical exploration.**

3. **Management of asymptomatic patients**

—with penetrating neck trauma generally depends on the zone injured.

a. **Zone I and III injuries**

—may initially be evaluated nonoperatively.

(1) For potential **vascular injuries,** use **angiography.**

(2) To assess potential injuries to the **oropharynx** and **esophagus,** perform **endoscopy.**

—Endoscopic evaluation of the larynx and tracheobronchial tree should also be performed to rule out potential injuries to these structures.

b. **Zone II injuries**

—are traditionally managed by performing an **urgent neck exploration,** although some centers are now evaluating some of these patients nonoperatively.

B. **Aortic arch injuries**

1. The need for **further evaluation of aortic arch injuries** should be done if

—there is **radiographic evidence of injury.**

—the **mechanism of injury** warrants further evaluation (i.e., fall from higher than 12 feet or high-speed motor vehicle accident).

2. **Chest radiograph findings** suggestive of **thoracic vessel injuries** include

   —**widened mediastinum.**

   —first rib fracture.

   —apical pleural capping.

   —loss of aortic contour/knob.

   —depression of left main stem bronchus.

   —nasogastric (N/G) tube/trachea deviation.

   —pleural effusion.

3. **A normal chest radiograph**

   —will appear in 10% of patients with aortic arch injuries.

4. An **aortogram**

   —is the gold standard for evaluating potential arch injuries.

5. **Chest computed tomography (CT) scans**

   —are now being used by some centers to evaluate for arch injuries.

C. **Penetrating injury to the "box" (Figure 8-5)**

1. **Hemodynamically unstable patients**

   —require **immediate exploration** of the pericardial space **via a left lateral thoracotomy or sternotomy.**

2. **Otherwise, patients with penetrating injuries**

   —to this area generally require exploration of the pericardial sac via a **subxiphoid window.**

3. If there is **gross blood in the pericardium**

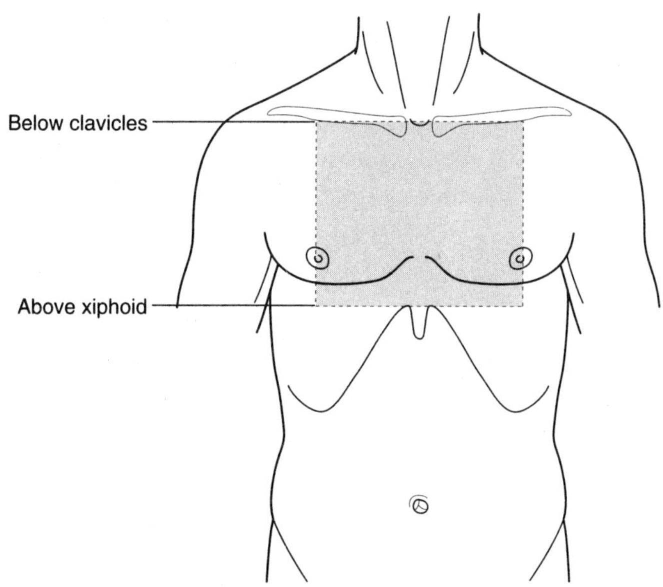

Figure 8-5. The anatomical "box."

—a sternotomy is indicated to assess for injuries to the pericardium, heart, or major vessels.

D. Abdominal injuries

1. Blunt abdominal injury

a. Suspect this type of injury in patients

—involved in significant **deceleration accidents.**

—when the abdominal examination is unreliable (e.g., ethyl alcohol [EtOH] intoxication).

b. Indications for **immediate surgical exploration** without further diagnostic evaluation of the abdomen include

—peritonitis.

—hypotension with a distended abdomen.

c. Both **CT** and **diagnostic peritoneal lavage (DPL)**

—may be used to evaluate patients with suspected abdominal injury (**Table 8-4**).

d. Diagnostic peritoneal lavage

(1) A **Foley catheter and N/G tube** must be placed before performing DPL.

(2) A **catheter** is placed into the peritoneal cavity below the umbilicus and the contents aspirated.

—If **gross blood or succus** are initially aspirated, **surgical exploration is indicated.**

—If initial syringe **aspiration is negative,** 1 L of crystalloid is infused through the catheter and then the fluid is drained.

(3) The **criteria for surgical exploration** based upon the **analysis of the DPL fluid** are listed in **Table 8-5.**

e. Rapid ultrasound evaluation

—of the abdomen may also be used in this setting.

2. Penetrating abdominal trauma

a. Penetrating injury to the thorax

—at or below the **fourth intercostal space** (at the nipple in men) needs to be evaluated for concomitant abdominal injury.

—The diaphragm may extend to that level during expiration.

Table 8-4. Diagnostic Peritoneal Lavage (DPL) versus Computed Tomography (CT) Scan for Assessment of Potential Abdominal Injuries

	Advantages	Disadvantages
DPL	Faster Can be done at the bedside Very sensitive	Invasive Results in approximately 15% nontherapeutic laparotomies Cannot evaluate retroperitoneum
CT	Greater specificity Allows visualization of retroperitoneal structures Allows evaluation of solid organ injuries Noninvasive	Requires more time Patient must be transported Patient must be stable More costly and requires more personnel Poor sensitivity for early hollow viscus injury

Table 8-5. Findings of a Positive Diagnostic Peritoneal Lavage (DPL)

Immediate or Macroscopic Findings	Delayed or Microscopic Findings
5 mL **gross blood** on aspirate	Classic: inability to read newsprint through the lavage fluid in the tube
Enteric or **succus** on aspiration	**RBC > 100,000 mm³**
Lavage fluid noted to be draining from	**WBC > 500/mm³**
Chest tube (diaphragm injury)	Elevated amylase
Foley catheter (bladder injury)	**Bile** present
N/G tube (injury to viscera)	**Bacteria** present
	Vegetable matter present

RBC = red blood cells; WBC = white blood cells; N/G = nasogastric.

b. Stab wounds

(1) In a **hemodynamically unstable patient**

with a stab wound to the abdomen, **immediate surgical exploration** is indicated.

(2) Stable, asymptomatic patients may undergo local wound exploration.

—After **wound exploration,** laparotomy or laparoscopy is performed if the fascia has been violated or if the tract cannot be visualized.

c. Abdominal gunshot wounds (GSWs)

(1) GSWs to the **abdomen** require **immediate exploratory laparotomy.**

(2) The **amount of damage** caused is related to the **kinetic energy** (K.E. = $\frac{1}{2}MV^2$) and the surface area of the bullet.

3. Specific abdominal organ injuries

a. The **small bowel**

—is the most commonly injured organ in penetrating trauma.

(1) Minor injuries can be repaired primarily with simple suture closure.

(2) Larger injuries can be resected and repaired with a primary anastomosis.

b. The **spleen and liver**

—are the most commonly injured organs in **blunt trauma.**

(1) Minor injuries in stable and asymptomatic patients may be managed with bedrest, followed by 6 weeks of limited activity.

(2) Symptomatic or large injuries to the **liver** require immediate repair or packing.

(3) Symptomatic or large **splenic** injuries generally require **splenectomy** (see Chapter 17).

—**Postsplenectomy sepsis** may occur in 1%–5% of patients after splenectomy.

c. Colon injuries

—are managed according to several factors.

(1) These include

—size of the injury.

—location of the injury.

—amount of fecal soilage.

—presence of associated injuries.

—hemodynamic stability of the patient.

(2) **Small injuries** with minimal associated injuries **in stable patients** can be repaired primarily.

(3) **Unstable patients** or patients with multiple associated injuries will likely require a **colostomy** following resection of the injured bowel.

(4) Larger injuries to the **right or transverse colon** with minimal associated injuries can be repaired with **resection and primary anastomosis.**

(5) **Large left-sided colon injuries** generally require performance of a colostomy after resection of the injured bowel.

d. Rectal injuries

—are generally caused by penetrating injury.

—may require a proximal diverting colostomy, placement of a presacral drain, and repair of the injury if possible.

e. Pancreatic and duodenal injuries

—are frequently missed and can be the most complicated injuries to repair.

(1) **Isolated small** duodenal injuries can be repaired by primary closure.

(2) **Larger injuries** may require **duodenal resection** and gastric diversion.

(3) Injuries to the **pancreatic duct** distal to the head of the pancreas can be managed with a **distal pancreatectomy.**

(4) Severe injuries to the **head of the pancreas** with severe associated duodenal injuries may need a pancreaticoduodenectomy (Whipple's operation).

VI. Pelvic Injuries

A. Pelvic injuries

—are common in victims of blunt trauma (see *BRS Surgical Specialties,* Chapter 5).

B. Fractures

—can cause **retroperitoneal or preperitoneal hematomas** that are large enough to cause hemodynamic instability.

C. Treatment depends mainly on

—the **hemodynamic stability** of the patient.

—the **presence or absence of intra-abdominal bleeding.**

1. Pelvic fixation

—is important to reduce bleeding in unstable fractures.

2. Patients who are **hemodynamically unstable**

—with a grossly negative DPL may undergo **angiography** to evaluate for pelvic arterial bleeding, which may be controlled with **embolization.**

3. A **grossly positive DPL**

—in association with a pelvic injury still requires immediate exploratory laparotomy.

—With pelvic injuries, DPL should be performed above the umbilicus.

VII. Burns

A. Anatomy

1. Depth

a. First degree burns

—involve damage to the **epidermis only.**

(1) The skin is erythematous and **very tender** (e.g., minor sunburn).

(2) There is no blistering and **no permanent damage** to the underlying dermal layer.

b. Second degree, or **partial-thickness** burns

—are intradermal injuries.

—can be further subdivided into superficial and deep.

(1) In **superficial partial-thickness burns**

—the hair follicles, the sweat glands, and the sebaceous glands are intact.

—the areas affected are **very painful** and hypersensitive to touch.

—the wound appears red and mottled with edema and blistering.

—the surface is typically moist and weepy.

(2) Deep partial-thickness burns

—have necrosis well into the dermis and **skin appendages are involved.**

—are slightly tougher and firmer, and are less sensitive to touch.

c. Third degree, or **full-thickness** burns

—involve **the entire depth of the dermis.**

(1) All dermal elements are destroyed including **nerve endings,** dermal appendages, and blood vessels.

(2) The wound surface appears waxy-white or gray, dark and leathery, or charred.

(3) The affected area is often dry, and thrombosed vessels may be visible.

(4) The lesions are **painless and insensate to touch.**

2. Extent of injury

a. The **severity of burn damage**

—is also based on the percent of total body surface area (TBSA) involved.

(1) TBSA is determined in **adults** by the "**rule of nines.**"

—The proportions in **infants** and children are slightly different (**Figure 8-6**).

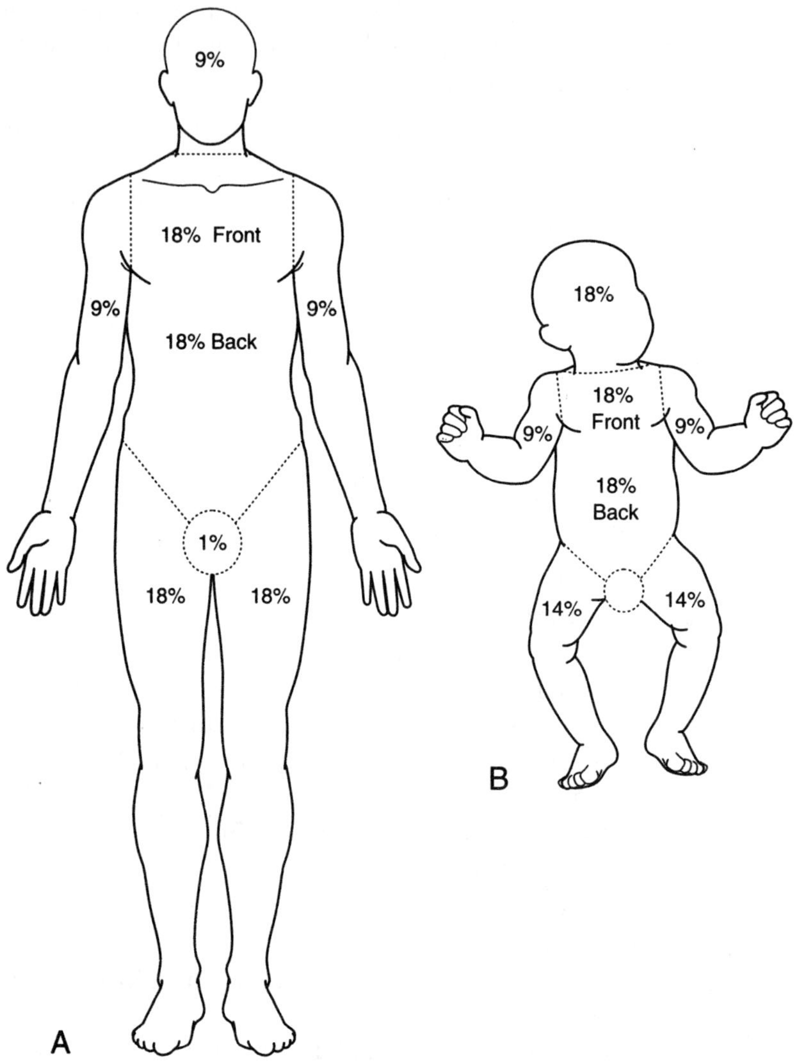

Figure 8-6. Estimation of percent of body surface area affected by burn injury. (*A*) In adults, each designated area is divisible by 9 ("rule of nines"). (*B*) The estimates are slightly different in infants because of the proportionately larger head. (Adapted with permission from Lawrence PF: *Essentials of General Surgery,* 2nd ed. Baltimore, Williams & Wilkins, 1992, p 163.)

(2) The genitalia and **palm** are roughly equivalent to **1% TBSA** each.

b. Burns are considered serious

—regardless of the total extent of the burn in certain locations such as **the face, hands, perineum, and joints.**

B. Initial management

1. Airway

a. Evaluation for signs suggestive of inhalation injury **(Table 8-6)** is absolutely necessary.

—One must have a very low threshold for intubation.

(1) Early intubation is essential because airway management be-

Table 8-6. Evidence of Possible Inhalation Injury

Confinement in a closed space
History of explosion
History of **decreased level or loss of consciousness**
Charring or **carbon deposits around the mouth, nose, or in the oropharynx**
Carbonaceous sputum
Dyspnea
Inflammatory changes to the oropharynx
Facial burns
Singed facial or nasal hair
Circumferential burns of the trunk
Alteration in the patient's voice
Low oxygen saturation

comes more difficult as **swelling rapidly increases over the first 24 hours.**

(2) Sloughing of the mucosa with occlusion of the airway can also occur.

b. **Bronchoscopy**

—may also be used in the initial evaluation of the airway.

2. **Breathing**

a. **Arterial blood gas**

—should be obtained in severely burned patients.

b. **Carbon monoxide levels**

—should be obtained if there is a history of **exposure to noxious fumes or smoke inhalation.**

(1) **Carboxyhemoglobin** of greater than 10% is considered significant.

(2) **Treatment** involves administration of 100% oxygen.

3. **Circulation**

a. **Early and aggressive volume resuscitation** is essential.

(1) The **"Parkland Formula"** is an **estimate** of the **volume of crystalloid** (lactated Ringer's) necessary for resuscitation in the **first 24 hours:**

$$\textbf{Volume} = \textbf{\% TBSA burned} \times \textbf{body weight (kg)} \times \textbf{4 mL.}$$

—TBSA of second and third degree burns are used in this calculation.

(2) **Half of the estimated volume** should be given in the first 8 hours after injury.

—The remainder is given over the next 16 hours.

b. **Measurement of urine output**

—via a Foley catheter is the most sensitive indicator of the adequacy of volume resuscitation.

(1) **Adult patients** should have a minimum urine output of **0.5 mL/kg/hour.**

—Children should have an output of 1–2 mL/kg/hour.

(2) **Adjustments to the rate** estimated by the Parkland formula may be necessary to achieve these goals (see VII B 3 a).

c. **Monitoring central venous and pulmonary capillary pressure**
   —may be necessary in the severely injured patient.

d. **After the first 24 hours**
   —colloid (e.g., albumin solution) may be used, as **capillary permeability returns to near baseline.**

e. **Distal pulses must be monitored**
   —especially in the presence of circumferential burns, because swelling may compress vessels.

   (1) **Escharotomies** are performed to prevent circulatory compromise of the extremity.

   (2) This involves making longitudinal incisions through the eschar to healthy adipose tissue with a scalpel or electrocautery (**Figure 8-7**).

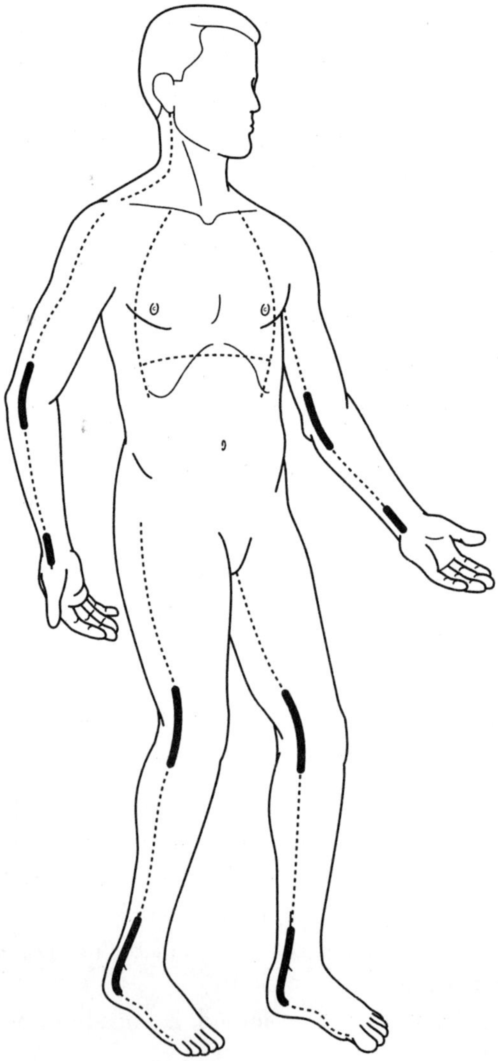

Figure 8-7. Escharotomy lines represented by the dark lines. (Adapted with permission from Sabiston D: *Textbook of Surgery: The Biological Basis of Modern Surgical Practice,* 15th ed. Philadelphia, WB Saunders, 1997, p 230.)

f. **Truncal escharotomies**

—may be necessary in circumferential chest burns to prevent inhibition of inspiratory capacity and respiratory compromise.

4. **After the initial ABC's, determine**

—the mechanism of injury.

—if other disabilities or injuries exist.

5. It is also **essential to ensure that the burning process has been stopped.**

a. **Clothing,** especially synthetic fabrics, may continue to burn or smolder.

—Clothing **must be extinguished and removed.**

b. **Other hot adherent substances** such as grease or tar need to be removed.

c. **Chemical burns or corrosive injuries** require copious irrigation.

6. **Burn patients are at a significant risk**

—for **severe heat loss** and hypothermia.

—Care should be taken to maintain normothermia (see II E 3).

C. **Criteria for hospitalization**

—or transfer to a specialized burn treatment center are outlined in **Table 8-7.**

D. **Burn wound care**

1. **First degree burns**

—can be treated by applying bacitracin to the area.

a. **Analgesics**

—may be needed for pain.

b. **Healing is complete**

—and without scar formation or skin discoloration.

2. **Superficial partial-thickness burns**

—are initially cleaned with an antiseptic soap to remove foreign material and dead skin.

a. **Blisters** are generally unroofed.

Table 8-7. Admission Criteria for Burn Injured Victims

All burns > 10 % TBSA in children and the elderly
Any suspected inhalation injury
All burns of **face, hands, feet, and perineum**
Full-thickness burns > 10% TBSA
Partial-thickness burns > 20% TBSA
Partial- or full-thickness burns of major flexion creases
Burns with associated trauma
Electrical burns
Chemical burns
If there are reasons to believe that the burn injury was a result of abuse

TBSA = total body surface area.

—Topical antibiotics are applied before dressing the wounds.

b. These wounds can be **very painful**

—and require treatment with analgesics.

c. There is **little or no scar formation**

—with **no major change in skin pigmentation.**

3. **Deep partial-thickness burns** and **full-thickness burns**

a. These are **initially managed** like superficial second degree burns with

—cleansing.

—topical antibiotic agents.

—dressing changes.

b. However, these **wounds will need**

—frequent **surgical débridement and skin grafting** to minimize complications of the burn injury.

c. **Complications include**

—**contracture formation.**

—**infection.**

—severe scar formation.

—prolonged hospitalization.

d. **Excision of wounds and coverage**

—should be performed **early.**

(1) Excision and coverage **within 72 hours decreases the rate of development of burn wound sepsis.**

—Early excision and coverage also allows for early mobilization and rehabilitation, improved joint function, and shorter hospitalization.

(2) Delay excision if the patient is **hemodynamically unstable.**

(3) Burns are tangentially excised until a healthy bed of tissue is reached.

e. **Wound closure**

—is best accomplished immediately after excision.

(1) The **gold standard** of burn wound closure is **split-thickness skin graft** (autograft-skin obtained from a nonburned area on the patient).

(2) Reasons to **delay closure** may include

—**inadequate recipient tissue bed** (e.g., persistent infection).

—unwillingness to create donor sites.

—**insufficient donor sites** available for autograft coverage.

(3) **Other choices** used to close excised burn wounds include temporary and permanent coverings.

(a) **Grafts** (See Chapter 6)

—**Allograft** is a cadaveric skin graft from an individual of **the same species.**

—**Xenograft** is a skin graft from a **different species** (e.g., pig, shark).

(b) Silastic and other commercially produced **membranes** are also available, but are used less commonly.

(c) **Permanent covers** include cultured epithelial autografts and composites of Silastic and collagen.

(d) All of these tend to be more costly than autografts, with inferior results.

E. Other aspects of the burn care

1. **Nutrition**

—is very important in treating the burn patient (see Chapter 3).

a. A **burn patient is in a hypermetabolic state**

—that is unsurpassed by any other form of trauma or illness.

b. **Recommended protein requirements**

—are **1.5–3.0 g of protein/kg/day.**

c. **Early enteral feeding**

—is essential and is favored over parenteral nutrition.

2. **Prophylaxis against gastrointestinal ulceration**

—is important (e.g., H2-blockers) because burn patients are at an increased risk of developing acute erosive gastritis **(Curling's ulcer)**.

3. **Electrolytes abnormalities** frequently occur.

—Close monitoring and adequate treatment are essential.

4. The **burn patient** is at **high risk**

—for infectious complications.

a. **Pneumonia**

—Aggressive pulmonary toilet is important to minimize the risk of developing pneumonia.

—N/G decompression is important because of the increased risk of developing **gastric ileus,** which can potentially lead to aspiration.

b. **Burn wound infections**

—can lead to sepsis and death.

(1) The **most common infectious organisms are**

—*Staphylococcus aureus.*

—*Pseudomonas* species.

—*Streptococcus* species.

—*Candida albicans.*

(2) The **diagnosis** can be confirmed by culturing a biopsy section of the wound for quantitative burn wound bacterial count.

—More than 10^5 organisms/g of tissue is considered significant.

—Organism identification can also be determined.

(3) **Specific signs** of burn wound infection include

—the **conversion of second degree burns to full-thickness burns**

—green pigmentation.

—discoloration or change of burned areas.

Review Test

Directions: Each of the numbered items or incomplete statements in this section is followed by answers or by completions of the statement. Select the ONE lettered answer or completion that is BEST in each case.

1. A 20-year-old man presents to the emergency room after being involved in a bar fight. Other than some abrasions on his face and hands, the patient has a laceration on the side of his neck. Exploration of this wound at the bedside reveals a large superficial laceration that does not penetrate the platysma muscle. Which of the following is most appropriate in the initial management of this patient?

(A) Immediate surgical neck exploration
(B) Angiography to evaluate for vascular injury
(C) Aggressive irrigation and local wound care
(D) Evaluation of the esophagus via endoscopy
(E) Evaluation of the esophagus via esophagography

2. A 16-year-old man is brought to the emergency room after his clothes caught on fire. He has severe burns to both his upper extremities. What signs would indicate the need for an escharotomy?

(A) Circumferential burns with severe blistering and erythema
(B) Circumferential burns with severe pain over the affected area
(C) Circumferential partial-thickness burns over the elbow joint
(D) Circumferential burns with an absence of the left radial pulse
(E) Circumferential superficial burns over the elbow joint

3. A 58-year-old woman presents to the emergency room after a motor vehicle accident. Despite 2 liters of intravenous fluid, her heart rate is still 130 beats per minute and her systolic blood pressure is 86 mm Hg. Her chest radiograph reveals normal lung fields with no evidence of pneumothorax or hemothorax, although there is a small amount of air noted between the diaphragm and the liver. Pelvic radiograph also reveals a fracture of the pubic symphysis and the right sacroiliac. Which of the following is most appropriate initial step in the evaluation and treatment of this patient?

(A) Obtain an immediate angiogram of the pelvis.
(B) Obtain an abdominal/pelvis computed tomography scan.
(C) Perform immediate diagnostic peritoneal lavage.
(D) Perform abdominal ultrasound and pelvic fixation.
(E) Perform immediate exploratory laparotomy.

4. An 18-year-old man is admitted to the hospital after sustaining a burn injury from a gasoline fire. His entire anterior trunk, left upper extremity, and both complete anterior thighs are affected. All areas appear to be at least partial-thickness burns. What is the estimated total body surface area of burn injury involvement?

(A) 18%
(B) 27%
(C) 36%
(D) 55%
(E) 60%

5. After being hit on the left side, a 24-year-old football player becomes unconscious. He regains consciousness and is brought emergently to the hospital. After initial resuscitation, performance of an abdominal computed tomography (CT) scan reveals a splenic injury involving the vessels within the hilum with significant intraperitoneal bleeding. Which of the following statements is true regarding the management of this patient?

(A) Nonoperative management with bedrest is indicated for this splenic injury.
(B) This patient will need to be immunized with vaccines against *Haemophilus, Pneumococcus,* and *Neisseria.*
(C) If a splenectomy is performed, this patient will require lifelong antibiotic therapy.
(D) This injury is a grade 1 splenic injury because of the involvement of the hilum.
(E) If nonoperative treatment is performed, this patient could return to play football in 2 weeks.

6. A 46-year-old woman suffered a full-thickness burn to 10% of her body, a partial-thickness burn to 30% of her body, and first degree burns to an additional 20% of her body. She weighs 50 kg and the burn occurred just before admission. What is the estimated amount of fluids she will need for the first 24 hours?

(A) 2 liters
(B) 3.6 liters
(C) 8.0 liters
(D) 12.4 liters
(E) 14.4 liters

7. A 27-year-old man sustains a gunshot wound to the abdomen with a small caliber handgun. There is a small entrance wound in the right lower quadrant and an exit wound on the back directly posterior to the entrance wound. His blood pressure is 120/60 mm Hg and his heart rate is 95 beats per minute. Exploratory laparotomy reveals a 1.5-cm laceration on the antimesenteric border of the ascending colon with no other injuries discovered. There is minimal fecal leakage. Which statement is true regarding the management of this patient?

(A) A pelvic angiogram should be performed postoperatively.
(B) A right colectomy and a diverting ileostomy should be performed.
(C) A completely diverting colostomy should be performed.
(D) This patient's injury can be managed with primary repair.
(E) If hematuria is present a nephrectomy should be performed.

8. A 19-year-old cross country runner presents to the emergency room after falling off a 9-foot ridge and landing on his right side. He is complaining of some tenderness over his right lower ribs with no abdominal tenderness to palpation. His blood pressure is 128/74 mm Hg with a pulse of 96 beats per minute. An abdominal computed tomography (CT) scan is performed, which reveals a grade III liver injury with intra-abdominal bleeding. Which statement is true regarding this patient?

(A) Hypotension and tachycardia are often late findings of shock in young athletes.
(B) Hepatic arteriography is the preferred examination in the evaluation of liver injuries.
(C) A 9-foot fall is not sufficient enough to cause a severe liver injury.
(D) The lack of abdominal tenderness is inconsistent with intra-abdominal bleeding.
(E) A diagnostic peritoneal lavage should be performed to confirm bleeding.

9. An elderly male is involved in a motor vehicle accident. He states he was going approximately 45 mph when his car struck a car that stopped abruptly in front of him. His blood pressure is 110/74 mm Hg, with a heart rate of 87 beats per minute. After thorough examination his only injuries include a nondisplaced right femur fracture with intact peripheral pulses and some minor abrasions. Which of the following would be appropriate to confirm the absence of a cervical spine injury in this patient?

(A) A normal lateral neck film with no cervical tenderness or pain during examination
(B) A normal anterior posterior film with no cervical tenderness or pain during examination
(C) A normal computed tomography (CT) scan of the cervical spine with pain upon lateral neck motion
(D) Lateral, anterior-posterior, and odontoid views with no cervical tenderness or pain during examination
(E) Physical examination alone with no cervical tenderness or pain during examination

10. A 4-year-old girl is brought in by her parents after she apparently was burned during her bath. Her feet, buttocks, and perineum are badly scalded with blistering skin. Her legs have no blistering, but are mildly red and somewhat tender to the touch. Which of the following is true regarding admission criteria for burn injured victims?

(A) Children with deep partial-thickness burns on ≤ 30% total body surface area (TBSA) can be managed as outpatients with close follow-up.
(B) Patients with full-thickness burns to the perineum only can be managed as outpatients with close follow-up.
(C) Children with full-thickness burns to the feet only can be managed as outpatients with close follow-up.
(D) All patients with superficial burns to the entire torso region and both lower extremities require inpatient treatment.
(E) All children with burn injuries and a concern of possible abuse should be admitted for inpatient treatment.

11. A 43-year-old patient who has been in the intensive care unit for 7 days following a severe 70% total body surface area (TBSA) burn has become increasingly tachycardic and mildly hypotensive with a decrease in urine output. Based upon changes in the color and odor of the burn wound, you suspect burn wound sepsis. Which organisms are most likely to be involved?

(A) *Staphylococcus aureus, Pseudomonas* species, and *Bacteroides* species
(B) *Staphylococcus aureus, Streptococcus* species, and *Pseudomonas* species
(C) *Candida albicans, Bacteroides* species, and *Escherichia coli*
(D) *Candida albicans, E. coli,* and *Proteus* species
(E) *E. coli, Bacteroides* species, and *Clostridium difficile*

12. A patient is complaining of shortness of breath after falling off his tractor and getting run over by the rear wheel. Physical examination reveals a blood pressure of 82/40 mm Hg, a heart rate of 122 beats per minute, short shallow respirations, breath sounds louder on the left than on the right, and tracheal shifting toward the patient's left. What is the most likely diagnosis?

(A) Right tension pneumothorax
(B) Left tension pneumothorax
(C) Cardiac tamponade
(D) Severe tracheal injury
(E) Right flail chest

13. A 49-year-old man presents to the emergency room after being hit by a car while walking down the road. Minimal history is available from the emergency medical technicians. He is conscious upon arrival and moving all 4 extremities. The most appropriate initial step in the evaluation of this patient is to

(A) Remove all clothing and inspect for injuries.
(B) Ask the patient his name.
(C) Place a Foley catheter after a rectal examination.
(D) Evaluate the patient's pupils.
(E) Obtain chest and pelvis radiographs.

14. A 17-year-old woman is seen in the emergency room with severe burns to both of her hands. She seems very responsible, and is with her parents who are very willing to help take care of her at home. She is not complaining of any pain and wonders if she can be treated as an outpatient. Which of the following statements is true regarding the management of this patient?

(A) This patient can be adequately managed as an outpatient with close follow-up.
(B) Skin grafting should be performed in 1–2 months to provide the best outcome.
(C) Her burns are likely to be superficial partial-thickness burns.
(D) Early skin grafting (within days) will decrease contracture formation.
(E) Wound cleansing and application of antibiotic ointment is adequate treatment.

15. A 52-year-old, 60-kg woman is admitted to the hospital immediately after being involved in a house fire. She has approximately 50% total body surface area (TBSA) burns that are at least partial-thickness burns. She has not received any intravenous (IV) fluids up to this point. Which of the following is the most appropriate IV fluid and rate of administration that should initially be given to this patient?

(A) Lactated Ringer's at 500 mL/hr
(B) 5% Dextrose in H_2O at 750 mL/hr
(C) Lactated Ringer's at 1000 mL/hr
(D) 5% Dextrose in H_2O at 1000 mL/hr
(E) Lactated Ringer's at 750 mL/hr

Answers and Explanations

1-C. A stab wound that does not penetrate the platysma needs no further evaluation. Meticulous wound care and local irrigation are needed, however significant injury to the deep structures of the neck is unlikely without penetration of the platysma. If the stab wound did penetrate the platysma, evaluation and treatment would be determined by the zone of the neck injured, as well as the presence or absence of signs suggestive of an injury to vital structures. Such signs include frank arterial bleeding, hematoma formation, bruit, cerebral changes indicative of an ischemic or embolic event, stridor, dysphonia, hemoptysis, hematemesis, dysphagia, odynophagia, or subcutaneous air.

2-D. An escharotomy is a procedure that involves placement of full-thickness longitudinal incisions over sites of severe burn injury to prevent and treat vascular compromise and ischemia secondary to swelling and edema formation at the burn site. Full-thickness incisions to the level of healthy adipose tissue are necessary for adequate compartmental decompression. Indications for escharotomy in an extremity include circumferential burns with absent distal pulses or with significant neurologic changes. Superficial burns generally do not result in such an injury and the presence of partial-thickness burns over a joint does not mandate performance of an escharotomy. Blistering, erythema, and pain are not indications for escharotomy.

3-E. Free air seen under the diaphragm after a motor vehicle accident is an indication for immediate surgical exploration of the abdomen because of the likelihood of a visceral injury. Performance of an abdominal computed tomography (CT) scan, abdominal ultrasound, or diagnostic peritoneal lavage is not necessary when free air is present in the abdomen. Operative pelvic fixation and angiography of the pelvis may be important in the management of this patient but should not precede performance of a laparotomy.

4-C. Total body surface area (TBSA) estimates used to quantify the extent of burn injuries in adults is based on the "rule of nines." The anterior trunk is equal to 18%. The left upper extremity is equal to 9%. Each lower extremity is equal to 18%, thus each anterior thigh is approximately 4.5%, and making a total of 9% TBSA involved in the lower extremity. Therefore $18 + 9 + 2(4.5) = 36\%$.

5-B. A severe splenic injury involving the splenic hilum requires immediate splenectomy and should not be managed with observation and bedrest. Some minor splenic injuries can be managed nonoperatively with bedrest and observation if there is no hemodynamic instability or significant intraperitoneal hemorrhage. Conservative treatment of minor splenic injuries with strict bedrest for 5 days would still require avoidance of contact sports with limited activity for approximately 6 weeks. Patients undergoing a splenectomy should receive immunization against encapsulated organisms, specifically *Haemophilus, Pneumococcus,* and *Neisseria.* Grading of splenic injuries is complex although grade 1 injuries are characterized by small (< 1 cm) lacerations not involving the capsule while grade V injuries include those with complete devascularization or avulsion of the spleen or a completely shattered spleen.

6-C. Resuscitation fluid is determined using the Parkland formula, which estimates the volume of fluid to be administered during the first 24 hours after a severe burn injury. The formula is: volume = (% TBSA burned) × (weight in kg) × (4 mL), where TBSA = total body surface area. It is important to calculate the TBSA in this formula using only second and third degree burns. First degree burns are not used in calculating fluid resuscitation. So for this patient, the calculation is volume = (10% [full-thickness] + 30% [partial-thickness]) × 50 kg × 4 mL = 8000 kg/mL, which = 8.0 L.

7-D. Historically, a colostomy was performed in most patients with colonic injuries to avoid anastomotic leaking and wound infection. Recently, it has become evident that for many colon injuries a colostomy is not required. Patients with small injuries, especially to the right-sided colon, with minimal fecal soilage, and who are hemodynamically stable are appropriately managed with primary repair or closure of the injured segment. A pelvic injury is not indicated based on the clinical and intraoperative findings. Hematuria alone would not be an indication for nephrectomy, although the renal system and kidney should be carefully inspected intraoperatively for potential injury after a gunshot wound (GSW) to this area. The absence of other injuries at exploratory laparotomy warrant no further surgery or radiologic tests.

8-A. Because of the well-adapted cardiovascular response, young athletes may frequently develop significant hypotension and tachycardia only as a late finding even in the presence of severe hypovolemia or blood loss. Patients on β blockers also can have a blunted tachycardic response to hypovolemia. The fact that abdominal tenderness was not present is not abnormal. Acute bleeding in the abdomen does not always cause peritoneal irritation. Hepatic arteriography may be used in some situations to treat hepatic injuries, however it is generally not preferred over computed tomography (CT) scan for evaluation. There is no need to perform diagnostic peritoneal lavage when bleeding is seen on CT scan.

9-D. To adequately confirm the absence of a cervical spine injury in a patient at a potential risk for such injury (i.e., high-speed motor vehicle accident) radiographs must be performed. To rely on the physical examination alone, the patient must be alert and oriented and have no distracting injuries (e.g., femur fracture) or be under the influence of drugs. Radiographs needed to evaluate the cervical spine are a lateral, anterior-posterior, and open mouth odontoid views. It is important to visualize all seven cervical vertebrae. If a physical examination is reliable and negative for tenderness or pain with full range of motion, no further evaluation needs to be performed. Even with a normal computed tomography (CT) scan, however, the presence of pain during range of motion testing should prompt an evaluation for a potential ligamentous injury.

10-E. Partial-thickness burns to the face, perineum, hands, or feet are criteria for admission and inpatient management. The total body surface area (TBSA) burned in this patient is greater than 10% and she is only 4 years old. This is also criteria for admission. Although this could simply be an unintentional accident, the question of abuse or neglect needs to be addressed and is an adequate indication for admission in any child regardless of extent of injury. Patients with superficial burns (e.g., minor sunburn) generally do not require inpatient treatment and can be managed appropriately as outpatients.

11-B. Changes in burn wound color and odor may occur when burn wound sepsis is occurring. The most common organisms involved in burn wound infections include *Staphylococcus aureus, Pseudomonas* species, *Streptococcus* species, and *Candida albicans.* Confirmation of significant burn wound infection requires performing quantitative cultures of a biopsy specimen of the affected burn area.

12-A. The most likely diagnosis in this patient is a tension pneumothorax. Injury to the lung parenchyma caused by rib fractures from blunt chest trauma may result in development of a pneumothorax. As air continues to enter the pleural space with each inspiration, the intrapleural pressure continues to rise, resulting in lung collapse and even compression of vascular structures within the mediastinum (e.g., superior vena cava). This results in decreased venous return to the heart and rapid development of shock. This may also cause shifting of mediastinal structures such as the trachea away from the side of the pneumothorax. Cardiac tamponade is not associated with unilateral decreased breath sounds. Tracheal injuries are rare after blunt trauma to the chest. A flail chest can cause shallow respirations and unilateral decreased breath sounds but it is not always associated with development of a pneumothorax.

13-B. Although all of the procedures listed are important in the evaluation of the traumatized patient within the first few minutes, it is essential to proceed systematically with the ABC's (Airway, Breathing, Circulation), in that order. One of the easiest ways to assess for airway patency in a conscious patient is by determining the patient's ability to talk. If a patient can verbalize normally, the airway is likely patent.

14-D. The fact that these burns are painless makes it highly likely that they are a full-thickness burn. Any burn of that degree to the hands requires inpatient treatment. If left untreated, deep partial-thickness and full-thickness burns will heal slowly with significant scar formation and contracture formation. The gold standard is to do a split-thickness skin grafting within days after adequate excision and débridement of the burn.

15-E. The Parkland formula is used to calculate an estimated volume of intravenous (IV) fluids to administer during the first 24 hours after a burn. Thus, 12 liters of IV fluids will need to be given to this patient during the first 24 hours. However, half of the fluid needs to be given in the first 8 hours after the injury; this means that approximately 6 liters will need to be given over an 8-hour period (750 mL/hr). Initial losses are isotonic, and therefore need to be replaced with an isotonic crystalloid such as lactated Ringer's.

9

Acute Abdominal Pain

Steven M. Fiser

I. Clinical Approach to Acute Abdominal Pain

A. Surgical intervention is indicated

—for most causes of severe acute abdominal pain.

—for any worsening condition.

B. Early diagnosis and treatment

—is essential in improving outcome.

C. A thorough history and physical examination

—is key in determining which patients require surgery.

D. A brief period of close observation (6–12 hours) and frequent examination may be necessary in some situations where the etiology of pain is initially unclear.

II. History

A. Anorexia, nausea, and vomiting

—commonly occur with inflammatory processes and proximal obstructions.

B. Changes in bowel habits

1. Bloody stools or melena may indicate

—inflammation.

—infection.

—ischemia.

—diverticulosis.

—arterial-venous malformation.

—cancer.

—ulcers.

—esophageal varices.

—other source of hemorrhage.

2. **Obstipation, constipation, or diarrhea**

—can occur with inflammation, obstruction, and infection.

C. **Pain**

1. **Onset of pain** can be gradual or abrupt.

2. **Characteristics of pain**

a. **Visceral pain**

—arises from the visceral peritoneum and capsule of solid organs.

—is **poorly localized, deep,** and **dull.**

b. **Somatic pain**

—arises from the parietal peritoneum after it becomes inflamed.

—is **localized, sharp,** and **constant.**

—gives rise to either local or diffuse **peritoneal signs.**

c. **Colicky pain**

—comes in **waves.**

—is caused by obstruction of a hollow lumen.

(1) **This type of pain is seen in**

—bowel obstructions.

—nephrolithiasis.

—biliary colic.

(2) **Patients will often have**

—**intense writhing movements** in an attempt to alleviate the pain, with other periods during which they are relatively asymptomatic.

d. **Referred pain**

—typically arises from deep structures (**Table 9-1**).

—is **sharp and constant.**

e. **Pain that awakens the patient at night or is incapacitating** is also considered significant.

3. **Factors that may attenuate pain and other symptoms** include

—antibiotics.

—narcotics.

—steroids.

—immunosuppressive agents.

—age greater than 65 years.

—diabetes.

—immunodeficiency [e.g., acquired immunodeficiency syndrome (AIDS)].

4. **Location of pain**

a. Pain can be localized, diffuse, or shifting (e.g., appendicitis).

Table 9-1. Location of Referred Pain

Small bowel:	epigastrium and periumbilical area
Large bowel:	suprapubic area
Gallbladder:	right shoulder/scapula
Kidney/ureters:	groin, genitalia, and flank
Pancreas:	lumbar area and left shoulder/scapula
Ulcer disease:	shoulders

b. **Pain in different areas** may be associated with different etiologies (**Table 9-2**).

D. **Other parts of a patient's history**

—may also yield clues to the diagnosis (**Table 9-3**).

III. Physical Examination and Laboratory Evaluation

A. Cardiovascular and pulmonary assessment

1. **It is important to rule out pulmonary and cardiac causes for pain,** such as pneumonia and myocardial infarction.
2. **In the presence of shock, potential diagnoses** include

   —sepsis.

   —pancreatitis.

   —peritonitis.

   —mesenteric ischemia.

   —ruptured abdominal aortic aneurysm (AAA).

   —aortic dissection.

   —coronary thrombosis.

   —ruptured ectopic pregnancy.

   —aortoenteric fistula.

B. Abdominal examination

1. **Narcotics** should generally be withheld until surgical evaluation is performed.

Table 9-2. Etiology of Localized Tenderness Based on Location

Location	Etiology
RUQ	Acute cholecystitis, biliary colic, perforated duodenal ulcer
LUQ (uncommon)	Pancreatitis, perforated gastric ulcer
RLQ	Appendicitis, PID
LLQ	Diverticulitis, volvulus, PID
Epigastric	Pancreatitis, perforated ulcer
Suprapubic	PID, ruptured appendix or diverticula

RUQ = right upper quadrant; LUQ = left upper quadrant; RLQ = right lower quadrant; LLQ = left lower quadrant; PID = pelvic inflammatory disease.

Table 9-3. Components of a Complete History

Prior episodes	Previous pregnancies
Previous illness	Menstrual history
Previous surgery	Social history
Medications	Family history
Ill contacts	Sexual history
Recent travel	Urinary habits
Weight loss	

2. Examination of the abdomen may reveal **peritoneal signs.**
   a. **Patient remains motionless** with the legs and knees flexed.
   b. **Pain may be increased by**
      —gentle percussion or with any movement.
      —quickly releasing pressure after palpation (**rebound tenderness**).
   c. **Guarding** (voluntary or involuntary)
      —is caused by severe pain and peritoneal inflammation, respectively.
   d. **Rigidity** (local or diffuse)
      —is another significant finding.

C. Rectal examination

—may show fecal impaction, masses, tenderness, or blood.

D. Gynecologic examination

—may reveal masses, cervical motion tenderness, parauterine discomfort, or discharge.

E. Genitalia examination

—in males may show tenderness or masses.

F. Laboratory evaluation

1. **Initial evaluation** should include
   —a complete blood count with differential.
   —urinalysis.
   —amylase.
   —**beta-human chorionic gonadotropin (β-HCG) in women of child-bearing age.**
2. **Assessment of electrolytes and renal function** is also important to identify potential abnormalities in metabolic and hydration status.
3. **Liver function tests** may be necessary with upper abdominal pain or suspected liver or biliary disease.
4. **Chest (posterior–anterior and lateral) and abdominal (upright and supine) radiographs** may frequently provide useful information in the initial evaluation.
5. **Abdominal computed tomography (CT) scanning** is frequently used when the diagnosis is unclear.

IV. Gastroenteritis

A. Overview

1. **Gastroenteritis can be related to** specific food intake or recent respiratory infection.
2. **Often other family members or close contacts** will have a similar illness.

B. Etiologies include

—*Escherichia coli.*

—*Shigella* species.

—*Salmonella* species.

—*Yersinia.*

—*Campylobacter.*

—viruses.

—alcohol.

—drugs.

C. Signs and symptoms include

—**dull, gnawing, epigastric discomfort,** typically lasting 6–12 hours.

—marked **nausea, vomiting, and diarrhea** (usually occurring before the onset of pain).

D. Treatment primarily involves adequate hydration.

V. Appendicitis (see Chapter 13)

A. Overview

1. **Appendicitis most commonly occurs** in patients between 20–35 years of age.
2. In **young children and the elderly** perforation rates are higher because there is generally a delay in the diagnosis, related to a lack of classic findings in these patients.
3. It is the most common cause of an **acute abdomen** in the **second and third trimesters of pregnancy.**

B. Signs and symptoms

1. **Pain**

   —The onset of pain **occurs 3–4 hours before nausea and vomiting,** unlike with gastroenteritis, in which the converse is true. The pain worsens over time.

   —**Visceral, periumbilical pain** may shift to somatic right lower quadrant (RLQ) pain as local peritonitis develops.

2. **Loss of appetite** is common.

3. **Low-grade fever and leukocytosis** with a left shift are common.
4. **High temperatures** may be associated with perforation, but is a nonspecific finding.
   —Chance of perforation 48 hours after onset of pain is 75%.
   —Patients with free perforation frequently have generalized peritonitis.
5. **McBurney's point** will often be the point of maximal tenderness.
   —Patients will generally have guarding, rigidity, and rebound in this area **once local peritonitis develops.**
6. **The psoas sign**
   —indicates inflammation of the psoas muscle beneath the appendix.
   —is elicited when the thigh is flexed against resistance.
7. **The obturator sign**
   —indicates inflammation of the obturator muscle.
   —is elicited when the thigh is flexed and internally rotated.
   —is often positive with a retrocecal appendix.
8. **Rovsing's sign**
   —occurs when the patient feels pain in the RLQ after palpation to the left lower quadrant (LLQ).
9. **A retrocecal appendix**
   —may cause only mild tenderness and rigidity in the RLQ with less nausea and vomiting than usual.
10. **A pelvic appendix**
   —may give rise to minimal abdominal pain but can be painful on rectal examination.

C. Radiographic studies

—are generally unnecessary in uncomplicated appendicitis because the diagnosis is generally based on clinical findings alone.

D. A CT scan or ultrasound

—is sometimes useful when the diagnosis is unclear or when complications are suspected.

E. Definitive therapy

—generally involves appendectomy.

VI. Cholecystitis (see Chapter 16)

A. Overview

1. **In the elderly** there is an increased incidence of bile duct obstruction and cholangitis.
2. **Biliary colic,** secondary to **temporary cystic duct obstruction** from passage of a gallstone, usually resolves after 4–6 hours.

—**Cholecystitis,** however, will progress.

—In addition, fever and leukocytosis are characteristically absent in patients with biliary colic.

B. Major risk factors include

—**obesity.**

—**being female.**

—**age over 40 years.**

—Native American descent.

—rapid weight loss.

—ileal resection.

—total parenteral nutrition (TPN).

C. Signs and symptoms

1. **Signs and symptoms of cholecystitis** include

   —visceral **epigastric pain** that gradually progresses to somatic, **right upper quadrant (RUQ) pain.**

   —**referred pain** to the right shoulder and scapula.

   —**nausea, vomiting,** and **loss of appetite.** Attacks frequently occur after eating, especially a **fatty meal.**

   —**tenderness** and rigidity in the RUQ.

   —**Murphy's sign,** when the patient resists inspiration after deep palpation to the RUQ, secondary to pain.

2. **Patients with acute cholecystitis**

   —can have fever and mild jaundice.

3. **Cholangitis is indicated by Charcot's triad** (fever/chills, RUQ pain, and jaundice).

   a. These findings plus hypotension and mental status changes (**Reynolds pentad**) indicate severe septic shock secondary to cholangitis.

   b. Cholangitis secondary to common duct obstruction requires antibiotics and early surgical or endoscopic intervention to relieve the obstruction.

D. Laboratory evaluation

1. **Leukocytosis with a left shift** is frequently present.

2. **Liver function tests**

   a. **Alkaline phosphatase**

      —is often elevated with obstruction and inflammation of the biliary tree.

   b. **Aspartate aminotransferase** (AST) and **alanine aminotransferase** (ALT) are usually normal or slightly increased.

      —If significantly elevated, primary liver pathology may be present (e.g., hepatitis).

c. **Total bilirubin** higher than 3.0 is associated with a retained common bile duct stone, which will need extraction.

E. **Diagnostic studies**

1. **Ultrasound** can be used to identify

—gallstones.

—gallbladder changes (e.g., wall thickening, pericholecystic fluid).

—bile duct stones.

—primary liver pathology.

2. **Air in the portal system** can indicate **cholangitis** or **erosion of a gallstone** through the gallbladder or biliary system into the gastrointestinal tract.

3. **Hepatobiliary iminodiacetic acid (HIDA) scans**

—can provide images of the liver and biliary tree when the diagnosis of cholecystitis is unclear.

F. **Definitive treatment** generally involves cholecystectomy (see Chapter 16).

VII. Intestinal Obstruction (see Chapter 13)

A. **Causes of bowel obstruction**

1. The most common causes of **large bowel obstruction** are cancer, diverticulitis and volvulus.

2. The most common causes of **small bowel obstruction** are adhesions from prior surgery, hernias, and cancer.

3. **Crohn's disease and ulcerative colitis** can also cause obstruction in addition to fulminant colitis (toxic megacolon).

B. **Signs and symptoms**

1. **General intestinal obstruction**

a. **Symptoms vary according to the**

—**portion of gut involved.** More proximal obstructions are associated with worse symptoms.

—**degree of obstruction** (partial versus complete). Partial obstructions manifest less severe symptoms and may display profuse watery diarrhea but no flatus.

—presence of **complications.**

b. **Pain**

—is intermittent.

—is caused by violent peristalsis at the site of obstruction in an attempt to move intraluminal contents.

c. **Vomiting**

—progresses from bilious to brown intestinal contents to feculent particulate matter the more distal the obstruction.

d. **Bowel ischemia associated with obstruction (strangulation) frequently presents with**

—severe, persistent pain.
—nausea.
—vomiting.
—fever.
—tachycardia.
—leukocytosis.
—Acute rigidity and peritoneal signs **are generally absent unless gangrene or perforation has occurred.**

e. **Shock and signs of massive fluid loss**
—can frequently occur with obstruction.

2. **Small bowel obstruction**
   a. **Pain**
   —is generally a **sudden, severe, colicky type pain in the periumbilical region.**
   (1) The patient may adopt a **flexed body position** in an attempt to alleviate pain.
   (2) **Intensity and frequency of pain paroxysms** are increased with higher obstructions.
   b. **Significant nausea and vomiting**
   —usually occurs.
   (1) Severity depends on the location of the obstruction.
   (2) More proximal obstructions result in increased severity.
   c. **Patients may initially have bowel movements**
   —but will eventually fail to pass flatus or stool.
   d. **Abdominal distension**
   —is generally more severe with more distal obstructions.
3. **Large bowel obstruction**
   a. Patients typically pass no stool or flatus 1–2 days before seeking medical attention.
   —Patient may also give a history of constipation or changed bowel habits in the preceding weeks.
   b. **Colicky, suprapubic pain**
   —is generally minimal until complications occur.
   c. **Nausea and vomiting**
   —**are minimal** until late in the course; however, anorexia is common.
   d. **A history of small caliber and blood-streaked stools** with a history of worsening constipation and weight loss is suggestive of cancer.
   e. Symptoms of a small bowel obstruction
   —can occur with an incompetent ileocecal valve.
   f. Examination will reveal **significant distension and minimal tenderness.**

C. **Laboratory evaluation**
1. **White blood cell count** is usually normal unless perforation or ischemia has occurred.
2. **Laboratory data** may also reveal hypovolemia secondary to dehydration and intestinal "third-spacing" of fluid.

D. Diagnostic studies

1. Abdominal series

a. **Significant findings** include
—multiple air-fluid levels.
—distended loops of large or small bowel.
—distal decompression.

b. **Closed loops**
—as seen with intestinal volvulus are at high risk for rupture.

c. **Cecal diameter** larger than **10–12 cm**
—is a significant risk factor for rupture.

d. **Toxic megacolon** is massive nonmechanical colonic dilation associated with the onset of acute colitis.
—**Perforation is imminent in this situation.**

e. **Pneumatosis intestinalis**
—is air in the bowel wall.
—is associated with ischemia and dissection of air through areas of mucosal injury.

f. **Air in the portal system**
—usually represents infection or necrotic tissue in the large or small bowel.
—is an ominous sign.

2. Contrast studies

a. **A barium or diatrizoate meglumine (Gastrografin) enema**
—can be high yield in large bowel obstruction if the diagnosis is uncertain.
—Ischemic or gangrenous bowel may produce "**thumbprinting**" in the bowel wall.

b. **Swallow studies**
—are usually low yield in the initial evaluation of these patients unless gastric outlet obstruction or duodenal obstruction is suspected.

3. Endoscopy
—can be useful in the diagnosis of large bowel obstruction.
—can also be therapeutic in cases of intestinal volvulus.

E. Treatment depends on the primary cause of obstruction (see Chapters 13 and 14).

VIII. Diverticulitis (see Chapter 14)

A. Overview

1. **Around 90% of diverticula** are found in the sigmoid colon.
2. **Complications occur in 25% of patients with diverticulitis** and include
—**abscess formation** (most common).

—fistula formation.

—perforation.

—obstruction.

B. Signs and symptoms

1. Patients with diverticulitis

—generally have increasing **LLQ pain and constipation** occurring over several days.

—may also have pain on defecation and diarrhea.

—frequently have **chills and a mild fever.**

—infrequently have nausea, vomiting, and anorexia.

2. **Examination reveals**

—tenderness in the LLQ.

—a palpable mass, occasionally.

3. **Complicated cases** may include

—high fever.

—leukocytosis.

—abdominal distension.

—peritoneal signs.

C. Diagnostic studies

1. **CT scan** is necessary if diagnosis is uncertain or complications are suspected.

2. **Barium enema and colonoscopy** are **not recommended during the acute attack** because of the potential risk of perforation.

D. Initial management depends on the presentation (see Chapter 14), while resection of the diseased bowel is definitive therapy.

IX. Volvulus

A. Overview

1. Volvolus is more common in nursing homes and psychiatric facilities.

2. Sigmoid volvulus is more common than cecal volvulus, which is very rare.

B. Risk factors include

—elderly age.

—immobility.

—adhesions.

—pregnancy.

—laxative or enema abuse.

C. Complications include

—perforation and gangrene.

D. **Signs and symptoms**

1. In **nonstrangulated cases**

—the **presentation is similar to diverticulitis.**

—symptoms include **pain, constipation,** and **abdominal distension.**

2. **Strangulation is associated with**

—severe LLQ pain.

—rapid distension.

—obstipation.

3. **Cecal volvulus**

—is associated with an earlier onset of pain.

—frequently presents as a distal small bowel obstruction.

4. **The white blood cell count** can be normal or elevated depending on whether or not a complication, such as ischemia or gangrene, has occurred.

E. **Diagnostic studies**

1. **Plain abdominal radiographs**

—may show a massively dilated colon.

2. **A water soluble contrast enema**

—may show a tapered colon (**"bird's beak"**).

3. **Sigmoidoscopy**

—**can be diagnostic or therapeutic,** with a 75% success rate. Fifty percent of the time, however, the volvulus will recur.

X. Ulcers

A. **Risk factors** include

—**being male** (more common in men).

—smoking.

—alcohol.

—nonsteroidal anti-inflammatory drug (NSAID) use.

—*H. pylori* infection.

—uremia.

—stress (trauma or burns).

—steroids.

—sepsis.

—chemotherapy.

B. **History of antacid use**

—is also suggestive of the diagnosis.

C. Signs and symptoms include

—**epigastric burning and back pain relieved with meals.**

—mild nausea and vomiting with pain.

—melena or guaiac-positive stools.

D. Perforation

—is associated with a 5%–10% mortality.

—can additionally cause pancreatitis or bleeding from the gastroduodenal artery.

1. Initial period

a. Patients generally complain of sudden, sharp, epigastric pain. Other significant findings include

—anxiety.

—pallor.

—vomiting.

—shallow respirations.

b. Patients may attempt to remain motionless, with the supine position providing some relief from pain.

c. Pain

—may radiate to the flanks or lower quadrants if drainage occurs in the colic gutters.

—may rarely be referred to the right shoulder with duodenal perforations and to both shoulders with stomach perforation.

2. An intermediate period

—may occur 2–12 hours after onset, during which the **patient feels better.**

a. Acidic fluid from the perforation

—becomes diluted with leakage from the irritated intestinal wall.

b. Pain

—and nausea subside.

—will still be increased with movement.

c. The abdominal wall

—will still have "board-like" rigidity and tenderness.

3. Late in the course

—(more than 12 hours), renewed nausea and vomiting along with distension, extensive peritoneal signs, and signs of shock can occur as **generalized peritonitis develops.**

E. Diagnostic studies

1. An upright chest radiograph (Figure 9-1) will show **free air 75% of the time** after rupture.

a. Free air is more common with anterior duodenal ruptures.

b. The patient needs to be upright for free air to appear under the diaphragm.

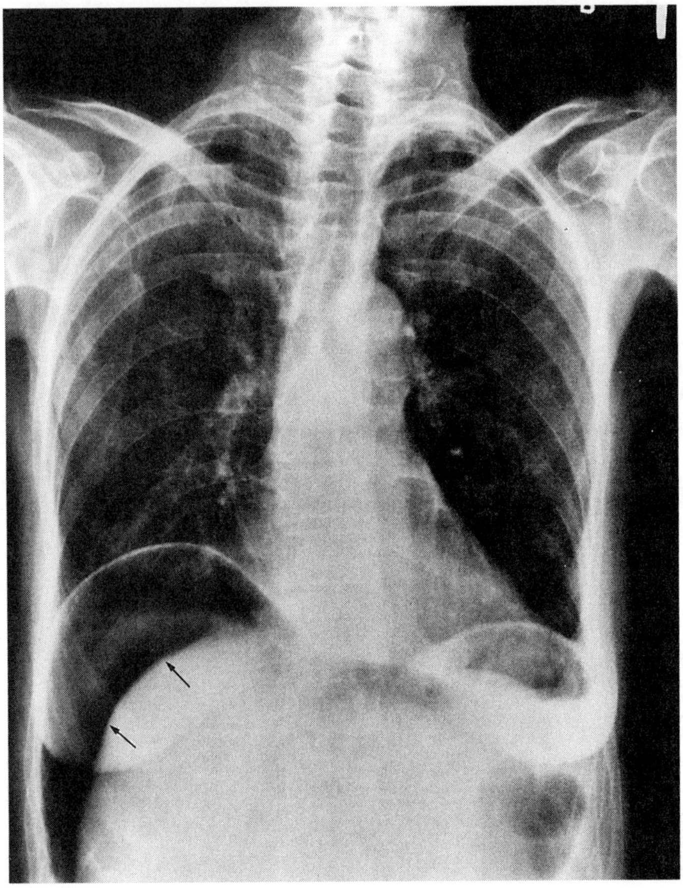

Figure 9-1. Chest radiograph showing air beneath the diaphragm (*arrows* indicate liver edge). (Reprinted with permission from Daffner RH: *Clinical Radiology: The Essentials,* 2nd ed. Baltimore, Williams & Wilkins, 1999, p 267.)

2. **An abdominal series**
   —may also show free air.
3. **A Gastrografin swallow**
   —will show the presence of ulcers and leakage if perforation has occurred, although this is generally not necessary.
4. **Upper endoscopy**
   —may also identify ulcers.

F. **Treatment** depends on the presentation (see Chapter 12).

XI. Pancreatitis (see Chapter 17)

A. **Etiologies** include

—**alcohol and gallstones** (responsible for 90%).

—**trauma.**

—**hyperlipidemia.**

—**hypercalcemia.**

—endoscopic retrograde cholangiopancreatography (ERCP).

—medications (thiazide diuretics, H-2 blockers, erythromycin, tetracycline, acetaminophen, sulfonamides, steroids, and azathioprine).

—scorpion bite (exotic islands).

B. Complications

1. **General complications** include

   —**pseudocyst formation.**

   —**hemorrhage.**

   —**necrosis** of the pancreas (necrotizing pancreatitis).

2. **Significant systemic complications** include

   —coagulopathy.

   —hemorrhage.

   —shock.

   —sepsis.

   —acute respiratory distress syndrome.

C. Morphine should probably be avoided

—for pain relief because it **contracts the sphincter of Oddi,** potentially contributing to obstruction of biliary and pancreatic drainage.

D. Signs and symptoms

1. **Epigastric pain**

   —is usually **sudden, constant, and excruciating.**

   —is referred to the lumbar area and left scapula/shoulder.

   —Patients often have epigastric tenderness and rigidity on examination.

2. **Pain**

   —**can also originate from** the left upper quadrant (LUQ).

   —is generally **exacerbated by food.**

   —**An upright posture** may offer some relief.

3. **Common signs** include

   —fever.

   —anorexia.

   —persistent nausea and vomiting.

4. **Slight jaundice occurs**

   —in 50% secondary to stone obstruction or a swollen pancreas, causing impaired biliary drainage.

5. **Shock**

   —can occur rapidly and massive volume replacement may be necessary.

6. **Grey-Turner sign**

—is associated with hemorrhagic pancreatitis.

—occurs when ecchymosis is found in the flank region.

7. **Cullen's sign**

—is periumbilical ecchymosis caused by hemorrhage.

E. **Laboratory evaluation**

1. **Amylase and lipase** will be elevated in most patients with the exception of some patients with chronic pancreatitis.
2. **Leukocytosis** with a left shift is frequently present.
3. **Hyperglycemia** and hyperlipidemia may also be present.

F. **Diagnostic studies**

1. **CT scan**
   a. **CT scan is necessary when** the diagnosis has not been firmly established and significant complications are felt to have occurred.
   b. Significant findings include **hemorrhage, necrosis,** and **edema.**
2. **Radiographs**

—An abdominal series may show a sentinel loop.

—A left-sided pleural effusion may also be present on chest radiograph.

G. **Treatment** is nonsurgical in most cases (see Chapter 17).

XII. Intestinal Ischemia

A. **Overview**

1. **This anemia characteristically occurs** in the elderly and patients with atherosclerosis, heart disease, arrhythmias, vasculitis, or hypercoagulable syndromes.
2. **The pathogenesis involves**

—embolization.

—thrombosis.

—low flow states.

a. **Patients suffering from embolization often have a history of**

—**atrial flutter/fibrillation.**

—endocarditis.

—angiography.

—recent myocardial infarction.

b. **Patients with low flow states usually have a history of**

—prolonged shock.

—prolonged heart bypass procedure.

—myocardial infarction.

—congestive heart failure.

—prolonged bowel wall distension.

—strangulated hernia.

—use of digoxin (causes splanchnic vasoconstriction).

B. Signs and symptoms

1. The **most common complaints** are

   —**midabdominal pain.**

   —**bright red rectal bleeding.**

   —diarrhea.

   —vomiting.

2. **Patients with atherosclerotic thrombosis** may have

   —**food fear** secondary to pain after eating (intestinal angina).

   —associated **weight loss.**

3. **Venous occlusion occurs** most often in **hypercoagulable syndromes.**

4. **Pain is often out of proportion to physical examination findings** early on.

5. **The bowel wall** can rapidly become **gangrenous.**

   —At this time **perforation** and **peritonitis** will occur, followed by shock.

6. **Leukocytosis**

   —suggests that tissue necrosis or perforation have occurred.

C. Diagnostic studies

1. **CT scan can show**

   —bowel wall thickening.

   —intramural gas.

   —portal venous gas.

   —vascular occlusion.

2. **Early angiography**

   —is essential to confirm the diagnosis and plan operative intervention.

XIII. Aortic Dissection (see *BRS Surgical Specialties,* Chapter 2)

A. Risk factors include

—hypertension.

—Marfan's syndrome.

—atherosclerosis.

—coarctation.

B. Complications include

—cardiac tamponade.

—aortic insufficiency.

—occlusion of aortic branches.

—tearing or occlusion of coronary arteries.

—aortic rupture.

—The majority of complications are caused by **ascending aortic dissections.**

C. Signs and symptoms

1. Pain

—is **usually tearing-like and severe.**

—usually migrates from the **chest and back to the abdomen.**

2. Patients may have

—unequal pulses.

—blood pressure in the upper extremities.

—associated hemiplegia or paraplegia.

—new heart murmurs.

D. Diagnostic studies

1. **CT scan** will almost always show the dissection.

2. **Aortogram and transesophageal echocardiography** may also be useful.

E. Management

—Because hypertension is frequently present and can lead to continued dissection and rupture, **early blood pressure control** with **nitrates or β blockers** is essential.

XIV. Abdominal Aortic Aneurysm (AAA)

—Mortality with rupture is approximately 40%–50%.

A. Risk factors include

—atherosclerosis.

—hypertension.

—being male.

—smoking.

—family history.

—elderly age.

B. Signs and symptoms

1. A **palpable abdominal mass** is common.

2. Patients may have **profound hypotension or shock** if rupture has occurred.

3. Patients are **usually asymptomatic;** however, they may have a history of progressively increasing **abdominal or back pain.**

C. **Diagnostic studies**

1. **It should be emphasized that patients should be taken directly to surgery without diagnostic studies if they have**

—**hypotension.**

—**abdominal pain.**

—**a pulsating abdominal mass or a history of an AAA.**

2. **CT scan**

—gives a very accurate measurement of the size of the aneurysm.

3. **Ultrasound**

—can provide a rapid diagnosis in urgent situations.

XV. Obstetric/Gynecologic Causes of Acute Abdominal Pain

A. Several **gynecologic and obstetrical causes of acute abdominal pain** are listed in Table 9-4.

B. **Ultrasound** is effective in diagnosing disorders of the female reproductive tract.

C. **Pain accompanying menstrual period** is suspicious for threatened early abortion or tubal gestation.

D. **Pelvic inflammatory disease** (PID)

1. **A significant risk factor**

—is numerous sexual partners.

2. **This disease commonly occurs**

—in the first half of the menstrual cycle.

3. **Complications of PID** include

—persistent pelvic pain.

Table 9-4. Gynecologic and Obstetrical Causes of Acute Abdominal Pain

Gynecologic Causes	Pain Related to Pregnancy
Pelvic inflammatory disease (PID)	Ruptured uterus
Endometriosis	Ovarian torsion
Ectopic pregnancy	Splenic artery aneurysm rupture
Ovarian tumor, torsion, cyst, or abscess	Placental abruption
Rupture of follicular or luteal cyst	Ectopic pregnancy
Mittelschmerz	Normal intrauterine pregnancy
Pelvic adhesions	Miscarriage
Vaginitis	Endometritis
Uterine fibroids	Pulmonary embolism
Menstrual cramps	Urologic infections

—infertility.

—ectopic pregnancy.

4. **Patients commonly have**

—hypogastric pain.

—fever.

—nausea and vomiting.

—vaginal discharge.

5. **Cervical cultures**

—frequently demonstrate the causative organisms.

6. **Adnexal and cervical motion tenderness**

—are common (**chandelier sign**).

E. **Ectopic pregnancy**

1. **Risk factors** include

—previous tubal manipulation.

—PID.

—previous ectopic pregnancy.

2. **Patients may have**

—a history of a **missed period.**

—pain and abnormal uterine bleeding (most common complaints). Pain is usually sharp and persistent without associated vomiting.

3. **Because significant hemorrhage and shock can occur**

—this diagnosis should always be considered when evaluating a premenopausal female with abdominal pain.

4. **Pelvic examination may show**

—blood.

—an enlarged uterus.

—cervical motion tenderness.

—a blue-tinged cervix.

5. An **ultrasound** may also be useful for confirming the presence of an intrauterine pregnancy.

XVI. Urologic Causes of Acute Abdominal Pain (see *BRS Surgical Specialties,* Chapter 6)

A. **Infection**

1. **Potential sources of pain** include

—pyelonephritis.

—cystitis.

—urethritis.

2. **Symptoms**

—Fever and dysuria are common.

—**Costovertebral tenderness** is typical of pyelonephritis.

3. **Urinalysis may demonstrate the presence of**

—**nitrates.**

—**leukocyte esterase.**

—**bacteria.**

—**white blood cells.**

—minimal hematuria.

B. **Kidney stones**

1. **Signs and symptoms** include

—**severe colicky-type pain due to ureteral obstruction.**

—extreme **restlessness** secondary to the pain.

2. **Urinalysis**

—usually shows **stones or hematuria.**

3. **Intrascrotal causes of acute abdominal pain** include

—associated testicular tenderness and pain from trauma.

—venous thrombosis.

—epididymitis.

—seminal vesiculitis.

—Testicular torsion may be present.

XVII. Abdominal Pain in Pediatric Populations (Table 9-5)

Table 9-5. Causes of Acute Abdominal Pain in Infants and Children

Intussusception	Urologic causes
Pyloric stenosis	Viral/bacterial enteritis
Meconium ileus	Appendicitis
Necrotizing enterocolitis	Strangulated hernia
Hirschsprung's disease	Trauma
Malrotation	Child abuse
Volvulus (midgut)	Poisoning
Gastroesophageal reflux disease	Psychosomatic illness
Incarcerated hernia	Mesenteric cysts
Meckel's diverticulum	Pancreatitis
Annular pancreas	Pneumonia
Small bowel atresia	Ruptured tumors
Duodenal webs/bands	Inflammatory bowel disease
Gastric/intestinal duplication syndromes	

XVIII. Nonsurgical Causes of Abdominal Pain (Table 9-6)

Table 9-6. Other Causes of Acute Abdominal Pain Not Requiring Surgery

Cardiac	Myocardial infarction (typically inferior), pericarditis
Pulmonary	Pneumonia, pulmonary embolism, pneumothorax, empyema
Other thoracic	Reflux disease
Endocrine	Adrenal insufficiency, diabetic ketoacidosis
Metabolic	Acute intermittent porphyria, uremia, hypercalcemia
Toxic	Venom from snakes and scorpions, lead poisoning, drugs, alcohol
Hematologic	Hemolytic crisis (sickle cell anemia), rectus sheath hematoma (warfarin use)
Neurogenic	Herpes zoster, spinal cord/nerve root compression from tumor or abscess, tabes dorsalis
Infection	Gastroenteritis, pseudomembranous colitis, hepatitis, spontaneous bacterial peritonitis, tuberculosis peritonitis, malaria, numerous bacterial/viral infections
Congenital	Familial Mediterranean fever
Musculoskeletal	Vertebral compression of abdominal wall nerves
Vascular	Splenic infarction

Review Test

Directions: Each of the numbered items or incomplete statements in this section is followed by answers or by completions of the statement. Select the ONE lettered answer or completion that is BEST in each case.

1. A 65-year-old woman with a long history of atrial fibrillation presents to the emergency department with a history of sudden onset of constant, severe abdominal pain. After the onset of the pain, she vomited once and had a large bowel movement. No flatus has passed since that time. Her vital signs are: heart rate, 124 beats/min (irregular); respiration, 18/min; blood pressure, 140/60 mm Hg; temperature, 38.0°C. Physical examination reveals a mildly distended abdomen that is mildly tender diffusely. There are no peritoneal signs. Electrocardiogram reveals the patient to be in atrial fibrillation but otherwise normal. Chest radiograph is unremarkable. Ten years ago, this patient underwent a vaginal hysterectomy. Which of the following would be most appropriate in the subsequent evaluation of this patient?

(A) Abdominal ultrasound
(B) Upper gastrointestinal endoscopy
(C) Abdominal computed tomography scan
(D) Mesenteric vessel arteriogram
(E) Upper gastrointestinal contrast study

2. A 44-year-old, obese woman presents to the emergency department with a history of acute onset of severe epigastric pain radiating toward the back. The pain began several hours after dinner. The patient has no significant past medical history and denies any previous surgery. She takes no medications. On examination, the patient has marked epigastric tenderness with guarding and hypoactive bowel sounds. Her vital signs are: heart rate, 110 beats/min; blood pressure, 120/50 mm Hg; respiration, 28/min; temperature, 38.0°C. Amylase level is 2500 units. Which of the following is the most likely cause of this patient's pain?

(A) Gallstones
(B) Alcohol abuse
(C) Hyperparathyroidism
(D) Hyperlipidemia
(E) Peptic ulcer disease

3. A 40-year-old man presents with significant right flank pain radiating down to his testicle. The pain is intermittent and severe in nature. Microscopic hematuria is present on urinalysis, but there are no white blood cells. Leukocyte esterase and nitrates are negative. His vital signs are: heart rate, 88 beats/min; blood pressure, 130/60 mm Hg; respiration, 20/min; temperature, 37.2°C. Which of the following is the most appropriate next step in the management of this patient?

(A) Intravenous antibiotics
(B) Immediate laparotomy
(C) Intravenous fluids and pain medication
(D) Computed tomography (CT) scan of the abdomen
(E) Immediate orchiopexy

4. A 50-year-old woman presents to the emergency department with abdominal pain and jaundice. Her vital signs are: heart rate, 80 beats/min; blood pressure, 130/72 mm Hg; respiration, 18/min; temperature, 37.0°C. Examination reveals tenderness in the right upper quadrant (RUQ) and a positive Murphy's sign. Which of the following statements regarding this patient is true?

(A) Referred pain would likely be to the right shoulder or scapula.
(B) This disease is characterized by Charcot's triad.
(C) Jaundice is rarely present in these patients.
(D) Etiology of the pain would likely be present on abdominal film.
(E) Morphine is the most appropriate analgesic to use in this patient.

5. A 23-year-old man presents to the emergency department complaining of scrotal pain. The pain began 4 days ago but has gradually worsened. The patient now feels hot and his scrotum is too tender to allow for examination. His vital signs are: heart rate, 90 beats/min; respiration, 20/min; blood pressure, 120/60 mm Hg; temperature, 38.5°C. Which of the following is the most likely diagnosis?

(A) Testicular torsion
(B) Hydrocele
(C) Epididymitis
(D) Urethritis
(E) Spermatocele

6. A 50-year-old woman presents to the emergency room with ripping chest pain that is now radiating into the abdomen. The patient has unequal pulses in the upper extremities. Her vital signs are: heart rate, 125 beats/min; respiration, 20/min; temperature, 36.5°C. Which of the following statements is true?

(A) The patient will most likely be hypotensive on presentation.
(B) S-T segment elevation in the anterior leads is diagnostic.
(C) Coronary artery disease is the likely etiology of the pain.
(D) Magnetic resonance imaging of the chest is usually used to make the diagnosis.
(E) A new heart murmur can be associated with this disease.

7. A 60-year-old man presents to the emergency room with sudden abdominal pain and an expanding, pulsatile abdominal mass on examination. His vital signs are: heart rate, 130 beats/min; blood pressure, 70/20 mm Hg; respiration, 30/min; temperature, 36.0°C. Which of the following is the most appropriate next step in the management of this patient?

(A) Emergency computed tomography (CT) of the abdomen
(B) Emergency CT of the chest
(C) Emergency aortogram
(D) Emergency laparotomy
(E) Volume resuscitation and observation

Directions: Each set of matching questions in this section consists of a list of four to twenty-six lettered options followed by several numbered items. For each numbered item, select the appropriate lettered option(s). Each lettered option may be selected once, more than once, or not at all.

Questions 8–12

(A) Small bowel obstruction
(B) Large bowel obstruction
(C) Cholecystitis
(D) Ureteral calculi
(E) Pyelonephritis
(F) Pancreatitis

For each clinical description, select the most likely diagnosis(es).

8. A 39-year-old man presents to the emergency room with severe vomiting and increasing abdominal pain. Abdominal radiograph shows multiple dilated loops of small bowel and air-fluid levels throughout the abdomen. The patient underwent an emergent splenectomy 1 year ago after a motor vehicle accident. (SELECT 1 DIAGNOSIS)

9. A 48-year-old woman presents to the emergency room with severe epigastric pain radiating to the lumbar area. The pain is somewhat relieved with upright posture. The patient has had severe nausea and vomiting since the onset of pain. Chest and abdominal films are unremarkable. Urinalysis is normal. (SELECT 2 DIAGNOSES)

10. A 60-year-old man presents with epigastric pain after eating. The pain seems to radiate to the right scapula. Examination reveals tenderness in the epigastric area, but no rebound or guarding are present. Amylase and lipase are normal. Chest and abdominal films are unremarkable. (SELECT 1 DIAGNOSIS)

11. A 35-year-old man presents with flank pain radiating to the ipsilateral testicle. The pain came on suddenly 2 hours ago. Urinalysis shows red blood cells. Chest and abdominal films are unremarkable. Laboratory values are unremarkable. Vital signs are normal. (SELECT 1 DIAGNOSIS)

12. A 65-year-old man presents with gradually increasing abdominal pain and obstipation over the past several weeks. The patient denies any nausea or vomiting. Vital signs are normal. Examination reveals abdominal distension and guaiac-positive stools. (SELECT 1 DIAGNOSIS)

Questions 13–16

(A) Take the patient to the operating room.
(B) Admit for medical treatment and observation.
(C) Perform an abdominal ultrasound.
(D) Perform a computed tomography (CT) scan of the chest and abdomen.
(E) Perform a magnetic resonance imaging scan of the abdomen.
(F) Discharge the patient with close follow-up.

For each clinical scenario, select the most appropriate management plan(s).

13. A 65-year-old man presents to the emergency room with abdominal pain for the past 12 hours. The patient has nausea and has vomited once. The patient also has anorexia. On examination, a midline abdominal scar is noted and the pain is noted to be poorly localized. Plain films show some air–fluid levels but there is air and stool distally. The small bowel appears dilated. (SELECT 1 MANAGEMENT PLAN)

14. A 45-year-old man presents with nausea and vomiting 1 hour after eating. The patient now has developed dull, epigastric discomfort, and watery diarrhea 5 hours later, although the vomiting has ceased and the patient is able to drink liquids. Abdominal films and labs are unremarkable. Past medical history is unremarkable and the patient does not take any medications. The patient tells you that his daughter has also started having diarrhea. (SELECT 1 MANAGEMENT PLAN)

15. A 60-year-old man presents with tearing-like chest pain radiating to his back and abdomen. Electrocardiogram is normal. The patient is hypertensive and tachycardic but is otherwise alert and oriented. (SELECT 1 MANAGEMENT PLAN)

16. A 54-year-old woman with a past medical history significant for ulcerative colitis presents to the emergency room with severe abdominal pain, rebound, guarding, and abdominal distention. Supine plain films show a transverse colon diameter of 13 cm. (SELECT 1 MANAGEMENT PLAN)

Answers and Explanations

1-D. The triad of a cardiac arrhythmia, sudden onset of severe abdominal pain, and gut emptying is classic for embolic mesenteric ischemia. This patient's pain is also out of proportion to the physical examination, another classic sign of mesenteric ischemia. In this setting, the most appropriate initial diagnostic study should be an arteriogram of the mesenteric arterial supply to characterize the extent and location of disease. Abdominal ultrasound, computed tomography scanning, and upper endoscopy are useful in other situations in which the clinical findings are more subtle or suggestive of other specific intra-abdominal diagnoses.

2-A. The history, physical examination, and elevated amylase are all consistent with pancreatitis. Gallstones and alcohol account for 90% of the cases of pancreatitis in the United States. A high amylase level (over 1000) suggests gallstones over alcohol abuse. Age in the 40s, being female, and obesity are also risk factors for gallstones. Hyperparathyroidism and hyperlipidemia are rare causes of pancreatitis. A ruptured peptic ulcer could present in a similar manner but the elevated amylase suggests pancreatitis. A history of epigastric discomfort or antacid use would also suggest ulcer disease.

3-C. Urinary tract calculi classically present with flank pain that is colicky in nature with radiation to the ipsilateral testicle and red blood cells and stones in the urine. Appropriate treatment of an initial episode of this disease generally involves administering intravenous fluids to assure appropriate hydration and to provide adequate pain control [e.g., nonsteroidal anti-inflammatory drugs (NSAIDs)] during passage of the stone. Ultrasound and intravenous pyelogram (IVP) are the tests of choice in diagnosing patients with recurrent or complicated urinary tract stones. A computed tomography scan could also show stones but is not as sensitive as ultrasound or IVP. The patient's clinical presentation, in addition to the urinalysis findings of no white blood cells, nitrates, leukocyte esterase, or bacteria, makes infection possible, but less likely. Immediate orchiopexy would be appropriate if testicular torsion were suspected. This generally presents with acute abdominal pain and extreme tenderness in the affected testicle.

4-A. Cholecystitis is caused when a gallstone is impacted in the cystic duct. Referred pain is to the right shoulder and scapula. Jaundice may be present, despite the fact that there is no obstruction of the common bile duct. Charcot's triad is associated with ascending cholangitis, which results from bacterial infection of the biliary tree after a gallstone is impacted in the common bile duct. Only 15% of gallstones are radio-opaque, thus an abdominal film is not likely to show the etiology of the pain. Morphine should probably be avoided in patients with cholecystitis as it theoretically contracts the sphincter of Oddi, which will prevent stone passage and possibly increase the risk of complications such as pancreatitis.

5-C. This patient most likely has acute epididymitis. The patient does not complain of penile discharge or dysuria, making urethritis less likely. Spermatocele and hydrocele are generally not associated with testicular tenderness. Testicular torsion can present with severe testicular pain and is a surgical emergency. However, torsion is generally associated with a more acute onset of pain (within minutes to hours) and is not commonly associated with fever.

6-E. Thoracic aortic dissection is most commonly a complication of hypertension. Patients most commonly present with hypertension and chest pain radiating to the back, although dissections involving the lower thoracic or abdominal aorta may also cause abdominal pain. S-T segment changes can occur with aortic dissections, but are not diagnostic because they may also occur with myocardial infarction. Coronary artery disease can present with similar chest pain in addition to abdominal pain, although this scenario is most likely associated with aortic dissection. A computed tomography (CT) scan of the chest or aortogram are usually used to make the diagnosis. Magnetic resonance imaging could also make the diagnosis but is generally too time consuming in this setting. New heart murmurs may occur with ascending aortic dissections, causing aortic valve incompetence.

7-D. The triad of acute abdominal pain, a pulsatile abdominal mass, and hypotension is classic for a ruptured abdominal aortic aneurysm (AAA). This patient should be taken to the operating room immediately. Performing a computed tomography (CT) scan or aortogram in this situation would only delay definitive operative treatment and is not indicated in this patient.

8-A. A small bowel obstruction characteristically presents with nausea, vomiting, abdominal pain, and eventually failure to pass stool or gas. Adhesions after surgery are the most common cause of small bowel obstruction in the United States. Abdominal films typically show multiple fluid levels. The clinical presentation in association with a history of previous abdominal surgery is more consistent with a small bowel obstruction than a large bowel obstruction.

9-C, F. Gallstones and alcohol are the major causes of pancreatitis. These patients typically present with severe epigastric pain radiating to the lumbar area or left shoulder and with nausea, vomiting, and anorexia. Pain is sometimes relieved with upright posture. Amylase is generally elevated in these patients. Cholecystitis may also present with similar signs and symptoms. These patients frequently have an elevated alkaline phosphatase. Biliary ultrasound is often diagnostic.

10-C. Cholecystitis is caused by gallstones and typically presents with vague epigastric pain that eventually progresses to somatic pain in the right upper quadrant (RUQ). Alkaline phosphatase is generally elevated. Pancreatitis can present with epigastric pain; however, amylase is usually elevated.

11-D. Ureteral calculi typically present with severe pain in the flank region with radiation to the ipsilateral testicle. Urinalysis generally shows hematuria and possibly stones or crystals. Pyelonephritis could present with flank pain; however, these patients generally have a fever along with red and white blood cells in their urine. The pain from pyelonephritis is gradual in nature and is not as acute as that found with ureteral calculi.

12-B. Large bowel obstructions typically present with gradually increasing abdominal distension and eventual failure to pass gas or stool. Abdominal films commonly show dilated loops of large bowel, and possibly dilated loops of small bowel, depending on whether or not the ileocecal valve is competent. Cancer is the most common cause of large bowel obstruction. A history of guaiac-positive stools and obstipation is very suspicious for adenocarcinoma of the colon.

13-B. Nausea, vomiting, anorexia, and abdominal pain associated with air–fluid levels on abdominal plain film are signs of small bowel obstruction. The presence of stool and air distal to the site of obstruction is suggestive of a partial obstruction. In some patients with a partial small bowel obstruction and previous abdominal surgery, a course of inpatient management with bowel rest, volume resuscitation, and nasogastric tube decompression may be attempted. No additional diagnostic tests are necessary at this time.

14-F. Nausea and vomiting preceding abdominal pain, watery diarrhea, and epigastric discomfort following a meal is classic for gastroenteritis. Often, other family members will have similar symptoms. In this setting additional diagnostic tests are unnecessary. Computed tomography (CT) scan and ultrasound of the abdomen are likely to be poor yield in this patient. This patient does not require immediate surgery. Whether or not to discharge or admit a patient to the hospital can be a difficult decision. Because the patient is able to tolerate liquids, outpatient management with close follow-up is appropriate.

15-D. This patient may potentially have a dissection of the thoracic aorta descending into the abdomen. A computed tomography (CT) scan of the chest or an aortogram are appropriate diagnostic studies for confirming a dissection, although a transesophageal echocardiogram can also provide for excellent visualization of this portion of the aorta and may frequently be used to diagnose a suspected thoracic aortic dissection. Surgery and admission to the hospital may eventually be necessary; however, a diagnostic study is the most appropriate next step. Ultrasound could possibly detect a dissection but it is not as sensitive as the other studies noted.

16-A. This patient most likely has toxic megacolon. This is a complication of ulcerative colitis and is manifested by rapid distention, usually of the transverse colon. Initial management of uncomplicated toxic megacolon includes aggressive fluid resuscitation and administration of steroids. However, when associated with signs and symptoms of peritonitis or perforation, this becomes a surgical emergency. No further diagnostic studies are necessary at this point, based on the patient's medical history and current abdominal findings.

10

Hernias and Lesions of the Abdominal Wall

Traves D. Crabtree

I. Overview

A. An abdominal hernia

—is generally defined as a congenital or acquired defect in the fascia and musculature of the abdominal wall that may allow for protrusion of a peritoneal sac and structures within the peritoneum (e.g., bowel).

B. Epidemiology

1. **The overall prevalence**

   —of spontaneous abdominal wall hernias is approximately 5%–10% over a lifetime.

2. **The distribution of hernias**

   a. **Inguinal hernias**

   —**account for 80%** of all spontaneous hernias.

   b. **Umbilical hernias**

   —account for approximately 15% of all hernias.

   c. **Femoral hernias**

   —account for approximately 5%.

   d. All **other types of hernias** are very rare.

C. Definitions

1. **A hernia is reducible**

   —when the **contents of the hernia sac (e.g., intestines) can be returned to their normal anatomic domain**.

2. **A hernia is incarcerated**

—**when the contents of the hernia sac cannot be reduced,** trapping the contents of the hernia sac.

—Incarceration can lead to intestinal obstruction in the absence of ischemia.

3. **A strangulated hernia**

—results when the contents of an incarcerated hernia become **ischemic** secondary to tissue swelling and compromise of the blood supply.

4. **A sliding hernia (Figure 10-1)**

—occurs when the **hernia sac is partially formed by the wall of an organ** without peritoneal covering (e.g., posterior cecum, ovary, bladder, sigmoid).

5. **A Richter hernia (Figure 10-2)**

—represents a **partial herniation** of the antimesenteric wall **of the intestine**.

a. This **rare hernia can result in**

—**strangulation and necrosis in the absence of intestinal obstruction**.

b. This is a **dangerous hernia**

—because inadvertent reduction of the necrotic segment during hernia repair may result in **perforation** and **peritonitis.**

6. A **hernia sac** may rarely contain a **Meckel's diverticulum (Littré's hernia**).

—These hernias are similar to Richter's hernias in that strangulation and necrosis can occur in the absence of intestinal obstruction.

D. Anatomy of the abdominal wall (Figure 10-3)

1. **The rectus sheath**

—Superiorly in the midline of the abdomen the rectus abdominis muscles are ensheathed in a thick anterior and posterior fascia known as the **rectus sheath**.

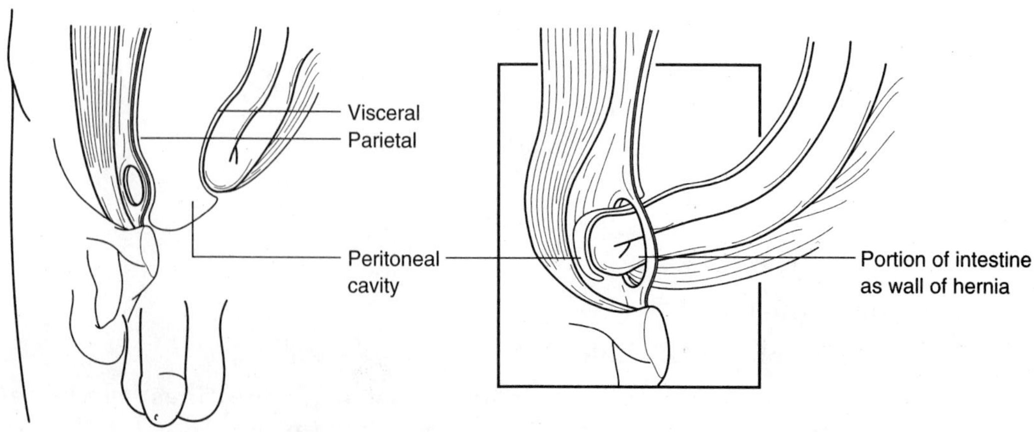

Figure 10-1. Right-sided sliding inguinal hernia. (Adapted with permission from Way LW: *Current Surgical Diagnosis and Treatment,* 10th ed. Stamford, CT, Appleton & Lange, 1994, p 717.)

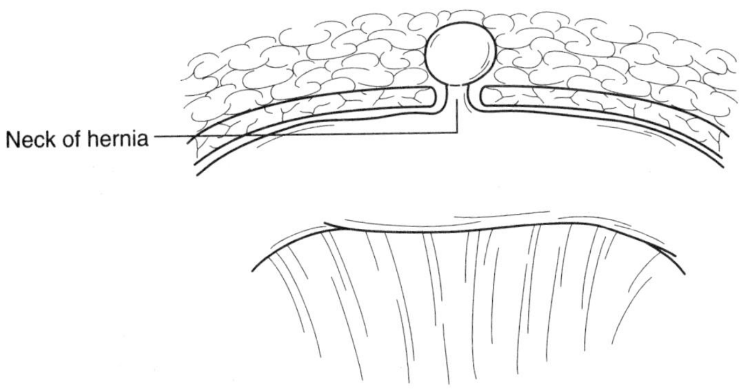

Figure 10-2. Richter hernia. (Adapted with permission from Greenfield L: *Surgery: Scientific Principles and Practice,* 2nd ed. Philadelphia, Lippincott Williams & Wilkins, 1997, p 1218.)

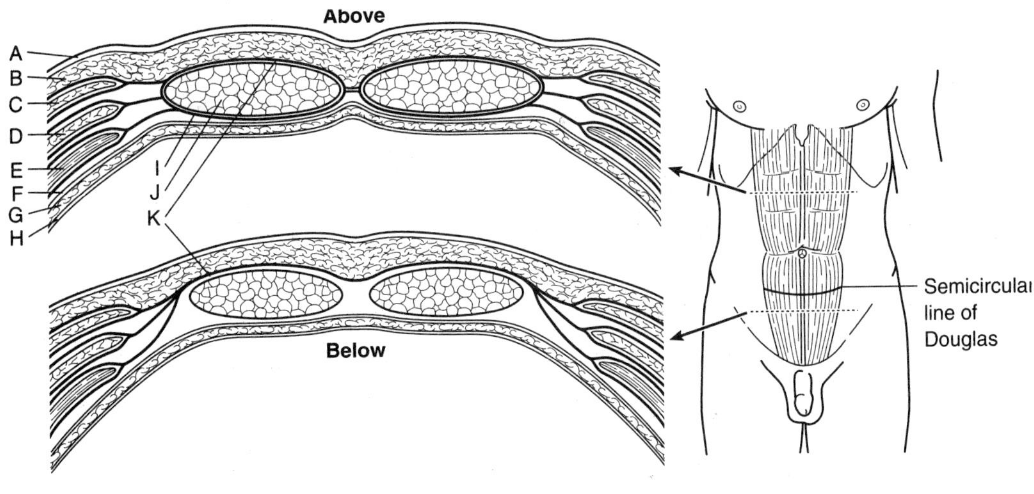

Figure 10-3. Fascial layers of the abdominal wall. *Above* and *Below* indicate placement about the semicircular line of Douglas. *A* = skin; *B* = subcutaneous fat; *C* = external oblique muscle; *D* = internal oblique muscle; *E* = transversus abdominis muscle; *F* = transversalis fascia; *G* = preperitoneal fat; *H* = peritoneum; *I* = posterior layer of rectus sheath; *J* = rectus abdominis muscle; *K* = anterior layer of rectus sheath. (Adapted with permission from Lippincott Williams & Wilkins. Gray and Skandalakis: *Atlas of Surgical Anatomy for General Surgeons.* Baltimore, Williams & Wilkins, 1985, p 91.)

2. Above the semicircular line of Douglas

a. The **anterior rectus sheath**

—is composed of the aponeurosis of the external oblique muscle and the anterior aponeurosis of the internal oblique.

b. The **posterior rectus sheath**

—is composed of the aponeurosis of the transversalis muscle and the posterior aponeurosis of the internal oblique.

3. Below the semicircular line of Douglas

—all of the aponeuroses join to form the anterior rectus sheath with no fascia covering the rectus muscles posteriorly.

II. Inguinal Hernias

A. Overview

1. Inguinal hernias

—occur with a **male predominance (7:1)**.

2. The pathogenesis

—of inguinal hernias is incompletely understood.

a. A **persistently patent processus vaginalis**
—may contribute to the pathogenesis of indirect inguinal hernias.

b. Other **contributing factors** may include
—intrinsic abnormalities of collagen formation.
—chronic trauma.
—overstretching of fascial layers.
—chronic increases in intra-abdominal pressure (e.g., chronic cough or obstipation associated with an obstructing colon cancer).

B. Anatomy of the inguinal canal (Figure 10-4)

1. Indirect inguinal hernias

—**originate at the deep inguinal ring.**
—are most frequently located anteromedial to the cord structures.
—pass **lateral to the inferior epigastric vessels**.

2. Direct inguinal hernias

—occur directly through the abdominal wall without passing through the deep inguinal ring (see Figure 10-4*B*).

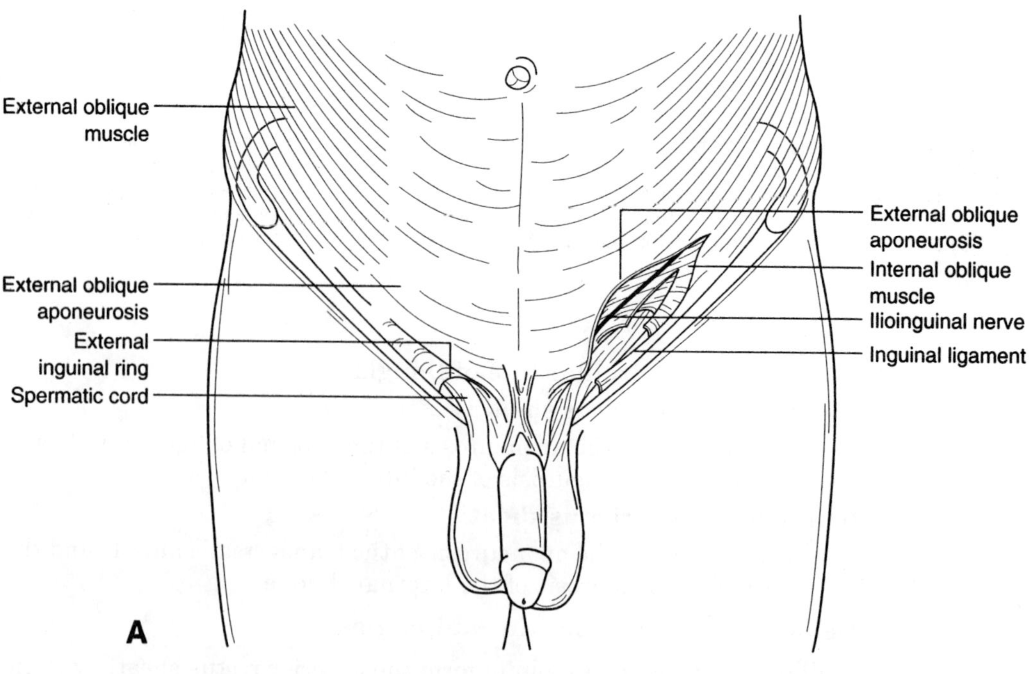

Figure 10-4. Anatomy of the inguinal region. (*A*) Superficial layer of the inguinal region.

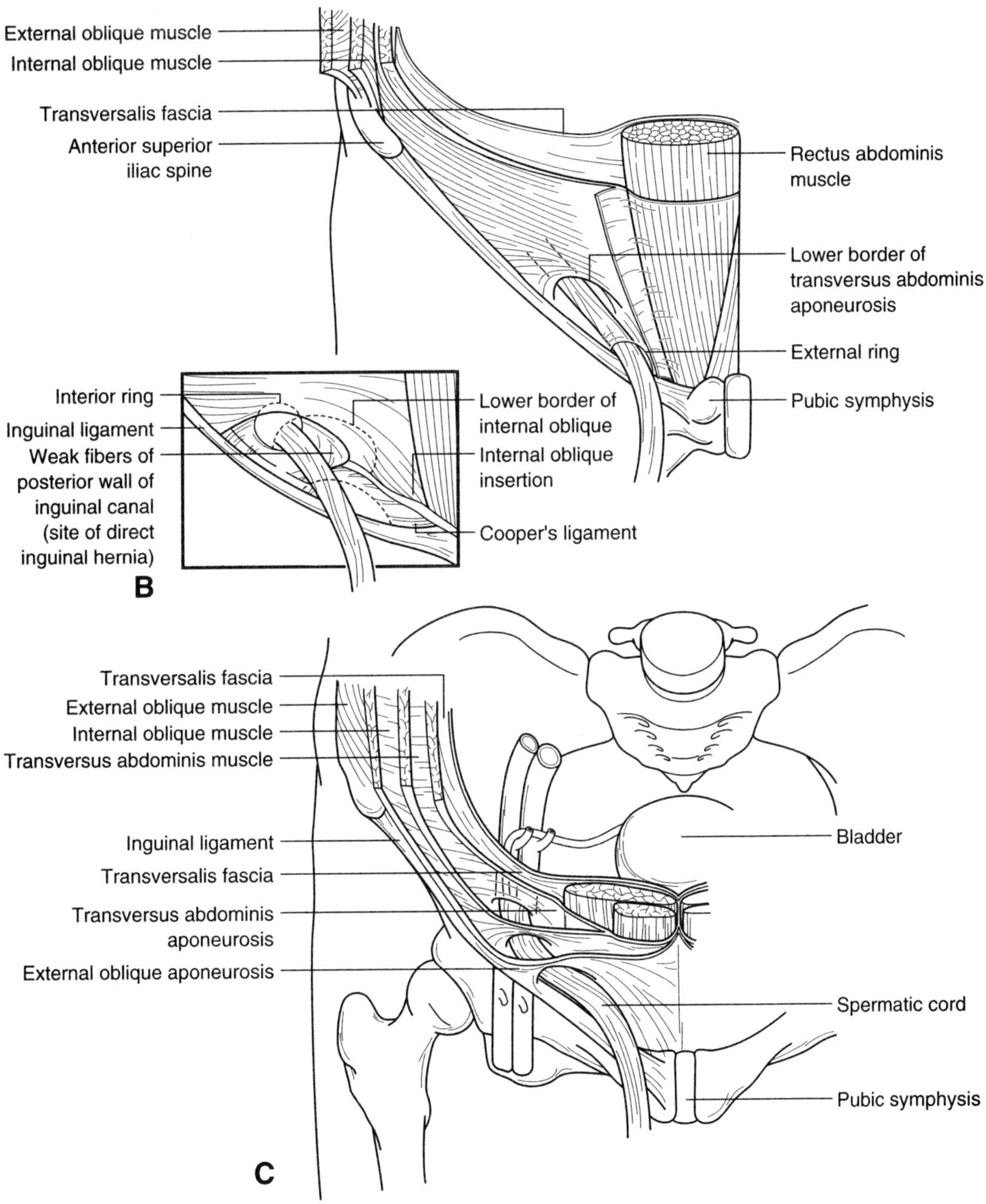

Figure 10-4 (*continued*). (*B*) Deep layers with external oblique fascia removed. (*C*) View of all fascial layers as the cord traverses the inguinal canal. (Adapted with permission from Lippincott Williams & Wilkins. Gray and Skandalakis: *Atlas of Surgical Anatomy for General Surgeons*. Baltimore, Williams & Wilkins, 1985, pp 93–95.)

a. Direct hernias occur through Hesselbach's triangle (Figure 10-5), and are bound

—medially by the lateral border of the rectus.

—laterally by the inferior epigastric vessel.

—inferiorly by the inguinal ligament (Poupart's ligament).

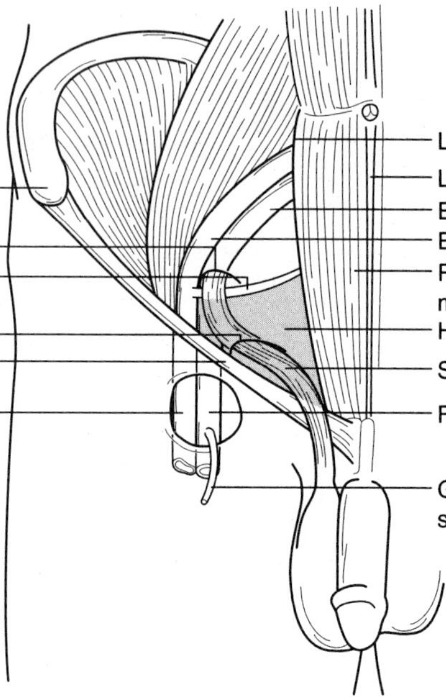

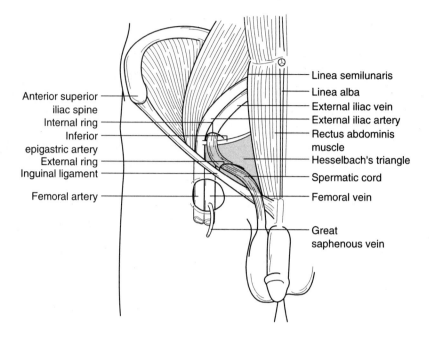

Figure 10-5. Hesselbach's triangle. (Adapted with permission from Lippincott Williams & Wilkins. Gray and Skandalakis: *Atlas of Surgical Anatomy for General Surgeons.* Baltimore, Williams & Wilkins, 1985, p 96.)

b. **Direct hernias pass**
—**medial to the inferior epigastric vessels.**

3. **A pantaloon hernia**
—is characterized by a hernia with **both a direct and an indirect component,** surrounding the inferior epigastric vessels.

4. **The conjoined tendon**
—is composed of the medial aponeuroses of the internal oblique and transversus abdominis muscles.
—runs along the inferolateral border of the rectus muscle to attach to the pubic tubercle.
—A true conjoined tendon only occurs in approximately 25% of individuals.

C. **Risk factors** include
—advancing age.
—severe obesity.
—heavy exercise or lifting.
—chronic cough associated with chronic obstructive pulmonary disease (COPD).
—chronic constipation (e.g., associated with an obstructing colon cancer).
—chronic straining for urination (e.g., benign prostatic hyperplasia).
—ascites.

—pregnancy.

—peritoneal dialysis.

D. Signs and symptoms

1. Many hernias are **asymptomatic** and **are found during routine physical examination**.
2. **Other signs** include

   —a nontender groin mass.

   —sudden onset of a painful mass after straining.

   —scrotal pain or discomfort.
3. **Hernias may present**

   —with signs and symptoms of a small bowel obstruction.
4. **Indirect hernias**

   —are more likely to become incarcerated or strangulated compared with direct hernias.

E. Diagnosis

—of a hernia is based on identification during **physical examination.**

1. **No other specific diagnostic tests** are required for the diagnosis.

   —**Fever and or leukocytosis,** along with abdominal pain, **may suggest the presence of strangulation** of bowel.
2. In general, it is **difficult to distinguish**

   —a direct hernia from an indirect hernia on physical examination.
3. The **differential diagnosis** may include

   —femoral hernia.

   —lipoma of the spermatic cord.

   —hydrocele of the cord (may transilluminate on examination).

   —communicating hydrocele.

   —congenital undescended testis (absence of testis in scrotum).

   —varicocele.

   —lymphadenopathy.

   —hematoma formation.

F. Indications for surgery

1. **Inguinal hernias**

   —require surgical repair because of the significant risk of complications associated with incarceration, obstruction, and strangulation.
2. A **reducible hernia**

   —should be **repaired electively**.

   a. The **most effective measure of reduction**

      —is application of slow, constant pressure over the hernia sac.

   b. **Abdominal relaxation**

—can be facilitated by placing the patient in the supine position with the knees slightly flexed.

c. **Mild anesthesia**

—or sedation may also be beneficial.

3. **Incarcerated hernias**

—**require urgent surgical repair** with reduction of the hernia sac because of the risk of subsequent obstruction or strangulation.

G. **Methods of surgical repair**

1. **Indirect hernias in children and young adults** may be repaired by

—reduction of the hernia contents.

—**high ligation and resection of the hernia sac** near the deep inguinal ring.

—simple tightening of the ring to reduce the potential space for herniation (**Marcy repair**).

2. **Inguinal hernias in adults** are repaired

—by reduction of the hernia sac along with **formal repair of the inguinal floor** by several techniques.

a. The **superficial Bassini repair (Figure 10-6) involves approximation of the** conjoined tendon and transversalis fascia (superior) **to the free edge of the inguinal ligament** (inferior).

b. The **deeper McVay repair** (**Cooper's ligament repair**) **(Figure 10-7)** approximates **the conjoined tendon and transversalis fascia to Cooper's ligament** (lateral).

—This repair requires placement of a relaxing incision in the anterior rectus sheath because of the significant tension associated with this repair.

c. A **Lichtenstein repair (Figure 10-8)** involves **insertion of synthetic mesh** (e.g., polypropylene) over the hernia defect.

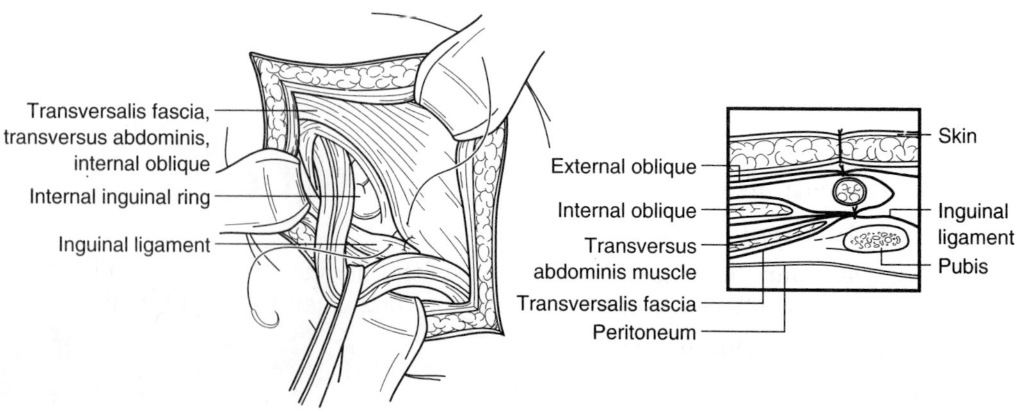

Figure 10-6. Bassini repair of an inguinal hernia. The transversalis fascia is approximated to the inguinal ligament. (Adapted with permission from Schwartz S: *Principles of Surgery.* 5th ed. New York, McGraw Hill, 1989, p 1538.)

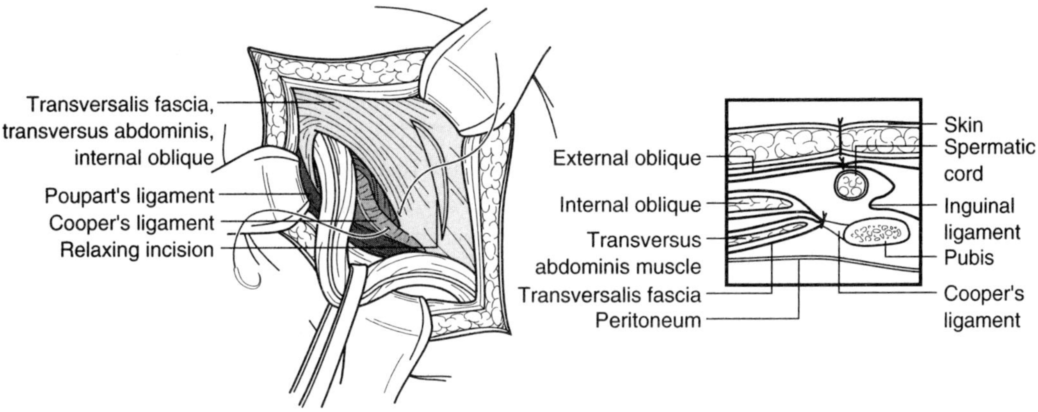

Figure 10-7. McVay repair (Cooper's ligament repair) of an inguinal hernia. The transversalis fascia is approximated to Cooper's ligament. (Adapted with permission from Schwartz S: *Principles of Surgery,* 5th ed. New York, McGraw-Hill, 1989, p 1538.)

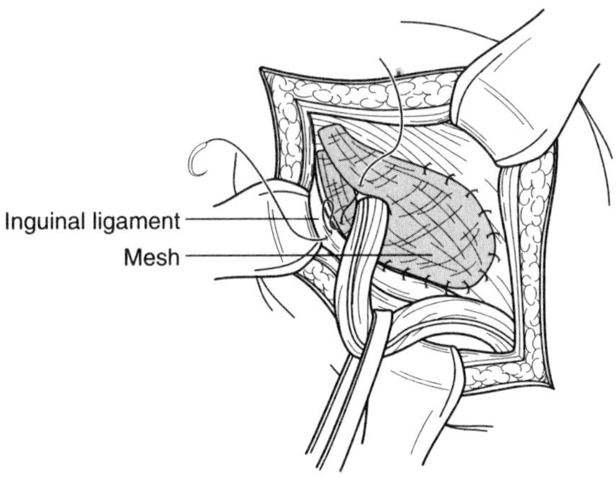

Figure 10-8. Lichenstein repair of an inguinal hernia. Mesh is sewn to the transversalis fascia and the inguinal ligament to close the defect. (Adapted with permission from Cameron J: *Current Surgical Therapy,* 6th ed. St. Louis, Mosby, 1998, p 558.)

d. **The choice of repair**

—is generally based on surgeon preference with no definitive data demonstrating a distinct advantage of one procedure over another.

3. **Laparoscopy**

—may also be used to insert synthetic mesh over the hernia defect intraperitoneally via a transabdominal approach or via a preperitoneal approach.

—may be particularly useful in patients with recurrent or bilateral hernias.

—Laparoscopic hernia repair is currently being investigated to compare the benefit of this procedure over other repair techniques.

4. In **all hernias, abdominal exploration**

—should be considered to assess bowel viability and the need for resection **if the presence of necrotic bowel is suspected**.

a. **Signs suggestive of necrotic bowel** include

—leukocytosis.

—the presence of dark or bloody fluid within the peritoneal sac.

b. **Signs or symptoms of peritonitis**

—represent an **absolute indication for abdominal exploration.**

c. In rare instances **when surgery cannot be performed** (e.g., patient refusal), a truss may be strapped in over the defect to attempt to prevent herniation.

—This technique is unreliable and may result in significant scarring, making subsequent repair difficult.

H. Postoperative complications

1. **Recurrence of the hernia**

—after repair is estimated to occur in 3%–10% of patients.

2. **Temporary urinary retention**

—with difficulty urinating is common.

3. **Wound infection**

—occurs in 1%–3% of patients postoperatively.

—is a particularly difficult problem to manage when synthetic mesh is directly involved in the infection.

4. **Injury**

—**to the ilioinguinal, iliohypogastric, and genital branch of the genitofemoral nerves** rarely occurs and may result in paresthesias in their distribution of innervation.

—This may present with paresthesias in the scrotum and medial or anterior thigh.

5. **Inadvertent injury**

—to the structures of the spermatic cord rarely occurs.

—Injury to the vas deferens may be repaired primarily.

6. **Seroma and hematoma**

III. Other Hernias

A. Femoral hernia (Figure 10-9)

1. **Femoral hernias pass under the inguinal ligament,** passing medially to the femoral artery, nerve, and vein.

2. **These hernias occur much more frequently in women.**

—Inguinal hernias, however, are still the most common among women.

3. **Characteristically, femoral hernias**

—are **prone to incarceration and strangulation** because of the **narrow neck of the femoral canal.**

4. **Signs and symptoms**

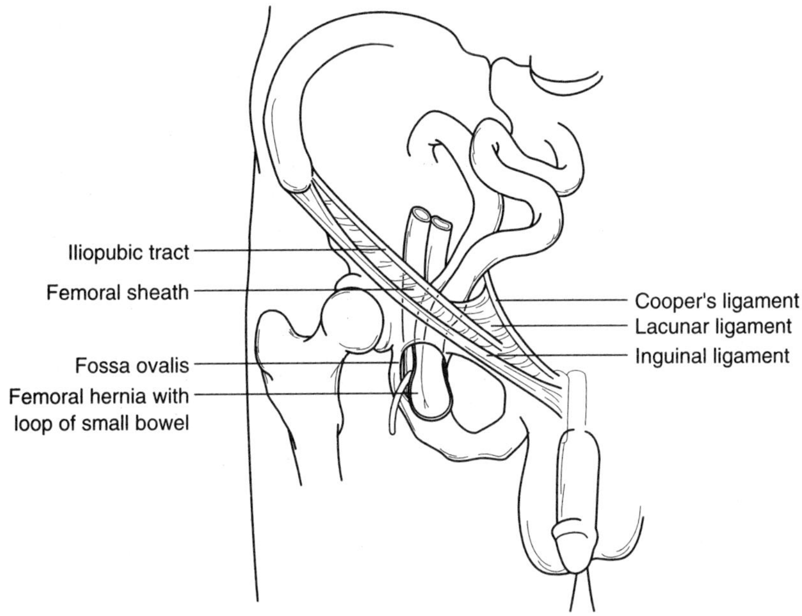

Figure 10-9. Femoral hernia. (Adapted with permission from Lippincott Williams & Wilkins. Gray and Skandalakis: *Atlas of Surgical Anatomy for General Surgeons.* Baltimore, Williams & Wilkins, 1985, p 97.)

a. These hernias are **frequently asymptomatic** until obstruction or strangulation occurs.

—Abdominal pain and manifestations of intestinal obstruction may be present in the absence of localized symptoms in the groin.

b. A **characteristic bulge**

—in the anteromedial thigh, below the inguinal ligament may be present.

c. Femoral hernias may be confused

—with inguinal hernias if the femoral hernia is deflected over the inguinal ligament through the fossa ovalis femoris.

5. Treatment

a. Femoral hernias are generally repaired

—through an inguinal approach.

b. Reduction of the hernia sac

—is often difficult.

—may be facilitated by division of the inguinal ligament, if necessary.

c. A Cooper's ligament or McVay repair

—is necessary to assure adequate closure of the femoral canal.

d. Given the high incidence of strangulation

—a surgeon should have a low threshold for abdominal exploration if strangulation is suspected.

e. Blood in the hernia sac

—is **characteristic of strangulation**.

B. Umbilical hernias (see *BRS Surgical Specialties,* Chapter 3, for umbilical hernias in children)

1. **In adults**

—gradual weakening of the periumbilical fascial tissue may result in hernia formation over time.

2. **These hernias occur**

—**more frequently in women** than in men.

3. **Risk factors** include

—multiparity.

—obesity.

—ascites.

—large intra-abdominal tumors.

4. **Appropriate treatment** involves

—primary surgical repair of the defect.

—insertion of synthetic mesh for large defects.

C. Incisional hernias (ventral hernia)

1. **Of patients undergoing abdominal operations**

—approximately 5%–10% will develop an incisional hernia.

2. **Poor surgical technique**

—with inadequate fascial closure or excessive tension is the most common cause of incisional hernia formation.

3. **Other risk factors** include

—postoperative wound infection.

—increasing age.

—obesity.

—malnutrition.

—pulmonary disease with persistent coughing postoperatively (e.g., smokers).

4. **Treatment** involves

—careful dissection of the hernia sac with primary fascial repair of small defects.

—insertion of synthetic mesh for large defects to avoid undue tension and potential recurrence.

D. Other rare hernias

—of the abdominal wall are characterized in **Table 10-1.**

IV. Other Lesions of the Abdominal Wall

A. Rectus sheath hematoma

—is characterized by formation of a hematoma within the muscular layers of the abdominal wall.

Table 10-1. Abdominal Wall Hernias

Hernia	Location	Characteristics
Indirect inguinal	Through deep inguinal ring; lateral to inferior epigastric vessels	Most common hernia in children and adults
Direct inguinal	Directly through defect in transversalis fascia; through Hesselbach's triangle medial to inferior epigastric vessels	Borders of Hesselbach's triangle: inferior epigastric vessels, lateral border or rectus, inguinal ligament
Pantaloon	Inguinal hernia with both direct and indirect components	Hernia sac straddles inferior epigastric vessels
Femoral	Below inguinal ligament medial to femoral vessels	Seen more commonly in women; high rate of incarceration and strangulation
Umbilical	Through defect in umbilical ring	Increased risk with obesity, ascites, pregnancy
Incisional (ventral)	Through fascial defect in previous incision	Occurs in 5%–10% of patients with abdominal incision
Epigastric	Primary defects in linea alba above umbilicus	May be multiple; recurrence rate is 10%–20%
Spigelian	Through linea semilunaris (where aponeurosis join to form the rectus sheath just lateral to the rectus muscles); most commonly at the level of the semicircular line of Douglas.	Pain may be present over defect without palpable mass; CT scan or ultrasound may be diagnostic
Lumbar	Through superior (Grynfeltt's) and inferior (Petit's) lumbar triangles in the posterior abdominal wall	Although rare, they occur most commonly in young athletic women
Obturator	Through obturator canal with obturator nerve and blood vessels	Often presents as obstruction; high mortality; pain in medial thigh increased by extension or abduction of leg (Howship-Romberg sign)
Internal	Through defect in visceral structure (e.g., defect in mesentery)	May occur after bowel resection if mesenteric defects not repaired
Perineal	Through floor of perineum	Most frequently occurs following pelvic surgery
Interparietal	Hernia sac contents migrate between layers of the abdominal wall	Rare; high rate of strangulation; ultrasound or CT scan often diagnostic
Sciatic	Herniation through greater sciatic foramen	Rare; high rate of strangulation

CT = computed tomography.

1. **Hematoma formation**

—may be precipitated by mild trauma.

—**may occur spontaneously** in association with **disorders of coagulation or platelet function**.

2. **Abdominal pain**

—is the most frequent presenting symptom.

3. **Physical examination**

—often reveals a very **painful abdominal wall mass**.

a. Upon **flexion of the rectus abdominis muscles**

—**the mass becomes more prominent and painful** (**Fothergill's sign**).

b. **Intra-abdominal masses**

—often disappear upon flexion of the rectus muscles.

c. **Ecchymosis**

—over the abdomen may also be present.

4. A **computed tomography (CT) scan** or **ultrasound** may demonstrate the hematoma.
5. The hematoma will **usually resolve without surgical intervention**.
6. **Evacuation of the clot** with adequate hemostasis

—may be performed in patients with severe, persistent pain.

B. **Tumors of the abdominal wall**

1. **Most tumors of the abdominal wall are benign**.
2. **Examples** include lipomas, hemangiomas, and fibromas.

—These may be resected if symptomatic.

3. **Desmoid tumors**

—are also benign lesions, although they may resemble low-grade fibrosarcomas.

—may infiltrate adjacent tissues but never metastasize.

—Effective treatment of desmoid tumors involves resection or radiation therapy.

4. **Malignant lesions of the abdominal wall**

—are most often metastatic lesions from an intra-abdominal source.

Review Test

Directions: Each of the numbered items or incomplete statements in this section is followed by answers or by completions of the statement. Select the ONE lettered answer or completion that is BEST in each case.

1. A 35-year-old man presents to the office with complaints of a recurrent right tender groin mass. He states that he most frequently notices the mass after working all day but that it usually goes away by morning. On physical examination, there is a palpable mass noted upon insertion of the index finger into the scrotal region. The mass is soft and becomes more prominent when the patient performs a Valsalva maneuver (e.g., cough). In this patient, this mass passes through

(A) The deep inguinal ring
(B) Hesselbach's triangle
(C) The femoral canal
(D) The obturator foramen
(E) The superficial inguinal ring

2. A 35-year-old man undergoes an uneventful elective right inguinal Lichtenstein hernia repair. The patient presents 10 days later with a complaint of severe pain over the incision site. On physical examination, the incision site is noted to be erythematous and there is significant purulent drainage coming from the wound. There is also a significant reducible soft mass in the wound suggestive of a recurrence of the hernia. Which of the following is the most appropriate treatment strategy for this patient?

(A) Wound exploration, mesh removal, and repair of hernia with new mesh
(B) Discharge, administration of antibiotics, and close follow-up
(C) Wound exploration, mesh removal, and perform a McVay repair
(D) Discharge and wet to dry dressing changes 3 times a day
(E) Insertion of a drain, administration of antibiotics, and close observation

3. A 65-year-old man with no previous abdominal surgery presents with severe abdominal pain over the right lower quadrant (RLQ). His past medical history is significant for a previous aortic valve repair and the patient is on chronic coumarin (Coumadin) anticoagulant therapy. On physical examination there is an exquisitely tender mass noted in the RLQ just lateral to the umbilicus. When the patient attempts to sit up the mass remains palpable and the pain associated with the mass increases. Of the following, which is most appropriate in the management of this patient?

(A) Incision and drainage with wound packing
(B) Immediate exploratory laparotomy
(C) Local exploration and biopsy of the mass
(D) Performance of an abdominal computed tomography (CT) scan
(E) Colonoscopy to rule out colon cancer

4. A 59-year-old, obese woman presents to the emergency room with a painful right groin mass below the inguinal ligament. Aggressive attempts to reduce the mass are unsuccessful. Intraoperatively, the patient is confirmed to have an incarcerated femoral hernia although the viability of the bowel appears intact. Attempted intraoperative reduction of the hernia sac is unsuccessful as well. Which of the following is the most appropriate next step in the management of this patient?

(A) Resection of the herniated bowel and primary reanastomosis
(B) Division of the inguinal ligament with reduction of the hernia contents
(C) Performance of an enterotomy and decompression of the herniated bowel
(D) Performance of a laparotomy with traction of the herniated bowel intraperitoneally
(E) Performance of a McVay repair despite the inability to reduce the hernia sac

5. After a routine left inguinal hernia repair, a 45-year-old man presents to the office complaining of numbness over a portion of the left side of his scrotum and over the anteromedial portion of his left thigh. Very anxious about these findings, the patient also asks if this is associated with sexual dysfunction. Which of the following is an appropriate explanation with regards to the patient's inquiry?

(A) There is a significant risk of erectile dysfunction associated with this complication
(B) Erectile function remains unaffected although the patient may be sterile
(C) The hernia has probably recurred and will require reoperation
(D) This probably represents an inadvertent injury to the iliohypogastric nerve
(E) This probably represents an inadvertent injury to the ilioinguinal nerve

Directions: Each set of matching questions in this section consists of a list of four to twenty-six lettered options followed by several numbered items. For each numbered item, select the appropriate lettered option(s). Each lettered option may be selected once, more than once, or not at all.

Questions 6–12

(A) Indirect inguinal hernia
(B) Direct inguinal hernia
(C) Umbilical hernia
(D) Spigelian hernia
(E) Pantaloon hernia
(F) Littré's hernia
(G) Richter's hernia
(H) Obturator hernia
(I) Incisional (ventral) hernia
(J) Femoral hernia
(K) Epigastric hernia
(L) Lumbar hernia

Choose the hernia(s) associated with each patient scenario.

6. A 55-year-old woman with no history of previous abdominal surgery presents with signs and symptoms suggestive of a small bowel obstruction. There are no groin masses noted upon physical examination. The patient notes pain in the medial thigh, which worsens upon extension of the leg. (SELECT 1 HERNIA)

7. A 35-year-old man presents with a tender right scrotal mass. Upon physical examination, a soft mass is palpated at the level of the external inguinal ring. (SELECT 3 HERNIAS)

8. A 34-year-old woman with no previous abdominal surgery presents with complaints of a tender mass in the midline of the abdomen above the level of the umbilicus. Upon physical examination, there are 2 small midline soft masses noted above the level of the umbilicus. (SELECT 1 HERNIA)

9. A 42-year-old woman presents with signs and symptoms suggestive of a small bowel obstruction. She has had no previous abdominal surgeries. There are no palpable abdominal masses or masses in the groin region, however there is a localized point of tenderness over a small region inferior to the umbilicus and lateral to the rectus abdominis muscle. (SELECT 1 HERNIA)

10. A 42-year-old woman with a previous open cholecystectomy presents to the emergency room with signs and symptoms suggestive of a small bowel obstruction. On physical examination, there is a palpable soft mass noted just below the right inguinal ligament. (SELECT 1 HERNIA)

11. A 42-year-old man presents with a very painful right groin mass. The mass is reduced preoperatively. Intraoperatively, the hernia sac is noted to be lateral to Hesselbach's triangle and a McVay hernia repair is performed. Of note, there was bloody fluid noted within the hernia sac. (SELECT 3 HERNIAS)

12. A 65-year-old, obese man has had a previous colon resection for colon cancer through a midline abdominal incision. He now presents with a nontender soft mass in the midline approximately 4 cm above the umbilicus. (SELECT 1 HERNIA)

Answers and Explanations

1–E. It is very difficult to differentiate a direct hernia (through Hesselbach's triangle) from an indirect (through the deep inguinal ring) hernia on physical examination. Identification of a hernia sac in the scrotum merely confirms that an inguinal hernia has passed through the superficial inguinal ring into the scrotum. Hernias through the femoral canal or obturator canal would not present with a scrotal mass.

2–C. A wound infection with an early recurrence of the hernia in the presence of synthetic material requires prompt exploration with drainage and removal of the infected mesh. Repair of the hernia with new mesh would not be indicated in the presence of an infected wound, thus a repair without mesh, such as the McVay repair, would be indicated in this situation. Discharging the patient would be inappropriate in this setting. Insertion of a drain and antibiotic therapy would not be adequate treatment for an infection in this setting.

3–D. Increasing pain and persistence of the mass with flexion of the rectus abdominis muscles (Fothergill's sign) is a characteristic finding of a rectus sheath hematoma. Coumarin (Coumadin) anticoagulant therapy is also a significant risk factor for the development of a rectus sheath hematoma. Despite these suggestive findings, an abdominal computed tomography (CT) scan would help to rule out other potential causes such as an abdominal wall hernia, tumor, or abscess. Local exploration or incision and drainage is not necessary before performing the CT scan. Because the mass appears to be within the abdominal wall, an exploratory laparotomy is not indicated at this time, although if a hernia is identified on CT scan, exploration may be indicated. This lesion is not likely to be associated with a colon cancer and thus colonoscopy is not indicated.

4–B. Because of the narrow neck of the femoral canal, femoral hernias frequently present with incarceration. Some femoral hernias are even difficult to reduce intraoperatively, in which case the inguinal ligament can be divided and repaired following reduction of the hernia sac. If the bowel is viable, resection is not indicated. Performance of an enterotomy is not indicated because of the risk of contamination. A laparotomy would not be necessary in this situation and repair of the hernia without reduction of the hernia sac would be impossible.

5–E. Although uncommon, injury of the iliohypogastric, ilioinguinal, and genital branch of the genitofemoral nerve may occur during inguinal hernia repairs. As in this patient, ilioinguinal nerve transection generally presents with paresthesias and numbness in the scrotum and anteromedial thigh region. This nerve provides cutaneous sensory fibers and injury would not be associated with erectile dysfunction or sterility. These symptoms are also not consistent with recurrence of the hernia. Injury to the iliohypogastric nerve generally presents with paresthesias in the region of the lower abdomen below the umbilicus and the anterolateral thigh.

6–H. Any patient that presents with a small bowel obstruction without previous abdominal surgery should be suspected of having a hernia. Although rare, an obturator hernia may present as a small bowel obstruction without other significant findings. Pain noted in the medial thigh that worsens upon extension or abduction of the leg is a characteristic finding (Howship-Romberg sign) of an obturator hernia.

7–A, B, E. Palpation of a hernia sac at the level of the external inguinal ring suggests the presence of either a direct or an indirect hernia, or both (pantaloon hernia). Simple palpation of a hernia sac at this level does not differentiate between these hernias.

8–K. In the absence of previous abdominal surgery, hernias in the midline above the level of the umbilicus probably represent epigastric hernias. These hernias occur through defects in the linea alba and may be multiple.

9–D. Spigelian hernias occur through defects in the linea semilunaris, where the aponeuroses of the abdominal muscles converge to form the rectus sheath just lateral to the rectus abdominis muscles. The most common site is at the level of the semicircular line of Douglas just below the umbilicus where the posterior rectus sheath ends. Because the hernia sac may track between the layers of the abdominal muscles, a mass may not be palpable. There may, however, be pain noted over the site of herniation. Ultrasound or computed tomography (CT) scan may be diagnostic when these lesions are suspected.

10–J. Signs and symptoms of a small bowel obstruction with a hernia palpated below the level of the inguinal ligament should suggest the presence of an incarcerated femoral hernia. The defect associated with a femoral hernia is small, therefore these hernias are prone to incarceration and strangulation.

11–A, F, G. Indirect inguinal hernias occur lateral to the inferior epigastric vessels through the deep inguinal ring. Bloody fluid noted within the hernia sac suggests the presence of strangulated bowel. Two types of hernias that may present with strangulation without previous signs or symptoms of bowel obstruction include Richter's hernia and Littré's hernia. A Richter's hernia is characterized by partial herniation of the antimesenteric border of the intestinal wall. Littré's hernia is characterized by herniation of a Meckel's diverticulum. A significant risk associated with these two hernias is reduction of a strangulated portion of intestine.

12–I. Identification of a hernia sac at the site of a previous incision probably represents a ventral or incisional hernia. These hernias occur in 5%–10% of patients undergoing abdominal surgery. Umbilical hernias generally occur directly around the umbilicus.

11

The Esophagus

James W. Thiele

I. Anatomy and Physiology

A. General anatomy (Figure 11-1)

1. **The esophagus**
   —is a midline structure divided into 3 anatomical segments.
   a. **The cervical esophagus**
      —extends approximately 5 cm from the cricoid cartilage, where it is firmly attached, to the second thoracic vertebrae.
   b. **The thoracic esophagus**
      —is approximately 20 cm long.
      —extends from the thoracic inlet to the diaphragmatic esophageal hiatus.
   c. **The abdominal esophagus**
      —is 2 cm long.
      —is anchored by an extension of the transversalis fascia called the **phrenoesophageal membrane.**
      —extends from the diaphragm to the gastroesophageal junction.
2. **Esophageal sphincter function**
   a. **The upper esophageal sphincter (UES)** is a distinct anatomic structure defined by the **cricopharyngeus muscle.**
      (1) **Relaxation of the UES**
          —allows swallowed material propelled by a pharyngeal swallow to enter the upper esophagus.
      (2) **Contraction of the UES**
          —0.5 seconds later **prevents regurgitation.**
   b. **The lower esophageal sphincter (LES)** is a physiologic sphincter.
      —Its competence is determined by a variety of factors (see IV A 1).
3. **Areas of normal anatomic narrowing**

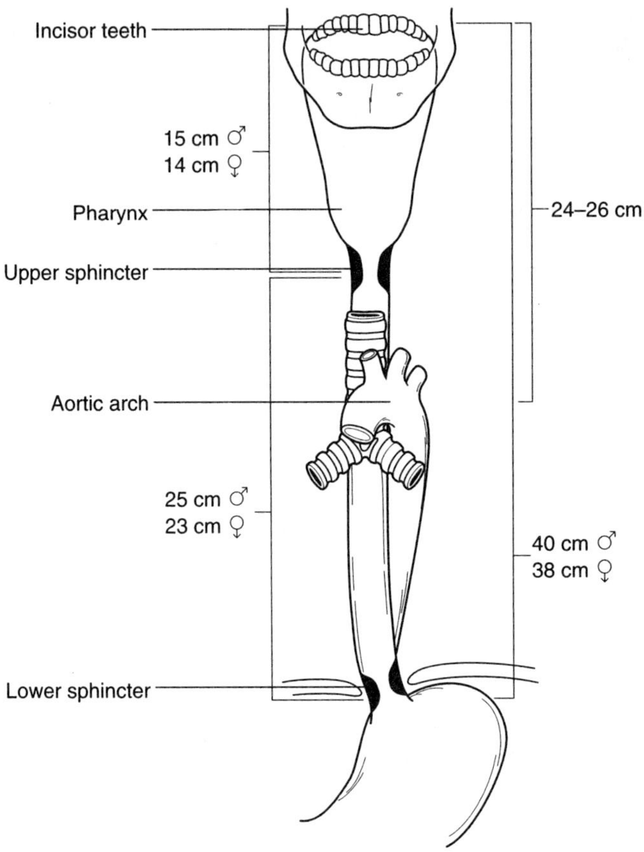

Figure 11-1. General anatomy of the esophagus. Measurements indicate clinically important endoscopic landmarks as measured from the incisors in adults. (Reprinted with permission from Shields TW: *General Thoracic Surgery,* 4th ed. Baltimore, Williams & Wilkins, 1994, p 1361.)

a. **Cervical constriction**

—occurs at the **cricopharyngeus muscle.**

b. **Broncho-aortic constriction**

—is located at the fourth thoracic vertebrae.

—is secondary to the aortic arch and left mainstem bronchus crossing over the esophagus at this level.

c. **Diaphragmatic constriction**

—occurs as the esophagus passes through the diaphragm.

4. **The surgical approach to the esophagus**

a. **The cervical esophagus**

—is best approached via a **left thoracotomy** owing to left-sided deviation of the esophagus in this region.

b. **The mid-thoracic esophagus**

—is best approached via a **right thoracotomy,** because this approach avoids the aortic arch.

c. The **lower thoracic esophagus**

—is best approached via a left thoraco-abdominal incision.

B. Histologic characteristics

1. **The entire esophagus is lined** by stratified squamous epithelium.
2. **Muscular layers consist of** inner circular and outer longitudinal muscle.
3. **The upper 2–6 cm of the esophagus contains** only striated muscle fibers.
   —Smooth muscle fibers become more predominant more distally in the esophagus.
4. **There is no serosal covering** in the esophagus.

C. Arterial supply and venous drainage (**Figure 11-2**)

1. **The cervical esophagus**
   —receives arterial blood from **the inferior thyroid artery.**
   —Venous blood from this region drains into the **inferior thyroid veins.**
2. **The thoracic esophagus**
   —receives arterial blood from **bronchial arteries** and directly from the **aorta.**
   —Venous blood in this region drains into either **bronchial veins** or into the **azygos** or **hemiazygos** systems.

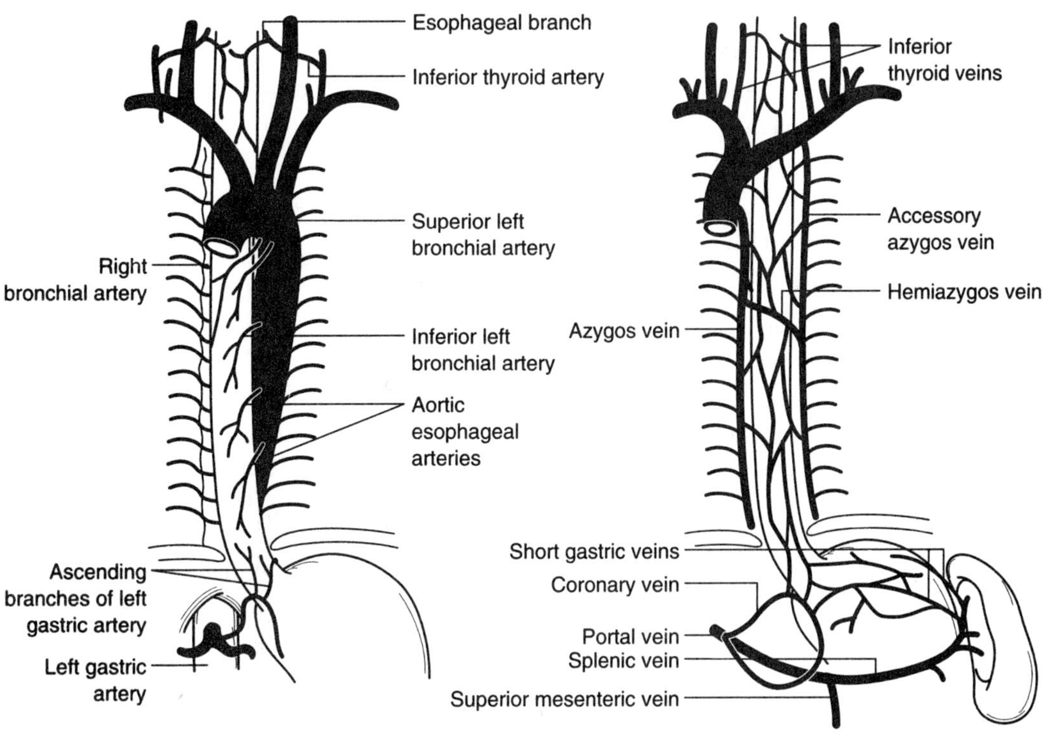

Figure 11-2. Arterial supply and venous drainage of the esophagus. (Reprinted with permission from Shields TW: *General Thoracic Surgery,* 4th ed. Baltimore, Williams & Wilkins, 1994, p 1368.)

3. **The abdominal esophagus**
   - —receives arterial blood from the **left gastric** and **inferior phrenic arteries.**
   - —Venous blood from this region drains into the **coronary vein.**

D. Nervous supply and lymphatic drainage

1. **Innervation**
   a. **Parasympathetic innervation is**
      - —via the left and right vagus nerves.

   b. **Sympathetic innervation is**
      - —from branches of the sympathetic chain
      - —via the **celiac ganglion.**

2. **Lymphatic drainage**
   - —As a general rule, the lymphatic drainage of the **upper two thirds of the esophagus** is **cephalad.**
   - —That of the **lower third** is **caudad.**

E. Physiologic function of the esophagus

1. **Peristaltic waves in the esophagus** are grouped into three types.
   a. **Primary peristalsis**
      - —is progressive.
      - —follows a voluntary swallow.

   b. **Secondary peristalsis**
      - —is progressive.
      - —is generated by esophageal distention or irritation.

   c. **Tertiary contractions**
      - —are nonprogressive.
      - —may occur either after voluntary swallows or between swallows.

2. **Relaxation of the LES**
   - —occurs 1.5–2.5 seconds after a voluntary swallow.
   - —allows food propelled by primary and secondary peristalsis to enter the stomach.

   a. **Factors that induce LES relaxation** include
      - —secretin, cholecystokinin, vasoactive intestinal peptide, progesterone, α-adrenergic antagonists, anticholinergic agents, nicotine, ethanol, chocolate, fatty meals, and gastric acidification.

   b. **Factors that inhibit LES relaxation** include
      - —gastrin, motilin, vasopressin, glucagon, α-adrenergic agonists, cholinergic agents, and gastric alkalinization.

II. Tests of Esophageal Anatomy and Function

A. Barium esophagram with static radiographs

1. **This is the test of choice**

—to evaluate **structural changes** in the esophagus.

—to **define surgical anatomy.**

2. **Generally, it is the initial test of choice** for evaluating patients with

—dysphagia.

—suspected esophageal mass lesions.

B. Endoscopic ultrasound is useful for evaluation and staging of patients with mass lesions of the esophagus.

C. A cinematographic esophagram

—differs from a standard esophagram in that the entire examination is videotaped.

1. **Videotape review**

—allows for a closer inspection of esophageal function.

2. It is **useful for detecting motility disorders** and is the **only test that can adequately evaluate the oropharyngeal phase of swallowing.**

3. Its **sensitivity** in detecting small mucosal abnormalities is **low.**

D. Esophageal manometry

—is used to evaluate the effectiveness of esophageal body and sphincter contractile function.

1. **Pressure sensitive transducers** measure both the amplitude of contraction and the progression of the peristaltic wave.

2. **It can also evaluate** the major components of LES function (resting pressure, intra-abdominal length, and total length).

E. Esophageal pH probe monitoring

—can be used to evaluate the degree of acid reflux into the distal esophagus.

1. **A pH probe** is placed 5 cm above the manometrically determined LES. Data is collected via a portable recorder.

2. **The distal esophageal pH** is recorded every second over a 24-hour period. The data are analyzed to determine if pathologic reflux is present.

F. Esophagoscopy

—is used to directly visualize the esophageal mucosa.

1. **Flexible endoscopy**

—can be performed with sedation.

—can be used to evaluate esophageal mucosal abnormalities and obtain biopsies.

2. **Rigid endoscopy**

—requires general anesthesia.

—is better than flexible endoscopy for retrieving swallowed foreign objects.

III. Disorders of Esophageal Motility

A. Achalasia

—is the most common esophageal motility disorder.

1. **This disorder is characterized by**
   —**esophageal aperistalsis** and **dilation**
   —**failure** of the **LES to relax.**
2. **Patients typically present** in the third to fifth decades of life.
3. Men and women are equally affected.
4. **Symptoms** include
   —**dysphagia** involving both solids and liquids.
   —**regurgitation of undigested food.**
5. **Underlying pathology** involves
   —degenerative changes in the ganglia of **Auerbach's plexus (myenteric)** in the esophagus.
   a. **These degenerative changes** result in a hypertensive LES.
   b. **Failure of the LES to relax with swallowing results in**
      —increased intraluminal pressure.
      —dilation.
      —eventual loss of peristalsis.
   c. **In Third World countries**
      —infection with *Trypanosoma cruzi* (Chagas' disease) produces similar degenerative changes.
6. **Patient evaluation** should include esophageal manometry to evaluate esophageal function and document LES hypertension.
   —Contrast radiographs may reveal a characteristic "bird's beak" appearance with proximal esophageal dilation.
7. **Treatment**
   —can be medical, mechanical, or surgical.
   a. **Medical treatment**
      —with **nitrates** and **calcium channel blockers** can be used in very mild cases of achalasia, but has poor long-term success (less than 20%).
   b. **Dilation of the LES**
      —with rigid or pneumatic devices has had better (60%–80%) long-term success than medical therapy.
      (1) Dilation may be repeated multiple times if symptoms recur.
      (2) The main risk is **rupture** of the esophagus.
   c. **Surgical therapy**
      —involves muscle division (**myotomy**) to mechanically disrupt the hypertensive LES and lower esophageal smooth muscle.

B. Esophageal spasm syndromes

—involve disturbances in the coordination of normal esophageal peristalsis.

1. **Named disorders include** nutcracker esophagus, diffuse esophageal spasm, and hypertensive LES. Each syndrome differs in the type of peristaltic disturbance seen (**Table 11-1**).
2. **The hallmark symptoms of these disorders are**
   —**chest pain** that may radiate to the back, neck, ears, jaw, or arms.
   —**dysphagia** for both liquids and solids.
3. **Diagnosis**
   —**Esophageal manometry** is the **gold standard for diagnosis.**
   —Video esophagogram and endoscopy may also be useful.
4. **Treatment**
   a. **Medical therapy includes**
      —**nitrates** and **calcium channel blockers.**
      —sedatives and muscle relaxants.
   b. **Surgical therapy**
      —consists of a long esophageal myotomy.
      —is generally reserved for those patients with incapacitating dysphagia.
      (1) **Surgical myotomy**
         —results in a loss of high amplitude contractions.
      (2) **Palliation of dysphagia**
         —is reported in 80%–90% of patients.

C. Scleroderma

—is a disease that affects esophageal motility in 80% of patients.

1. **The effects in the gastrointestinal tract are characterized by**
   —smooth muscle atrophy.
   —collagen deposition.
2. **Diagnosis**
   —is made manometrically.
   a. **Normal peristalsis**

Table 11-1. Manometric Findings Noted in Esophageal Spasm Disorders

Disorder	Manometric Findings
Nutcracker esophagus	**Normal LES;** mean amplitude of esophageal contractions in the lower esophagus is > 180 mm Hg, but **peristalsis is normal.**
Diffuse esophageal spasm	LES relaxation is often inadequate; **simultaneous contractions** greater than 20% of the time, often with high amplitude contractions. **Intermittent normal peristalsis** is present.
Hypertensive LES	**Elevated LES pressure** (> 26 mm Hg) with complete relaxation. Peristalsis in the esophageal body is normal.

LES = lower esophageal sphincter.

—is seen in the proximal esophagus owing to the predominance of striated muscle.

b. **Peristaltic function**

—diminishes more distally in the esophagus as the smooth muscle content increases.

3. **Symptoms are related to**

—gastroesophageal reflux secondary to a weak LES and poor clearance of refluxed acid because of diminished lower esophageal peristalsis.

4. **Treatment** (either medical or surgical)

—The goal of management is to prevent the associated gastroesophageal reflux (see IV).

D. Diverticuli of the esophagus

—may be either pulsion or traction in origin.

1. **Pulsion divertuculi or pseudodiverticuli**

—develop as a result of increased intraluminal esophageal pressure.

—do not involve all layers of the esophageal wall (hence they are considered pseudodiverticula).

a. **A pharyngeo-esophageal or Zenker's diverticulum**

—is the most common diverticulum in the esophagus.

(1) **This type of diverticulum**

—occurs just proximal to the **cricopharyngeus muscle.**

—is most common in the fifth to eighth decades of life.

(2) **Symptoms** include

—dysphagia.

—regurgitation of undigested food.

—choking.

—halitosis.

(3) **Diagnosis**

—is made by barium esophagram.

—endoscopy (careful to not rupture diverticulum).

(4) **Treatment** involves

—a **cricopharyngeal myotomy** to relieve intraluminal pressure in addition to resection of large (> 2 cm) diverticuli.

b. **An epiphrenic diverticulum**

—is rare and is **usually associated with an esophageal motility disorder.**

(1) **These can occur** anywhere, but are **most prevalent in the distal 10 cm** of the esophagus.

(2) **Many patients are asymptomatic**

—but common presenting symptoms include dysphagia and regurgitation.

(3) **Diagnosis**

—Both esophagram and esophageal manometry are necessary to define any underlying motility disorder.

(4) **Treatment** involves

—diverticulectomy and long esophageal myotomy on the side opposite the diverticulectomy.

2. **Traction diverticuli**

—result from inflammation in surrounding tissues.

a. **These diverticuli**

—are generally **midesophageal** and are considered true diverticuli because they involve all layers of the esophageal wall.

b. **Most are asymptomatic**

—but rare complications include fistula formation between the trachea or great vessels.

c. **Treatment**

—consists of excision of the inflamed tissue and primary closure of the esophagus.

IV. Gastroesophageal Reflux Disease (GERD) and Esophageal Hernia

A. GERD is characterized by

—the loss of the normal gastroesophageal barrier to reflux of stomach contents.

—decreased clearance of refluxed materials from the distal esophagus.

1. **Pathologic reflux**

—is caused by the loss of mechanical competency of the LES. This is defined by three parameters, all of which can be measured manometrically:

a. **A resting pressure greater than 6 mm Hg** is associated with a competent LES.

b. **Overall length of more than 2 cm** is also associated with a competent LES.

c. **Intra-abdominal length of more than 1 cm** results in transmission of the positive abdominal pressure to the LES and facilitates competence.

2. **Symptoms of GERD**

a. Heartburn and epigastric pain

b. Recurrent pneumonia and chronic cough from recurrent aspiration

c. Sour taste in the mouth upon waking ("water brash") and choking sensations

d. Symptoms are worse when the patient is lying or bending down, and after meals.

3. **Evaluation of patients with severe GERD**

a. **Esophageal pH probe monitoring**

—documents the presence of prolonged or repeated exposure of the distal esophagus to acid reflux.

b. **Manometry** both evaluates the competency of the LES and documents the peristaltic ability of the esophagus.

(1) **Distal esophageal dysfunction** can accompany GERD.

(2) **The type of surgical procedure** may be altered in the face of severe esophageal dysfunction (see IV A 4 b).

c. **Endoscopy** documents and evaluates the complications of GERD, such as

—stricture.

—ulcerations.

—Barrett's esophagus (see VI A).

4. **Therapy**

—for these patients may be medical or surgical depending on the severity of symptoms and the presence of complications.

a. **Medical therapy**

(1) Medical therapy is generally used in patients with new onset disease or those with mild symptoms.

(2) **Therapy** includes

—**H2-blockers,** such as famotidine.

—**proton pump inhibitors,** such as omeprazole.

—**prokinetic agents,** such as metoclopramide or erythromycin.

—**antibiotic therapy,** for patients with *H. pylori.*

b. **Indications for surgery** in patients with severe GERD include:

(1) **Failure of medical therapy** to control symptoms.

(2) **Recurrence of symptoms** after medical therapy is stopped.

(3) **The presence of complications** of the disease, such as

—esophageal stricture.

—pulmonary insufficiency secondary to aspiration.

c. **The surgical procedure**

—of choice for GERD is a **fundoplication.**

(1) **This procedure** is done by wrapping the gastric fundus around the distal esophagus to increase LES pressure (**Figure 11-3**). Fundoplication serves to re-establish the reflux barrier.

(2) **Operations**

(a) **A full 360° (Nissen) operation**

—is used in patients with normal esophageal function.

—can be performed via an open procedure laparoscopically.

(b) **A partial 270° (Belsey Mark IV operation) or loose wrap**

—is used **for patients with dysmotility** to **avoid dysphagia.**

(3) **It is imperative** that the **fundus** and not the body of the stomach be used for the wrap. Otherwise, it will relax after swallowing, as does the LES.

(4) **Any defect in the esophageal hiatus** should also be repaired.

B. **Esophageal hernias (Figure 11-4)**

1. **A type I or sliding esophageal hernia**

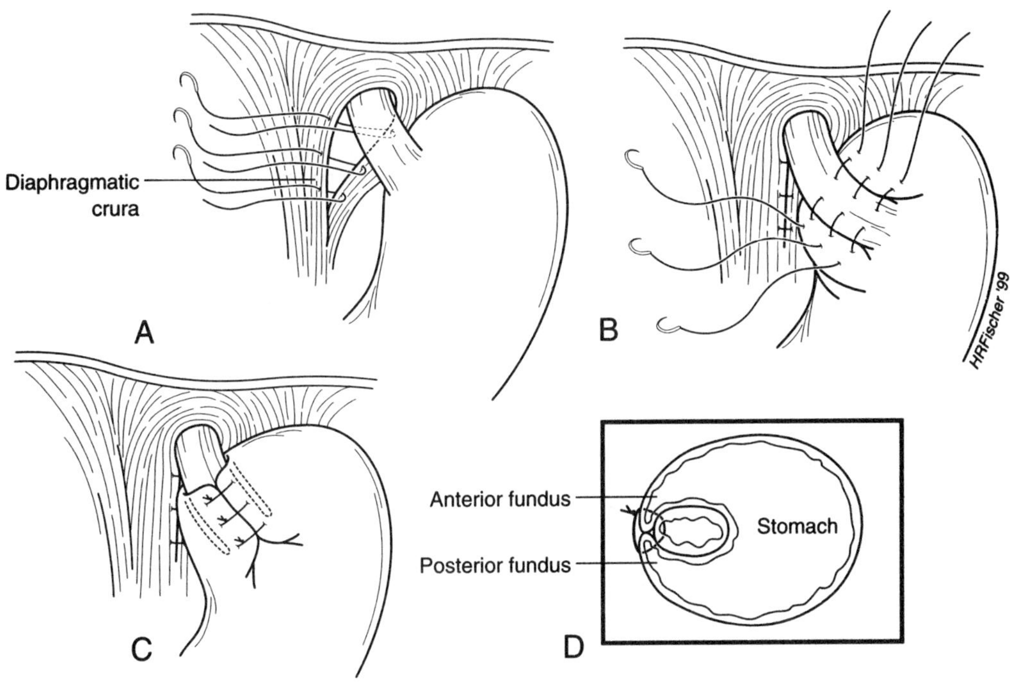

Figure 11-3. Nissen fundoplication procedure for gastroesophageal reflux disease. *(A)* Approximation of diaphragmatic crura. *(B)* Sites of stitches for fundoplication. *(C)* Complete fundoplication. *(D)* Cross-section of completed fundoplication. (Adapted with permission from Lippincott Williams & Wilkins. Zuidema GD: Surgical Treatment: abdominal approach. In *Gastroesophageal Reflux and Hiatal Hernia.* Edited by Skinner DB, Belsey RH, Hendrix TR. Boston: Little, Brown, 1972, p 154.)

—occurs when the gastroesophageal junction moves cephalad from the stomach into the chest.

—is the most common type of esophageal hernia.

a. **This type of hernia** is often associated with GERD.

b. **Indications for surgical repair** include

—**severe refractory symptoms.**

—**severe esophageal mucosal dysplasia** (e.g., Barrett's esophagus) resulting from GERD.

2. **A type II or rolling (paraesophageal) esophageal hernia**

—The gastroesophageal junction is in its normal position (intra-abdominal).

—A hernia sac containing gastric fundus and body develops along the side of the esophagus.

a. **Reflux is rarely present because of**

—pressure from the herniated stomach.

—the normal position of the gastroesophageal junction.

b. **Symptoms** include

—postprandial chest pain.

—dysphagia.

—early satiety.

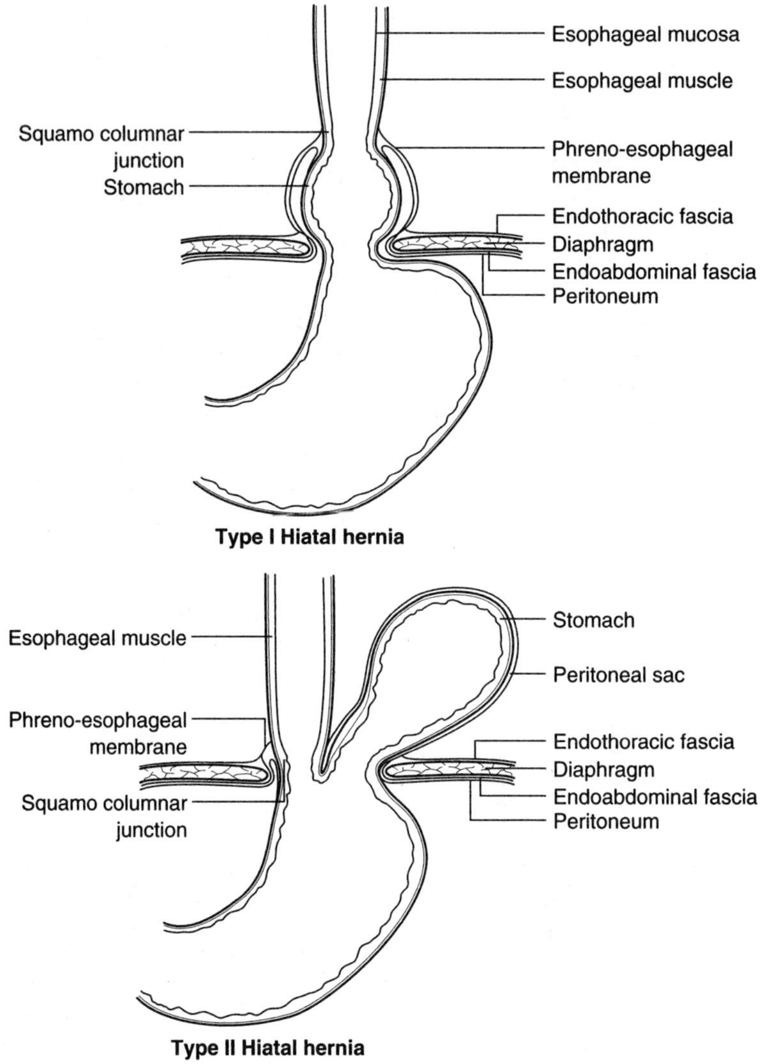

Figure 11-4. Hiatal hernias. (Reprinted with permission from Cameron J: *Current Surgical Therapy,* 6th ed. St. Louis, Mosby, 1998, p 14.)

c. **Surgical repair**

—is indicated for **all patients with type II hernias** because gastric **obstruction** as well as **strangulation** and **necrosis** of the stomach can occur in as many as **30% of patients.**

3. **Type III esophageal hernias**

—**are combinations of type I** and **type II.**

—should be treated as a type II.

4. **Evaluation** should include

—endoscopy to evaluate the position of the gastroesophageal junction.

—a barium esophagram to define hernia type.

5. **Surgical therapy**

—differs for each type of hernia.

a. **Type I hernias are repaired with**
   —fundoplication.
   —closure of the hiatal defect.

b. **Type II and III hernias are repaired by**
   —returning the stomach to the abdomen.
   —closing the hiatal defect.
   —fundoplication, if there was evidence of reflux disease pre-operatively.

V. Benign Lesions of the Esophagus

A. Schatzki's ring

—is a thin submucosal circumferential ring in the distal esophagus at the gastroesophageal junction.

1. **Almost all patients with a Schatzki's ring**

   —will have an associated sliding hiatal hernia.

2. The upper surface of the ring is covered by squamous epithelium, while the lower surface is covered by columnar epithelium.

3. **Patients usually present clinically**

   —with short episodes of dysphagia usually after a hurried swallow.

4. **Treatment**

   —**Symptomatic patients** usually respond to dilation of the ring.

   —Coexisting reflux symptoms, however, may require antireflux therapy or surgery.

5. **Esophageal webs**

   —are similar lesions occurring in the upper esophagus.

   a. **Plummer-Vinson syndrome is characterized by**
      —the presence of esophageal webs.
      —associated **iron deficiency anemia.**

   b. **Treatment**
      —involves administration of iron supplements.

B. Leiomyomas

—are the **most common benign tumors of the esophagus.**

—can occur throughout the esophagus, but are **rare in the neck.**

1. **These tumors**

   —are submucosal.

   —generally occur between the ages of 20 and 50.

   —are solitary in approximately 90% of cases.

2. **The most common presenting symptom** is dysphagia, however, most are asymptomatic.

3. **Diagnosis**

—is generally made by esophagogram.

a. **These masses appear** as smooth, concave defects with sharp borders.

b. **Endoscopy**

—is indicated to rule out carcinoma.

c. **Endoscopic ultrasound**

—is also useful for characterizing the lesion.

d. **Biopsy is not recommended**

—**if leiomyoma is suspected** because scarring from the biopsy site will make excision more difficult.

4. **Asymptomatic lesions**

—can be followed with serial esophagrams; whereas, symptomatic lesions warrant resection.

a. **Esophageal leiomyomas**

—can generally be carefully dissected away from the underlying tissues **without esophageal resection.**

b. **Recurrence** of these lesions is rare.

C. **Esophageal polyps**

—are the second most common benign esophageal tumors.

1. **These lesions** are most common in older men.

—Eighty percent are found in the cervical esophagus.

2. **Large lesions** may be regurgitated into the mouth.

3. **Additional symptoms** include

—dysphagia.

—hematemesis or melena.

4. **Resection**

—**Small** polyps can be resected endoscopically.

—**Larger** lesions require resection through a cervical incision.

VI. Premalignant and Malignant Lesions of the Esophagus

A. **Barrett's esophagus**

—is a premalignant lesion of the distal esophagus caused by chronic gastroesophageal reflux.

1. **This condition involves replacing the normal squamous epithelium with gastric epithelium** in the distal esophagus.

a. **Injury to the distal esophagus**

—results in metaplasia of the distal esophageal mucosa.

b. **The diagnosis of Barrett's esophagus**

—is made when the gastric epithelium extends **more than 2 cm** into the tubular esophagus.

2. **Metaplasia may progress** to **dysplasia or adenocarcinoma** of the esophagus if the chronic acid reflux is allowed to continue.

3. **Initial management** includes

—medical therapy with acid suppression.

—prokinetic agents.

—life-long endoscopic surveillance of the distal esophageal mucosa.

a. **Fundoplication** (see IV A 4 c)

—may be necessary in those patients who continue to have reflux symptoms while on medical therapy.

b. **Although fundoplication will halt further progression** of the Barrett's, those **changes that have already taken place will not regress.**

c. **Endoscopic surveillance**

—is necessary to monitor the Barrett's mucosa.

(1) **Mild or moderate dysplastic changes**

—may be monitored with frequent endoscopic surveillance and biopsy.

(2) **Severe dysplastic or cancerous changes**

—**require esophageal resection.**

B. **Malignant lesions of the esophagus**

1. **Squamous cell carcinoma and adenocarcinoma**

—are the two most common types of esophageal cancer.

a. **Squamous cell carcinoma**

—of the esophagus accounts for 60% of esophageal cancers.

(1) **Risk factors are diverse** and include

—**smoking.**

—**alcohol consumption.**

—long-standing **achalasia.**

—previous **caustic injuries.**

—**human papilloma virus infection.**

—nitrosamines.

(2) **These lesions are more common** in the **proximal two thirds** of the esophagus.

b. **Adenocarcinoma**

—was once an unusual diagnosis.

—now accounts for 40% of all esophageal cancers in Western countries.

(1) **The most important risk factor**

—is **Barrett's esophagus.**

(2) **Patients with Barrett's esophagus**

—are 40 times more likely than those without the condition to develop adenocarcinoma of the esophagus.

(3) **Adenocarcinoma is more common** in the **distal third** of the esophagus.

2. **Common symptoms** include
   —dysphagia.
   —weight loss.
   —anemia.
3. **Staging is based on**
   —the depth of invasion of the primary tumor.
   —the presence of lymph node and distant metastasis **(Table 11-2).**
   a. **Endoscopic ultrasound** is useful for staging.
   b. **Patients with upper or middle third lesions**
      —should undergo **bronchoscopy** to determine if there is tracheal or bronchial invasion, which is a contraindication to esophagectomy.
   c. **Distant metastasis**
      —documented by computed tomography (CT) scan **also precludes curative resection.**
4. **Treatment**
   a. **Resection of the esophagus**
      —may be performed through an abdominal incision combined with ei-

Table 11-2. The TNM* Staging Criteria for Esophageal Cancer

Criteria			
Primary tumor (T)			
T1	Tumor < 5 cm long, noncircumferential, without obstruction, and without extraesophageal spread		
T2	Tumor without spread beyond the muscularis propria, but with the presence of obstruction, a circumferential lesion, or a lesion > 5 cm		
T3	Evidence of extraesophageal spread of the tumor		
Nodal status (N)			
N0	No involvement of regional lymph nodes		
NX	Regional lymph nodes cannot be assessed		
N1	Palpable, mobile, unilateral nodes		
N2	Palpable, mobile, bilateral nodes		
N3	Fixed lymph nodes		
Distant Metastases (M)			
M0	No distant metastases		
M1	Distant metastases		
Staging			
Stage I	T1	N0	M0
Stage IIA	T2	N0	M0
	T3	N0	M0
Stage IIB	T1	N1	M0
	T2	N1	M0
Stage III	T3	N1	M0
	T4	Any N	M0
Stage IV	Any T	Any N	M1

*TNM = tumor-node-metastasis.

ther a **right thoracotomy** (Ivor-Lewis approach) or a **cervical/transhiatal approach.**

(1) Ivor-Lewis approach

—is preferred if the tumor is adherent to structures in the chest because much of the thoracic dissection is blind in the transhiatal approach.

(2) A transhiatal approach

—prevents the need for thoracotomy. An Ivor-Lewis approach, however, allows for more thorough lymph node sampling.

(3) Re-anastomosis

—is generally performed by pulling the stomach into the chest or neck and attaching it to the proximal esophagus.

(4) Alternative approaches to re-anastomosis include

—the use of either a colon or small bowel interposition graft.

b. Chemotherapy or radiation therapy alone

—**does not appear to affect survival** of these patients.

c. Combined modality

—(combination chemotherapy and radiation therapy) appears to have some promise; its effect on survival remains to be determined.

d. Five-year survival

—for **stage I** lesions is only 50%–70%.

—for **stage IV** lesions is generally less than 5%.

e. Palliation therapy

—for nonresectable patients generally centers on **relief of dysphagia** and **nutritional support.**

(1) Transient relief of dysphagia can be provided by

—endoscopic laser fulguration of the tumor mass.

—placement of esophageal stents.

—palliative resection or bypass.

(2) Nutritional support

—can be provided by gastrostomy or jejunostomy tubes.

VII. Other Considerations in Esophageal Disease

A. Esophageal perforation

1. The **most common causes** are

—iatrogenic rupture.

—spontaneous rupture.

—trauma.

a. Iatrogenic rupture

—related to interventions such as endoscopy and dilation of the esophagus is the **most common cause of rupture.**

—accounts for 50% to 75% of all cases.

b. Spontaneous rupture (Boerhaave's syndrome)

—typically accounts for 15% of all cases.

—is caused by straining.

(1) **Rupture after forceful vomiting**

—is the most common cause.

(2) **Perforation can also be induced by**

—childbirth.

—straining with defecation (especially in young children).

c. **Trauma**

(1) accounts for 20% of spontaneous ruptures.

(2) **Traumas** include

—blunt or penetrating trauma.

—caustic injuries.

—ingested foreign bodies.

2. **Diagnosis**

a. **Signs and symptoms** may include

—chest pain.

—fever.

—tachycardia.

—respiratory distress.

—hypotension.

—odynophagia.

—mediastinal emphysema.

—pneumothorax.

—Hamman's sign (mediastinal "crunch" associated with mediastinal emphysema).

b. A **water-soluble** or **barium contrast study** can help to characterize the location and severity of the perforation.

3. **Treatment**

—**largely depends on the duration of symptoms prior to presentation and treatment.**

a. Perforation is frequently fatal if not diagnosed and treated early.

b. **Immediate treatment for all patients** includes

—**stopping all oral intake.**

—**instituting intravenous hydration.**

—starting **broad spectrum antibiotics.**

—placing a **nasogastric tube** for stomach decompression.

c. **For a perforation less than 24 hours old, patients are generally treated with**

—débridement.

—primary repair of the defect.

—reinforcement of the area with autologous tissue (e.g., intercostal muscle).

d. **Patients presenting more than 24 hours after rupture may be treated with**

—débridement.

—primary repair.

—Some patients, however, will require esophageal exclusion and diversion to allow the rupture site to heal (**Figure 11-5**).

B. Caustic injuries of the esophagus

1. These injuries are most commonly a result of

—accidental ingestion in children younger than 5 years old.

—suicide attempts in adults.

2. Acid and alkali burns

—have different characteristics and clinical courses.

a. Acids cause a **coagulative type necrosis.**

—This necrosis is more superficial and less likely to penetrate beyond the submucosa.

b. Alkalis cause **liquefactive type necrosis.**

—This necrosis results in the destruction of surface lipoproteins and penetration deep into muscle and surrounding tissues.

3. Management

a. Induction of vomiting is contraindicated

—because it may re-expose the esophagus to the inciting agent.

b. Nasogastric tube placement is contraindicated

—because of the possibility of perforation of the friable, injured mucosa.

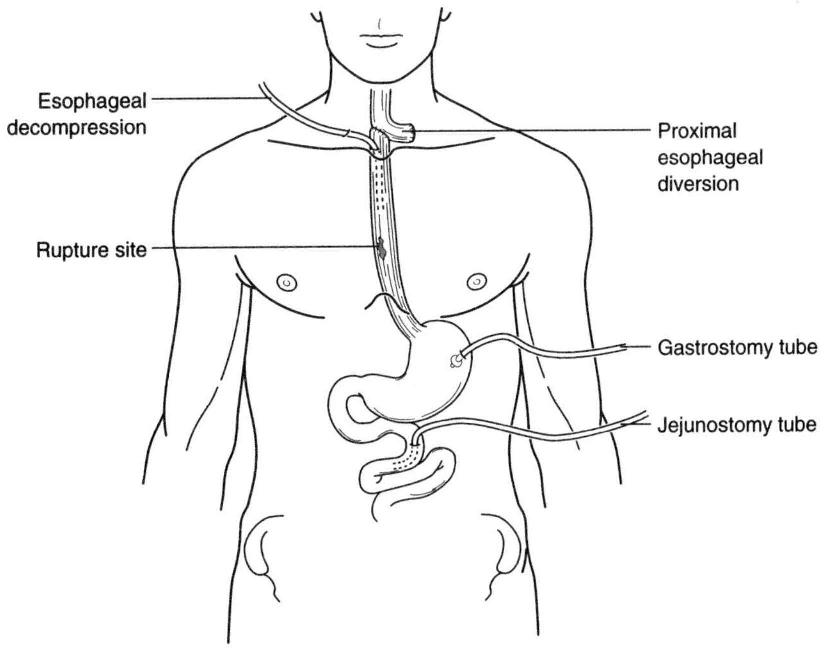

Figure 11-5. Esophageal diversion procedure for an esophageal perforation. (Reprinted with permission from Cameron J: *Current Surgical Therapy,* 6th ed. St. Louis, Mosby, 1998, p 14.)

Table 11-3. Classification and Treatment of Esophageal Burns

Grade	Findings on Endoscopy	Treatment
I	Mucosal edema and hyperemia	**Observation** for 24–48 hours, then discharge if stable
II	Mucosal ulcerations, **pseudomembrane formation,** sloughing	Patient is kept **NPO** for several days and **parenteral nutrition** is started. Esophagram is obtained in 2–4 weeks to look for stricture formation.
III	**Deep ulcerations** with eschar formation; severe edema with obliteration of the lumen	Treatment is similar to grade II injuries in the absence of complications such as bleeding or perforation.

NPO = nothing by mouth.

c. **Early endoscopy is indicated**
   —to evaluate and grade the injury, which helps to determine treatment (**Table 11–3**).

d. **Surgical indications** include
   —continued bleeding.
   —free mediastinal or peritoneal air.
   —evidence of peritonitis or mediastinitis.

e. **Delayed complications** include
   —stricture.
   —a **500-fold increase in the risk of esophageal cancer.**
   —development of an aortoesophageal fistula.

Review Test

Directions: Each of the numbered items or incomplete statements in this section is followed by answers or by completions of the statement. Select the ONE lettered answer or completion that is BEST in each case.

1. A 52-year-old man is referred for evaluation of dysphagia. Endoscopy reveals an ulcerated mass near the gastroesophageal junction and biopsies of this lesion are positive for adenocarcinoma. Which of the following statements is true?

(A) Most esophageal cancers are diagnosed early
(B) Neither chemotherapy nor radiation therapy alone have been shown to improve survival in these patients
(C) Smoking and alcoholism are important risk factors for development of this lesion
(D) With surgical resection, the 5-year survival for patients with esophageal cancer approaches 75%
(E) Cancers in the gastroesophageal junction tend to metastasize to cervical lymph nodes

2. A 47-year-old man presents with complaints of dysphagia when eating solid food. He denies any history of weight loss and is not anemic on laboratory evaluation. A barium swallow reveals a smooth, nonulcerated filling defect in the middle third of the esophagus that is highly suspicious for a leiomyoma. Which of the following statements is true regarding this patient?

(A) Endoscopy and biopsy is indicated before proceeding with surgical resection
(B) These tumors can generally be enucleated without the need for esophageal resection
(C) Multiple lesions are noted in at least 50% of cases
(D) Resection is indicated even in small, asymptomatic lesions due to malignant potential
(E) Dysphagia is an uncommon presenting symptom

3. A 51-year-old woman presents for evaluation of postprandial epigastric pain associated with intermittent episodes of gastroesophageal reflux. Upper gastrointestinal contrast study reveals a type III esophageal hernia and Barrett's changes are noted on endoscopic examination of the distal esophagus. Of the following statements, which most appropriately pertains to this patient?

(A) The presence of a type III esophageal hernia is an indication for surgery
(B) Type III esophageal hernias are the least common type
(C) Fundoplication is not indicated in this patient
(D) Complications occur in less than 5% of patients with this type of hernia
(E) Manometry is not necessary before proceeding with fundoplication in this patient

4. A 40-year-old man presents with a 6-month history of dysphagia for both solids and liquids, as well as regurgitation of undigested food after meals. Esophagram shows a dilated esophagus with a significant "bird's beak" narrowing at the lower esophageal sphincter (LES). Manometry reveals poor esophageal peristalsis and a very hypertensive LES. Which of the following statements is true regarding this patient's condition?

(A) Medical treatment with nitrates and calcium channel blockers is successful in most cases
(B) The surgical procedure of choice for this disorder is a long esophageal myotomy
(C) Although dysphagia is common, regurgitation is unusual in these patients
(D) Rigid or pneumatic LES dilation can offer a long-term success rate as high as 80%
(E) Manometry is not indicated if the patient has the classic presenting symptoms and esophagram findings

5. A 33-year-old man presents to the emergency room 30 minutes after having ingested alkaline drain cleaner. He is currently stable and exhibits no signs of respiratory distress. Examination of the oropharynx reveals only mild erythema of the posterior pharynx. Which of the following statements is true regarding the treatment of this patient?

(A) Induction of vomiting is indicated if the ingestion occurred less that 1 hour ago
(B) Alkali ingestion tends to cause a less serious injury because the stomach acid largely neutralizes it
(C) Early endoscopy is indicated to evaluate the extent of injury
(D) The lack of severity of the oropharyngeal injury indicates that the esophageal injury is not likely to be severe and endoscopy is not indicated
(E) There is a 2- to 4-fold increase in the risk of esophageal cancer in these patients

6. A 70-year-old man presents with dysphagia, occasional regurgitation of undigested food, and chronic halitosis. Manometric studies are normal but a barium esophagram reveals a 4-cm Zenker's diverticulum. Which of the following statements is true?

(A) This is the least common diverticulum of the esophagus
(B) A Zenker's diverticulum is a true diverticulum
(C) This type of diverticulum is most common in the third and fourth decades of life
(D) A Zenker's diverticulum occurs just distal to the cricopharyngeus muscle
(E) The procedure of choice in this patient would be a cricopharyngeal myotomy and diverticulectomy

7. A 42-year-old woman with scleroderma presents with symptoms of gastroesophageal reflux disease (GERD) that have persisted despite 6 months of adequate medical therapy. Which of the following statements best describes her condition?

(A) Further medical therapy is warranted before surgical intervention is considered
(B) Therapy is generally aimed at controlling gastroesophageal reflux
(C) Because this disease affects primarily the distal esophagus, resection of this segment is curative
(D) The risk of esophageal cancer is higher in these patients
(E) No further work-up is needed in this patient before proceeding with surgery

8. A 47-year-old man presents with a 6-month history of intermittent chest pain and dysphagia for both solids and liquids. Cardiac work-up is negative and standard barium esophagram was unremarkable. Esophageal manometry reveals high amplitude contractions and intermittent normal peristalsis with simultaneous contractions 40% of the time. Which of the following statements is true regarding this patient's condition?

(A) Surgery is the treatment of choice
(B) Medical therapy includes nitrates and H2-blockers
(C) In patients with incapacitating dysphagia, 80%–90% report palliation of their symptoms with surgical intervention
(D) Esophagram is the gold standard for identification of this disorder
(E) Surgical therapy consists of a distal esophageal myotomy

Directions: Each set of matching questions in this section consists of a list of four to twenty-six lettered options followed by several numbered items. For each numbered item, select the appropriate lettered option(s). Each lettered option may be selected once, more than once, or not at all.

Questions 9–12

(A) Gastroesophageal reflux disease
(B) Esophageal leiomyoma
(C) Zenker's diverticulum
(D) Type I esophageal hernia
(E) Type II esophageal hernia
(F) Type III esophageal hernia
(G) Esophageal cancer
(H) Caustic ingestion
(I) Nutcracker esophagus
(J) Boerhaave's syndrome
(K) Achalasia
(L) Diffuse esophageal spasm
(M) Barrett's esophagus

Match the following case scenarios with the most appropriate cause(s).

9. A 40-year-old man presents with a 1-year history of progressive dysphagia. He first noted difficulty swallowing only solids but his symptoms recently progressed to liquids as well. Esophagram reveals a distal esophageal stricture that is benign by biopsy. (SELECT 2 CAUSES)

10. A 56-year-old woman presents with progressive dysphagia for solids and liquids as well as intermittent chest pain. She noticed some relief in her symptoms after she was recently started on a calcium channel blocker for hypertension but her symptoms have recently returned. (SELECT 3 CAUSES)

11. A 58-year-old man presents with a history of dysphagia and intermittent regurgitation of undigested food. (SELECT 2 CAUSES)

12. A 56-year-old man presents with a history of 4 episodes of right lower middle lobe pneumonia in the past year. He also reports the presence of a persistent, dry cough. Pulmonary work-up, including bronchoscopy, has been negative and he is a nonsmoker. A barium esophagram recently obtained was normal. (SELECT 1 CAUSE)

Answers and Explanations

1–B. Most esophageal cancers grow to a significant size before producing symptoms of dysphagia because the esophagus lacks a serosa, thus permitting the smooth muscle in the esophagus to stretch and accommodate the enlarging mass. Because of this, most esophageal cancers present at an advanced stage that often precludes cure. The overall 5-year survival rate for patients with esophageal cancer after attempted curative resection is only 40%–50%. While smoking and alcohol abuse are important risk factors for squamous cell cancers, Barrett's esophagus is the most important risk factor for the development of adenocarcinoma. Tumors in the distal third of the esophagus tend to metastasize to caudad lymph nodes.

2–B. Esophageal leiomyomas are generally asymptomatic until they grow large enough to produce dysphagia, which is the most common presenting symptom. They are solitary in approximately 90% of cases and small, asymptomatic lesions can generally be followed with serial examinations, because these lesions have almost no malignant potential. Endoscopy is indicated to rule out malignancy, but if leiomyoma is suspected biopsy is contraindicated because it may make subsequent resection much more difficult due to scarring at the biopsy site.

3–A. Because of the risk of complications such as gastric volvulus and ischemia associated with type II and type III esophageal hernias, it is generally recommended that these defects be surgically repaired once they are identified. Complications can occur in as many as 30% of patients with type I and type II esophageal hernias. Fundoplication is not always indicated in these patients, because many will have no signs or symptoms of gastroesophageal reflux disease. However, if the patient complains of reflux symptoms, has signs of reflux on esophagogastroduodenoscopy (e.g., Barrett's changes), or if there is evidence of an incompetent lower esophageal sphincter on manometry, then a fundoplication is indicated.

4–D. This patient presents with the classic symptoms and manometric findings associated with achalasia. Regurgitation is common in patients with long-standing disease as they often retain undigested food in the dilated proximal esophagus. Medical therapy has a long-term success rate of less than 20% and is reserved for those patients with mild disease. The surgical treatment of choice in these patients is a lower esophageal myotomy designed to disrupt the lower esophageal sphincter, not a long esophageal myotomy. Manometry is always indicated in the work-up of any patient who presents with symptoms of esophageal dysmotility.

5–C. Early endoscopy is indicated to evaluate and grade the injury, which helps to determine treatment. The induction of vomiting after ingesting either acid or alkaline substances is contraindicated because further injury to the esophagus may occur as the caustic substance is expelled. Alkaline substances result in liquefactive necrosis in the wall of the esophagus and stomach, which causes deeper burns and thus a more significant injury. The severity of the oropharyngeal injury can be a poor indicator of the severity of the more distal gastrointestinal tract. The risk of esophageal cancer in these patients is increased 500-fold.

6–E Zenker's diverticula are the most common diverticula of the esophagus and are generally seen in the fifth to eighth decades of life. This is a pulsion type of diverticulum and is considered a pseudodiverticulum because it does not involve all layers of the esophageal wall. Zenker's diverticula occur just proximal to the cricopharyngeus muscle and the surgical procedure of choice to repair these defects is a cricopharyngeal myotomy. A diverticulectomy should also be performed if the diverticulum is greater than 2 cm.

7–B. Scleroderma is a disease that affects primarily smooth muscle resulting in atrophy and collagen deposition. The distal esophagus is composed entirely of smooth muscle and is thus affected to a greater degree than the proximal esophagus, which is primarily striated muscle. The presence of scleroderma does not change the evaluation and treatment of symptomatic gastroesophageal reflux disease (GERD). Treatment in these patients is aimed at preventing gastroesophageal reflux and the basic treatment and evaluation is the same as for patients without scleroderma. When symptoms are refractory to medical therapy, fundoplication is usually the next recommended step in treatment. Resection of the distal esophagus is not indicated unless there is evidence of severe dysplasia or adenocarcinoma of the distal esophagus secondary to the effects of chronic GER. The risk of esophageal cancer in these patients is the same as in any patient with chronic GER.

8–C. Patients with diffuse esophageal spasm usually present with chest pain and dysphagia for both solids and liquids. Although surgical intervention consisting of a long esophageal myotomy can be very successful in treating these patients, it is reserved only for those patients who have incapacitating dysphagia. Medical therapy consists of nitrates and calcium channel blockers as well as sedatives and muscle relaxants. H2-blockers have no role in the treatment of esophageal spasm. Although video esophagram may be included in the work-up of these patients, manometry is the gold standard in identifying all of the esophageal spasm disorders.

9–A, H. In addition to Barrett's changes in the distal esophagus, gastroesophageal reflux disease (GERD) can also result in stricture formation secondary to repeated injury to the esophageal mucosa. Stricture formation is also a late complication of ingesting a caustic substance and can occur years after the original injury. It is imperative that any newly diagnosed esophageal stricture be biopsied to rule out malignancy. Multiple biopsies should be obtained from the involved mucosa because foci of malignancy could easily be missed if only a single biopsy is obtained.

10–I, K, L. Dysphagia for both solids and liquids accompanied by intermittent chest pain is the typical presentation of patients suffering from esophageal spasm disorders. The only way to effectively distinguish these syndromes from one another is to evaluate the patient with esophageal manometry. Achalasia can also be associated with dysphagia and occasional chest pain that may be relieved with nitrates or calcium channel blockers.

11–C, K. Both achalasia and a Zenker's diverticulum should be suspected in a patient who presents with a history of dysphagia as well as the regurgitation of undigested food. The history of this type of regurgitation is important in differentiating these disorders from other causes of dysphagia. In achalasia, swallowed food is unable to pass into the stomach because of poor peristalsis and a hypertensive lower esophageal sphincter (LES). The proximal esophagus eventually dilates and serves as a reservoir for undigested food that is eventually regurgitated by the patient. Patients with a Zenker's diverticulum generally report regurgitation symptoms that are less severe as the diverticulum is a smaller reservoir. A Zenker's can be documented by esophagram, which may also show the esophageal changes of achalasia. Manometry is the gold standard in the diagnosis of achalasia.

12–A. Some patients with symptomatic gastroesophageal reflux disease (GERD) have an absence of gastrointestinal complaints. Other symptoms such as recurrent pneumonia caused by occult aspiration and chronic cough from reflux irritation of the upper airway should prompt a full work-up for GERD. Significant GER can often be missed on barium esophagram and definitive tests—including upper endoscopy, manometry, and 24-hour pH probe—should be performed to evaluate the lower esophagus as well as the lower esophageal sphincter, and to document the presence of reflux.

12

Stomach and Duodenum

Stewart Long

I. Anatomy and Histology

A. Topographic anatomy of the stomach (Figure 12-1)

1. **The anterior surface**
   —is adjacent to the left hemidiaphragm and the left hepatic lobe.
2. **The posterior surface**
   —is adjacent to the left hemidiaphragm, left kidney, left adrenal, and the pancreas.
3. **The greater curvature**
   —is adjacent to the transverse colon inferiorly and the spleen laterally.
4. **Risks of percutaneous placement of gastrostomy tubes** include **hemorrhage or perforation** given the proximity of the **liver and colon,** respectively.
   —Gastrostomy tubes pass through the anterior abdominal wall to the stomach lumen to provide enteral nutrition or allow for decompression of the stomach.

B. Topographic anatomy of the duodenum

—The duodenum spans 20 to 30 cm from the pyloric sphincter to the **ligament of Treitz** and is divided into **four parts.**

1. The **first portion [i.e., the duodenal bulb (cap)]** overlies the common bile duct and is the site of over **90% of duodenal ulcers.**
2. The **second (i.e., descending) portion** is attached to the pancreas and is retroperitoneal. The common bile duct and main pancreatic duct merge to form the **ampulla of Vater,** which **enters this portion of the duodenum.**
3. The **third (i.e., transverse) portion** is attached to the uncinate process of the pancreas and is wedged between the superior mesenteric artery anteriorly and the aorta posteriorly.

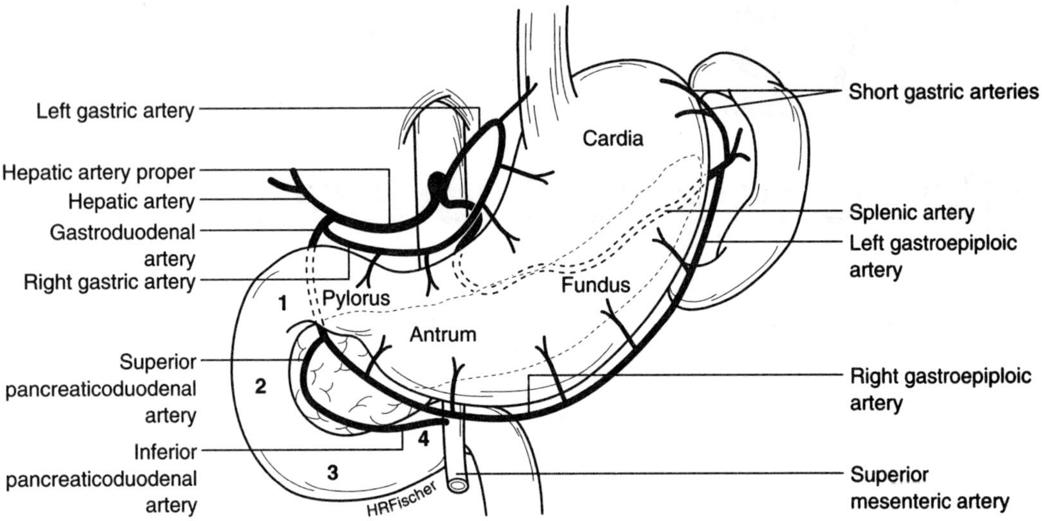

Figure 12-1. The major topographic areas of the stomach and major arteries supplying the stomach and duodenum. (Adapted with permission from Lawrence P: *Essentials of General Surgery.* Baltimore, Williams & Wilkins, 1992, p 176.)

4. The **fourth (i.e., ascending) portion** enters the jejunum at the **ligament of Treitz.**

C. **Arterial and venous supply**

1. **Gastric arterial blood supply** is primarily from the **celiac trunk.**
   a. **The lesser curve**
      —is supplied by the **right** and **left gastric arteries.**
   b. **The greater curve**
      —is supplied by the **right** and **left gastroepiploic arteries.**
   c. **The fundus**
      —is also supplied by the **short gastric arteries** branching from the distal splenic artery.
   d. **The pylorus**
      —is supplied by direct branches of the **gastroduodenal artery.**
   e. **Ligation**
      —of all but one of these major vessels may be performed without necrosis of the stomach wall.
2. **Duodenal arterial blood supply** stems primarily from the gastroduodenal artery and the superior mesenteric artery.
   a. **The superior pancreaticoduodenal branch**
      —of the **gastroduodenal artery** supplies the duodenal bulb and the descending portion.
   b. **The inferior pancreaticoduodenal branch**
      —of the **superior mesenteric artery** supplies the third and fourth portions of the duodenum.
   c. **These branches may communicate** to provide collateral flow between the celiac trunk and the superior mesenteric artery.

3. Venous and lymphatic drainage parallel each other.

a. Venous drainage

—is predominantly through the **splenic and superior mesenteric veins.**

b. Lymphatic drainage

—**Frequent communications between lymph channels** allow for easy spread of neoplastic disease through local lymph nodes.

D. Innervation

1. **The vagus nerves** are the major nerve supply.
2. The **left (anterior) vagus branches into** the

—**hepatic division.**

—anterior gastric wall branch.

3. **The right (posterior) vagus branches into** the

—celiac branch.

—posterior gastric wall branch.

4. **Gastroduodenal pain**

—is sensed via afferent sympathetic fibers from T5–T10.

E. Histology

1. The **stomach comprises**

—an external serosa.

—muscle layers.

—submucosa.

—muscularis mucosa.

—a mucosa.

2. The **proximal third of the stomach** contains **three layers of smooth muscle:** the outer longitudinal, the middle circular, and the inner oblique.
3. The **distal two thirds of the stomach** contains a **single longitudinal layer.** This layer demonstrates spontaneous, repeated electrical discharges for peristalsis.
4. The **mucosa** is lined by simple columnar epithelium with surface mucous cells.

a. The **proximal cardiac glands**

—secrete mucus.

b. The **fundus and body**

—contain oxyntic glands with parietal and chief cells.

(1) Parietal cells secrete

—**HCl** for digestion.

—**intrinsic factor** for vitamin B_{12} absorption in the terminal ileum.

(2) Chief cells secrete

—**pepsinogen** for protein digestion.

c. The **antrum contains**

—mucus-secreting cells.

—gastrin-producing G cells.

d. **The pyloric sphincter**

—is a thick circumferential layer of smooth muscle.

5. The **duodenum consists of**

—mucosal layers.

—submucosal layers.

—muscular layers.

—serosal layers.

—**Brunner's glands** unique to the duodenum secrete an **alkaline mucus.**

F. **Surgical anatomy of the stomach and duodenum**

1. **Vagotomy and pyloroplasty**

a. **Division of the main vagal trunks at the esophageal hiatus (truncal vagotomy)**

—ablates the cephalic phase of gastric acid secretion.

—desensitizes the parietal cells to gastrin.

b. **Denervation of the pylorus**

—also results in discordant gastric emptying, which causes rapid emptying of liquids and abnormal solid emptying.

c. **Division and reconstruction of the pylorus (pyloroplasty)**

—is performed with this procedure to facilitate gastric emptying (Figure 12-2).

d. **Diarrhea may occur after vagotomy**

—but generally resolves with time.

2. **Other types of vagotomy procedures** (Figure 12-3)

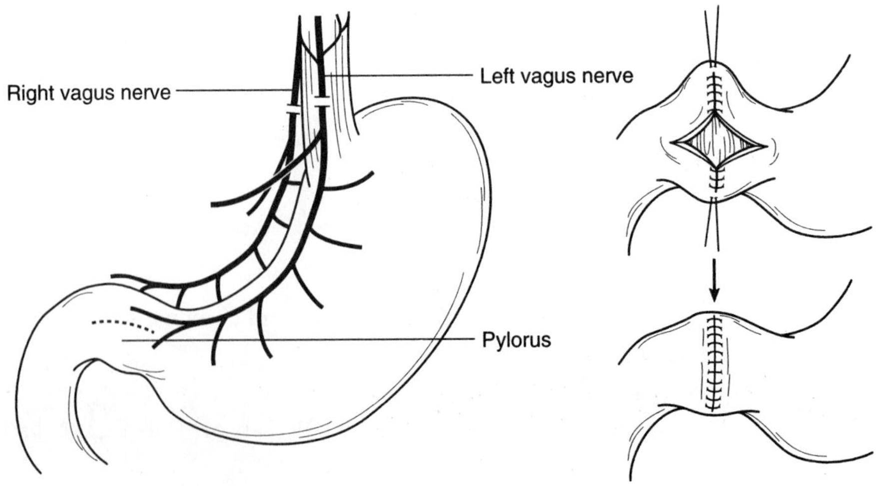

Figure 12-2. A Heineke-Mikulicz pyloroplasty. A longitudinal incision is made through the pyloric sphincter and then the duodenum is closed in a transverse manner. (Adapted with permission from Lawrence P: *Essentials of General Surgery.* Baltimore, Williams & Wilkins, 1992, p 195.)

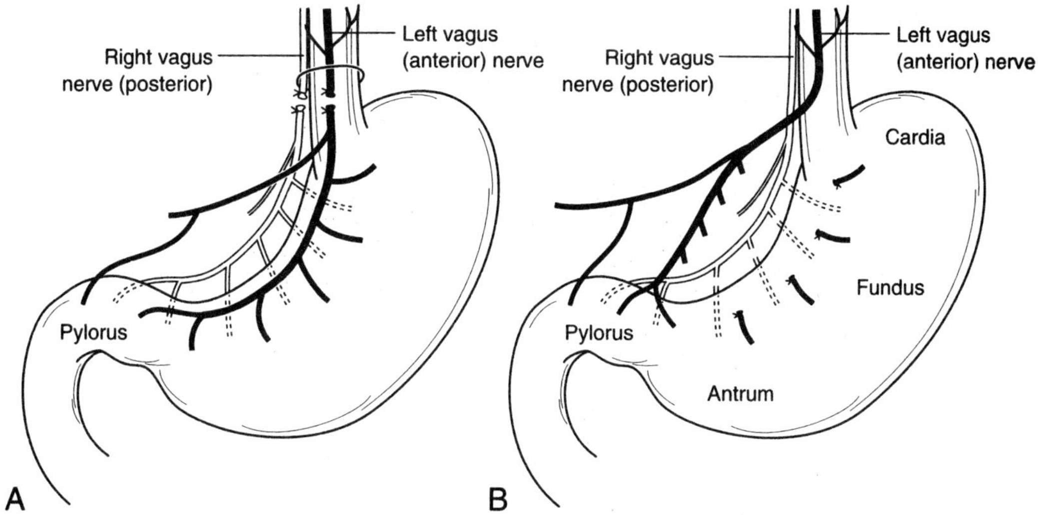

Figure 12-3. The truncal vagotomy and the proximal gastric vagotomy. (*A*) The main nerve trunks are both divided at the esophageal hiatus, denervating the entire abdomen of vagal innervation after truncal vagotomy. (*B*) A proximal gastric vagotomy or highly selective vagotomy only denervated the acid-producing parietal cell mass in the fundic region.

a. **Selective vagotomy**

—denervates the entire stomach, but preserves innervation to the hepatobiliary system and celiac ganglia.

b. **Proximal gastric vagotomy (parietal cell vagotomy or highly selective vagotomy)**

—denervates fibers to the acid-secreting fundic mucosa, preserving pyloric vagal innervation.

c. These procedures are associated with a **lower complication rate,** but have a **higher recurrence rate** of ulcer disease versus truncal vagotomy.

3. **Gastric resection and reconstruction**

a. **Antrectomy**

—consists of removing the gastric antrum for ulcer disease.

b. **Reconstruction**

—may be performed by a **Billroth I gastroduodenostomy** or a **Billroth II gastrojejunostomy** (Figure 12-4).

c. **Total gastrectomy**

—involves removing the entire stomach.

—may be performed for curative resection of gastric neoplasms, massive diffuse gastric bleeding, or palliation in Zollinger-Ellison syndrome.

II. Physiology

A. **Secretory factors of the upper gastrointestinal tract** (Table 12-1)

B. **Gastric acid secretion**

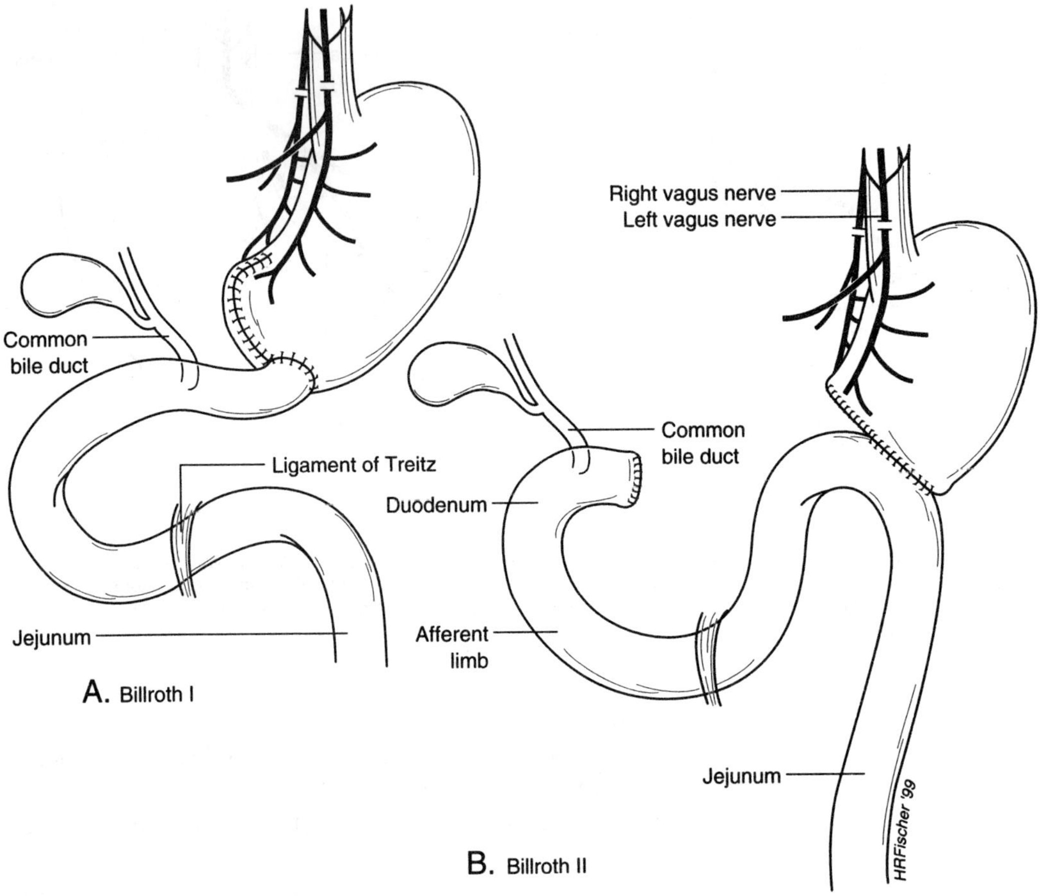

Figure 12-4. Billroth I and Billroth II. Both reconstructions follow vagotomy and antrectomy, which involves resection of the distal stomach. (*A*) In a Billroth I or gastroduodenostomy, the duodenum is reanastomosed to the stomach in physiologic continuity. (*B*) In the Billroth II or gastrojejunostomy, the duodenal stump is closed with a suture and a jejunal loop is reanastomosed to the remaining stomach. (Adapted with permission from Lawrence P: *Essentials of General Surgery.* Baltimore, Williams & Wilkins, 1992, p 193.)

1. **The basolateral membrane of parietal cells contains receptors for** histamine, gastrin, and acetylcholine.
   —These receptors decrease gastric pH through alterations in **ion transport.**
2. **During the cephalic phase**
   —acid secretion increases in response to the thought, sight, or smell of food via **vagal stimulation.**
3. **During the gastric phase**
   —acid secretion increases as food enters the stomach via **gastrin-mediated** stimulation.
4. **During the intestinal phase**
   —a decrease in stomach acidity is seen when acidified **chyme** enters the duodenum.

Table 12-1. Characteristics of Several Gastric and Duodenal Secretory Factors

Factor	Source	Stimulus	Action
Gastrin	G cells in antrum and duodenum	Meals, amino acids, gastric distension	Stimulates acid secretion and mucosal growth
Somatostatin	Pancreatic D cell	Intraluminal fat, PGE_2	Inhibits acid secretion and gastrin release
Histamine	Mast cells	Adrenergic stimuli	Stimulates acid secretion
Acetylcholine	Vagus nerve terminus	Vagal stimulation	Acid stimulation
Pepsin	Chief cells	Meals	Initiate protein digestion
Bicarbonate	Mucous cells, pancreatic ductal cells	Low mucosal pH, cholinergic stimuli	Neutralize acid
Intrinsic factor	Parietal cells	Meals, gastrin, histamine, acetylcholine	Bind vitamin B_{12} for terminal ileum absorption
Cholecystokinin	Duodenum and jejunum	Luminal fats and proteins	Gallbladder contraction, stimulates exocrine pancreatic secretion
Secretin	S cells of duodenum and jejunum	Duodenal acidification	Stimulates pancreatic secretion
Gastric inhibitory peptide	Duodenum and jejunum	Meals	Augments insulin response to enteral feedings
Motilin	Enterochromaffin cells of small intestine	Fasting state, erythromycin stimulates motilin receptors	Regulates migrating motor complex

PGE_2 = prostaglandin E_2.

C. Gastric motility

1. Increases in gastric volume

—lead to vagally mediated **receptive relaxation** of the stomach.

2. Meal ingestion

—stimulates proximal contraction and distal peristalsis.

3. The pylorus

—then closes 2–3 seconds before antral contraction, producing churning of chyme.

III. Upper Gastrointestinal Hemorrhage

—is defined as bleeding **proximal** to the **ligament of Treitz.**

A. Risk factors include

—previous upper gastrointestinal bleed.

—peptic ulcer disease.

—nonsteroidal anti-inflammatory drug (NSAID) use.

—alcohol abuse.

—smoking.

—liver disease.

—trauma or burn history.

—esophageal varices.

—sepsis.

—vomiting.

—splenic vein thrombosis.

B. **Potential causes** are characterized in Table 12-2.

—**Peptic ulcer disease** is the leading cause of upper gastrointestinal bleeding.

C. **Signs and symptoms** may include

—**hypotension/syncope/shock.**

—hematemesis/coffee ground emesis.

—melena/**guaiac-positive stools.**

—epigastric pain.

—fatigue.

D. **Diagnosis**

1. **Examination of the nasogastric (N/G) tube aspirate**

—can rapidly confirm the presence of upper gastrointestinal bleeding.

2. **Endoscopic esophagogastroduodenoscopy (EGD)**

—localizes most sources of upper gastrointestinal bleeding.

E. **Treatment**

1. **Initial treatment** involves

—**protection of the airway** if necessary (i.e., intubation).

—adequate **volume resuscitation.**

2. **Subsequent management** involves

—appropriate treatment of the specific cause of bleeding.

a. **Most** causes can be **treated endoscopically,** with surgery reserved for severe bleeding refractory to initial measures.

b. **Angiographic embolization** is used in some situations when the patient is a poor surgical candidate.

IV. Gastritis

A. **Overview**

1. **Gastritis consists of inflammatory changes in the mucosa** secondary to epithelial damage from **decreased mucosal defenses.**

2. **Clinically, gastritis is differentiated** as acute or chronic gastritis.

a. **Acute gastritis**

—is classified according to the cause (i.e., stress, *Helicobacter pylori* infection, NSAIDs).

Table 12-2. Causes of Upper Gastrointestinal Bleeding

Disease	Risks	Diagnosis	Treatment	Miscellaneous
PUD	*H. pylori* infection, alcohol abuse, smoking	EGD	EGD, medical therapy, surgery as indicated	Posterior duodenal ulcer erodes into gastroduodenal artery
Acute gastritis	Sepsis, CNS injury (Cushing's ulcer), trauma, severe burns (Curling's ulcer)	EGD	EGD, medical therapy	Mucosal superficial erosions in proximal stomach
Esophageal varices	Portal hypertension, alcohol abuse	EGD	Sclerotherapy, vasopressin infusion	Portal venous system is valveless
Mallory-Weiss tear	Severe retching, alcohol abuse	EGD	Majority spontaneously resolve	Linear mucosal tear at esophageal hiatus
Aorto-duodenal fistula	Abdominal aortic aneurysm, previous aortic surgery	Angiography	Emergent resection, repair hole in duodenum	Most present with a "sentinel bleed" before massive hemorrhage
Gastric neoplasm	Adenocarcinoma, lymphoma	EGD with biopsy	Resection	May mimic PUD
Hemobilia/hemosuccus pancreaticus	Prior history of hepatic/biliary trauma or chronic pancreatitis	EGD, selective angiography	Angiographic embolization	Arterial erosion into biliary or pancreatic ducts

CNS = central nervous system; EGD = esophagogastroduodenoscopy; *H. pylori* = *Helicobacter pylori;* PUD = peptic ulcer disease.

b. Chronic gastritis

—is classified as Type A (fundal) or Type B (antral).

B. Risk factors

1. Predisposing factors for acute erosive gastritis include

—NSAID use.

—cigarette smoking.

—alcohol abuse.

2. Predisposing factors for acute stress gastritis include

—multiple trauma.

—major burns.

—sepsis.

—brain injury.

—renal failure.

—adult respiratory distress syndrome (ARDS).

—hypotension.

—an extended stay in the intensive care unit.

3. Chronic gastritis

a. Type A (fundal) is associated with

—pernicious anemia.

—parietal cell antibodies.

—achlorhydria.

—autoimmune diseases.

b. Type B (antral) is associated with

—***H. pylori*** infection in almost 100% of cases.

C. Pathology

1. Acute erosive gastritis is characterized by

—a friable edematous mucosa with erosions and sites of bleeding that may be localized or diffuse.

—**Mucosal ischemia** is generally the inciting pathologic event.

2. Chronic gastritis typically is manifest

—by a patchy and irregular distribution of mucosal erosions.

D. Signs and symptoms of acute gastritis

1. Painless upper gastrointestinal bleeding

—is the hallmark of gastritis.

—is usually slow and intermittent, but can be profuse.

2. Other symptoms may include

—epigastric pain.

—nausea.

—vomiting.

3. **Other signs** include
—blood in the N/G tube aspirate.
—guaiac-positive stools.
—unexplained anemia.
—a drop in the hematocrit.

E. The diagnosis of acute gastritis
—is confirmed by **EGD.**

F. Treatment of acute gastritis

1. **Resuscitation**
—with crystalloid and appropriate blood products is essential.

2. **Antacids, H_2-blockers, and proton pump inhibitors (e.g., omeprazole)**
—are used to decrease gastric pH.

3. **Endoscopic electrocautery**
—may occasionally be used to treat a localized source of bleeding.

4. **Surgery for acute gastritis**
—is associated with a high mortality.
—is rarely necessary.
   a. **Vagotomy and pyloroplasty**
   —with oversewing of obvious bleeding points is recommended in most patients who require an operation.
   b. **Total gastric resection**
   —is reserved for diffuse bleeding not amenable to any other therapy.

V. Peptic Ulcer Disease

A. Ulcers are classified according to **location.**
—Common locations include the stomach, duodenum, esophagus, and jejunum (i.e., after gastrojejunostomy).

B. Duodenal ulcers most commonly occur in **middle-aged men.**
—Ninety-five percent occur **within 2 cm of the pylorus** in the first portion of the duodenum.

1. **Risk factors**
   a. The **primary risk factor**
   —is the **presence of *H. pylori*** in the upper gastrointestinal tract.
   b. **Other risk factors** include
   —cigarette smoking.
   —NSAID use.
   —delayed gastric emptying.
   —uremia.

—Zollinger-Ellison syndrome.

2. **Pathogenesis**
   a. ***H. pylori* infection**
      —plays a major role in the weakening of mucosal defenses and subsequent ulcer development.
   b. **Gastric acid secretion**
      —is usually **elevated** in patients with duodenal ulcers, in contrast to gastric ulcers.
3. **Signs and symptoms**
   a. **Epigastric pain**
      —is a cardinal feature.
      —is typically burning, stabbing, and gnawing.
      —may be **relieved by food or antacids.**
   b. **Other possible symptoms** include
      —nausea.
      —vomiting.
      —anorexia.
      —hematemesis.
      —melena.
   c. **Patients can present with**
      —guaiac-positive stools.
      —symptoms of hypotension secondary to hemorrhage (e.g., syncope).
4. **Diagnosis**
   a. **EGD is the preferred diagnostic method**
      —because it allows for visualization, biopsy, and possible treatment.
   b. ***H. pylori* infection can be confirmed with**
      —biopsy.
      —noninvasive techniques (e.g., breath test).
   c. **Contrast radiographs**
      —may demonstrate retention of contrast in the ulcer.
5. **Treatment**
   a. **Medical therapy** is primary in the treatment of uncomplicated duodenal ulcer disease.
      (1) **Frequently used agents** include
         —**H_2-blockers** (e.g., famotidine).
         —**proton pump inhibitors** (e.g., omeprazole).
      (2) **Antibiotic therapy (when *H. pylori* is present)** in addition to these agents heals more than 90% of ulcers.
   b. **Surgery** is required in a small minority of patients with ulcer disease.
      —Indications for surgery are listed in Table 12-3.

C. **Gastric ulcers** have many characteristics similar to duodenal ulcers.

1. **Clinical presentation**

Table 12-3. Indications for Surgical Therapy of a Duodenal Ulcer

Indication	Definition	Clinical Findings	Procedure
Perforation	Full-thickness erosion of ulcer through deuodenal wall	Severe epigastric pain, peritonitis, free air, 90% occur on anterior duodenal bulb (first portion)	Oversewing piece of omentum over perforation (Graham patch); may perform definitive ulcer operation depending on patient status
Hemorrhage	Blood transfusion (≥ 6 units), recurrent bleeding after endoscopic therapy	Severe hypotension or shock, hematemesis, blood from rectum (frequently associated with a posterior duodenal ulcer with erosion into the gastroduodenal artery)	Duodentomy and direct vessel oversewing followed by vagotomy and pyloroplasty
Obstruction	Obstructive symptoms secondary to scarring and edema	Nausea, vomiting, anorexia, pyloric channel ulcers	Vagotomy and antrectomy with Billroth II or vagotomy and drainage
Intractability	Recurrent or persistent ulceration despite ≥ 8 weeks of H_2-blockers or ≥ 6 weeks of proton pump inhibitors as well as adequate treatment for *Helicobacter pylori*	Persistent pain refractory to medical therapy; symptoms significantly interfere with daily activities	Parietal cell vagotomy

—**Gastric adenocarcinoma may mimic gastric ulcer disease;** therefore, care must be taken to rule out malignancy.

2. **Risk factors**

—The risk factors for gastric ulcer disease are generally the same as those for duodenal ulcer disease.

3. **Location**

   a. The location of the gastric ulcers plays an important role in determining the pathogenesis and treatment.

   b. **Classification of gastric ulcers** is based on their location (Figure 12-5).

   —Gastric ulcers most commonly occur on the **lesser curve** of the stomach.

   c. **Acid secretion** may not be elevated, unlike in duodenal ulcer disease.

4. **Signs and symptoms**

   a. **Epigastric pain** is generally gnawing, dull, and burning.

   —**Food may aggravate or precipitate pain** in contrast to duodenal ulcers.

   b. **Other possible symptoms** include nausea, vomiting, and anorexia.

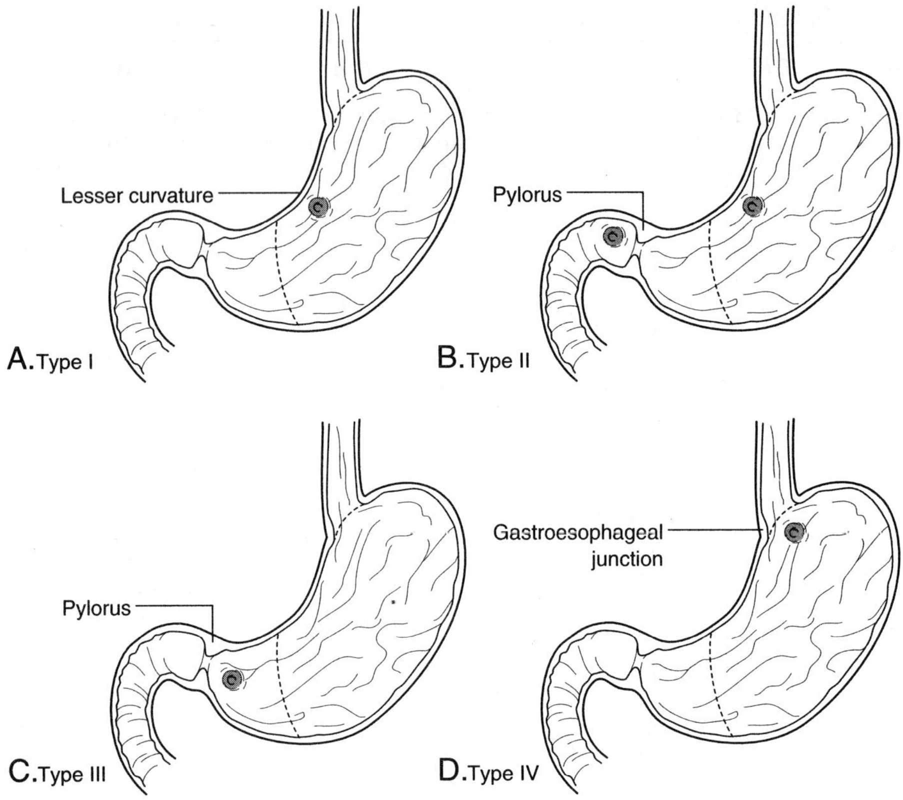

Figure 12-5. The location of the four types of gastric ulcer. (*A*) Type I occurs along the lesser curvature and is associated with large volumes of secretion. (*B*) Type II occurs in the body of the stomach and in combination with a duodenal ulcer. (*C*) Type III is simply a prepyloric ulcer. (*D*) Type IV is rare and occurs in close proximity to the gastroesophageal junction. (Adapted with permission from Blackbourne LH: *Advanced Surgical Recall.* Baltimore, Williams & Wilkins, 1997, p 375.)

c. **Perforation and severe hemorrhage**

—may also occur, as with duodenal ulcers.

5. **Diagnosis**

a. **Endoscopy**

—is the **most reliable** diagnostic tool.

—allows for **biopsy of the ulcer** to evaluate for carcinoma.

—**Indications for early endoscopy** include weight loss, obstructive symptoms, a palpable mass, guaiac-positive stools, and anemia.

b. **Barium contrast radiographs**

—may be useful if endoscopic evaluation is incomplete or contraindicated.

6. **Treatment**

a. **Medical therapy**

—is the **primary treatment,** like in duodenal ulcers.

—involves administration of acid-reducing agents with antibiotics when *H. pylori* is present.

b. **Indications for surgery** include

—intractability.

—severe hemorrhage.

—perforation.

—obstruction.

—These indications are identical to those for duodenal ulcers (see Table 12-3).

c. **Definitive surgical treatment**

—may vary depending on the site and pathogenesis of the gastric ulcer (Table 12-4).

d. **Gastric versus duodenal ulcers**

—A key difference in the approach to patients is the **appropriate recognition** and **management of malignancy** in patients with gastric ulcers.

VI. Gastric Neoplasms

A. Benign gastric neoplasms

1. Leiomyomas

—are the **most common benign gastric neoplasms.**

—are **usually asymptomatic,** but hemorrhage or obstruction can occur.

—are **submucosal lesions** that are **well-encapsulated.**

—Treatment involves **resection** of the lesion with margins of normal tissue.

2. Hyperplastic polyps

—account for 70%–80% of all gastric polyps.

—consist of histologically normal gastric epithelium.

—have **no malignant potential.**

3. Adenomatous polyps

—carry a 10%–20% **risk of carcinoma,** with an increased risk associated with increasing polyp size (e.g., > 2 cm).

a. **Treatment**

Table 12-4. Types of Gastric Ulcers

Type	Pathogenesis	Definitive Treatment
I	Decreased mucosal defense, low acid status	Distal gastrectomy with ulcer excision
II	High acid secretory status	Antrectomy with truncal vagotomy, vagotomy and pyloroplasty, or vagotomy and drainage
III	High acid secretory status	Vagotomy and antrectomy with ulcer excision in specimen
IV	High acid secretory status	Excision of ulcer or distal gastroectomy with vertical extension to include ulcer
V	Associated with nonsteroidal anti-inflammatory drugs	Usually responds to withdrawal of agent and medical treatment; surgery is rarely indicated

—consists of endoscopic resection of pedunculated lesions.

b. Operative excision may be required for

—sessile lesions larger than 2 cm.

—polyps with foci of invasive carcinoma.

—polyps complicated by pain or bleeding.

B. Malignant gastric neoplasms

1. Adenocarcinoma of the stomach

—is the most common malignant lesion of the stomach.

—occurs **more frequently in males** than females.

—is rare in the United States, although it is more common in Japan.

a. Risk factors include

—dietary nitrates.

—the presence of adenomatous polyps.

—exposure to *H. pylori.*

—chronic gastritis.

—pernicious anemia.

—achlorhydria.

b. Signs and symptoms

(1) The clinical presentation

—may be indistinguishable from peptic ulcer disease.

(2) Symptoms include

—**weight loss.**

—**pain.**

—nausea and vomiting.

—anorexia.

—dysphagia.

(3) Signs of advanced disease include

—supraclavicular adenopathy (**Virchow's node**).

—ovarian metastases (**Krukenberg's tumor**).

c. Diagnosis

(1) Endoscopy is the definitive diagnostic method with an accuracy of more than 95% when multiple biopsy specimens are obtained.

—Approximately 75% of patients have metastatic disease at the time of diagnosis.

(2) To characterize the extent of the disease use

—barium contrast studies.

—computed tomography (CT) scan.

—endoscopic ultrasound.

d. Staging and prognosis (Table 12-5)

e. Treatment

(1) Surgical resection

—Surgical resection may be curative, although most tumors are at an advanced stage at the time of diagnosis.

Table 12-5. Staging and Prognosis of Adenocarcinoma of the Stomach

Stage	Description	5-Year Survival Rate
I	Mucosal involvement	66%
II	Through muscularis propria without lymph node involvement	33%
III	Any lymph node involvement without distant metastases	10%
IV	Distant metastases or extension of primary tumor into adjacent structures (e.g., liver)	0%

—Procedures include a **subtotal or total gastrectomy** plus lymph node dissection for tumors amenable to curative resection.

(2) **Surgical palliation with gastric resection**

—is also frequently performed for incurable disease to provide relief of symptoms (e.g., dysphagia).

(3) **Radiation therapy and chemotherapy**

—play a minor role in the management of gastric cancer.

2. **Gastric lymphoma**

a. **Overview**

(1) **Non-Hodgkin lymphomas**

—account for 5% of malignant gastric tumors.

—occur most frequently in patients 60–70 years old.

(2) A subset of lymphomas associated with **mucosal-associated lymphoid tissue (MALT)** have a strong association with ***H. pylori*** infection.

b. **Signs and symptoms** include

—epigastric pain.

—weight loss.

—anorexia.

—nausea.

—vomiting.

—**occult bleeding and anemia** (50% of patients).

c. **Diagnosis**

(1) **Endoscopic biopsy**

—with brush cytology and ultrasound are 90% accurate.

(2) **Chest and abdominal CT scan and bone marrow biopsy**

—are used to identify systemic disease.

d. **Staging of gastric lymphomas** (Table 12-6)

e. **Treatment** is controversial.

(1) **The role of gastric resection**

—is controversial, with many advocating the use of chemoradiation therapy alone.

(2) **Gastrectomy allows for**

—accurate histological diagnosis.

—local cure.

Table 12-6. Gastric Lymphoma Staging

Stage	Definition
I	Tumor confined to stomach only
II	Spread to perigastric lymph nodes
III	Nodal spread beyond perigastric nodes (e.g., para-aortic nodes)
IV	Spread to other abdominal organs (e.g., liver, spleen)

—elimination of the risk of hemorrhage or perforation.

(3) **Combination chemoradiation therapy**

—**with or without surgical resection** is generally used to treat gastric lymphomas.

(4) **MALT-associated lymphomas**

—may regress with treatment of *H. pylori.*

f. **Overall survival** for all stages of gastric lymphoma is greater than or equal to 50%.

3. **Gastric leiomyosarcomas**

—require wide excision, although local recurrence and peritoneal involvement are common.

4. **Gastric carcinoids**

—are extremely rare.

VII. Surgical Treatment of Morbid Obesity

A. Overview

1. **Morbid (severe) obesity**

—is defined as more than 100 lb above ideal body weight, or a **body mass index greater than or equal to 35.**

—is also associated with an **increase** in overall **mortality.**

2. **Associated morbidity** includes

—cardiac and pulmonary dysfunction.

—diabetes mellitus.

—degenerative joint disease.

—sexual dysfunction.

3. **Dietary management**

—has not achieved uniform, long-term success for the treatment of morbid obesity.

—Ninety-five percent of patients will regain all weight lost through diets.

B. Results of surgical treatment

1. The average weight loss is **50%–67% of excess weight** within 1.5 years.

2. **Most patients requiring insulin**

—for non–insulin-dependent diabetes mellitus (NIDDM) preoperatively **will not require insulin after surgery.**

3. **Hypertension** resolves or improves in 80% of patients.
4. **Obstructive sleep apnea** usually resolves.
5. The patient's **self image** often improves.

C. Surgical options

1. **Gastroplasty**

—provides slightly less weight loss than gastric bypass.

a. **Mesh** used in the procedure **may erode into the stomach.**
b. **Gastroesophageal reflux** may also occur, which generally requires conversion to a gastric bypass.

2. **Gastric bypass** (Figure 12-6)

—involves formation of a small stomach pouch and a **gastrojejunostomy** to drain the pouch.

a. **Weight loss is regained**

—in 10%–15% of patients from excessive, constant nibbling of high-calorie foods.

b. **Operative mortality**

—with surgery is 0.5%.

D. Complications of gastric operations include

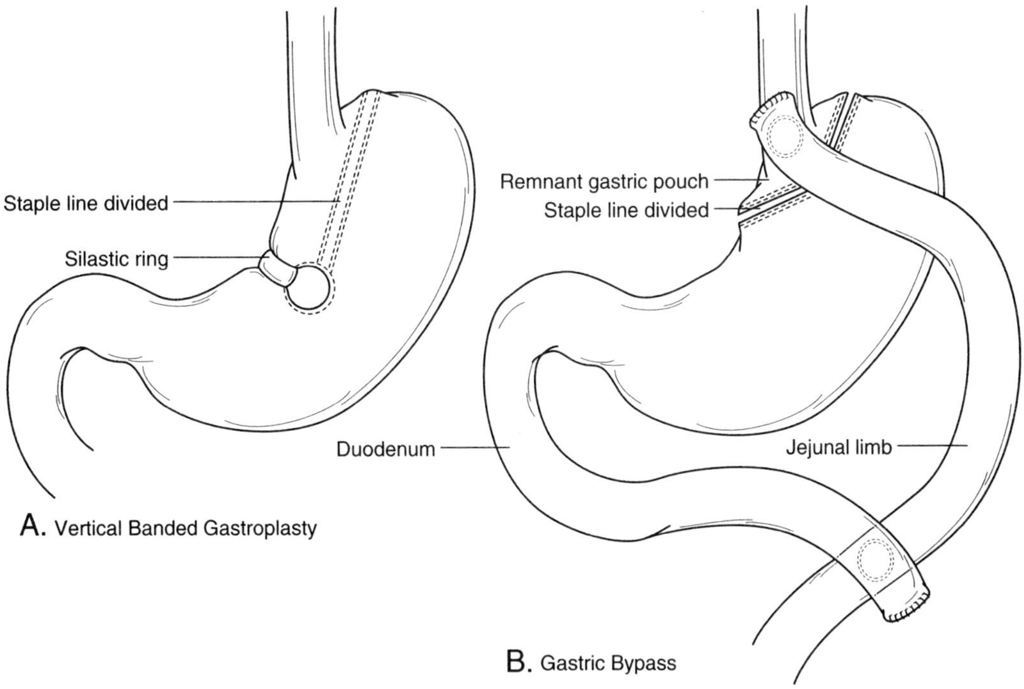

Figure 12-6. Surgical procedure for bariatric surgery. (*A*) Vertical banded gastroplasty consists of placing a Silastic ring near the incisura, creating an in-flow obstruction and limiting the volume of food consumed. Erosion of mesh into the stomach is a potential problem. (*B*) The proximal Roux-en-Y gastric bypass consists of the formation of a small gastric pouch anastomosed to a long jejunal limb. Typically, the staple line is divided. (Adapted with permission from Greenfield L: *Surgery: Scientific Principles and Practice,* 2nd ed. Philadelphia, Lippincott Williams & Wilkins, 1997, pp 791–792.)

—perforation or leak at anastomosis sites.

—necrosis of the distal stomach.

—ulcer formation at anastomosis sites (often responds to medical therapy).

—obstruction or stenosis (may be treated with endoscopic balloon dilation).

—vitamin B_{12} deficiency or anemia.

—**gallstone formation with rapid weight loss** (cholecystectomy may be performed at the time of operation).

VIII. Miscellaneous Disorders of the Stomach and Duodenum

A. Mallory-Weiss tear

—is a potential cause of upper gastrointestinal bleeding that results from a **longitudinal tear** of the mucosa and submucosa near the **gastro-esophageal junction.**

1. **Risk factors** include

   —severe retching or coughing.

   —alcohol abuse.

   —presence of a hiatal hernia.

2. **Symptoms** may include

   —epigastric pain.

   —substernal pain.

   —classically, **hematemesis after an episode of forceful retching.**

3. **Endoscopic evaluation**

   —can confirm the presence of a tear.

4. **Treatment**

   a. **Bleeding stops spontaneously**

      —in 90% of patients.

   b. **Persistent bleeding**

      —is managed with **endoscopic electrocautery.**

   c. **Refractory bleeding**

      —may require surgical repair of the laceration.

B. Dumping syndrome

1. **Symptoms**

   —generally occur after **rapid entry of a carbohydrate load** into the small bowel secondary to **bypass of the pylorus** (e.g., Billroth II).

   a. **Characteristic gastrointestinal and vasomotor symptoms** include

      —nausea.

      —vomiting.

      —abdominal pain.

—flatus.
—palpitations.
—dizziness.
—diaphoresis.

b. Early symptoms

—occur immediately after a meal.
—may occur 1–3 hours after a meal, secondary to reactive hypoglycemia (i.e., late dumping syndrome).

2. Treatment

a. Most cases resolve with time

—although dietary changes (i.e., small, low-carbohydrate meals) and somatostatin may be beneficial.

b. Severe cases

—may require conversion to a Roux-en-Y gastrojejunostomy (Figure 12-7).

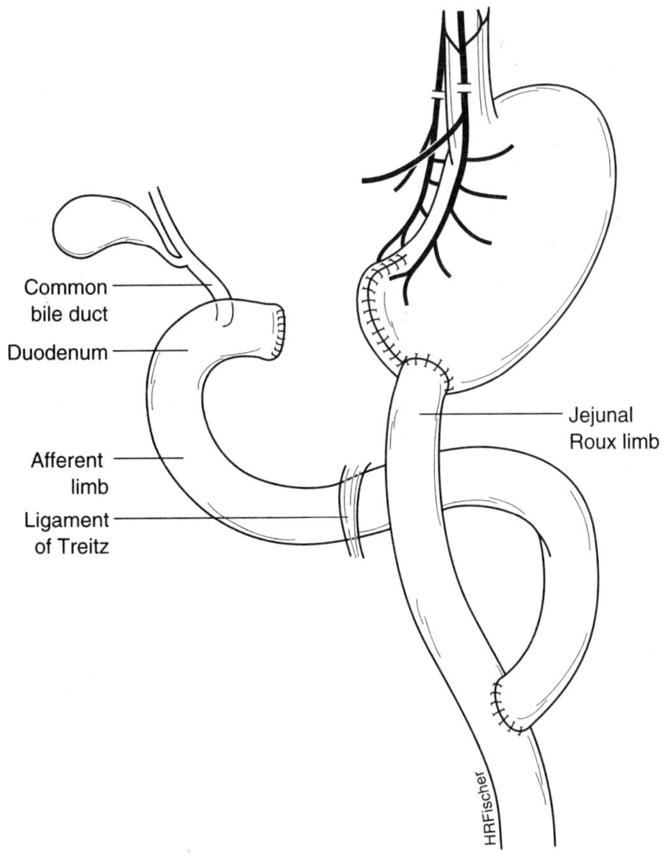

Figure 12-7. Truncal vagotomy with antrectomy and Roux-en-Y anastomosis. This anastomosis is particularly useful to correct many of the problems associated with vagotomy and Billroth I reanastomosis. It is particularly useful for alkaline reflux gastritis because reflux of small bowel contents into the stomach is reduced. (Adapted with permission from Lawrence P: *Essentials of General Surgery.* Baltimore, Williams & Wilkins, 1992, p 194.)

C. Afferent loop syndrome

—**results from obstruction of the afferent limb** after a Billroth II procedure (see Figure 12-6) with accumulation of biliary secretions.

1. **Over 66% present in the first postoperative week with**

—postprandial right upper quadrant (RUQ) pain.

—nonbilious vomiting.

—fever.

—steatorrhea.

2. **Diagnosis**

—Contrast radiographs, CT scan, and endoscopy may be useful.

3. **Treatment consists of**

—surgical reconstruction with a Roux-en-Y gastrojejunostomy or balloon dilation.

D. Alkaline reflux gastritis

—results from bile reflux into the stomach.

1. **Symptoms** include

—postprandial epigastric pain.

—nausea.

—vomiting.

2. **Diagnosis**

—is made with endoscopic confirmation of **bile reflux and biopsy-proven gastritis.**

3. **Treatment**

—**Sucralfate** may be used to bind bile.

—Surgery is rarely required.

E. Gastric volvulus

—is very rare.

—results from torsion of the stomach secondary to laxity of the ligamentous support to the stomach.

—is **frequently associated with** a **diaphragmatic hernia.**

—Treatment involves **emergent detorsion** and **fixation of the stomach.**

Review Test

Directions: Each of the numbered items or incomplete statements in this section is followed by answers or by completions of the statement. Select the ONE lettered answer or completion that is BEST in each case.

1. A 63-year-old woman underwent placement of a percutaneous endoscopic gastrostomy tube 1 day ago. Today she is tachycardic with a heart rate of 135 beats/min and a blood pressure of 95/45 mm Hg. Her abdomen is distended and notably tender. Abdominal plain film radiograph reveals a large amount of free air. A small amount of contrast added to the gastrostomy tube confirms appropriate placement within the stomach. Her hematocrit is 37% and her white blood cell count is within normal limits. Her calcium is 7.8 mg/dL. Which of the following is the most likely cause of this patient's symptoms?

(A) Injury to the esophagus during endoscope placement
(B) Injury to the liver during placement of the gastrostomy tube
(C) Injury to the transverse colon during placement of the gastrostomy tube
(D) Traumatic injury to the spleen during placement of the gastrostomy tube
(E) Acute pancreatitis caused by retrograde flow of gastric contents into the ampulla of Vater

2. A 35-year-old trauma victim with a severe closed head injury is post-trauma day 14. After surviving an eventful intensive care unit stay, he has recently undergone elective tracheostomy and percutaneous gastrostomy tube placement. Today he is febrile to 39°C (102.2°F) and tachycardic to 125 beats/min. He is comatose secondary to his head injury, but his abdomen is quiet and rigid to palpation. Which of the following is the most appropriate next step in the management of this patient?

(A) Esophagogastroduodenoscopy (EGD)
(B) Emergent laparotomy
(C) Barium swallow
(D) A barium enema to identify any source of colonic injury
(E) Immediate removal of the gastrostomy tube with observation

3. A 69-year-old, white woman with a history of chronic mesenteric ischemia has recently undergone superior mesenteric artery (SMA) saphenous vein bypass grafting after presenting with acute SMA occlusion. On postoperative day 3 she was returned to the operating room and underwent small bowel resection and reanastomosis with duodenojejunostomy. Now, 48 hours after her second surgery, she is passing large melanotic stools and her hematocrit has fallen from 32% to 20%. Despite aggressive resuscitation with crystalloid and 2 units of packed red blood cells (PRBCs), her hematocrit remains 21%. If an upper gastrointestinal source of bleeding is suspected, which of the following would be the most appropriate next step?

(A) Esophagogastroduodenoscopy (EGD)
(B) Emergent laparotomy
(C) Mesenteric vessel arteriography
(D) Vasopressin administration
(E) Placement of a Sengstaken-Blakemore tube

4. A 63-year-old man with no significant past medical history is admitted with an acute abdomen secondary to gastric perforation. If a definitive ulcer procedure is performed on this patient, which of the following procedures is associated with the lowest ulcer recurrence rate?

(A) Truncal vagotomy
(B) Truncal vagotomy and pyloroplasty
(C) Vagotomy and antrectomy
(D) Parietal cell vagotomy
(E) Gastric bypass

5. A thin, cachectic, 61-year-old woman presents to the office requesting a prescription for a "strong heartburn medicine." She complains of gnawing abdominal pain after meals. Upon further questioning she admits to an unwanted 25-pound weight loss over the previous 3 months. She is a nonsmoker. Physical examination is unremarkable except for some mild epigastric tenderness. Rectal examination is heme-negative. Which of the following would be the most appropriate definitive diagnostic test for this patient?

(A) Esophagogastroduodenoscopy (EGD) with biopsy
(B) Esophageal manometry
(C) Magnetic resonance image (MRI) of the abdomen
(D) Upper gastrointestinal barium swallow
(E) Angiography of mesenteric vessels

6. An obese, 45-year-old businessman comes to the office for a routine physical examination. He states that his father and grandfather have died from stomach cancer. He admits to smoking one pack of unfiltered cigarettes a day and to moderate alcohol consumption only on weekends. He also states that he takes an antacid pill after meals for heartburn. All of the following are considered risk factors for gastric adenocarcinoma EXCEPT:

(A) *Helicobacter pylori* infection
(B) Smoking
(C) High-fat diet
(D) Previous gastric surgery
(E) Alkaline reflux gastritis

7. A 42-year-old woman presents to the office with a 2-month history of increasing nausea and nonbilious vomiting associated with a 15-lb weight loss. Upon upper gastrointestinal endoscopy, biopsy reveals *Helicobacter pylori* and a low-grade lymphoma. Which of the following is the most appropriate statement regarding the management of gastric lymphoma?

(A) Treatment is limited to radiation therapy alone
(B) Treatment consists of surgery alone
(C) Some lymphomas may regress with treatment of *H. pylori*
(D) Overall 5-year survival is less than 20%
(E) Obstructive symptoms are a contraindication to surgery

8. A 62-year-old man with a history of alcoholic cirrhosis presents to the emergency room with a 4-hour history of hematemesis. His abdomen is soft. He is tachycardic with a heart rate of 121 beats/min and has a blood pressure of 98/58 mm Hg. Which of the following is the most appropriate step in the immediate management of this patient?

(A) Airway control and resuscitation
(B) Intravenous vasopressin infusion
(C) Placement of a Sengstaken-Blakemore tube
(D) Performance of a barium swallow
(E) Upright chest radiograph to evaluate for free air

9. A 68-year-old man presents to the emergency room complaining of severe intense abdominal pain that came on suddenly and quickly reached peak intensity. Upon evaluation, the patient is lying completely still, is tachycardic, and has an ashen-gray appearance. Upon further questioning he reveals that the pain began in his epigastric region and then moved down to the right quadrants. His abdomen is rigid and extremely tender. Laboratory investigation reveals a white blood cell count of 30,000 and a hematocrit of 44%. Which of the following is the most likely cause of this patient's clinical presentation?

(A) Mallory-Weiss tear
(B) Bleeding duodenal ulcer
(C) Acute gastritis
(D) Perforated peptic ulcer
(E) Gastric lymphoma

10. An 85-year-old man presents with a 3-day history of severe abdominal pain. The patient's temperature is 39.4°C (103°F), he is tachycardic with 130 beats/min, and he has a blood pressure of 80/40 mm Hg. The patient is becoming more tachypneic, and upon placement of a Foley catheter no urine is produced. His abdomen is rigid and plain abdominal film demonstrates free air under the right hemidiaphragm. His past medical history is significant for coronary artery disease, emphysema, chronic renal insufficiency secondary to insulin-dependent diabetes mellitus, as well as manic depression. Which of the following is the most appropriate operation to perform on this patient?

(A) Pyloromyotomy
(B) Omental patching with or without a vagotomy
(C) Gastrectomy
(D) Billroth II
(E) Vagotomy and antrectomy

Directions: Each set of matching questions in this section consists of a list of four to twenty-six lettered options followed by several numbered items. For each numbered item, select the appropriate lettered option(s). Each lettered option may be selected once, more than once, or not at all.

Questions 11–21

(A) Alkaline reflux gastritis
(B) Dumping syndrome
(C) Gastric volvulus
(D) Mallory-Weiss tear
(E) Hemobilia
(F) Duodenal ulcer
(G) Gastric ulcer
(H) Afferent loop syndrome
(I) Aortoduodenal fistula
(J) Cushing's ulcer
(K) Curling's ulcer

For each clinical scenario, select the most appropriate upper gastrointestinal disorder(s).

11. An elderly man with a history of an abdominal aortic aneurysm repair 10 years ago presents with a history of one episode of hematemesis. He is currently hemodynamically stable, but appears very anxious and scared. Upon endoscopy, there is no evidence of bleeding to the level of the pylorus. (SELECT 2 DISORDERS)

12. A 30-year-old woman presents with a 3–4-day history of bloody bilious emesis. The patient has no medical illnesses but did sustain a significant liver laceration treated with several weeks of bedrest after a high-speed motor vehicle accident 3 months earlier. Upper endoscopy does not reveal any evidence of gastric ulceration or gastritis. There is noted to be minimal blood-tinged bile around the region of the ampulla of Vater without obvious signs of duodenal ulceration or inflammation. (SELECT 1 DISORDER)

13. A 45-year-old motorcyclist suffered a severe closed head injury 2 days ago. Today he has an unexplained drop in his hematocrit from 43% to 25%, and his guaiac stool test is positive. Aspiration of the nasogastric tube contents are grossly positive for blood. (SELECT 3 DISORDERS)

14. A 56-year-old woman was caught in a house fire started by a kerosene heater. She was immediately brought to the surgical intensive care unit and resuscitated and débrided. Her total body surface area (TBSA) burn estimate is 40% partial and full thickness burns. Thirty-six hours after admission the patient's nasogastric tube drains 1 L of bright red blood over a 1-hour period. Endoscopy reveals diffuse mucosal bleeding. (SELECT 1 DISORDER)

15. A 48-year-old woman with severe rheumatoid arthritis reports dull epigastric pain aggravated by food. She ingests 2400 mg of ibuprofen daily. Her vital signs are stable. She is guaiac-negative. Abdominal examination reveals moderate epigastric pain, but no rebound tenderness. You empirically discontinue her nonsteroidal anti-inflammatory drug (NSAID) therapy and the symptoms resolve within 6 weeks. (SELECT 2 DISORDERS)

16. A 50-year-old man complains of epigastric pain relieved by antacids. Endoscopic biopsy of the antral mucosa is positive for *Helicobacter pylori*. A barium swallow shows enlarged gastric mucosa and evidence of duodenal bulb spasm. (SELECT 1 DISORDER)

17. An elderly man who has been debilitated in a nursing home for the past 6 years and who has a history of paraesophageal hernia presents to the emergency room complaining of sudden, severe, substernal chest pain. The patient is febrile with a temperature of 39°C (102.2°F) and his white blood cell count is 25,000. After proper placement of a nasogastric tube, the tip is noted to be in the left hemithorax upon chest radiograph. (SELECT 1 DISORDER)

18. A 43-year-old, previously healthy woman presents to the emergency room with a 3-hour history of hematemesis. The patient states that she has had the "stomach flu" for 3 days and has been vomiting bilious emesis during her illness. She notes that the emesis became bloody after an episode of "dry heaves" this morning. (SELECT 1 DISORDER)

19. A 52-year-old woman with a recent Billroth I reconstruction (gastroduodenostomy) after ulcer surgery reports that within minutes after eating a meal she experiences weakness, palpitations, dizziness, diaphoresis, and a strong desire to lie down. You advise her to eat smaller meals and to avoid liquids with her meals. She returns in 4 weeks reporting improvement in her symptoms. You reassure her that most likely all of her symptoms will resolve with time. (SELECT 1 DISORDER)

20. A 59-year-old man is 1 week postoperative from a Billroth II reconstruction (gastrojejunostomy) performed after antrectomy and vagotomy for chronic gastric outlet obstruction secondary to duodenal ulcer disease. He has been eating regular food for 1 day, although he now reports intermittent colicky right upper quadrant (RUQ) pain relieved by bilious vomiting. His abdomen is distended. Plain abdominal film reveals a single dilated segment of bowel in the RUQ. (SELECT 1 DISORDER)

21. A 46-year-old woman is 2 months postoperative from a gastroduodenostomy (Billroth I) performed to treat her ulcer disease. She complains of severe upper abdominal pain that is burning in nature. She reports that the pain usually occurs just after eating a large meal. Endoscopic examination reveals a "beefy red" gastric mucosa. Biopsy demonstrates both acute and chronic inflammation. (SELECT 1 DISORDER)

Answers and Explanations

1–C. Although rare, major complications associated with gastrostomy tube placement may occur, given the proximity of several major organs. Hemorrhage secondary to inadvertent placement of the percutaneous needle may be secondary to lacerations of the liver (superomedial), spleen (lateral), or major vessels along the greater or lesser curvature of the stomach. In addition, the proximity of the colon inferiorly makes colon perforation a significant risk factor. Given the scenario of an acute abdomen associated with free air on the abdominal film, injury to the transverse colon is most likely. Although simultaneous injury to other organs with associated hemorrhage is possible, the most likely primary origin of this patient's clinical findings is perforation of the transverse colon. Acute pancreatitis may occur with endoscopic manipulation of the biliary tree, but is rarely a complication of gastrostomy tube placement.

2–B. Given this patient's scenario with severe diffuse abdominal pain and a suspected bowel perforation, an exploratory laparotomy with appropriate surgical management of the injury is indicated. Other potential life-threatening injuries associated with an acute abdomen may also be identified at the time of operation. Endoscopy, barium swallow, or a barium enema would simply delay therapy for potential life-threatening intra-abdominal injuries that may exist in this patient and are therefore not indicated in this situation. Barium studies may actually worsen the situation by introducing barium into the peritoneal cavity.

3–A. After initial resuscitative efforts, esophagogastroduodenoscopy (EGD) would be the most appropriate diagnostic, and frequently therapeutic measure for this patient. Most causes of upper gastrointestinal bleeding can be diagnosed by endoscopy. In addition, several therapeutic techniques for upper gastrointestinal bleeding can also be performed endoscopically (e.g., electrocautery, banding of varices). Given this presentation, exploratory laparotomy or angiography are not indicated at this point in the work-up. Angiography may be indicated when a gastrointestinal source of bleeding is suspected but not confirmed by endoscopic techniques. Both administering vasopressin and placing a Sengstaken-Blakemore tube are useful for variceal bleeding; however, without confirming variceal bleeding as the source of hemorrhage, these techniques would not be indicated.

4–C. Among the choices provided, vagotomy with a simultaneous antrectomy has the lowest ulcer recurrence rate. However, this procedure is associated with a higher morbidity secondary to anastomotic complications (e.g., leak or stricture) or problems associated with denervation of the proximal stomach and distal bowel. Complications include postvagotomy diarrhea, dumping syndrome, delayed gastric emptying, and alkaline reflux gastritis.

5–A. A recent 25-lb unintended weight loss should raise suspicion for a possible malignancy in any patient. This patient's symptoms of epigastric pain in association with the weight loss should raise suspicion for an upper gastrointestinal malignancy such as gastric carcinoma. Among the choices above, endoscopy with biopsy of any suspicious lesions would be the most appropriate definitive diagnostic examination.

Findings on upper gastrointestinal barium swallow may be suggestive of ulcerative disease or malignancy, but endoscopic biopsy would allow for histologic verification of suspicious lesions. Angiography would not provide adequate information for definitive diagnosis. Esophageal manometry is useful for diagnosis of esophageal dysmotility disorders but would not be useful in this situation. Magnetic resonance imaging (MRI) would not allow for biopsy and tissue diagnosis.

6–C. A diet high in saturated fats is associated with a relative increased risk for developing colon adenocarcinoma but has not been shown to be associated with gastric adenocarcinoma. A diet that includes nitrates is a significant risk factor for gastric adenocarcinoma. Other significant risk factors include *H. pylori* infection, smoking, previous gastric surgery, and chronic alkaline reflux gastritis.

7–C. There is a small subset of lymphomas that are specifically associated with the presence of *Helicobacter pylori.* These lesions arise from mucosal-associated lymphoid tissue (MALT). There is evidence suggesting that many of these lesions may regress with eradication of *H. pylori.* Overall management of gastric lymphomas remains controversial. Treatment generally involves a combination of chemotherapy, radiation therapy, and surgery, although recent studies have suggested that chemoradiation therapy alone may be adequate. Overall survival for all stages of gastric lymphoma is greater than or equal to 50%. Obstructive symptoms may frequently be an indication for surgery, rather than a contraindication.

8–A. Whatever the cause of bleeding in this patient, the first and foremost important step in his management is securing a functional airway (e.g., endotracheal intubation) and adequate volume resuscitation (e.g., crystalloid and blood products when necessary). Administering intravenous vasopressin or placing a Sengstaken-Blakemore tube are appropriate in the management of esophageal varices but should not precede initial resuscitative measures. Although a chest radiograph should be performed early in the course of management to rule out potential pulmonary pathology and to identify a pulmonary source of hemorrhage, it should not precede resuscitation. A barium swallow is not indicated in this situation.

9–D. Gnawing epigastric pain that suddenly progresses to severe intense epigastric pain is frequently associated with perforated peptic ulcer disease. Patients may rapidly develop peritonitis and tend to lie very still to prevent further peritoneal irritation. A Mallory-Weiss tear is generally precipitated by forceful retching or coughing before development of pain. Although pain associated with acute gastritis may come on rapidly, it is generally not associated with rupture and peritoneal irritation. Gastric lymphoma may present with a perforation but is a rare occurrence relative to perforated peptic ulcer disease. Although a bleeding duodenal ulcer is a possibility despite a normal hematocrit, perforation and hemorrhage from peptic ulcer disease rarely occur simultaneously and bleeding ulcers are unlikely to cause peritonitis unless bleeding is directly into the peritoneum.

10–B. Given this patient's other comorbidities and the persistence of severe hypotension, the most appropriate operation would be one that effectively treats the perforation and minimizes the time the patient is in the operating room. Omental patching of a perforated ulcer involves oversewing the greater omentum directly over the perforated intestine. Additionally, a vagotomy may be done quickly as an acid-reducing procedure. If *Helicobacter pylori* is identified, appropriate treatment is also important to prevent recurrence postoperatively. A gastrectomy or antrectomy with a Billroth I, Billroth II, or Roux-en-Y gastrojejunostomy are effective in the treatment of this disease but would likely significantly increase the operative time and would not be the best choice given this scenario.

11–F, I. Despite the history of a previous abdominal aortic aneurysm repair, this patient could still potentially have a duodenal ulcer, which remains one of the most frequent causes of upper gastrointestinal bleeding in this population. Although rare (0.05%), one must always suspect aortoenteric fistula in any patient with a history of an abdominal aortic aneurysm repair or a history of aortic surgery. This patient may have experienced what is known as a "sentinel bleed," which is usually followed by massive hemorrhage within 48 hours. The most accurate means of diagnosis is angiography, although preparations for emergent surgery should be made immediately upon diagnosis in case rebleeding occurs during the evaluation. Treatment involves closure of the duodenum and reconstruction of the aortic graft.

12–E. Hemobilia is another rare cause of massive upper gastrointestinal bleeding that must be considered when the source cannot be localized to the stomach or duodenum. Pseudoaneurysms resulting from blunt trauma to the liver may erode into the lumen of the biliary tract, leading to bilious bloody emesis. This may also be seen with chronic pancreatitis, which may cause erosion of a peripancreatic artery into the pancreatic duct. Endoscopy may demonstrate arterial blood from the ampulla of Vater. Angiography is frequently used for diagnosis and embolization therapy.

13–F, G, J. The most likely diagnosis would be Cushing's ulcer, which is the eponym for acute gastritis associated with severe neurologic injury. Classically, Cushing's ulcer is solitary and can be located anywhere from the distal esophagus to the fourth portion of the duodenum. Perforation is the most common complication. The pathogenesis may be related to centrally mediated gastric hypersecretion. Cushing's ulcers generally occur in the stomach but can also occur in the duodenum. Additionally, the patient could have had peptic ulcer disease previously with the presentation of gastric or duodenal ulcers at this time.

14–K. Curling's ulcer is a variant of acute gastritis associated with a thermal burn injury of greater than 35% of total body surface area (TBSA). Curling's ulcer is usually found in the duodenum and also has the tendency to perforate. Endoscopy may be both diagnostic and therapeutic.

15–F, G. This patient most likely has a gastric ulcer as a result of her nonsteroidal anti-inflammatory drug (NSAID) use, although she could still potentially have a duodenal ulcer. Only endoscopy or barium swallow would differentiate these two possible diagnoses. Gastric ulcers typically present with dull, gnawing epigastric pain that may be precipitated or aggravated by food. Type V gastric ulcers can be located anywhere in the stomach and are usually associated with the use of NSAIDs. Treatment is medical therapy and withdrawal of the offending agent if possible. Surgery is rarely indicated, however one should be suspicious for carcinoma should the ulcer persist.

16–F. This patient has a classic presentation of a duodenal ulcer. Over 90% of duodenal ulcers are associated with *Helicobacter pylori*. Eradication of *H. pylori* heals the ulcer in over 90% of patients. Characteristic radiographic findings include demonstration of an ulcer crater and associated duodenal spasm. Typically, duodenal ulcer pain is relieved by ingestion of antacids or food.

17–C. Although rare, gastric volvulus typically occurs in patients who have herniation of the stomach through the diaphragm (e.g., paraesophageal hernia, traumatic diaphragmatic hernia). Gastric volvulus results from spontaneous torsion of the stomach compromising tissue perfusion, which may lead to necrosis, as suggested by this patient's elevated temperature and white blood cell count. Patients often present with chest pain, although cardiac evaluation is generally unremarkable. The diagnosis should be suspected when the chest radiograph reveals a retrocardiac air bubble or demonstrates the presence of the tip of the nasogastric tube in the hemithorax above the level of the diaphragm. Treatment involves emergent laparotomy and resection or detorsion of the affected stomach, depending on the presence or absence of necrosis.

18–D. Mallory-Weiss syndrome is the result of a linear tear in the mucosa of the gastric cardia, which typically results from violent retching or vomiting. Often a history of alcohol abuse or recent binge drinking is obtained, although this syndrome may occur in other clinical settings as well (e.g., severe coughing). The typical presentation involves initial nonbloody emesis followed later by hematemesis. Usually, the bleeding is painless. Evaluation with endoscopy allows for accurate diagnosis and rules out other sources of hematemesis. The majority of patients heal spontaneously without surgical intervention.

19–B. Dumping syndrome is divided into early and late dumping. This patient is experiencing the more common early dumping syndrome often termed "early vasomotor dumping," which is caused by the rapid onset of cardiovascular symptoms. Typical symptoms include nausea, vomiting, abdominal pain, excessive flatus, palpitations, dizziness, and diaphoresis. Symptoms can follow any meal, but worst offenders are foods high in carbohydrates and sugars. Over 90% of patients are successfully treated with dietary manipulation and time. Somatostatin analogs such as octreotide may be used before meals if dietary manipulations fail. Surgery is rarely indicated. When necessary, surgical reconstruction to a Roux-en-Y gastrojejunostomy may provide excellent relief of symptoms.

20–H. Afferent loop syndrome is present only after Billroth II reconstructions and is caused by intermittent obstruction of the afferent limb. The classic symptoms are intermittent right upper quadrant (RUQ) or epigastric pain that is relieved by bilious vomiting. Evaluation consists of radionucleotide scanning, which may demonstrate a massively dilated afferent limb. Severe dilation of the afferent loop can result in rupture and peritonitis, thus urgent surgical intervention is generally required. Conversion to a Roux-en-Y gastrojejunostomy is an appropriate surgical option.

21–A. Alkaline reflux gastritis is largely a diagnosis of exclusion. Patients complain of severe upper abdominal burning and often bilious vomiting. One must exclude marginal ulceration, afferent loop syndrome, chronic gastroparesis, and anastomotic stricture first. Endoscopy typically reveals marked gastritis and a "beefy red" appearance in the presence of bile reflux into the stomach. Radionucleotide scanning may demonstrate this bile reflux. Diagnosis is often made with biopsy that demonstrates acute and chronic inflammation of the mucosa. There is no specific medical treatment, although there has been some success with the use of sucralfate. Surgery is rarely necessary.

13

Small Bowel and Appendix

Santosh Krishnan

I. Structural and Functional Anatomy of the Small Intestine

A. Anatomy

1. The small intestine is

—approximately 280 cm long or 160% of body height.

a. **The jejunum begins** at the ligament of Treitz, but there is no clear demarcation between the jejunum and ileum.

b. **The jejunum is characterized by**

—long vasa rectae.

—large plicae.

—thick walls.

—a transparent mesentery.

c. **The ileum is characterized by**

—short vasa rectae.

—small plicae.

—thin walls.

—fat in the mesentery.

2. Mesentery

—is the tissue that attaches the small intestine to the posterior abdominal wall.

—contains blood vessels, nerves, lymphatics, lymph nodes, and fat.

3. Lymph tissue

—known as **Peyer's patches** are abundant in the **ileum.**

4. The arterial supply (Figure 13-1)

—is from the **superior mesenteric artery (SMA).**

—The SMA supplies the midgut structures (duodenum distal to the am-

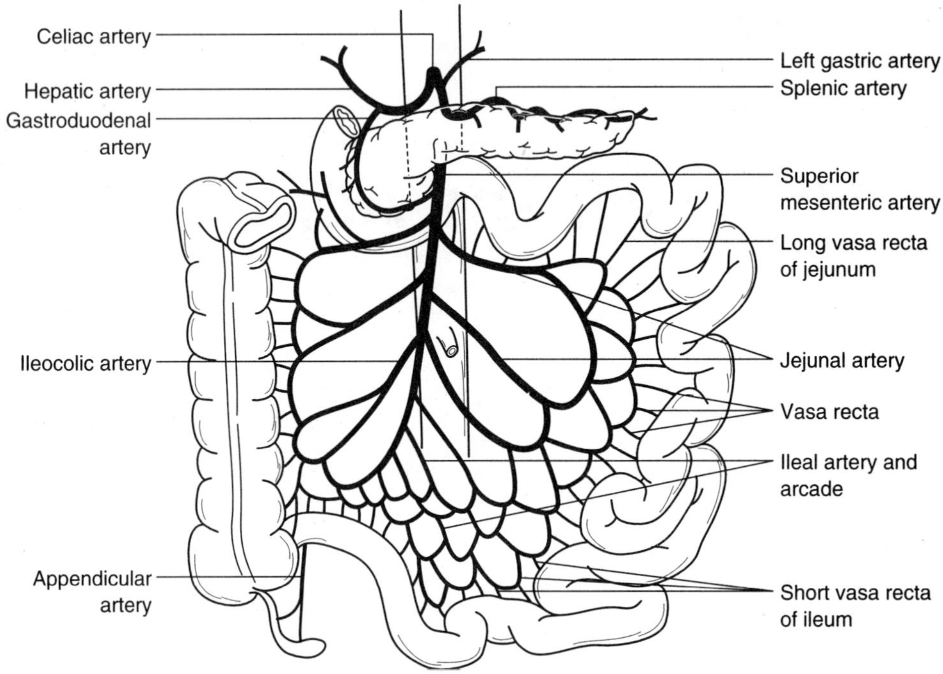

Figure 13-1. Arterial supply of the small intestine. (Adapted with permission from Nelson RL, Nyhus LM: *Surgery of the Small Intestine.* Norwalk, CT, Appleton & Lange, 1987, p 16.)

pulla of Vater, pancreas, small intestine, and the ascending and transverse colon).

5. Venous drainage

—is by the **superior mesenteric vein.**

B. Histology

—The small bowel consists of four layers.

1. **Mucosa** consists of epithelium, lamina propria, and muscularis mucosa.

   —Epithelium turns over every 3–7 days.

2. **Submucosa** contains vessels, nerves, lymph nodes, and the **nervous plexus of Meissner.**

   —This layer provides the major strength when suturing the small intestine.

3. The **muscularis** consists of an outer longitudinal layer and an inner circular layer of muscle fibers.

   —The muscularis contains the **nervous plexus of Auerbach** (myenteric).

4. The **adventitia** is a layer of visceral peritoneum.

II. Physiology

A. Carbohydrate absorption

1. The daily carbohydrate load

—is about **350 g** of starch, lactose, and sucrose.

2. **Initial enzymatic digestion**

   —is by pancreatic and salivary **amylase.**

3. **Carbohydrates**

   —are subsequently broken down by the microvilli into monosaccharides.

B. Protein absorption

1. **The jejunum**

   —is responsible for 80%–90% of **protein absorption.**

2. **Proteins are converted**

   —by acid and pepsin from the stomach to polypeptides.

3. **Acid is neutralized**

   —and pepsin is inactivated as chyme enters the duodenum.

4. **Trypsinogen from the pancreas is activated**

   —to trypsin by enterokinase in the duodenum.

5. **Trypsin activates**

   —chymotrypsin and elastase, which further digest polypeptides.

6. **Amino acids and dipeptides are absorbed**

   —by specific transporters.

C. Fat absorption

1. **Emulsification begins**

   —in the stomach.

2. **Fat enters the duodenum**

   —where pancreatic and biliary secretions mix.

3. **Lipase breaks down fats**

   —into monoglycerides, which are then absorbed by diffusion.

4. **In epithelial cells**

   —triglycerides are resynthesized.

   —chylomicrons are formed and enter the lymphatic system through small lacteals.

5. **Bile salts are absorbed**

   —in the **ileum.**

6. **Most of the excreted fat**

   —comes from desquamated cells and bacteria.

D. Water, electrolytes, vitamins, and mineral absorption

1. **Iron**

   —is absorbed mainly in the **duodenum.**

2. **Most minerals and water-soluble vitamins**

   —are absorbed in the **jejunum.**

3. **Vitamin B_{12}**

—is absorbed only in the **terminal ileum.**

4. **Of the 5–10 liters**

—entering the small bowel, only 500 mL enter the colon.

E. **Consequences of small bowel resection**

—frequently improve with time.

—can often be adequately treated with **dietary changes and antiperistaltic agents.**

1. **Diarrhea** can result from

—water overload of the colon.

—malabsorption (**steatorrhea**).

—irritation of colonic mucosa by bile salts.

2. **Bacterial overgrowth in the small intestine** may occur after resection of the ileocecal valve and can lead to deconjugation of bile salts in the small intestine.

a. **Alterations in water and electrolyte transport** result in net secretion instead of net absorption.

b. **Fermentation of carbohydrates** leads to gas production.

c. These factors lead to bloating, diarrhea, and steatorrhea.

3. **Nutritional deficiencies**

—**B_{12} supplementation** should be provided after resecting the terminal ileum.

4. **Short bowel syndrome**

—is characterized by inadequate length of intestine.

—generally occurs when more than 50% of the small bowel is resected or if less than **100 cm** remains.

—leads to diarrhea, steatorrhea, weight loss, nutritional deficiency, and hypergastrinemia.

—**If the terminal ileum and ileocecal valve** are retained, 70% can be resected.

5. **Cholelithiasis**

—may result from bile acid malabsorption after ileal resections.

6. **Hyperoxaluria and nephrolithiasis**

—with calcium oxalate stones may also occur.

a. **Normally oxalate is excreted** in the stool as insoluble calcium oxalate.

b. **Fat malabsorption may lead to** calcium binding of fat in the colon.

—This leaves oxalate free to form water-soluble absorbable salts excreted in the urine.

F. **Hormones**

1. **Secretin**

—is released by duodenal cells in response to acid.

—stimulates water and bicarbonate secretion by the pancreas.

2. **Cholecystokinin (CCK)**

—is released by intestinal mucosa in response to fat and amino acids.

—stimulates gallbladder contraction, increased bile flow, pancreatic secretion, and relaxation of the sphincter of Oddi.

3. **Both CCK and secretin**

—inhibit gastrin secretion by the stomach.

G. Motility

—is inhibited by **epinephrine.**

—is increased by **acetylcholine.**

1. **Migrating myoelectric complex (MMC)**

—results in cyclic contractions occurring every 3 minutes during fasting.

—These cyclic contractions are thought to clean the intestine and may be regulated by **motilin.**

2. **The order of recovery of bowel function after surgery is**

—small bowel.

—colon.

—stomach.

III. Small Bowel Obstruction (SBO)

A. Pathophysiology of SBO

1. **Substances that accumulate proximal to the obstruction** include ingested fluids, digestive secretions, and swallowed air.

—Most air in dilated bowel is **swallowed air** and mainly nonabsorbable **nitrogen.**

2. **Fluid enters the lumen** because distention increases secretion ("third spacing" of fluid).

3. **Intravascular volume is reduced** resulting in oliguria and hypotension.

4. **Bacteria proliferate** in the normally sterile small intestine.

B. Signs and symptoms

1. **Symptoms** include

—crampy abdominal pain.

—bloating.

—nausea.

—vomiting.

—failure to pass flatus or stool.

a. **Proximal obstruction may present with**

—profuse vomiting without significant distention.

b. Distal obstruction may present with

—less vomiting, but the emesis may be feculent from bacterial overgrowth and distention.

2. Signs of obstruction include

—abdominal distension.

—high-pitched bowel sounds.

a. Signs of hypovolemia from **"third spacing"** of fluid may be present.

b. Identification of a hernia should raise suspicion of **incarceration.**

c. Surgical scars on the abdomen may suggest **adhesion** formation.

3. Signs of strangulation include

—fever.

—tachycardia.

—peritoneal signs (severe abdominal pain, guarding, rebound).

—leukocytosis.

—These signs suggest that bowel ischemia and necrosis may be present.

C. Causes of SBO (Table 13-1)

1. Mechanical obstruction

a. Adhesions

—are the most common cause of SBO in patients who have had a **previous abdominal operation.**

—are also the most common cause of SBO in the United States.

b. Hernias

—are the most common cause of SBO in patients who have not had a previous abdominal operation.

—are the most common cause of bowel obstruction in the world.

—may involve the abdominal wall or be internal (see Chapter 10).

c. Tumors

(1) Colon cancers

—are the most common tumors causing obstruction.

(a) Right-sided colon lesions

—may cause obstruction at the ileocecal valve.

(b) Metastatic lesions

—may cause obstruction anywhere along the small bowel.

(2) Other locally advanced intra-abdominal tumors

—may cause obstruction (e.g., ovarian tumors).

(3) Primary tumors of the small bowel

—may cause obstruction but are rare.

d. Other less common causes of mechanical obstruction include

—intussusception.

—ingested foreign body.

—gallstone ileus.

Table 13-1. Classification and Differential Diagnosis of Small Bowel Obstruction

Lesion	Risk Factors	Etiology	Characteristics	Treatment	Misc.
Adhesions	**Previous abdominal surgery**	Peritoneal inflammation & scarring	**Obstruction with Hx of previous abdominal surgery**	**NPO & N/G tube decompression;** lysis of adhesions if refractory	**Most common cause of obstruction in United States**
Incarcerated hernia	Presence of hernia	Incarceration of small bowel in hernia	**Obstruction with an unreduced hernia on exam**	Reduction of herniated bowel and hernia repair	**Most common cause of obstruction worldwide**
Neoplasm	Hx of malignancy	Primary tumors of small bowel, metastatic lesions to bowel	Mass on radiocontrast studies, + hemoccult, wt. loss	**Resection**	Right-sided colon cancers can mimic small bowel obstruction
Stricture	**Hx of Crohn's radiation,** or previous abdominal surgery	Chronic intestinal inflammation and scarring	**Multiple strictured segments** may be seen with Crohn's and radiation	Resection of segment; **strictureplasty for Crohn's strictures**	May occur at surgical anastamosis sites
Intussusception	**Lymphoid hyperplasia–children;** polyps or masses–adults	Abnormal segment enveloped by peristalsis of normal intestine	Intermittent crampy abdominal pain with peristalsis; **"currant jelly" stools in children**	**Children–initially barium enema; adults–exploration and resection**	Frequently **associated with malignancy in adults**
Ingested foreign body	Children, retardation, psychosis, abnormal gastric emptying	Undigested material; **trichobezoars—hair; phytobezoars—plant material**	Bezoars frequently cause **obstruction at the level of the stomach**	Surgical or endoscopic removal; enzymatic digestion of some types	Perforation may occur with some ingested objects

(continued)

Table 13-1. Classification and Differential Diagnosis of Small Bowel Obstruction (*continued*)

Lesion	Risk Factors	Etiology	Characteristics	Treatment	Misc.
Gallstone ileus	**Hx of cholecystitis/ cholelithiasis**	Obstructing gallstone originating from **cholecystoenteric fistula**	Gallstone frequently obstructs at **ileocecal valve**	Enterotomy and stone removal or resection; cholecystectomy and repair of fistula site	Cholecystoduodenal fistulas are most common
Volvulus	—	Twisting of bowel upon itself	Cecal volvulus may cause small bowel obstruction	Surgical reduction of volvulus; cecopexy	Volvulus may also be associated with other segments of bowel
Congenital lesions	See *BRS Surgical Specialties,* Chapter 3	Intestinal malrotation, annular pancreas, webs, intestinal duplication	Seen in small children without obvious source of obstruction	Treat individual causes	**Some lesions may not present until adulthood**
Ogilvie's syndrome (pseudo-obstruction)	Recent surgery, serious illness, anticholinergics, narcotics, advanced age	**Idiopathic colonic dilation**	**Massive proximal colonic dilation without obvious source of obstruction**	Nonsurgical decompression (i.e., colonoscopy)	Small bowel dilation may not be present

Hx = history; NPO = nothing by mouth; N/G = nasogastric; + = positive; wt. = weight.

—volvulus.

—congenital lesions (e.g., atresia, web).

2. **Nonmechanical causes of small bowel dilation**

a. **Paralytic ileus**

—refers to a **functional loss of intestinal motility** resulting in delayed transit of luminal contents.

—may also **mimic** SBO.

(1) **Paralytic ileus may result in** small bowel dilation and accumulation of fluid within the lumen ("third-spacing").

(2) **Causes** may include

—**surgery** (most commonly associated with abdominal operations).

—**electrolyte abnormalities** (e.g., hypokalemia).

—peritonitis.

—ischemia.

—trauma.

—drugs.

b. **Ogilvie's syndrome**

—is a form of paralytic ileus that may mimic SBO.

—involves **massive acute dilation of the colon** in the absence of mechanical obstruction in severely ill and debilitated patients.

(1) **Predisposing conditions** include

—recent surgery.

—infection.

—neurologic or cardiopulmonary disorders.

—metabolic abnormalities.

—drugs.

(2) **Treatment** involves

—transrectal decompression of the colon.

D. **Radiographic findings** (Figure 13-2)

1. **Plain films show**

—**gas-filled loops.**

—**air-fluid levels** with a "step-ladder" appearance.

—These findings may be subtle if the obstruction is proximal.

2. **Mechanical obstruction versus paralytic ileus**

a. **In mechanical obstruction**

—the bowel distal to the point of obstruction empties because the bowel retains its function.

—**high-pitched, active bowel sounds** may be present because peristalsis attempts to overcome the obstruction.

b. **In paralytic ileus**

—there is uniform gas in the stomach, small bowel, and colon because the bowel has lost its motility.

—bowel sounds are generally infrequent or absent.

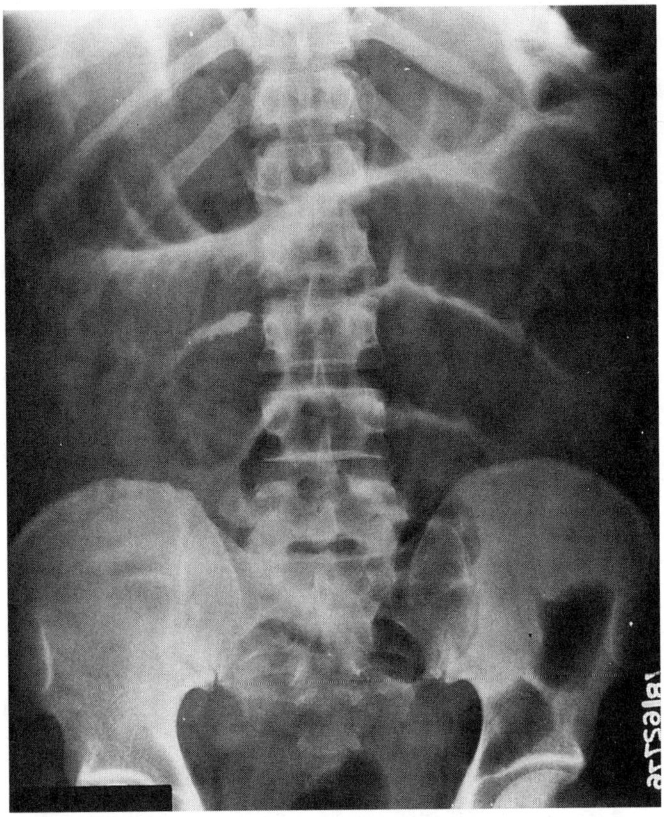

Figure 13-2. Radiograph of a small bowel obstruction. (Reprinted with permission from Daffner RH: *Clinical Radiology: The Essentials,* 2nd ed. Baltimore, Williams & Wilkins, 1999, p 260.)

E. **Treatment**

1. **Initial steps** include **fluid resuscitation** and correction of electrolyte abnormalities.
2. **Placement of a nasogastric (N/G) tube** and a Foley catheter should also be performed.
3. **Further management** involves identifying and surgically treating the primary cause of the obstruction.
4. **N/G tube decompression and bowel rest** are effective for some causes of obstruction (e.g., adhesions).
   —**If the obstruction does not begin to resolve** within 1–2 days, surgery should be directed at the cause of obstruction.
5. **Patients without previous surgery** with SBO require **urgent surgical intervention.**

IV. Crohn's Disease

—is a chronic, **transmural,** inflammatory process.
—is **also known as** regional enteritis, terminal ileitis, and granulomatous ileocolitis.

A. Incidence

1. Males and females are equally affected.
2. Peak age of onset is between the second and fourth decades.
3. Incidence in the United States is higher than in Japan.
4. Ashkenazi Jews have a higher incidence than African Americans do.

B. Etiology

—is unknown, but there are many hypotheses.

1. **Genetic basis**
   a. **HLA-DR2 and DRB1**
      —are closely associated with ulcerative colitis but not Crohn's disease.
   b. **A new marker**
      —is the MLH1 DNA repair gene.
2. **An infectious source**
   —has been proposed but never proven (i.e., mycobacterial infection).
3. **An inappropriate immune response**
   —may play a role because a favorable response is obtained from corticosteroids and immunosuppressive drugs such as cyclosporine.

C. Pathology

1. **Crohn's disease characteristically progresses** in a discontinuous manner with affected bowel interspersed with normal bowel (**"skip areas"**).
   a. **The most common gastrointestinal tract sites affected** include the
      —terminal ileum and cecum (40%).
      —colon only (35%).
      —small bowel only (20%).
      —perianal region (5%).
   b. **Anal involvement** may be characterized by fissures, abscesses, or fistulae.
   c. The disease may also affect **multiple sites** (18%).
2. **The mucosa** may have a **cobblestone** appearance.
3. **Transmural (full-thickness) inflammation** is the most consistent feature.
4. **Fibrosis** may lead to stricture formation with stiffening of bowel loops.
5. **Fistula formation** to other loops of bowel, bladder, vagina, or skin may occur.
6. **The serosa** may have a beefy-red appearance with **"creeping" mesenteric fat** seen over areas of greatest inflammation.
7. **Noncaseating granulomas** are found in **lamina propria** or **submucosa** in 50% of patients.

D. Clinical features (Table 13-2)

Table 13-2. Clinical Features of Crohn's Disease

Intestinal manifestations	Extraintestinal manifestations*
Diarrhea (90%)	Arthritis/arthralgia (parallels intestinal disease)
Abdominal pain (55%)	Erythema nodosum
Anorexia	Erythema multiforme
Nausea	Pyoderma gangrenosum
Weight loss	Pericholangitis/cholelithiasis
Perirectal disease (e.g., fistulae, fissure)	Renal calculi (calcium oxalate stones)
	Endocrine disorders (e.g., growth failure, amenorrhea)
	Ocular disease (e.g., uveitis, blepharitis, corneal ulcers)

*Extraintestinal manifestations should raise suspicion for Crohn's disease in patients with intestinal symptoms.

E. Diagnosis

1. The diagnosis is based on

—clinical presentation.

—radiologic findings.

—mucosal appearance.

—histology.

—exclusion of alternative etiologies.

2. Enteroclysis

—is an effective study for diagnosing Crohn's disease.

—helps to define small bowel disease occurring in 90% of patients.

a. Partial obstruction may be indicated by poststenotic dilation.

b. Strictures may be seen as a **"string sign"** of Kantor.

c. Thickening of mucosal folds appears as **"thumbprinting."**

3. Colonoscopy

—with biopsy of the colon and terminal ileum is also an effective diagnostic tool.

a. Intervening areas may be normal.

b. Biopsies must be obtained from multiple sites.

c. Histologic evidence of disease includes

—fibrosis.

—mononuclear cell and plasma cell infiltrates.

—granulomas.

—architectural distortion.

F. Complications include

—enteric fistulas (29%).

—pelvic abscesses (20%).

—obstruction (9%).

—gastrointestinal hemorrhage (2%).

—cancer (1%).

—intestinal perforation (1%).

—ureteral obstruction (1%).

—megaloblastic anemia from vitamin B_{12} or folate deficiency secondary to malabsorption.

G. Medical management

—is the primary treatment for Crohn's disease.

1. Sulfa drugs

—are generally first-line therapy for medical management of Crohn's disease.

a. Sulfasalazine

—is broken down to **5-aminosalicylic acid (5-ASA)** and sulfapyridine (sulfa antibiotic) by colonic bacteria.

b. 5-ASA

—**blocks prostaglandin release** and decreases inflammation associated with Crohn's.

2. Steroids

—are effective at treating disease refractory to sulfa drugs.

3. Immunosuppressive agents

—used with steroids in a small number of patients with refractory disease include azathioprine, 6-mercaptopurine, and methotrexate.

H. Surgical considerations

1. Surgical therapy for Crohn's has classically been **for treating complications.**

2. Indications for surgery include

—obstruction (complete or partial).

—perforation.

—fistula formation.

—the presence of tumor.

—hemorrhage.

—failure of medical management.

3. Surgical resection of small bowel for Crohn's disease

—is generally not considered curative.

—may be associated with a high rate of complications.

a. Short bowel syndrome may result from extensive resections.

b. An alternative to resection for stricture disease is **stricturoplasty.**

—This involves opening a stricture longitudinally and closing the bowel horizontally to increase the lumen size.

4. Generally the recurrence rate

—after surgical resection and primary anastomosis for Crohn's is 70%–75%.

—Approximately 35% of these patients will require additional surgery.

V. Small Bowel Fistulae

A. Overview

1. **Fistulae are abnormal connections** between a hollow viscus and another organ, including the skin.
2. **Most are iatrogenic** resulting from anastomotic leaks.
3. **Contributing factors**
   a. **Bowel inflammation** (e.g., Crohn's disease)
   —may lead to fistula formation.
   b. **Malnutrition**
   —may contribute to poor healing of fistulae.
   c. **Factors contributing to maintenance** of fistula patency are (FRIEND)
   —*f*oreign bodies.
   —*r*adiation therapy.
   —*i*nfection and inflammation (e.g., Crohn's disease).
   —*e*pithelialization of the fistula tract.
   —*n*eoplasm.
   —*d*istal obstruction (i.e., distal to fistula).
4. **Classification**
   a. **Descriptions are based on** the origin and termination site (e.g., enterocutaneous).
   b. **Proximal fistulae (e.g., jejunal)** are
   —generally **high output** (> 200 mL/day).
   —frequently resistant to closure with conservative therapy.

B. Management

1. **Replenish** lost **fluids** and **electrolytes.**
2. **Initiate local skin care** for enterocutaneous fistula.
3. **Identify the cause and location** of the fistula and treat if appropriate.
4. **Decrease output** with **proximal N/G tube decompression.**
5. **Provide appropriate nutrition** (i.e., parenteral or enteral beyond fistula).
6. **Nonsurgical therapy**
—Fifty percent will close with nonsurgical therapy.
7. **Refractory fistula require resection** in continuity with the diseased bowel.

VI. Neoplasms of the Small Bowel

A. Overview

1. **Small bowel tumors** are **rare** (1.5%–6.0% of all gastrointestinal tumors).
2. **Benign tumors** are **more common** than malignant tumors.

3. **Sites of occurrence** include the
   —duodenum (15%).
   —jejunum (25%).
   —ileum (60%).
4. **The most common clinical manifestations are bleeding and obstruction.**

B. Benign neoplasms

1. **Epithelial tumors**
   —include tubular adenomas, villous adenomas, and Brunner's gland adenomas.
   —are frequently **incidental findings.**
   —may cause bleeding or obstruction.
   a. **Duodenal lesions**
      —can generally be removed endoscopically.
   b. **Symptomatic jejunal or ileal tumors**
      —require segmental resection.
2. **Stromal tumors** include
   —lipomas.
   —leiomyomas.
   —neurogenic tumors (e.g., neurofibromas, schwannomas, gangliomas).
   —hemangiomas.
3. **Peutz-Jeghers syndrome**
   —is an **inherited syndrome** with mucocutaneous melanotic pigmentation and multiple gastrointestinal hamartomatous polyps.
   —is the **most common syndrome** affecting the **small intestine.**
   —is inherited in an **autosomal dominant** fashion.
   —generally presents with **bleeding** or **obstruction.**
   —is associated with a **high risk** of **extraintestinal malignancy.**

C. Malignant neoplasms

—are **rare** (Table 13-3).

1. **Adenocarcinomas** are the most common malignant neoplasm.
   a. **Sites of occurrence** include the
      —duodenum (40%).
      —jejunum (40%).
      —ileum (20%).
   b. **Wide segmental resection** including lymph **nodes,** is required.
   c. **Adenocarcinomas of the duodenum** may require a pancreaticoduodenectomy (**Whipple's** operation) [see Chapter 17].
2. **Leiomyosarcomas** occur most commonly in the **jejunum** and **ileum.**
   a. **Wide segmental resection** is required.
   b. **Node resection** is not required because these neoplasms spread hematogenously.

Table 13-3. Malignant Tumors of the Small Intestine*

Type	Site	Characteristics	Treatment	Miscellaneous
Adenocarcinoma	40% duodenum, 40% jejunum, 20% ileum	Weight loss and abdominal pain. Duodenal lesion–jaundice; jejunum/ileum–obstruction	Wide segmental resection with draining nodes	**Most common malignant tumor of small intestine**
Leiomyosarcoma	Jejunum, ileum	Weight loss, abdominal pain, perforation, obstruction, palpable mass	Wide segmental resection	Node resection not required because **spread is generally hematogenous**
Lymphoma	Ileum	GI lymphomas account for 5% of all lymphomas and are the most common extranodal lymphoma	Surgery and chemoradiation	Most are **non-Hodgkin B-cell** lymphomas
Carcinoid	**85% appendix,** 13% small intestine, 2% rectum	Weight loss, abdominal pain, carcinoid syndrome, may be incidental finding	Surgery, octreotide for carcinoid syndrome	**Ileal lesions more likely to metastasize** than appendiceal lesions

*Malignant tumors of the small intestine are very rare. GI = gastrointestinal.

3. **Lymphomas**

—are most commonly found in the ileum.

—are the **most common** form of **extranodal lymphoma.**

—are usually **non-Hodgkin B-cell lymphomas.**

—Treatment includes **surgery** and **chemoradiation therapy.**

4. **Carcinoid tumors** may also occur in the small intestine, especially the ileum.

VII. Miscellaneous Lesions of the Small Intestine

A. Mesenteric ischemia

—may occur with vascular disease of the visceral blood vessels (see *BRS Surgical Specialties,* Chapter 1).

B. Meckel's diverticulum

—is a congenital diverticulum caused by the failure of obliteration of the **omphalomesenteric duct.**

—contains all layers of the intestine.

—is found on the antimesenteric border.

—is usually found incidentally, although bleeding and obstruction may occur.

—Inflammation or infection of the diverticulum may mimic appendicitis.

1. **General characteristics** are described by the **"rule of 2s."**
   - **a.** They are generally found 2 feet from the ileocecal valve.
   - **b.** They are present in 2% of the population.
   - **c.** Only 2% are symptomatic.
   - **d.** Most present by age 2.
2. **A diagnostic Meckel's scan** uses technetium preferentially taken up by **gastric mucosa** frequently found in Meckel's diverticula.
3. **Other anomalies** include

   —**omphalomesenteric fistulae.**

   —cysts.

C. Other diverticula

1. **Jejunoileal diverticula**

   —are otherwise rare.

2. **Duodenal diverticula**

   —are relatively common.

   —may cause obstructive biliary symptoms if near the ampulla.

VIII. The Appendix

A. Anatomy (Figure 13-3)

1. **The appendix**

   —arises from the posteromedial cecal wall just distal to the ileocecal valve.

   —varies in length from 2–20 cm but the average length is 9 cm in adults.

   —may be located in the pelvis (35%) or it may be retrocecal (behind the cecum) [5%].

2. **The appendicular artery**

   —is a branch of the lower division of the ileocolic.

3. **Surface marking for the appendicular base**

   —is along a line connecting the umbilicus and the anterior superior iliac spine at a point two thirds the distance from the umbilicus (**McBurney's point**).

4. **The anterior taeniae coli of the colon**

   —leads to the base of the appendix.

B. Appendicitis

—can occur at any age but is **most common from 12–30 years.**

1. **Pathogenesis** involves

   —obstruction of the appendiceal lumen.

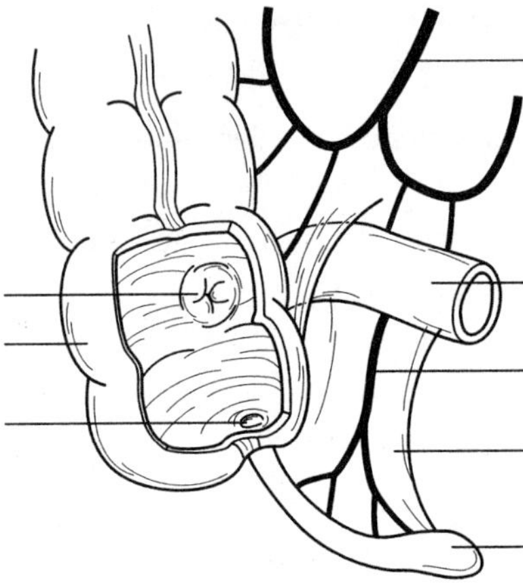

Figure 13-3. The appendix. (Adapted with permission from Moore K: *Essential Clinical Anatomy.* Baltimore, Williams & Wilkins, 1996, p 107.)

—increased luminal pressure.

2. **Causes of luminal obstruction** include
   —lymphoid hyperplasia (60%, primarily in children).
   —fecaliths (35%, primarily in adults).
   —foreign bodies (4%).
   —tumors (1%).
3. **This obstruction leads to**
   —**ischemia,** venous thrombosis (**gangrenous appendicitis**), and finally rupture (**perforated appendicitis**).
4. **Signs and symptoms of appendicitis**
   a. **Abdominal pain**
      —is the **classic sign.**
      —characteristically **precedes nausea and vomiting.**
      —begins in the **periumbilical** region.
      —localizes to the **right lower quadrant** (RLQ).
      (1) **Rovsing's sign** is pain in the RLQ with pressure in the left lower quadrant (LLQ).
      (2) **The psoas sign** is pain on extension of the thigh.
      (3) **The obturator sign** is pain on flexion and internal rotation of the thigh.
   b. **Other possible signs** include
      —fever.
      —anorexia.
      —increased white blood cell count.
   c. **Symptoms may be subtle**
      —in the **very young or very old.**
      —when the appendix is **retrocecal** or **pelvic.**

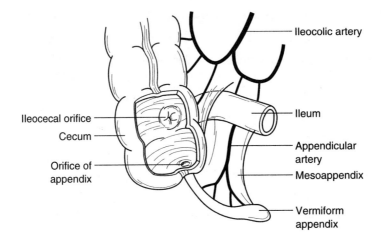

5. **Diagnosis of appendicitis**
   a. **Differential diagnosis** includes
      —Crohn's disease.
      —mesenteric adenitis.
      —ectopic pregnancy.
      —tubo-ovarian abscess.
      —pelvic inflammatory disease.
      —mittelschmerz.
   b. **Diagnosis is generally based on**
      —history.
      —physical examination findings.
   c. **Plain films may show**
      —a fecalith or a "sentinel loop"—a distended loop of small bowel in the RLQ.
   d. **In complex cases** an ultrasound or a computed tomography (CT) scan showing periappendiceal fluid or a thickened appendix may confirm the diagnosis.
      —**A negative study does not rule out appendicitis.**
   e. **For women**
      —a **pelvic examination** and **β-HCG must be performed.**
      —**ultrasound** may be helpful to evaluate gynecologic causes for abdominal pain that may mimic appendicitis.
6. **Management of appendicitis**
   a. **Intravenous (IV) fluids** and broad-spectrum antibiotics should be administered initially.
   b. **Immediate appendectomy** should be performed through an open or laparoscopic approach.
      (1) **McBurney's incision**
         —is parallel to the inguinal ligament through McBurney's point.
      (2) **A Rockey-Davis incision**
         —is also through McBurney's point but is transverse, thus providing a better cosmetic result.
      (3) **If there is rupture**
         —with generalized peritonitis, the appendix may be removed and IV antibiotics continued.
      (4) **Patients with a periappendiceal abscess**
         —can undergo delayed appendectomy 6 weeks or longer after treatment of the abscess.

C. Tumors of the appendix

1. **Carcinoid tumors**
   —arise from **Kultschitzky** cells (neural crest).
   —are the most common tumors of the appendix (0.5%).
   —are located in the appendix (85%), small intestine (ileum) [13%], and rectum (2%).

a. **Metastasis**

—Only 3% of appendiceal tumors metastasize versus 35% of ileal carcinoids.

—Tumors smaller than 1 cm rarely metastasize.

—The risk of metastases is 50% for 1- to 2-cm lesions, and 80%–90% for lesions larger than 2 cm.

b. **Presenting features** may include weight loss and abdominal pain.

—Many are diagnosed as incidental findings.

(1) **A desmoplastic reaction** can cause ischemia and obstruction.

(2) **Carcinoid syndrome** may occur with the presence of liver metastases.

(a) **Symptoms** may include

—flushing.

—diarrhea.

—asthma.

(b) **Patients may have valvular heart disease** of the **tricuspid** and **pulmonary** valves.

(c) **A useful diagnostic test is** measurement of urinary **5-hydroxyindoleacetic acid (5-HIAA),** a metabolite of serotonin.

(d) **Octreotide** may provide symptomatic relief.

c. **Appendectomy and resection**

—of the mesoappendix is adequate for carcinoids that have not metastasized.

d. **A right hemicolectomy should be performed**

—if nodes are involved or if the tumor is **larger than 2 cm.**

2. **Mucinous tumors of the appendix (0.2%)**

—can be benign or malignant.

—are rarely associated with **Trousseau's syndrome** (migratory thrombophlebitis).

—**Mucin from these tumors** may disseminate throughout the peritoneum (**pseudomyxoma peritonei**).

3. **Adenocarcinoma**

—is rare and behaves similarly to colon adenocarcinoma (see Chapter 14).

Review Test

Directions: Each of the numbered items or incomplete statements in this section is followed by answers or by completions of the statement. Select the ONE lettered answer or completion that is BEST in each case.

1. A 57-year-old woman with a history of thyroid resection for papillary thyroid carcinoma is admitted after 2 weeks of frequent vomiting. Her only medications include over-the-counter aluminum hydroxide taken occasionally for mild epigastric discomfort. On physical examination, the patient is notably dehydrated. Work-up shows complete small bowel obstruction. Her serum chloride is 90 mEq/dL (low), potassium is 2.9 mEq/dL (low), bicarbonate is 35 mEq/dL (high), and urine pH is low (acidic). Which of the following is the explanation for the alkalotic serum and acidic urine?

(A) Renal bicarbonate loss
(B) Use of aluminum-based antacids
(C) Renal conservation of potassium with hydrogen loss
(D) Stool losses of hydrogen
(E) Excess gastrointestinal absorption of bicarbonate

Questions 2–3

A 53-year-old man with a previous extensive resection of the terminal ileum for a strangulated hernia returns 2 years later without interim follow-up complaining of fatigue, malaise, and weakness. His stools are noted to be heme-negative on physical examination. He is eating without difficulty. His blood smear shows anemia with many hypersegmented neutrophils.

2. Which of the following is the most appropriate therapy for the primary cause of his anemia?

(A) Parenteral iron sulfate
(B) Blood transfusion
(C) Parenteral vitamin B_{12}
(D) Oral vitamin B_{12}
(E) Oral iron sulfate

3. Which of the following would most likely be associated with nutritional disorders similar to those seen with resection of the terminal ileum?

(A) Peptic ulcer disease
(B) Crohn's disease
(C) Diverticulosis
(D) Colonic ulcerative colitis
(E) Segmental jejunal resection

Questions 4–5

During an operation for presumed appendicitis, the patient's appendix is found to be normal. The terminal ileum, however, is found to be markedly thickened and feels rubbery to firm. The serosa is edematous and inflamed and the mesentery is thickened with fat growing about the bowel circumference.

4. Which of the following is the most likely diagnosis?

(A) Ileal Crohn's disease
(B) Meckel's diverticulitis
(C) Ulcerative colitis
(D) Ileocecal tuberculosis
(E) Ileal carcinoid

5. After identifying a normal appendix and inflammatory changes are noted to be limited to the terminal ileum, the surgeon plans to perform the appropriate operation. Intraoperatively, which of the following procedures would be the most appropriate to perform in this patient?

(A) Resection of the appendix only
(B) Resection of involved ileum and appendix
(C) Placement of peritoneal drains and appendectomy
(D) Enterotomy with inspection of the ileal mucosa
(E) Right hemicolectomy with lymph node dissection

6. A 65-year-old man undergoes a right hemicolectomy with a primary anastomosis for a stage II, right-sided, colon adenocarcinoma. Five months postoperatively the patient presents with a distal ileocutaneous fistula. Which of the following is the most appropriate initial therapy?

(A) Prompt exploration and interruption of the fistula tract
(B) Prompt exploration and bypass of the fistula
(C) A 4–6-week trial of low residue or elemental enteral nutrition or hyperalimentation
(D) Prompt exploration with resection of the involved ileum and primary anastomosis
(E) Ileostomy and ileocecal resection

7. A 49-year-old, white man presents to the emergency room with complaints of a 2- to 3-day history of worsening nausea and vomiting. The patient has undergone a previous small bowel resection for Meckel's diverticulitis. The patient's abdomen is distended but nontender. Initial resuscitative measures are taken. Which of the following radiologic studies would be most helpful in the initial evaluation of this patient?

(A) Intravenous (IV) pyelogram
(B) Barium enema
(C) Abdominal ultrasound
(D) Supine and upright abdominal films
(E) Abdominal and pelvic computed tomography (CT) scan

8. Which of the following is a frequent cause of paralytic ileus?

(A) Bezoars
(B) Annular pancreas
(C) Cecal volvulus
(D) Intussusception
(E) Peritonitis

9. A 20-year-old college student presents with right lower quadrant (RLQ) pain, fever, anorexia, and leukocytosis. He undergoes appendectomy. Pathological report reveals a 1-cm carcinoid at the tip of the appendix without involvement of the mesentery. Appropriate therapy includes which of the following?

(A) Reexploration and cecectomy
(B) Reexploration and right hemicolectomy
(C) Reexploration with mesenteric node biopsy
(D) Chemotherapy
(E) No further therapy

10. A 42-year-old woman is found to have a solid, irregular, asymptomatic lesion in the right lobe of her liver during an abdominal computed tomography (CT) scan performed for a trauma evaluation. One week later the patient undergoes percutaneous biopsy of the lesion, which reveals a carcinoid tumor. Efforts to identify the primary source of this lesion are undertaken. Which of the following is the most frequent site of carcinoid tumors?

(A) Jejunum
(B) Liver
(C) Ileum
(D) Appendix
(E) Colon

Directions: Each set of matching questions in this section consists of a list of four to twenty-six lettered options followed by several numbered items. For each numbered item, select the appropriate lettered option(s). Each lettered option may be selected once, more than once, or not at all.

Questions 11–20

(A) Adhesions
(B) Inguinal hernia
(C) Intussusception
(D) Cecal adenocarcinoma
(E) Paralytic ileus
(F) Crohn's disease
(G) Ogilvie's syndrome
(H) Midgut volvulus
(I) Bezoar
(J) Annular pancreas

For each clinical scenario, select the correct diagnosis(es).

11. A 1-year-old with a history of cystic fibrosis presents with 1 day of nausea, vomiting, and intermittent severe abdominal pain. Her mother states that the child has passed stools that are red with clots and mucus. (SELECT 1 DIAGNOSIS)

12. A 67-year-old with a history of thoracic aortic aneurysm repair presents with a 1-day history of bilious vomiting. Physical examination reveals a swollen right groin that is tender and erythematous. The patient is febrile with rebound and guarding. (SELECT 1 DIAGNOSIS)

13. A 35-year-old woman presents with a 2- to 3-week history of worsening nausea and vomiting. The patient also gives a history of chronic intermittent diarrhea, which she has "learned to live with." On physical examination the abdomen is distended with hyperactive bowel sounds. A small bowel follow-through reveals multiple consecutive strictures of the distal ileum. (SELECT 1 DIAGNOSIS)

14. A 47-year-old with a history of melanoma presents with a 2-day history of nausea; vomiting; and intermittent, crampy, abdominal pain. A right lower quadrant (RLQ) mass is noted on physical examination. (SELECT 2 DIAGNOSES)

15. A 72-year-old woman, 2 days postoperative from a laparoscopic cholecystectomy, presents with complaints of persistent nausea and vomiting. She denies abdominal pain. On physical examination, the abdomen is distended and without bowel sounds. Nasogastric tube placement and suctioning results in drainage of 1.5 L over the initial hour after placement. Her serum potassium is 2.9 mEq/dL. Abdominal radiograph reveals diffuse dilation of the small bowel. (SELECT 1 DIAGNOSIS)

16. A 12-year-old boy with severe mental retardation is brought from a group home with 1 week of nausea, poor feeding, and intermittent vomiting. On physical examination a palpable mass is noted above the umbilicus in the midline. Bowel sounds are normal. Plain films show an enlarged stomach with mottling but without evidence of small bowel dilation. (SELECT 1 DIAGNOSIS)

17. A 1-month-old presents with a 1-day history of bilious vomiting and abdominal pain. She has not been feeding well and her fontanelles are depressed. She is lethargic and has not had a wet diaper in more than 12 hours. Plain abdominal radiographs reveal a proximal small bowel obstruction. (SELECT 2 DIAGNOSES)

18. A 37-year-old man presents with complaints of worsening nausea, vomiting, and abdominal pain. His history is significant for a previous laparoscopic cholecystectomy for gangrenous cholecystitis 12 years ago. He states that he has had similar symptoms in the past, but they resolved on their own. Plain film of the abdomen shows multiple dilated loops of small bowel. (SELECT 1 DIAGNOSIS)

19. A 47-year-old man presents with a 2-week history of worsening nausea and vomiting. The patient has also noted a 10-lb weight loss over the past month. He has had no previous surgery and there are no masses noted on physical examination. Rectal examination reveals no masses, but shows heme-positive stools. Plain film of the abdomen shows multiple air-fluid levels in the small intestine and no air in the colon. (SELECT 1 DIAGNOSIS)

20. An 82-year-old, retired coal miner is hospitalized in the coronary care unit with an acute myocardial infarction. He has had no previous surgery and there are no masses noted on physical examination. Two days into his hospitalization he develops abdominal distention and crampy pain. Plain films reveal no evidence of small bowel dilation. Barium enema reveals a massively dilated right colon without obvious masses. (SELECT 1 DIAGNOSIS)

Answers and Explanations

1–C. Patients with vomiting of long duration frequently lose large amounts of potassium and hydrogen ions found in gastric secretions. In addition, dehydration leads to an aldosterone-mediated resorption of sodium in the distal tubules of the kidney in exchange for secretion of potassium and hydrogen ions into the urine. In the setting of dehydration and severe hypokalemia, hydrogen ions are preferentially secreted in the urine in exchange for sodium to prevent additional loss of potassium. This produces a "paradoxical" acid urine from a patient with hypokalemic metabolic alkalosis. Renal bicarbonate loss would produce serum acidosis rather than alkalosis. Stool losses of hydrogen ions are insignificant, although significant bicarbonate may be lost in patients with severe diarrhea. Aluminum-based antacids also will not cause this electrolyte abnormality.

2–C. The patient most likely has pernicious anemia secondary to vitamin B_{12} deficiency following ileal resection. Parenteral [intravenous (IV)] vitamin B_{12} obviates the absorption problem caused by terminal ileum resection. Oral B_{12} administration may be ineffective secondary to inadequate absorption. Blood transfusion would be inappropriate in this setting and would not address the likely cause of the anemia. Iron supplementation would be appropriate for patients with microcytic anemia secondary to iron deficiency and may provide some benefit in this patient if a concomitant iron deficiency exists. However, hypersegmented neutrophils represent a characteristic sign of B_{12} deficiency and may occasionally be present without obvious macrocytic changes in red blood cells. IV iron therapy is rarely indicated for treatment of iron deficiency.

3–B. Among the choices listed, Crohn's disease frequently affects the terminal ileum and may cause malabsorption of vitamin B_{12}. Peptic ulcer disease may be associated with blood loss anemia but not with vitamin B_{12} deficiency, although gastric resection for peptic ulcer disease may lead to a deficiency in intrinsic factor with subsequent B_{12} malabsorption and deficiency. Diverticulosis and ulcerative colitis may both be associated with significant blood loss anemia but are not characteristically associated with vitamin B_{12} deficiency. Jejunal resection will generally not affect vitamin B_{12} absorption.

4–A. Crohn's disease can present acutely, and when it involves the terminal ileum may clinically resemble appendicitis. The bowel in this patient has the characteristic gross findings and inflammatory changes of Crohn's disease including the "creeping fat" within the mesentery. Meckel's diverticulitis can mimic appendicitis but it presents as an inflammatory phlegmon located approximately 50 cm (2 feet) from the ileocecal valve and does not have the bowel changes seen in this patient. Ulcerative colitis is usually confined to the large bowel and, although it may occasionally be associated with inflammatory changes of the ileal mucosa (backwash ileitis), it is generally not associated with full-thickness changes described above. Tubercular ileitis is rare in the United States, although it can produce scarring and stenosis of the distal ileum with enlarged mesenteric lymph nodes. Demonstration of caseation and acid-fast bacilli on lymph node biopsy confirms the diagnosis. Ileal carcinoid would present as a mass in the ileum and would not be associated with the inflammatory changes seen in this patient.

5–A. When acute Crohn's disease is encountered during exploration for presumed appendicitis, the appropriateness of appendectomy is somewhat controversial. The incidence of enterocutaneous fistula after operation in patients with Crohn's disease is higher than in patients without it, but fistulae usually arise from the diseased ileum and not the appendiceal stump. Therefore, if the stump is not involved, many surgeons perform an appendectomy. This simplifies the differential diagnosis if right lower quadrant (RLQ) pain returns at a later date. The ileum should not be resected unless there is evidence of obstruction, perforation, or fistula formation. Drain placement is not indicated in this patient and may even increase the risk of fistula formation with extensive inflammatory changes in the ileum. In addition, performing an enterotomy may also increase the risk of fistula formation and would be of little, if any, benefit in the management of this patient.

6–C. Because most fistulas close with proper supportive care and hyperalimentation or low-residue elemental nutrition, this should be attempted before any operation. If needed, the preferred operation is resection of the fistula in continuity with the diseased segment of bowel, followed by reanastomosis. Bypass operations should be avoided, or operations that just resect the fistula or only the involved bowel are not appropriate. Ileostomy and ileocecal resection are not indicated at this point in the management of this patient.

7–D. The simplest test that will show the obstruction is the plain abdominal film. Plain films may show gas-filled loops and air-fluid levels. These findings may be more subtle if the obstruction is proximal. Gas in small bowel outlines valvulae conniventes, which run the entire transverse diameter of bowel. In mechanical obstruction, the distal bowel empties out past the point of obstruction because the bowel retains its ability to move. So a mechanical bowel obstruction has too much gas proximally, and distal to the obstruction it will empty. In paralytic ileus there is a uniform gas pattern in the stomach, small bowel, and colon because the bowel has lost its motility. Intravenous (IV) pyelogram, abdominal ultrasound, and abdominal computed tomography (CT) scanning may frequently be useful in evaluating patients with these symptoms, but they generally should not preclude acquisition of plain radiographs of the abdomen in the setting of a suspected obstruction.

8–E. Among the choices listed, peritonitis is the most likely cause of paralytic ileus. The most common cause of paralytic ileus is abdominal surgery. Bezoars frequently found in the stomach may cause a mechanical obstruction of the stomach. Annular pancreas may cause a mechanical obstruction of the duodenum, while cecal volvulus and intussusception may cause a mechanical obstruction of the small bowel.

9–E. Carcinoid tumors of the appendix usually require no more than simple appendectomy. Exceptions are lesions larger than 2 cm, lesions with nodal involvement or serosal spread, or lesions at the base of the appendix near the cecum; right hemicolectomy would be the correct operation for these situations. Cecectomy alone would not be sufficient if the carcinoid tumor met the criteria for further resection. Reexploration with biopsy is not needed because the site of the tumor is known. Chemotherapy is not used for treatment of carcinoid tumors, although medications, such as octreotide, are used to control symptoms of carcinoid syndrome.

10–D. The most common site of carcinoid tumors is the appendix. Hepatic metastases may lead to the carcinoid syndrome. One of 500 appendectomies will reveal carcinoid tumor. Carcinoid tumors may metastasize to the liver but are not usually primary. Eighty-five percent are found in the appendix, 13% in the small intestine (ileum), and 2% in the rectum.

11–C. Intussusception should be considered in any child younger than 2 years old with intermittent, colicky, abdominal pain. It occurs more commonly in males, and 75% of the cases are in children under 2 years old. At first the vomitus is only gastric contents but eventually becomes bilious. The stool is often described as "currant jelly" (i.e., purple clots with mucus and blood streaking). In most cases, definitive diagnosis and therapy can be effected by barium enema. If this is not successful, operative intervention with reduction of the "lead point" of the intussusception may be necessary.

12–B. Incarcerated hernias represent hernias that are not easily reducible by standard nonoperative means (i.e., mild sedation with application of steady, mild, constant pressure). Incarcerated hernias are the most common cause of small bowel obstruction in the world, with the inguinal region being a frequent site. If the incarcerated hernia has been present for only a few hours, gentle manual reduction may be possible. The presence of a hernia in association with fever, tachycardia, rebound tenderness, guarding, and erythema over the hernia suggests the presence of a strangulated hernia. Strangulation occurs when the perfusion of the incarcerated bowel is compromised, resulting in ischemia and necrosis. This is an indication for immediate operative intervention with resection of the affected bowel and repair of the hernia defect.

13–F. The finding of multiple consecutive strictures in the distal small bowel is very suggestive of Crohn's disease. Other characteristics of Crohn's may also be present, such as diarrhea, abdominal pain, and perianal disease. Stricture formation and small bowel obstruction is a frequent problem in patients with Crohn's disease.

14–C, D. Melanoma is the most common extraintestinal tumor to metastasize to the small intestine. Metastatic disease to the colon may present with small bowel obstruction (SBO). Obstruction may be secondary to a mass effect of the lesion, causing direct luminal obstruction, or the mass may result in intussusception. Intussusception may present with signs and symptoms of SBO and intermittent, crampy, abdominal pain. In adults with suspected intussusception, early surgical exploration is indicated because many are associated with malignancy. Colonic adenocarcinoma may also present as an SBO. Metastatic colon cancer can affect any part of the intestine while right-sided colon lesions can cause obstruction at the level of the ileocecal valve.

15–E. Among the choices provided, paralytic ileus is the most likely cause of this patient's symptoms. Although laparoscopic surgery is less likely to be associated with a persistent postoperative ileus versus open abdominal procedures, ileus may still occur. Dehydration with hypokalemia may also contribute to the persistence of a postoperative ileus.

16–I. A bezoar represents a cumulative mass of ingested nondigestible material [e.g., trichobezoar (hair), phytobezoar (plant material)]. Ingestion of such material may be seen in children or in patients with poor gastric emptying (i.e., after gastric surgery) and may also be associated with certain psychiatric disorders. Bezoars frequently cause obstruction at the level of the stomach and frequently require endoscopic or surgical removal, although some types of bezoars may respond to enzymatic digestion.

17–H, J. Malrotation with midgut volvulus is a surgical emergency. It usually occurs in infancy (75% in the first month of life). Common findings are bilious vomiting, vascular collapse, and blood from the rectum. An upper gastrointestinal study will best show malrotation. This condition occurs when there is incomplete rotation of the midgut around the superior mesenteric artery. The base of the mesentery is congenitally narrow and the entire midgut can twist on its blood vessels and result in vascular compromise of the bowel. If this condition is ignored, bowel necrosis can occur. In addition, constriction of the second portion of the duodenum by a circumferential segment of pancreatic tissue can cause a proximal obstruction in very young children. This annular pancreas is secondary to abnormal migration of the pancreatic bud during embryologic development. Although this could also cause the symptoms mentioned above, bilious vomiting in a newborn is **a malrotation with midgut volvulus until proven otherwise** given the severe consequences of this process.

18–A. In Western countries where abdominal operations are common, adhesions are the most common cause of intestinal obstruction. Peritoneal irritation from any cause causes local outpouring of fibrin and adhesion formation. Substances such as hyaluronidase, steroids, and fibrinolysis have been instilled into the peritoneum without success in preventing adhesions. Conservative management with nasogastric suction may be curative but operative lysis of adhesions may be necessary.

19–D. Right-sided colon cancers may occasionally mimic small bowel obstruction (SBO) by causing obstruction at the level of the ileocecal valve. Recent weight loss and heme-positive stools should raise suspicion for the diagnosis of colon adenocarcinoma. Although this is a rare cause of SBO, a water-soluble (e.g., gastrografin) enema may help rule out such pathology in the absence of signs of more common causes of obstruction.

20–G. The cause of Ogilvie's syndrome remains unclear but may be related to altered motility of the colon from imbalance of sympathetic and parasympathetic tone to the colon. It is seen mainly in patients hospitalized with severe illnesses. Bowel sounds are usually present and there may be diarrhea. Abdominal radiographs show massive dilation of the colon (predominantly right and transverse) with little or no small bowel dilation. Decompressive colonoscopy is the therapeutic procedure of choice. A generalized paralytic ileus characteristically affects the small bowel in addition to the colon while this variant, Ogilvie's syndrome, may frequently affect the colon without involving the small bowel.

14

Colon, Rectum, and Anus

James W. Thiele

I. Anatomic Considerations

A. Anatomy of the colon

1. **The colon is divided** into the cecum and the ascending, transverse, descending, and sigmoid colon.
   a. **The cecum**
      —is the first and largest segment (7.5 cm to 8.5 cm) of the colon.
      —**is the most common site of colonic rupture** because it has the largest radius and most wall tension for a given pressure.
      —The ileum joins on its posteromedial border and the appendix is attached just below the ileocecal valve.
   b. **The colonic wall**
      —is composed of mucosa, submucosa, inner circular muscle, outer longitudinal muscle, and serosa.
   c. **Teniae coli**
      —are three longitudinal muscular bands that converge proximally on the appendix and continue to the proximal rectum.
   d. **Haustra**
      —are sacculations between the teniae that are divided by **plicae semilunaris.**
2. **Blood supply of the colon**
   a. **Arterial supply (Figure 14-1)**
      (1) **The superior mesenteric artery**
         —branches into the ileocolic, right colic, and middle colic branches to supply the colon **from the cecum to the splenic flexure.**
      (2) **The inferior mesenteric artery**
         —branches into the left colic, sigmoidal, and superior rectal branches to supply the descending and sigmoid colon and the upper rectum.

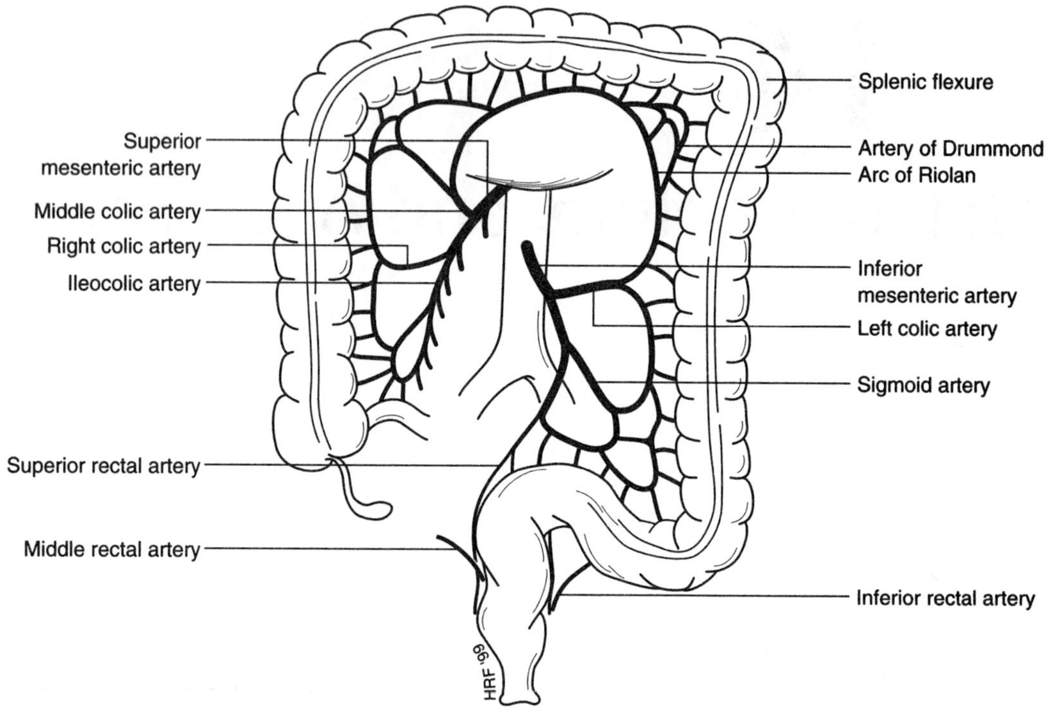

Figure 14-1. Arterial blood supply of the colon. The Arc of Riolan is the principle vessel that provides collateral blood flow between the superior and inferior mesenteric arteries. The splenic flexure is the watershed area of the colon, having distal blood supply from both of the mesenteric arteries. It is a common area of ischemia in states of low flow to the colon. (Reprinted with permission from Nora PF: *Operative Surgery: Principles and Techniques,* 3rd ed. Philadelphia, WB Saunders, p 613.)

(3) The arc of Riolan

—provides **collateral blood flow between the inferior** and **superior mesenteric arteries.**

b. Venous drainage

—of the colon and rectum is via the superior and inferior mesenteric veins, which parallel the arterial supply.

(1) The **inferior mesenteric vein** drains into the splenic vein.

(2) The **superior mesenteric vein** joins the splenic vein to form the portal vein.

3. Lymphatic drainage

a. Lymph channels are located in the submucosa and muscularis mucosa, but not in the mucosa.

—Thus, **mucosal cancers rarely metastasize.**

b. Lymph vessels parallel the arterial supply of the colon.

—Nodes are located in the wall of the colon (epicolic), along the inner margin (paracolic), near mesenteric vessels (intermediate), or around the main mesenteric arteries (main).

B. Anatomy of the rectum

1. The rectum extends from the sigmoid colon to the anal canal.

a. The proximal rectum

—is identified by the merging of the teniae coli into a single circumferential layer of longitudinal muscle.

b. The peritoneum

—**covers the upper third of the rectum** on the anterior and lateral surfaces and the middle third on the anterior surface only.

—The **lower third of the rectum is below the peritoneal reflection.**

c. Fascia

(1) Denonvillier's fascia (anterior)

—is the rectovesical fascia in men and the rectovaginal fascia in women.

(2) Waldeyer's fascia (posterior)

—is the rectosacral fascia in both genders.

2. Blood supply and drainage of the rectum (Figure 14-2)

a. Arterial supply

(1) The superior rectal branch of the inferior mesenteric artery and the middle rectal branch of the internal iliac artery supply the upper two thirds of the rectum and have collaterals between them.

(2) The inferior rectal branch of the pudendal artery supplies the

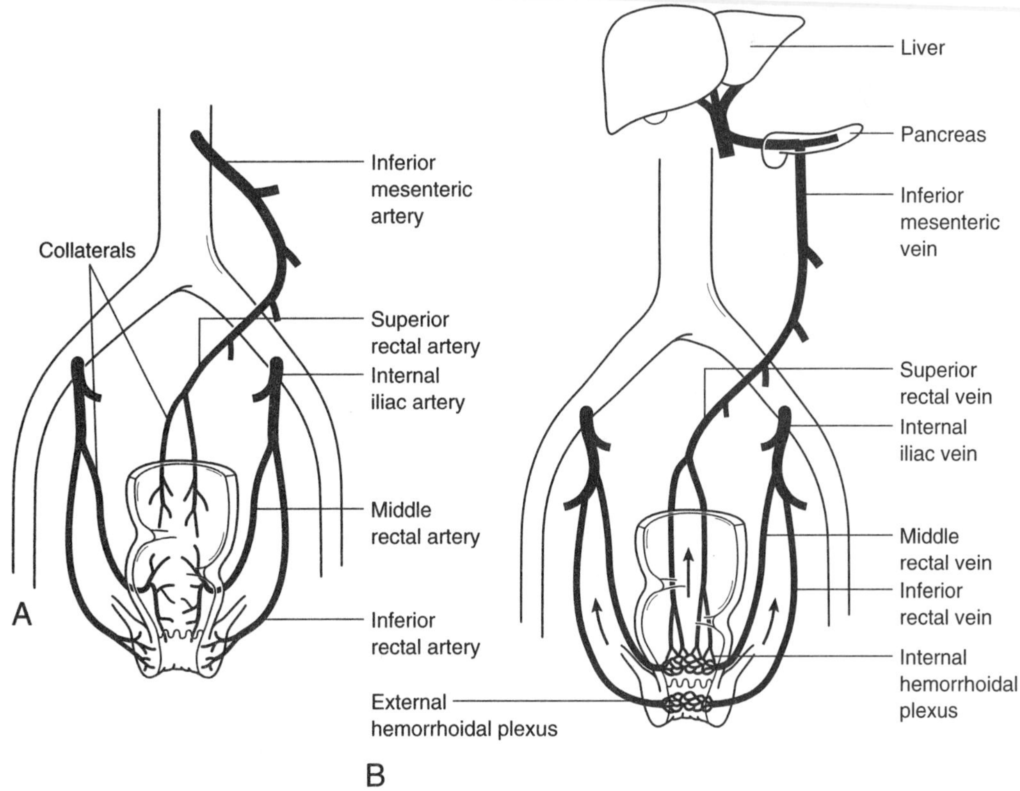

Figure 14-2. *(A)* Arterial supply and *(B)* venous drainage of the rectum. (Reprinted with permission from Schwartz S: *Principles of Surgery,* 7th ed. New York, McGraw-Hill, 1998, p 1270.)

lower third of the rectum and provides collaterals to the upper rectum.

b. **Venous drainage**

(1) **The upper two thirds**

—is drained by the superior and middle rectal veins, which empty into the portal system via the inferior mesenteric vein.

(2) **The lower third of the rectum**

—is drained by the inferior rectal vein, which empties into the caval system via the internal iliac veins.

3. **Lymphatic drainage of the rectum**

a. The upper two thirds of the rectum drains into the inferior mesenteric nodes.

b. The lower third of the rectum primarily drains into the **inferior mesenteric nodes** as well but can also drain via alternate routes into the **iliac nodes** and subsequently into the periaortic lymph nodes.

C. **General anatomy of the anal canal**

1. **The anal canal**

—extends from the levator ani muscle (pelvic diaphragm) to the anal verge.

—contains the **dentate line,** which is the **squamocolumnar junction** between the rectum and anus.

—is surrounded by a muscular sphincter.

a. **The internal sphincter**

—is **smooth muscle** and is contracted at rest.

—is a continuation of the inner circular muscle of the rectum.

—Activation of **sympathetic and parasympathetic** nerves causes **relaxation of this sphincter.**

b. **The external sphincter**

—is voluntary, striated muscle divided into subcutaneous, superficial, and deep portions.

—is a continuation of the levator ani muscle.

—**Innervation** is via the inferior rectal branch of the **pudendal nerve** and the perineal branch of the fourth **sacral nerve.**

2. **Arterial supply and venous drainage of the anus**

a. **Arterial supply** is via the inferior rectal artery.

b. **Venous drainage** above the dentate line is via the submucosal internal hemorrhoidal plexus, while that below the dentate line is via the communicating external hemorrhoidal plexus.

II. Benign Lesions of the Colon and Rectum

A. Adenomatous polyps

—are benign lesions with significant **malignant potential.**

1. **Tubular adenomas**

—constitute 60% to 80% of adenomatous polyps and are generally small, pedunculated masses with a branching, glandular histologic appearance.

a. The overall incidence of carcinoma in these polyps is 15%.

b. **Increasing size results in an increased incidence of cancer.**

2. **Villous adenomas**

—tend to occur more distally in the colon and are usually sessile with long, finger-like glandular projections.

—These polyps are generally **larger** than tubular adenomas and have a **greater propensity for malignant change.**

3. **Tubulovillous adenomas**

—have characteristics of both types of polyps and the degree of malignant potential is directly related to the **percentage of the villous component.**

B. **Benign lesions without malignant potential**

1. **Hyperplastic polyps**

—are smooth, rounded, usually sessile lesions found most frequently in the distal colon.

—are not premalignant and usually remain small or regress.

—These lesions may be indistinguishable from adenomas grossly.

2. **Inflammatory polyps**

—are benign lesions that arise in response to mucosal injury (e.g., ulcerative colitis).

3. **Juvenile polyps or hamartomatous polyps**

—are benign lesions frequently found throughout the entire gastrointestinal tract.

—may be a source of gastrointestinal bleeding.

—**Peutz-Jeghers syndrome** is an autosomal dominant syndrome associated with **multiple hamartomatous polyps** in addition to **melanin deposits in the buccal mucosa,** lips, nose, palms, and feet.

C. **Treatment of colonic polyps**

1. **Adenomatous polyps**

—are treated with **colonoscopic resection** with pathologic examination for foci of carcinoma.

a. For completely resected lesions, follow-up colonoscopy is performed in 3 to 5 years.

b. Incompletely resected lesions or lesions too large for colonoscopic resection generally require surgical resection of the affected colon.

2. **Asymptomatic hyperplastic, inflammatory, and juvenile polyps** generally do not require additional surveillance or therapy.

III. Malignant Neoplasms of the Colon and Rectum

A. Adenocarcinoma of the colon

1. **Risk factors**

a. **Genetic predisposition**

(1) **Nonpolyposis inherited colon cancer (Lynch syndrome)**

—is characterized by **right-sided colon cancer** in young patients without multiple polyps.

(a) Lynch syndrome I is **only associated with colon cancer.**

(b) Lynch syndrome II (family cancer syndrome) is associated with colorectal, endometrial, gastric, and other types of cancers.

(c) Both are **autosomal dominant,** linked to **chromosome 18.**

(2) **Familial adenomatous polyposis syndromes**

—are characterized by multiple colonic polyps occurring by age 30.

—exhibit **autosomal dominant** inheritance.

(a) Phenotypic subtypes include **familial polyposis coli, Gardner's syndrome** (epidermal inclusion cysts, colonic polyps, and osteomas), and **Turcot syndrome** (colonic polyps and brain tumors).

(b) **Chromosome 5 near q21** locus is the adenomatous polyposis coli **(APC) gene.**

(3) **Many familial colon cancers**

—are not associated with a well-defined genetic lesion as described with the above syndromes.

b. **A high-fat diet** is a significant risk factor.

—**Protective factors** may include **aspirin,** selenium, thioesters, carotenoids, and **high fiber.**

c. **Long-standing ulcerative colitis** is also a significant risk factor.

2. **Screening and diagnostic techniques**

a. **Current screening techniques**

—have generally not been shown to improve overall survival.

b. **The American Cancer Society's current recommendations** for screening in low-risk, asymptomatic individuals include:

(1) **Digital rectal examination** (DRE) and testing for occult blood annually beginning at age 40.

(2) **Flexible sigmoidoscopy** every 3 to 5 years after age 50.

c. **The colon can be inspected by**

—**DRE,** to inspect the distal 8 cm of colon.

—**flexible sigmoidoscopy,** to examine the distal 60 cm of colon.

—**proctosigmoidoscopy with a rigid proctoscope,** to inspect the distal 20 cm to 25 cm of colon; this test can be performed in the office.

—**colonoscopy,** to visualize the **entire colon and distal ileum.** This test **requires a full colonic preparation** and sedation for discomfort. Biopsy, polypectomy, and therapeutic measures for hemostasis can be performed.

3. **Staging of colon cancer (Tables 14-1 and 14-2)**

a. **The TNM (tumor-node-metastasis) classification** is currently the **preferred staging system.**

Table 14-1. TNM Classification System for Staging of Colon Cancer

Primary tumor (T)	
TX	Tumor cannot be assessed
T0	No primary tumor found
Tis	Carcinoma in situ
T1	Invasion into the submucosa
T2	Invasion into the muscularis propria
T3	Invasion through the muscularis and into the serosa or pericolic tissues
T4	Invasion into adjacent structures or organs
Regional lymph nodes (N)	
NX	Regional nodes cannot be assessed
N0	No regional node involvement
N1	Metastasis in 1 to 3 pericolic nodes
N2	Metastasis in 4 or more pericolic nodes
N3	Metastasis in any nodes along the course of named vascular trunks
Distant metastasis (M)	
MX	Presence of distant metastasis cannot be assessed
M0	No distant metastasis
M1	Distant metastasis

TNM = tumor, node, metastasis.

Table 14-2. Comparison of Staging Systems for Colon Cancer

Description of Cancer	Astler-Coller Modification of Dukes Staging	TNM Classification	AJCC/UICC	5-Year Survival Rate
		Tis/N0/M0	Stage 0	
Cancer limited to the mucosa but not through the muscularis propria and negative lymph nodes	A	T1 or T2/N0/M0	Stage I	90%
Limited to the muscularis propria, with negative nodes	B1	T3/N0/M0	Stage II	70%–75%
Full thickness invasion, with negative nodes	B2	T4/N0/M0		
Stage B1 invasion with positive nodes	C1	Any T/N1, N2, or N3/M0	Stage III	35%
Stage B2 invasion with positive nodes	C2			
Distant metastasis regardless of invasion	D	Any T/any N/M1	Stage IV	< 5%

AJCC = American Joint Committee on Cancer; UICC = International Union Against Cancer (Union International contre le cancre).

b. **The Astler-Coller modification of Dukes staging system** is based on the pathology of the resected specimen.

4. **Treatment of colon cancer**

   a. **Surgical intervention** consists of two different **resection** approaches:

(1) **Resection with primary anastomosis,** if a bowel preparation can be performed before surgery (single-stage procedure)

(2) **Resection with creation of a colostomy,** if a bowel preparation cannot be performed (two-stage procedure)

(a) Reanastomosis of bowel after a colostomy is generally performed at or after 6 weeks.

(b) This technique is generally used for obstructing lesions.

b. **Segmental resection** for colonic lesions depends on the **segmental distribution of the arterial supply** to the affected area.

(1) The mesenteric blood supply to the diseased segment is divided with resection of all accompanying mesenteric lymph nodes.

(2) Appropriate segmental resections for colonic tumors include

—**right hemicolectomy** for **cecal and ascending colon** tumors.

—**transverse colectomy** for tumors in the **transverse colon.**

—**left hemicolectomy** for tumors in the **splenic flexure and descending colon.**

—**sigmoid colectomy** for tumors in the **sigmoid colon.**

c. **Current chemotherapeutic agents**

—include 5-fluorouracil and levamisole used alone, or with other drugs.

(1) **Types of chemotherapy**

(a) **Adjuvant therapy**

—is administered after complete tumor resection to eliminate any microscopic metastatic disease.

(b) **Neoadjuvant therapy**

—is administered before other treatments to induce tumor shrinkage and eliminate occult metastatic disease.

(c) **Palliative therapy**

—is administered to patients with locally advanced disease not amenable to surgery.

(2) **Indications for chemotherapy**

(a) Chemotherapy improves survival in Stage III colon cancer and is recommended as adjuvant therapy in these patients.

(b) There is no efficacy for chemotherapy in Stage I or II cancers.

d. **Radiation therapy**

—**is generally not used in treating colonic adenocarcinoma.**

e. **Postoperative surveillance**

(1) Physical examination, laboratory tests (e.g., complete blood count, liver function tests), and tests for tumor markers [e.g., carcinoembryonic antigen (CEA)] are recommended every 3 months for the first 2 years, then less frequently thereafter.

(2) **Chest radiograph** should be performed annually for 5 years.

(3) **Barium enema or colonoscopy** is recommended every 3 years.

B. Special considerations for adenocarcinoma of the rectum

1. **Tumors confined to the pelvis usually make wide excision impossible.**
   a. The proximity of the sphincter mechanism poses potential problems with **incontinence.**
   b. A **permanent colostomy** may be necessary if the lesion is too close to the sphincter.
   c. The proximity to the organs and nerve supply of the urogenital tract may also lead to a high rate of **impotence** in men.
   d. There is a **greater risk of local and regional tumor recurrence** in the rectum versus the colon.
2. **Preoperative evaluation for suspected rectal cancer**
   a. **Local evaluation of the primary tumor**
      —**DRE** can estimate size and fixation.
      —**Rigid sigmoidoscopy** allows for adequate biopsy and reliable estimation of the distance of the tumor from the anal verge.
      —**Transanal ultrasound** may be used to determine depth of invasion.
   b. **Regional evaluation to determine resectability and local invasion**
      —The urogenital tract can be evaluated with ultrasound, computed tomography (CT), magnetic resonance imaging (MRI), or cystoscopy, as well as a pelvic examination in women
3. **Treatment of rectal cancer**
   a. **Surgical options** for the resection of rectal tumors (Figure 14-3)
      (1) Transanal local excision may be performed for small distal tumors confined to the mucosa.
      (2) **Low anterior resection** is used for **mid and upper rectal lesions.**
         —The distal colon and proximal rectum are resected with primary anastomosis performed above the levator ani muscle.
         —The sphincter mechanism is preserved.
      (3) **Abdominoperineal resection** is used for **lower rectal lesions.**
         —The anal canal below the level of the sphincter is excised along with the rectum with formation of a sigmoid colostomy.
   b. **Radiation therapy**
      —**has a role, unlike in colon adenocarcinoma.**
      (1) **Preoperative** radiation can be used to reduce tumor mass and potentially make an unresectable tumor resectable.
      (2) Radiation therapy can also allow for a less radical resection that will preserve the anal sphincter.
      (3) **Postoperative** radiation can be used to decrease the rate of local recurrence.
   c. **Chemotherapy regimens**
      —are similar to those used for adenocarcinoma of the colon (see III A 4 c).

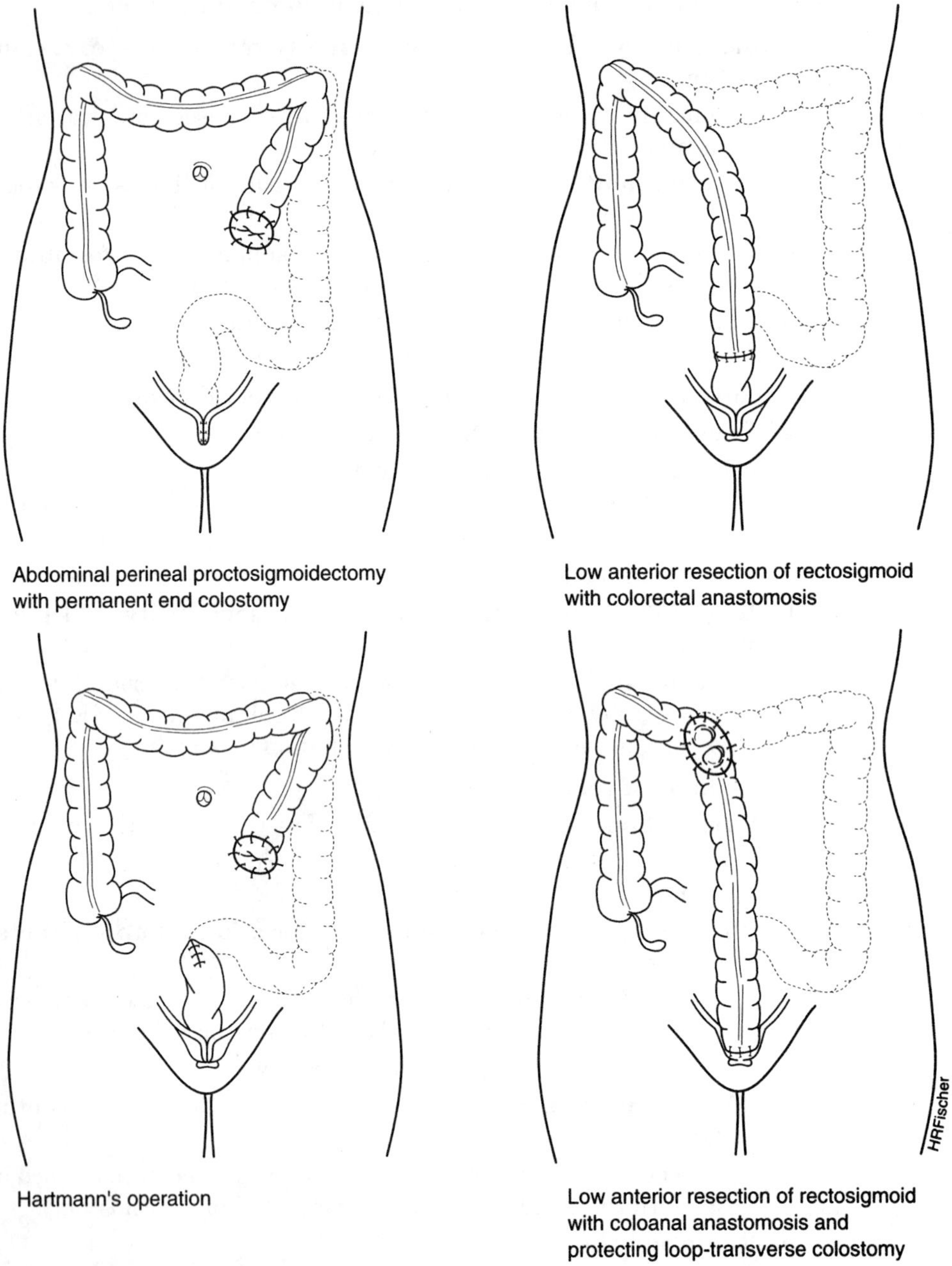

Abdominal perineal proctosigmoidectomy
with permanent end colostomy
Low anterior resection of rectosigmoid
with colorectal anastomosis
Hartmann's operation
Low anterior resection of rectosigmoid
with coloanal anastomosis and
protecting loop-transverse colostomy
HRFischer

Figure 14-3. Resections for low colonic and rectal cancer. The low anterior resection is used for cancers in the upper rectum or distal colon and consists of a distal resection with reanastomosis either immediately or at a later date after formation of a temporary colostomy (Hartmann's operation). The latter is generally used in emergent cases when the bowel is not prepared adequately. An abdominal perianal resection is used when the cancer is too distal to allow for future anastomosis. (Reprinted with permission from Schwartz S: *Principles of Surgery,* 7th ed. New York, McGraw-Hill, 1998, p 1357.)

IV. Neoplasms of the Anus

A. Squamous cell carcinoma

—of the anus generally presents **with pruritus, bleeding, and a palpable mass.**

1. Early lesions can be treated with **wide local excision.**
2. More advanced lesions that involve the sphincters can be treated with combined **chemoradiation** therapy.
3. Resection with **abdominoperineal resection** (APR) is reserved for persistent or recurrent disease.

B. Other rare neoplasms of the anus

—may mimic squamous cell carcinoma.

1. **Basal cell carcinoma** is treated with wide local excision.
2. **Bowen's disease, or squamous cell carcinoma in situ,** is also adequately treated with wide local excision.
3. Symptomatic **malignant melanoma** of the anus is usually associated with significant metastatic disease at the time of diagnosis.
4. **Perianal Paget's disease** is frequently associated with an **underlying large bowel malignancy.**
5. **Verrucous carcinoma,** also called giant condyloma or Buschke-Löwenstein tumor, is a large, wart-like lesion that is soft and slow growing.

V. Inflammatory Diseases of the Colon

A. Infections can cause or mimic surgical problems.

1. **Pseudomembranous colitis**

—secondary to ***Clostridium difficile*** infection can arise after antibiotic administration (see Chapter 4 III D 1).

2. **Mesenteric adenitis**

—secondary to viral infection or *Yersinia enterocolitica* infection can mimic appendicitis.

3. **Other inciting organisms**

—may include *Salmonella, Shigella,* and Cytomegalovirus.

4. **Neutropenic enterocolitis**

—(e.g., following chemotherapy) may also mimic surgical disease.

B. Inflammatory bowel disease (Table 14-3)

1. **Ulcerative colitis**

a. **Signs and symptoms**

—include bloody diarrhea, urgency, abdominal pain, fever, and weight loss.

b. **The rectum is always involved** and there is spread proximally in a continuous fashion **without "skip areas."**

—With proximal colonic involvement, the terminal ileum may be affected by a process called "**backwash ileitis.**"

c. **Mucosal and radiographic findings**

—Acute disease shows serrated mucosa.

—Chronic disease results in effacement of haustra and shortening of the colon causing a "**lead pipe**" appearance on barium enema.

d. **The risk of developing colon cancer**

Table 14-3. Features of Ulcerative Colitis and Crohn's Disease

	Ulcerative Colitis	Crohn's Disease
Distribution	Affects only the colon and rectum.	May affect any part of the bowel from mouth to anus
Histology	Crypt abscesses and psuedopolyps. Involves only the mucosa and submucosa.	Noncaseating granulomas. Involves the entire bowel wall.
Complications	Strictures and fistulas are rare. Toxic megacolon can occur.	Strictures and fistulas are common. Toxic megacolon can occur.
Pattern of progression	Always involves the rectum and progresses proximally in a continuous fashion.	Rectum may be spared. "Skip lesions" are common.
Cancer risk	Increased risk for cancer (10% at 20 years); greater than in Crohn's disease.	Increased risk for cancer, although not as great as in ulcerative colitis.
Role of surgery	Surgery can be curative.	Surgery is not curative and is reserved for treatment of disease complications.
Extracolonic manifestation	Arthritis and ocular manifestations often parallel severity of colonic disease. Erythema nodosum and pyoderma gangrenosum are also seen.	Erythema nodosum, iritis, uveitis, pyoderma gangrenosum, arthritis, spondylitis, sclerosing cholangitis, aphthous stomatitis, and pericholangitis.

—with ulcerative colitis is 1% per year after 10 years of disease (10% at 20 years).

e. **Medical management**

—is generally the **primary therapy** for uncomplicated disease.

(1) Maintenance with **sulfasalazine** is used to decrease relapse rates.

(2) Topical treatment (enemas) with **metronidazole or steroid therapy** may be used to treat acute exacerbations.

(3) Other immunosuppressive agents (e.g., azathioprine) may be used in some cases.

f. **Surgical indications for ulcerative colitis**

(1) **Emergency colectomy**

—is recommended for complications such as **hemorrhage and toxic megacolon** that do not respond promptly to medical management.

(2) **Elective colectomy**

—is recommended for disease **refractory to medical management** and **for cancer prophylaxis in long-standing disease** (> 10 years).

(a) The entire colon is resected and if rectal disease is mild, the rectum may be left in place and ileorectal anastomosis performed.

—This requires close follow-up surveillance of the rectal stump for evidence of cancer.

(b) If the rectum is removed, surgical options include a permanent ileostomy or creation of an ileal pouch with ileoanal anastomosis (Figure 14-4).

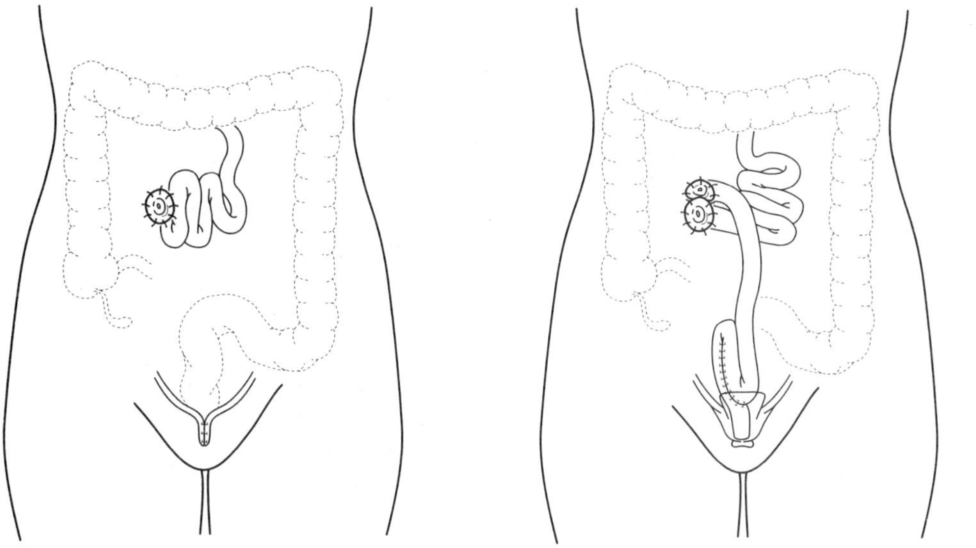

A Total abdominal perineal proctocolectomy (permanent ileostomy)
B Total abdominal colectomy, mucosal proctectomy, ileal pouch anal anastomosis (temporary ileostomy)

Figure 14-4. Surgical options in the treatment of ulcerative colitis. In the event that the entire colon is removed to provide a surgical cure for ulcerative colitis, two options are available postoperatively. *(A)* A permanent ileostomy may be performed following complete resection. *(B)* The ileal pouch with ileoanal anastomosis may provide the patient with more normal bowel function, although bowel movements may remain frequent and watery. The temporary ileostomy is used to divert the flow of small bowel content to protect the ileal anastomosis in the postoperative period. It is taken down at a later date. (Reprinted with permission from Schwartz S: *Principles of Surgery,* 7th ed. New York, McGraw-Hill, 1998, p 1322.)

(c) **Surgical therapy is curative if the entire colon and rectum are removed.**

2. **Crohn's disease** (see Chapter 13)

—A comparison of Crohn's disease and ulcerative colitis is summarized in Table 14-4.

VI. Diverticular Disease and Volvulus

A. Diverticular disease of the colon

1. Diverticuli

—are herniations of mucosa through the colon wall at the sites where arterioles enter the muscular wall.

a. They are **most prevalent in the sigmoid colon,** but can occur in any portion.

b. Increased intraluminal pressure forces the mucosa to herniate.

2. Diverticulosis

—is a **common cause of massive lower gastrointestinal bleeding.**

—usually presents as bright-red blood from the rectum, although there are many other potential sources (see Table 14-4).

a. **Hemorrhage** is the most common complication of **diverticulosis.**

Table 14-4. Causes of Gastrointestinal (GI) Bleeding Distal to the Ligament of Treitz (Lower GI Bleeding)

Diverticulosis (most common cause of massive bleeding from the rectum)
Angiodysplasia (frequent source of right-sided colonic bleeding)
Cancer (most common cause of occult blood loss)
Inflammatory bowel disease (i.e., ulcerative colitis and Crohn's disease)
Hemorrhoids
Small bowel tumors
Upper GI bleeding (may frequently present as bleeding from the rectum)
Infectious colitis
Benign colonic lesions (polyps)
Aortoenteric fistula (should be considered with a history of aortic aneurysm repair)
Ischemic colitis

b. The close association of the arteriole with the diverticulum can result in erosion into the vessel and massive hemorrhage.

3. Diverticulitis

—denotes infection and inflammation of the colonic serosa as well as the surrounding soft tissues.

a. Infection is a result of small perforations in the diverticulum with fecal contamination.

b. In most cases, spillage is minimal and infection is confined locally.

c. Symptoms include left lower quadrant (LLQ) abdominal pain, fever, chills, and alterations in bowel habit (constipation or diarrhea).

—Diverticulitis is usually not associated with bleeding.

d. A **CT scan** is a useful diagnostic test for **suspected diverticulitis.**

e. Most cases respond to medical management with antibiotics and bowel rest and do not require surgical intervention.

4. Complications of diverticular disease

—frequently require surgical intervention.

a. Uncontrolled hemorrhage

—secondary to **diverticulosis** should be approached with a full lower gastrointestinal bleed work-up even with known diverticular disease (Figure 14-5).

(1) Colonic bleeding will stop spontaneously in 85% of cases; however, resection of the diseased area may be necessary for refractory bleeding.

(2) The sites of bleeding should be localized if possible with a nuclear **bleeding scan or angiography.**

(3) If the bleeding site is identified, a segmental colectomy can be performed. If the site is not found, a subtotal colectomy for refractory bleeding may be required.

b. Complicated diverticulitis

—(e.g., abscess or fistula formation, perforation, obstruction) may require **emergent surgical resection.**

(1) The most common fistulas are between the bladder and colon in men, and the colon and vagina in women.

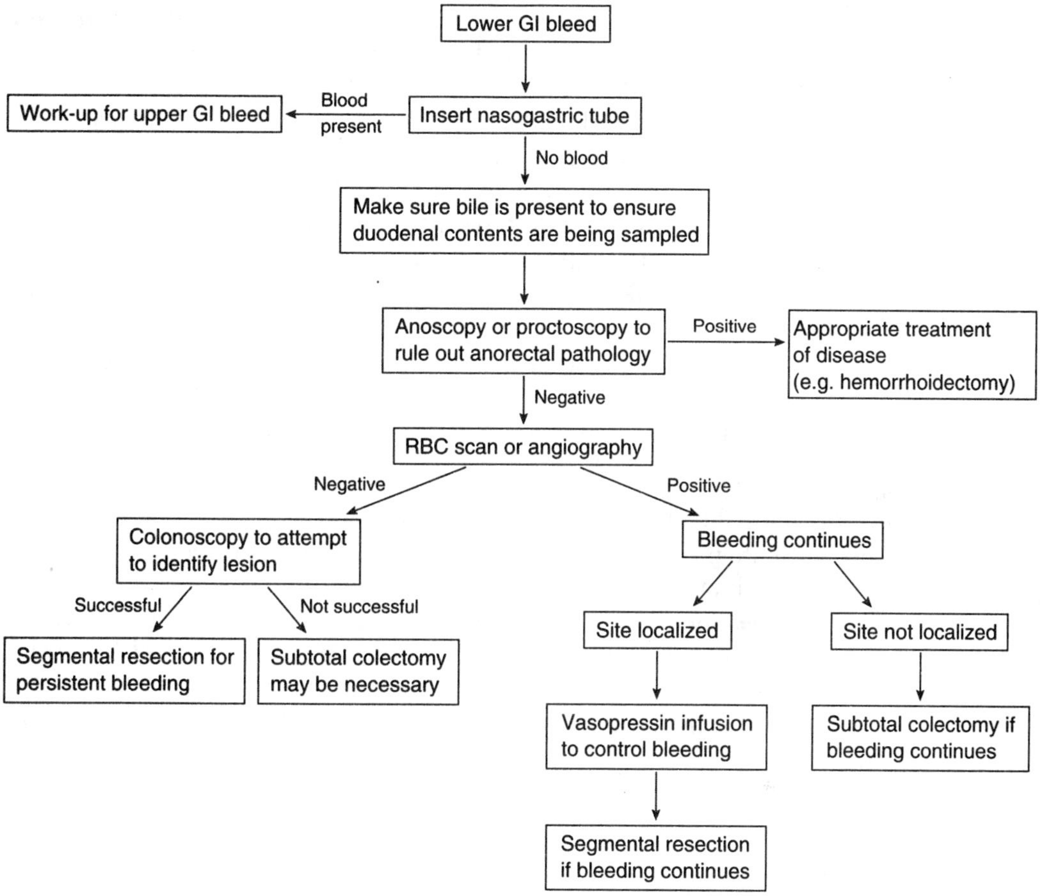

Figure 14-5. The work-up of acute lower gastrointestinal bleeding. *GI* = gastrointestinal; *NG* = nasogastric; *RBC* = red blood cell.

(2) Some abscesses can be drained percutaneously and the diseased segment of colon resected electively at a later date.

c. **Recurrent diverticulitis**

—may require surgical intervention.

(1) **Uncomplicated diverticulitis** is **treated with bowel rest and broad-spectrum antibiotic therapy** with a low recurrence rate after one episode.

(2) **Second attacks are associated with a 50% chance of recurrence** and elective resection is recommended after symptoms resolve.

B. Colonic volvulus

—involves twisting of the bowel and usually results in obstruction, with the sigmoid and cecum being the most common sites.

1. Sigmoid volvulus

—accounts for **about 80%** of colonic volvulus.

—is the most common cause of bowel obstruction in pregnancy.

a. Sigmoid volvulus is more common in **older and institutionalized patients** in whom a redundant sigmoid is often seen because of chronic constipation.

b. Patients present with abdominal pain, distention, and obstipation.

c. Plain radiographs of the abdomen reveal a dilated sigmoid that appears as a **U-shaped loop in the lower abdomen.**

d. **Sigmoidoscopy is often both diagnostic and therapeutic.**

e. Volvulus reduction and bowel decompression by sigmoidoscopy should be followed by elective sigmoid resection because there is a **40% rate of recurrence without operative intervention.**

f. If the volvulus cannot be reduced or if there are signs of bowel gangrene (e.g., peritoneal irritation, elevated white blood cell count, sepsis), the patient should be taken to surgery emergently.

2. **Cecal volvulus**

—accounts for **less than 20%** of colonic volvulus.

a. Patients present with symptoms of small bowel obstruction and may have a history of intermittent symptoms.

b. Plain radiographs of the abdomen reveal the **kidney bean–shaped, air-filled cecum located in the left upper quadrant (LUQ)** [Figure 14-6].

c. Operative detorsion with cecopexy (suturing the cecum in place) is associated with recurrence, and **right hemicolectomy is generally considered the treatment of choice** to avoid recurrence.

VII. Benign Anorectal Disease

A. An anal fissure

—is described as a split in the anoderm in either the anterior or **posterior (90%) midline.**

1. **Recurrent fissures**

—or fissures occurring laterally should raise suspicion of a contributing disease process (e.g., Crohn's disease).

2. **Symptoms associated with fissures**

—Patients generally complain of **painful defecation or bleeding from the rectum.**

—**Pain in the fissure** causes internal sphincter spasm and further tearing.

3. **Diagnosis and management**

a. **Inspection** of the perianal area may reveal the fissure.

b. **DRE** with adequate anesthesia may reveal a hypertrophied sphincter.

c. **Stool softeners, bulk laxatives, and warm sitz baths will heal 90% of cases.**

d. **Surgical intervention** for persistent fissures includes stretching or division of the distal internal sphincter (sphincterotomy).

B. Anorectal abscess

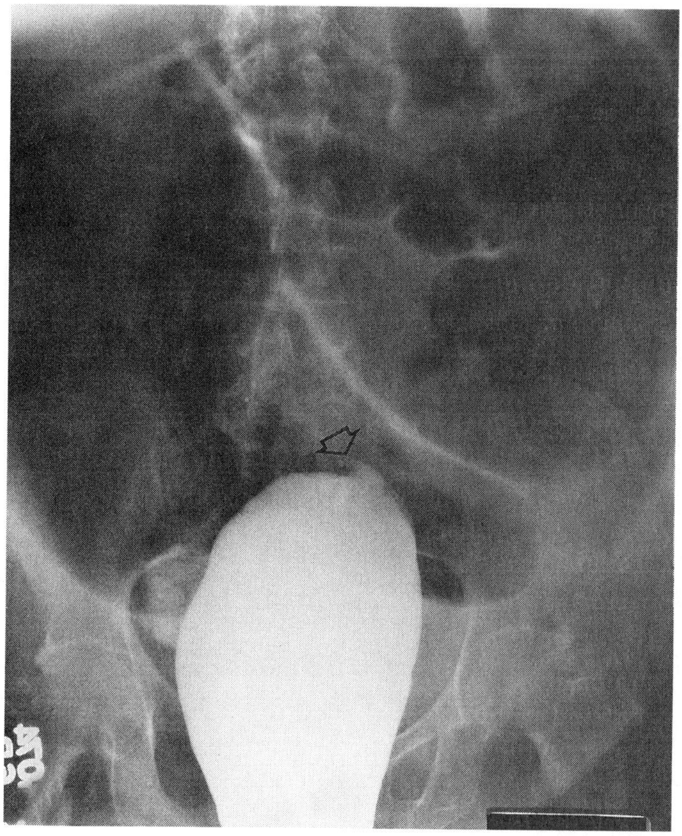

Figure 14-6. Barium enema demonstrating a sigmoid volvulus. Note loop of massively dilated colon and barium stopping at the point of obstruction. (Reprinted with permission from Daffner RH: *Clinical Radiology: The Essentials,* 2nd ed. Baltimore, Williams & Wilkins, 1999, p 261.)

1. **Potential spaces for abscess formation**

—include the perianal and intersphincteric spaces, the ischiorectal fossa, or above the levator ani muscles (supralevator) [Figure 14-7].

—The **ischiorectal and supralevator spaces** have a posterior communication that may allow for **"horseshoe" abscess** formation.

2. **Signs and symptoms**

—Symptoms include severe anal pain, fever, urinary retention, and occasionally sepsis.

—A palpable mass is often noted on DRE.

3. **Treatment**

—**Incision and drainage** should be performed as soon as possible.

—Perianal and ischiorectal abscesses can be drained through the overlying skin.

—Supralevator abscesses may be drained internally through the rectal wall.

C. Perianal fistula (fistula-in-ano)

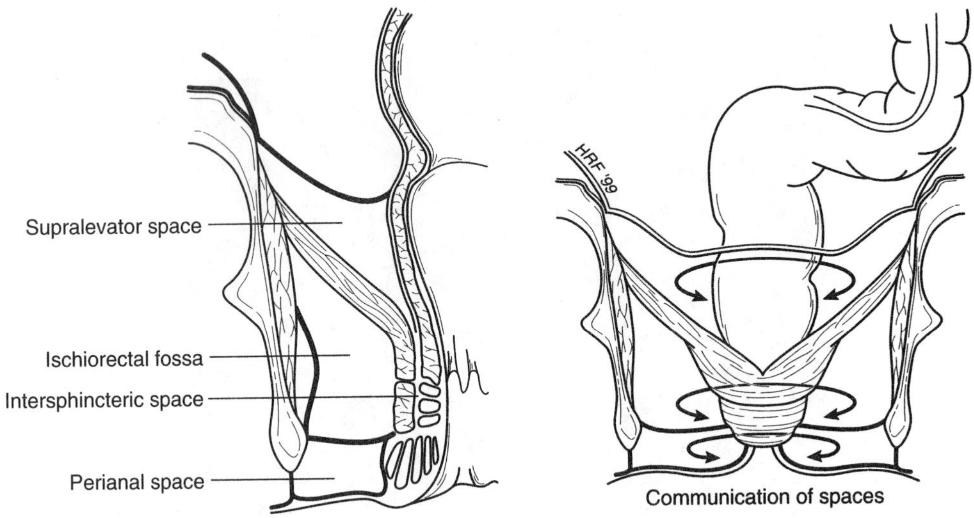

Figure 14-7. Perirectal spaces. (Reprinted with permission from Schwartz S: *Principles of Surgery,* 7th ed. New York, McGraw-Hill, 1998, p 1303.)

1. The **most common cause** of anal fistula formation is spontaneous drainage of an anorectal abscess, resulting in a persistently draining tract.

   —Other causes include Crohn's disease, trauma, and radiation.

2. **Diagnosis and treatment**

   a. Patients generally present with a chronically draining wound or recurrent anorectal abscesses.

   b. **Goodsall's rule** (Figure 14-8) divides the anus into anterior and posterior halves.

   —External openings in the **anterior half** will connect to an internal opening via a **direct fistula tract.**

   —External openings in the **posterior half** will connect to a posterior midline internal opening via a **curved tract.**

   c. Fistulas are generally treated by incising the fistula (fistulotomy) and curetting the tract. The wound then heals by secondary intention.

D. Pilonidal disease

—represents sinus or abscess formation in the skin and subcutaneous tissues over the **sacrococcygeal junction.**

1. These lesions are **more common in men** and infection may be secondary to fragmented hairs driven into the skin.
2. **Acute infection** presents with pain and swelling and incision and drainage should be performed.
3. After acute infection subsides, persistent sinus tracts should be excised.

E. Hemorrhoidal tissue

—is found at the right anterolateral and posterolateral positions and the left lateral position.

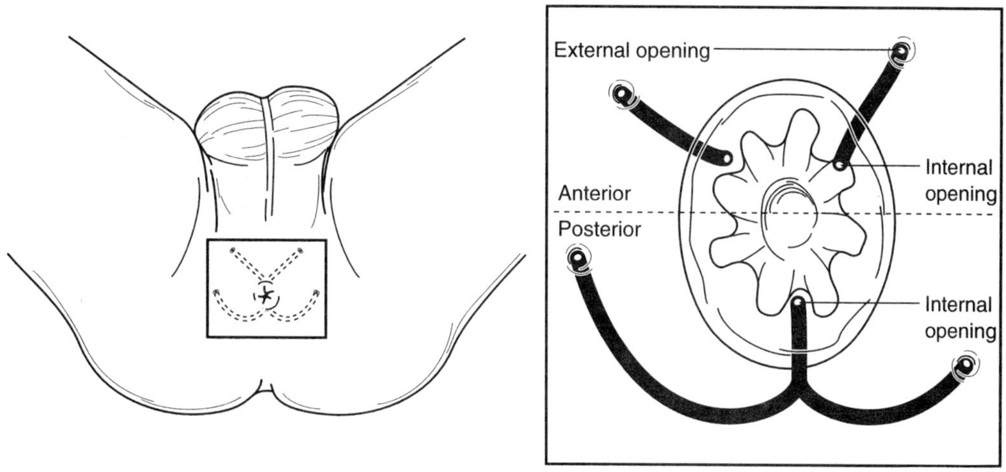

Figure 14-8. Goodsall's rule. Fistulae with an external opening posterior to the line bisecting the anorectum have internal openings in the midline. Those anterior to the line have internal openings that connect via a straight, radial line. (Reprinted with permission from Nyhus, LM: *Mastery of Surgery,* 3rd ed. Philadelphia, Little, Brown, 1997, p 1566.)

1. Internal hemorrhoids

—are above the dentate line (an insensate area) and are covered by mucosa.

a. These lesions **rarely cause pain** unless incarcerated.

b. Patients usually complain of painless bleeding or prolapse.

2. External hemorrhoids

—are distal to the dentate line and are covered by sensate squamous epithelium.

a. Common symptoms include perianal pain, itching, and swelling.

b. Acute pain and swelling is suggestive of acute thrombosis.

3. Treatment of hemorrhoids

—**Initial treatment** includes fiber diet, stool softeners, and avoidance of straining.

—**Insensate internal hemorrhoids** may be treated **by rubber-band ligation** resulting in necrosis and sloughing of the lesion.

—Sclerosis and cryosurgery are other techniques used to treat internal hemorrhoids.

—**Excisional hemorrhoidectomy** is the best choice for symptomatic hemorrhoids with a substantial **external component** or internal hemorrhoids refractory to banding.

F. Rectal prolapse

—is a complete **intussusception of the rectum through the anus.**

1. This process involves **all layers of the rectum** and appears as a large mass protruding from the anus.

2. Folds in the mucosa are circumferential as opposed to radial, which differentiates rectal prolapse from other conditions such as prolapsed hemorrhoid or rectal polyp.

3. Rectal prolapse is more common in **elderly women and institutionalized patients** and is associated with long-term anal outlet obstruction.

   —Patients are often incontinent of stool and have pudendal neuropathy.

4. Treatment involves **rectopexy (fixation of the rectum)** in the absence of a redundant sigmoid or low anterior resection of the rectosigmoid colon.

Review Test

Directions: Each of the numbered items or incomplete statements in this section is followed by answers or by completions of the statement. Select the ONE lettered answer or completion that is BEST in each case.

1. A 44-year-old woman with a 24-year history of ulcerative colitis presents with persistent melanotic, loose stools for the past 6 months. Her disease had been well controlled medically with steroids until her recent problems. Colonoscopic biopsy of a 6-cm mass in the descending colon reveals adenocarcinoma. After the proper procedure is performed in this patient, which of the following pathologic characteristics of ulcerative colitis might be seen in the resected segment?

(A) Full thickness involvement
(B) Sparing of the rectal segment
(C) Crypt abscesses
(D) "Creeping fat" around the affected bowel
(E) Segments of normal bowel between areas of disease ("skip areas")

Questions 2–3

An 83-year-old woman in a nursing home presents with a 24-hour history of obstipation and distended abdomen. Her vital signs and laboratory tests are normal. Plain abdominal film reveals a massively dilated loop of bowel in the lower abdomen.

2. Which of the following is the most likely diagnosis for this patient?

(A) Small bowel obstruction
(B) Fecal impaction
(C) Cecal volvulus
(D) Sigmoid volvulus
(E) Ogilvie's syndrome

3. Which of the following is the most appropriate next step in the treatment of this patient?

(A) Immediate surgery
(B) Flexible sigmoidoscopy
(C) Barium enema
(D) Admission and observation
(E) Discharge with laxatives

Questions 4–5

A 35-year-old truck driver presents with perianal pain and pain on defecation for 2 days. He has no prior history of medical problems and reports only a low-grade fever. Digital rectal examination (DRE) reveals a tender mass at the anal verge.

4. Which of the following is the most likely diagnosis for this patient?

(A) Perianal abscess
(B) Supralevator abscess
(C) Hemorrhoids
(D) Anal fissure
(E) Rectal cancer

5. Which of the following is the most appropriate next step in the management of this patient?

(A) Admission and antibiotics
(B) Incision and drainage
(C) Excisional hemorrhoidectomy
(D) Lateral sphincterotomy
(E) Colonoscopy

Questions 6–7

A 67-year-old man presents with sudden onset massive bleeding from the rectum. He has no prior history of gastrointestinal problems and denies any abdominal pain. He has been previously healthy and takes no medications. A nasogastric tube is placed and clear bile without blood is aspirated from the stomach.

6. All of the following would be an appropriate next step EXCEPT:

(A) Bleeding scan
(B) Type and crossmatch
(C) Colonoscopy
(D) Angiography
(E) Admission to the hospital

7. Which of the following is the most likely cause of the massive lower gastrointestinal bleeding in this patient?

(A) Hemorrhoids
(B) Cancer
(C) Peptic ulcer disease
(D) Diverticulosis
(E) Ischemic colitis

Questions 8–9

A 27-year-old woman presents with a history of chronic bloody diarrhea, abdominal cramping, and weight loss. The diagnosis of ulcerative colitis is made.

8. Which of the following is true regarding the management of this patient?

(A) High-dose steroids are used as a maintenance therapy to prevent relapse
(B) Surgery is rarely curative in this disease
(C) An appropriate surgical option would include a total proctocolectomy
(D) Barium enema is the diagnostic test of choice for this disease
(E) The risk of cancer is 70% after 20 years of active disease

9. Which of the following is true regarding the surgical management of this disease?

(A) Removal of the entire colon is rarely necessary
(B) If the rectum is removed it is impossible to provide anal continence for the patient
(C) Because the cancer risk is so high in this disease, subtotal colectomy is recommended as soon as the diagnosis is made
(D) This disease is confined to the colon and does not affect other parts of the bowel
(E) Surgery offers the best chance for cure in these patients

10. A 68-year-old woman was referred by her primary care physician who noted occult positive stools on routine physical examination. Barium enema subsequently revealed a mass in the ascending colon. The appropriate examination was performed and the lesion was found to be a poorly differentiated adenocarcinoma. At surgery, the mass was noted to invade through the entire thickness of the bowel with two positive nodes and no distant metastases. Which of the following is the stage of this cancer according to the Astler-Coller modification of Dukes staging system?

(A) D
(B) B1
(C) B2
(D) C1
(E) C2

Directions: Each set of matching questions in this section consists of a list of four to twenty-six lettered options followed by several numbered items. For each numbered item, select the appropriate lettered option(s). Each lettered option may be selected once, more than once, or not at all.

Questions 11–20

(A) Ulcerative colitis
(B) Crohn's disease
(C) *Salmonella* enterocolitis
(D) *Yersinia* enterocolitis
(E) Cytomegalovirus enterocolitis
(F) Neutropenic enterocolitis
(G) Pseudomembranous colitis
(H) Internal hemorrhoids
(I) External hemorrhoids
(J) Tubular adenoma
(K) Villous adenoma
(L) Hyperplastic polyp
(M) Rectal adenocarcinoma
(N) Colonic adenocarcinoma

For each patient description, select the most appropriate diagnosis.

11. A 45-year-old man presents with persistent diarrhea 3 weeks after hospitalization for sepsis. (SELECT 1 DIAGNOSIS)

12. A 32-year-old woman presents with 4 months of chronic diarrhea, which is occasionally bloody. Rigid proctoscopy is normal. (SELECT 1 DIAGNOSIS)

13. A 52-year-old renal transplant patient presents with bloody diarrhea and elevated liver enzymes. Colonoscopy reveals mucosal ulcerations and submucosal hemorrhage. (SELECT 1 DIAGNOSIS)

14. A 45-year-old leukemic patient who is currently undergoing chemotherapy presents with abdominal pain. Abdominal films reveal air in the wall of the cecum. (SELECT 1 DIAGNOSIS)

15. A 16-year-old man presents with right lower quadrant (RLQ) abdominal pain and fever. The appendix is normal at operation. (SELECT 1 DIAGNOSIS)

16. A 67-year-old woman has a small polyp removed by colonoscopy. Pathology reveals thickened mucosa without atypia. (SELECT 1 DIAGNOSIS)

17. A 69-year-old man presents with decreased caliber of stools and blood from the rectum. A firm mass is noted on rectal examination. (SELECT 1 DIAGNOSIS)

18. A 58-year-old man with a history of occult positive stools has a 3-cm polyp removed. Pathology reveals a long, finger-like glandular arrangement. (SELECT 1 DIAGNOSIS)

19. A 43-year-old woman presents with blood from the rectum after bowel movements. Rectal examination reveals a soft, spongy mass just above the dentate line. (SELECT 1 DIAGNOSIS)

20. A 31-year-old woman presents with 6 months of chronic diarrhea. Colonoscopy reveals areas of cobblestoning of the colonic mucosa dispersed between areas of normal mucosa. (SELECT 1 DIAGNOSIS)

Answers and Explanations

1–C. Of the listed gross and microscopic pathologic findings, only crypt abscesses are characteristic of ulcerative colitis. The remaining findings are typically seen in Crohn's disease. Ulcerative colitis involves only the mucosa and submucosa and virtually always involves the rectum and spreads proximally. "Creeping fat" is not unique to Crohn's disease and can be seen in any full thickness inflammatory process involving the bowel.

2–D. Sigmoid volvulus is most common in elderly and institutionalized individuals and usually presents with acute obstruction, abdominal distention, and obstipation. Plain films reveal a U-shaped, dilated loop of bowel in the lower abdomen. Ogilvie's syndrome, or colonic pseudo-obstruction, usually involves the entire large bowel. Small bowel obstruction would appear as "stair stepping" of loops of small bowel on plain film examination. Cecal volvulus appears as a bean-shaped loop of bowel in the left upper quadrant (LUQ) of the abdomen.

3–B. Sigmoidoscopy is usually both diagnostic and therapeutic in cases of sigmoid volvulus. Decompression should be followed by elective sigmoid resection to prevent recurrence of the volvulus. A barium enema study would be helpful in confirming the diagnosis but would not be therapeutic and is not the best choice in treating this patient. Immediate surgery is not indicated because the volvulus may be reduced by colonoscopy, allowing for an adequate bowel preparation and elective sigmoid resection with a primary anastomosis. Should colonoscopic reduction of the volvulus not be possible, emergent surgical resection with formation of a colostomy would be indicated.

4–A. Perianal abscess is the most likely etiology of acute-onset perianal pain with fever. A supralevator abscess would be higher in the rectum and would not likely be palpable on digital rectal examination (DRE). Hemorrhoids are not generally tender unless thrombosed nor do they present with fever. An anal fissure would not likely be associated with fever or a tender mass. Rectal cancer would be unlikely in this patient and generally presents as an ulcerated mass that is usually not painful.

5–B. Incision and drainage without delay is the most appropriate treatment for a perirectal or perianal abscess. Attempts to treat with antibiotics in the absence of drainage are generally unsuccessful. Colonoscopy is generally not indicated unless there is concern of some underlying colonic pathology such as ulcerative colitis or Crohn's disease. Lateral sphincterotomy is the treatment for anal fissures that are refractory to conservative therapy.

6–C. The patient should be admitted, typed and crossmatched for blood, and observed for further bleeding. Bleeding scan and angiography can locate the area in question if the patient is actively bleeding (at least 0.5 mL/min for bleeding scan and 1.0 mL/min for angiography). However, colonoscopy is usually not useful because the large amount of bleeding in the colon usually makes visualization of the colonic mucosa impossible. Colonoscopy would be an appropriate diagnostic step if the bleeding stopped and if the colon could be adequately prepped.

7–D. The most common causes of massive lower gastrointestinal bleeding in adults are diverticular disease and angiodysplasia. Although not a choice in this question, angiodysplasia consists of arteriovenous malformations of the mucosa that are a frequent cause of right-sided colonic bleeding. Angiodysplasia can frequently be treated by colonoscopic coagulation of the lesion. Hemorrhoids and colon cancer rarely cause massive lower gastrointestinal bleeding although colon cancer is a frequent cause of occult gastrointestinal bleeding. Ischemic colitis may cause lower gastrointestinal bleeding but is characteristically associated with severe abdominal pain.

8–C. Appropriate surgical options for ulcerative colitis include total proctocolectomy with an end ileostomy or with an ileoanal anastomosis. Subtotal colectomy with ileorectal anastomosis can also be performed in patients with ulcerative colitis if rectal disease is mild. This provides a better chance for rectal continence and more normal bowel function. However, the rectum should be monitored closely because cancers can still arise in this segment. Surveillance is easily done in the office with a rigid proctoscope. Steroids are used to treat acute exacerbations of the disease and are not used for maintenance therapy. Colonoscopy is generally considered to be the most appropriate diagnostic test for identifying ulcerative colitis. The risk of developing colon cancer is 10% at 20 years.

9–E. If the entire colon and rectum are removed, surgery is essentially curative. Surgery is not indicated at the time of diagnosis if there is no sign of dysplasia on biopsy and symptoms can be controlled with medical therapy. Close follow-up is necessary to detect cancers or areas of dysplasia early. Either of these noted on colonoscopic biopsy is an indication for surgical resection. Although ulcerative colitis does not affect other parts of the bowel primarily, the distal ileum can become inflamed if the proximal colon is involved, a condition termed "backwash ileitis."

10—E. Nodal disease automatically makes this lesion a Dukes stage C in the Astler-Coller modification system. Full thickness invasion places it in the C2 category, worsening the prognosis.

11–G. This patient likely received multiple antibiotics during his recent admission for sepsis. Thus, antibiotic-associated pseudomembranous colitis caused by *Clostridium difficile* is the most likely cause of those listed. It is important to remember that pseudomembranous colitis can follow the administration of any antibiotic and the onset of symptoms can be as many as 6 weeks after discontinuing antibiotic therapy.

12–B. Although both Crohn's and ulcerative colitis can present in this manner, Crohn's would be a more likely diagnosis in the absence of rectal involvement. Further work-up of this patient should include colonoscopic survey of the entire colon to look for pathology and obtain biopsy as needed.

13–E. Cytomegalovirus enterocolitis generally affects immunocompromised patients such as those with acquired immune deficiency syndrome (AIDS) and transplant patients. Cytomegalovirus can also involve other organs, and the elevated liver enzymes in this patient may indicate hepatic involvement. Cytomegalovirus enterocolitis can mimic surgical problems and should be considered in any immunocompromised patient. Treatment is with gancyclovir.

14–F. Neutropenic enterocolitis generally affects patients receiving high-dose chemotherapy. Plain films usually reveal the appearance of obstruction with air in the wall of the bowel (pneumatosis intestinalis). These patients can be managed conservatively unless perforation of the bowel occurs. Such a complication would require emergent laparotomy and resection of the diseased segment.

15–D. *Yersinia enterocolitica* infection can cause mesenteric adenitis, which will produce symptoms identical to acute appendicitis in the absence of a diseased appendix.

16–L. A colonic polyp that exhibits thickened mucosa without atypia on pathologic examination is a benign hyperplastic polyp and requires no further follow up.

17–M. A firm mass in the rectum that is large enough to cause a decreased caliber of stools but is otherwise asymptomatic is likely to be a rectal cancer in a 69-year-old man. Although benign adenomas can become large enough to cause such symptoms, they generally have a rubbery consistency and do not tend to be firm on examination. Treatment would likely consist of abdominoperineal resection with subsequent chemotherapy and radiation therapy depending on the stage of the disease.

18–K. Villous adenomas have a long, finger-like glandular arrangement on pathologic examination. They also tend to be larger than tubular adenomas, with 60% being larger than 2 cm. Villous adenomas have a higher incidence of harboring foci of cancer and should be excised either through a colonoscope or by laparotomy and segmental resection of the involved bowel.

19–H. Internal hemorrhoids are located just above the dentate line, are covered by mucosa, and have a soft, spongy consistency. They can prolapse and bleed but do not generally cause pain or itching. Red blood from the rectum only after bowel movement is a common complaint with internal hemorrhoid disease. Treatment consists of either rubber-band ligation or surgical excision.

20–B. Cobblestoning of the mucosa and "skip lesions" are typical of Crohn's disease and can be seen on colonoscopy. Ulcerative colitis tends to involve the colon in a continuous manner, starting with the rectum and moving proximally.

15

Liver

Traves D. Crabtree

I. Structural and Functional Anatomy

A. Major structures and landmarks (Figure 15-1)

1. **Glisson's capsule**

—is the peritoneal covering that surrounds the liver.

a. **The bare area**

—is an area on the posterior superior surface of the liver that is not covered by Glisson's capsule.

—is where Glisson's capsule reflects onto the parietal peritoneal covering of the inferior surface of the diaphragm.

b. **The coronary ligaments**

—are the actual reflections of peritoneum on the posterior superior surface of the liver.

c. **The triangular ligaments**

—are the lateral extensions of the coronary ligaments on each side of the liver.

2. **The falciform ligament**

—attaches the liver to the anterior abdominal wall.

—extends from the umbilicus to the diaphragm and contains the obliterated **remnant of the umbilical vein.**

a. The pathway of the **ligamentum teres,** known as the umbilical fissure, extends from the falciform ligament on the undersurface of the liver.

b. The ligamentum teres contains the extension of the **obliterated remnant of the umbilical vein.**

3. **The liver is functionally divided into eight segments** based on arterial and portal venous inflow and biliary drainage (**Figure 15-2**).

a. **Segment I**

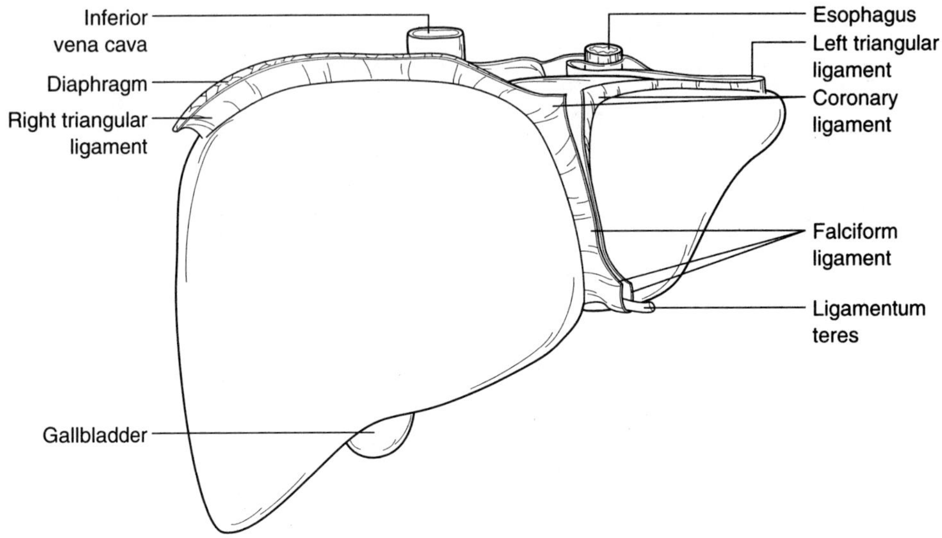

Figure 15-1. Major landmarks of the liver. (From Gray SW, Skandalakis JE: *Atlas of Surgical Anatomy for General Surgeons.* Baltimore, Williams & Wilkins, 1985, p 183.)

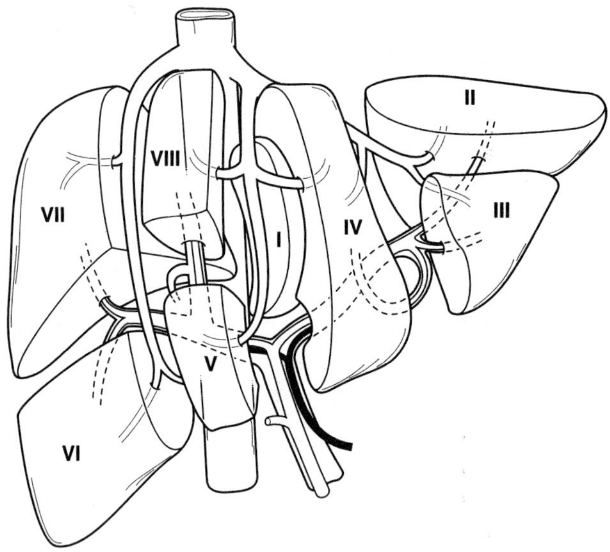

Figure 15-2. Functional segments of the liver. (From O'Leary JP: *The Physiologic Basis of Surgery,* 2nd ed. Baltimore, Williams & Wilkins, 1996, p 442.)

—is the **caudate lobe** of the liver.

b. Segments II to IV

—are segments of the **left lobe** resected during left hepatic lobectomy.

c. Segments V to VIII

—are segments of the **right lobe** resected during right hepatic lobectomy.

(1) The **falciform ligament does not divide the right** and **left lobe.**

(2) **The portal fissure, or Cantlies line,**

—is a plane passing from the left side of the gallbladder fossa to the left side of the inferior vena cava.

—defines the division of the physiologic right and left lobes of the liver.

d. **A right trisegmentectomy**

—includes resection of the right lobe and segment IV (**Figure 15-3**).

e. **A left lateral segmentectomy**

—includes resection of segments II and III to the left of the falciform ligament.

f. **Resection of 80% of parenchyma**

—in a normal liver is compatible with life.

B. Arterial supply and venous system

1. The portal vein

—**is a valveless vein** formed at the junction of the superior mesenteric vein and the splenic vein behind the head of the pancreas.

—passes posteriorly to the bile duct and the hepatic artery in the hepatoduodenal ligament.

—provides 75% of the liver's blood supply.

2. The common hepatic artery

—arises from the celiac artery and becomes the proper hepatic artery after the gastroduodenal artery branches.

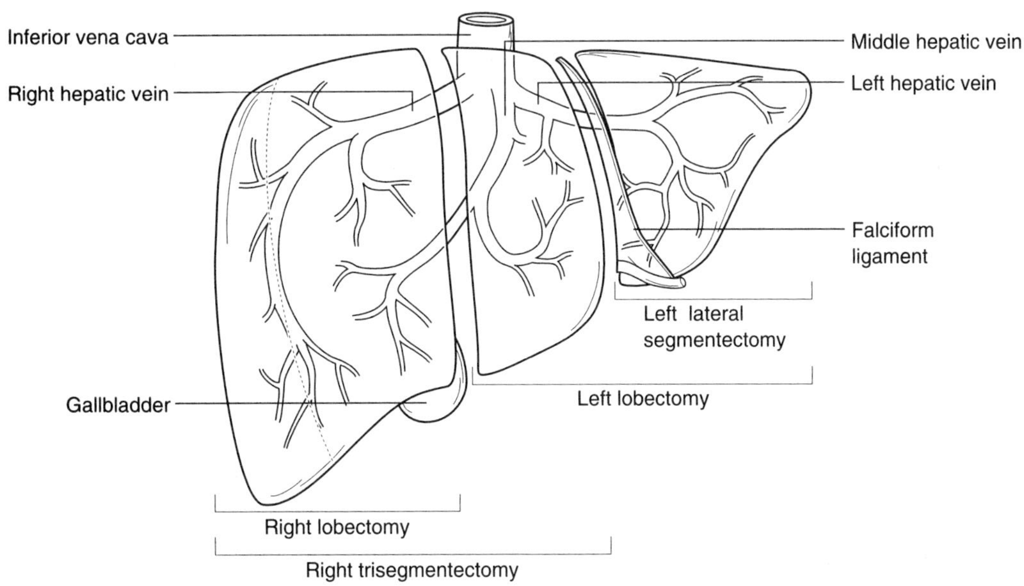

Figure 15-3. Surgical resection of the liver. (From Greenfield L J, et al: *Surgery: Scientific Principles and Practice.* Philadelphia, Lippincott, 1993, p 849.)

—passes medial to the common bile duct and anterior to the portal vein in the hepatoduodenal ligament.

—bifurcates into the right and left hepatic arteries within the hilum of the liver.

3. **Hepatic arterial anatomy** has many common variants:

—The **right hepatic artery** may arise from the superior mesenteric artery.

—The **left hepatic artery** may arise from the left gastric artery.

4. **The "Pringle maneuver"**

—is used occasionally during hepatic surgery.

—involves **compression** of the structures within the **hepatoduodenal ligament.**

—Compression of the **portal vein** and **hepatic artery** within the hepatoduodenal ligament helps to control hemorrhage during hepatic surgery.

5. **Hepatic drainage**

—The **left** and **right hepatic veins** drain directly into the inferior vena cava posteriorly.

—The **middle hepatic vein** characteristically drains into the left hepatic vein.

C. **Histology of the liver**

1. **The hepatic arteriole, portal venule,** and **bile ductule**

—run together to form the three components of the **portal triad (Figure 15-4)**.

2. **A hepatic lobule**

—contains a central hepatic vein with the portal triads along the periphery of the lobule.

—Radially dispersed hepatocytes and sinusoids perfused by the portal venules and hepatic arterioles are located around the central vein, forming the lobule.

3. **Endothelial cells within the sinusoids**

—comprise over 50% of nonhepatocyte cells within the liver.

4. **Kupffer cells**

—are leukocytes attached to the luminal surface of endothelial cells within the liver that **resemble macrophages.**

II. Infections of the Liver (Table 15-1)

A. **Pyogenic liver abscesses**

—account for approximately 80% of all hepatic abscesses.

1. **The major routes of infection** include

—the portal venous system.

—ascending biliary tree infections.

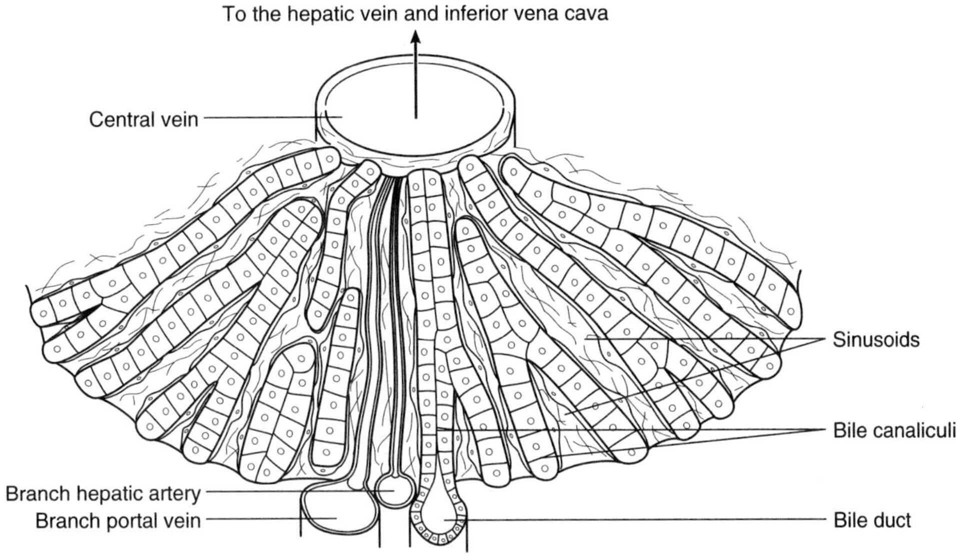

Figure 15-4. Functional hepatic lobule. (Adapted from Simmons RL, Steed DL: *Basic Science Review for Surgeons.* Philadelphia, WB Saunders, 1992, p 247.)

—bacteremia via the hepatic artery.

—direct extension from adjacent infection (i.e., appendicitis, diverticulitis).

—primary infection after hepatic trauma.

2. **Etiology**
   a. Frequently, there is **no obvious identifiable source** of bacterial infection leading to the development of these abscesses.
   b. **Intra-abdominal infections** are the most common **identifiable source** of bacteria for pyogenic liver abscesses.
      (1) **Biliary tract disease** and **colonic infections**
      —are the most common associated intra-abdominal infections.
      (2) **Sources include**
      —cholangitis.
      —cholecystitis.
      —appendicitis.
      —diverticulitis.
      —malignant biliary obstruction.
      —regional enteritis.
      —generalized sepsis.
      —pelvic inflammatory disease.
      —cryptogenic sources.
3. **Abscesses most often contain**
   —enteric gram-negative aerobic rods (i.e., *Klebsiella, Proteus, Escherichia coli*) and/or anaerobes (i.e., *Bacteroides*).
4. **Common signs and symptoms** include

Table 15-1. Hepatic Infections

	Organisms	Primary Source	Signs and Symptoms	Diagnosis	Initial Treatment
Pyogenic abscess	Enteric gram-negative rods with or without anaerobes	Cryptogenic or intra-abdominal infections	Fever, chills, RUQ pains, ↑ WBC, sepsis	CT scan, ultrasound	Radiologic or surgical drainage and antibiotics
Amebic liver abscess	*Entamoeba histolytica*	Recent intestinal infestation	Fever, chills, RUQ pain, ↑ WBC, hepatomegaly	CT scan, ultrasound, serum antibody to *E. histolytica*	Metronidazole (surgical drainage if rupture or secondary bacterial infection)
Hydatid liver cyst	*Echinococcus granulosus, Echinococcus multilocularis*	Fecal/oral contamination from animal carriers	Vague abdominal pain, jaundice, fever, eosinophilia	CT scan, serum ELISA for echinococcal antibody	Surgical drainage and injection of hypertonic saline and resection of cyst wall

CT = computed tomography; ELISA = enzyme-linked immunosorbent assay; RUQ = right upper quadrant; WBC = white blood cell.

—fever.

—chills.

—weight loss.

—right upper quadrant (RUQ) pain.

—leukocytosis.

—elevated liver function tests.

—sepsis.

5. **Treatment**

—should include broad spectrum **antibiotics and** either surgical or radiologically guided **drainage** of the abscess.

B. Amebic liver abscesses

1. **Etiology**

a. The parasite *Entamoeba histolytica*

—**causes** these abscesses.

—is transported via the portal venous system **after an intestinal infestation** with this organism.

—Its immature form—the trophozoite—is usually ingested and transported via the portal system.

b. **Tropical climates and areas of poor sanitation**

—have a higher incidence of amebic liver abscesses.

c. **Intestinal infestation**

—often precedes the abscess by several weeks.

2. **Pathology**

a. The abscess usually contains **necrotic tissue and blood,** giving the classic "**anchovy-paste**" aspirate.

b. Secondary bacterial infection may occur in 10%.

c. Most abscesses occur in the right lobe (75%–90%) and are solitary lesions (80%).

3. **Signs and symptoms** may include

—fever.

—chills.

—nausea.

—RUQ abdominal pain or tenderness.

—hepatomegaly.

—jaundice.

—leukocytosis.

4. **Diagnosis**

—Computed tomography (CT) scan or ultrasound may help with the diagnosis; however, it is difficult to discern pyogenic versus amebic abscesses.

—A serum test for antibody to *E. histolytica* is highly specific.

5. **Treatment** is initially nonsurgical.
   a. Most abscesses resolve upon initiation of the antibiotic of choice, **metronidazole.**
   b. Surgical drainage is indicated if there is suspected **rupture** or **secondary bacterial infection.**

C. **Hydatid liver cysts** (i.e., echinococcal cysts)

—are rare liver cysts.

—are caused by the parasite *Echinococcus granulosus* or, less commonly, *Echinococcus multilocularis.*

—most commonly occur in the **right lobe** of the liver.

1. **Endemic areas** include
   —most of Europe.
   —Australia.
   —New Zealand.
   —South America.
   —Africa.
2. **A major risk factor**
   —is contact with dogs that eat carrier animals (i.e., sheep).
3. **Most patients present with**
   —vague abdominal pain.
   —jaundice, fever, and nausea (more rare).
4 **Diagnosis**
   a. **Serum enzyme-linked immunosorbent assay (ELISA) test** for antibody against *Echinococcus* is accurate > 90% of the time.
   b. **Eosinophilia** is present in **10%–30% of patients.**
   c. Liver function studies may be abnormal in 25% of patients.
   d. A **CT scan**
      —may show the **characteristic calcified wall** of the cyst peripherally.
5. **Treatment**
   —is with **surgical drainage** of the cyst.
   —is followed by **injection of hypertonic saline** to kill the remaining organisms, then **resection of the cyst wall.**
   —Antibiotic therapy with mebendazole or albendazole may be used in conjunction with surgical drainage.
6. **Complications**
   —**Spillage of the cyst contents into the peritoneal cavity** during drainage can rarely result in a life-threatening **anaphylactic reaction.**

III. Benign Tumors of the Liver (Table 15-2)

A. Hemangiomas

—are the **most common benign tumors of the liver.**

Table 15-2. Hepatic Tumors

	Risk Factors	Signs and Symptoms	Diagnosis	Treatment	Pearls
Hemangioma	Female > male	Most asymptomatic; pain, nausea, vomiting, palpable mass	CT scan, ultrasound, **tagged-red blood cell scan,** arteriogram	Surgical excision if symptomatic	Rarely associated with Kasabach-Merritt syndrome
Hepatic adenoma	**Oral contraceptive,** diabetes, type 1 GSD	Most asymptomatic; RUQ pain, palpable mass, **hypotension secondary to rupture**	CT scan, ultrasound	Trial of discontinuation of oral contraceptives, surgical excision	10% may undergo **malignant transformation** to HCC
Focal nodular hyperplasia	Female > male	Often asymptomatic	**Central stellate scar** on CT scan, sulfur colloid radionuclide scan	Surgical excision only if symptomatic	Often confused radiographically with adenomas
Simple liver cysts	Female > male	Often asymptomatic; RUQ pain, palpable mass	CT scan, ultrasound	Surgical excision and oversewing cyst wall if symptomatic	Characteristic **blue hue** on gross examination
Polycystic liver disease	Childhood form—autosomal recessive; adult form—autosomal dominant	RUQ pain, palpable mass	CT scan, ultrasound with multiple cysts in liver (> 10)	Treat like simple cysts if symptomatic	Prognosis related to associated **polycystic kidney disease**
Hemangioendothelioma	**Infants < 2 years**	Palpable mass, CHF secondary to AV shunting, hepatomegaly, hypotension secondary to spontaneous rupture and hemorrhage	CT scan	If symptomatic, medical treatment of CHF, steroids; surgical excision for medical failures	Half may develop **Kasabach-Merritt syndrome;** associated with cutaneous hemangiomas

AV = arteriovenous; CHF = congestive heart failure; CT = computed tomography; GSD = glycogen storage disease; RUQ = right upper quadrant.

—are more common in **women (60%–80%).**

—generally present between the ages of 40 and 60.

1. **Histologically**

   —these tumors are simply dilated endothelial-lined vascular spaces.

2. **Presentation**

   a. **Most hemangiomas are asymptomatic,** although symptoms of pain, nausea, and vomiting may be present, especially with giant hemangiomas (> 4 cm).

   b. **Rupture** of a hemangioma is very rare.

   c. **Kasabach-Merritt syndrome** is a rare sequelae of hemangiomas associated with **thrombocytopenia** secondary to sequestration of platelets within the tumor.

3. **Diagnosis** can often be made

   —by characteristic CT scan findings.

   —with a **tagged-red blood cell scan.**

   —**Needle biopsy** is generally avoided because of the **risk of hemorrhage.**

4. **Treatment**

   —is by **surgical excision.**

   —is generally only indicated when symptoms are present, or when the diagnosis of hemangioma is indeterminate.

B. Hepatic adenoma

—is a **benign liver tumor seen almost exclusively in women 30–50 years old.**

1. **Risk factor**

   a. The greatest risk factor is the use of **oral contraceptives.**

   b. Other risk factors include

      —diabetes.

      —type I glycogen storage disease.

      —use of anabolic steroids.

2. **Lesions are**

   —made of hepatocytes.

   —generally solitary.

   —found in the right lobe of the liver.

3. **Signs and symptoms** may include

   —RUQ pain.

   —a palpable mass.

   —hepatomegaly.

   —As many as one third of patients may present acutely **with abdominal pain and hypotension secondary to rupture of the tumor.**

4. **Complications** include

—**malignant transformation** to hepatocellular carcinoma, which may occur in as many as 10% of adenomas.

—**rupture.**

5. **Diagnosis**

—is often made by CT scan or by ultrasound.

6. **Treatment**

a. **The risk of rupture** and the potential for **malignant transformation** are generally considered indications for **surgical excision** of asymptomatic lesions.

b. Occasionally, adenomas may regress after a trial of discontinuing oral contraceptives or steroids in patients with small, asymptomatic tumors or in the high-risk surgical patient.

C. **Focal nodular hyperplasia (FNH)**

—is **typically found in women 20–50 years old.**

—is **not associated with oral contraceptive use,** unlike hepatocellular adenomas.

1. **Diagnosis**

—FNH is usually **asymptomatic** but is often confused radiographically with adenomas.

—FNH is not associated with malignant transformation or rupture.

—A **central stellate scar** on CT scan is characteristic of FNH.

—A **sulfur colloid radionuclide scan** characteristically identifies the **Kupffer cells** within the FNH nodule.

2. **Treatment**

—Surgical resection is not indicated unless the lesion is symptomatic or if the diagnosis is indeterminate.

D **Benign cystic lesions of the liver**

1. **Simple cysts**

—are generally solitary cysts occurring more frequently in women.

a. The cyst walls have a characteristic blue hue.

—They histologically contain **von Meyenburg complexes,** islands of biliary ductal epithelium.

b. Most are found incidentally by CT scan or ultrasound.

c. **Treatment** is by surgical resection or unroofing of the cyst and oversewing the cyst wall.

d. **Indications for resection** include the presence of

—symptoms.

—rupture.

—hemorrhage.

—infection.

—indeterminate diagnosis.

2. **Polycystic liver disease**

—includes both adult and childhood forms.

a. **Childhood polycystic disease**

—is an **autosomal recessive** disorder with cyst formation in both the liver and kidney.

—High mortality in infancy and early childhood is attributed to progressive renal failure.

b. **Adult polycystic disease**

—is an **autosomal dominant** disorder seen more commonly in **women 30–80 years old.**

(1) Approximately half of the patients with polycystic livers will have polycystic kidneys.

(2) Prognosis is generally related to the level of kidney involvement and subsequent **renal impairment.**

(3) There is a rare association between adult polycystic disease and the development of cerebellar aneurysms.

E. Other rare lesions of the liver

1. **Mesenchymal hamartomas**

—are rare, benign, cystic tumors found in infants and children.

2. **Hemangioendotheliomas**

—are benign vesiculiform tumors seen in **infants younger than 2 years old.**

a. Arteriovenous (A/V) shunting within the tumor may cause congestive heart failure.

b. Medical treatment with steroids is appropriate.

—Surgery is reserved for medical failures.

3. **Intrahepatic bile duct adenomas**

—are generally small, benign lesions that require no treatment.

IV. Malignant Tumors of the Liver (Table 15-3)

A. Hepatocellular carcinoma (HCC)

—is the most common primary malignant tumor of the liver.

—is **4–9 times more common in men,** generally presenting at age 40–70.

1. **Risk factors**

a. The **most common risk factors** are

—**cirrhosis** (macronodular type).

—**hepatitis B infection.**

b. **Other risk factors** include

—**hepatitis C infection.**

—exposure to **carcinogens** [e.g., thorotrast, carbon tetrachloride, aflatoxins (*Aspergillus flavus*)].

—hemochromatosis.

—tyrosinemia.

Table 15-3. Malignant Hepatic Lesions

	Risk Factors	Signs and Symptoms	Diagnosis	Treatment	Pearls
Hepatocellular carcinoma	Males > females, cirrhosis, HBV and HCV	Malaise, anorexia, weight loss, abdominal pain, ascites, palpable mass	CT scan, ultrasound, occasionally MRI or intraoperative ultrasound for improved localization	Partial hepatic resection for resectable tumors	Associated with ↑ AFP
Fibrolamellar hepatocellular carcinoma	More common in adolescents and young adults	Abdominal mass, RUQ pain	CT scan, ultrasound	Partial hepatic resection for resectable tumors	No clear association with cirrhosis; AFP usually not elevated
Liver metastases	Primary lesion elsewhere (colon, breast, lung)	Often related to primary disease	CT scan, clinical history of primary lesions elsewhere, increased CEA	Partial hepatic resection for isolated colorectal metastases; chemotherapy	Resection for other metastatic lesions more controversial
Hepatoblastoma	Seen in children < 2 years, male > female	Palpable mass, nausea, vomiting, precocious puberty or virilization (rare)	CT scan, AFP elevated in > 90%	Partial hepatic resection and chemotherapy for resectable lesions; just chemotherapy for unresectable lesions	Associated with hemihypertrophy and Beckwith-Wiedemann syndrome

AFP = α-fetoprotein; CEA = carcinoembryonic antigen; CT = computed tomography; HBV = hepatitis B virus; HCV = hepatitis C virus; MRI = magnetic resonance imaging; RUQ = right upper quadrant.

—glycogen storage diseases.
—Wilson's disease.
—α_1-1 antitrypsin deficiency.
—porphyria cutanea tarda.
—hepatic adenoma.
—schistosomiasis.
—blood group B.

2. **Symptoms** may include
—fatigue.
—malaise.
—anorexia.
—weight loss.
—abdominal pain.
—shoulder pain.
—ascites.

3. **Diagnosis**

a. **α-Fetoprotein (AFP)**
—is a tumor marker that may be elevated in 40%–70% of patients with HCC.
—may also be elevated with teratocarcinomas, yolk sac tumors, and with hepatic metastases.

b. **Ultrasound, CT scan, and MRI**
—are generally very reliable at identifying tumors as small as 1 cm.

4. **Treatment**

a. **Surgical management of resectable tumors**
—provides 5-year survival of 31%.

(1) Without treatment, mean survival from the onset of symptoms is 1–4 months.

(2) The mean perioperative mortality rate is 11% and is much higher in cirrhotics.

(3) Cirrhosis is a major limiting factor in the surgical resection of liver tumors.

(4) Total hepatectomy with liver transplantation may benefit a select group of patients not amenable to partial hepatic resection although the rate of recurrence may be as high as 50%.

b. **Systemic chemotherapy**
—**has shown little benefit** in the treatment of HCC.
—Transarterial chemoembolization, and percutaneous ethanol injection of tumors may provide some survival benefit in unresectable tumors.

B. **Fibrolamellar hepatocellular carcinoma (FHCC)**

—is a variant of HCC seen most commonly in **adolescents** and **young adults.**

—is not clearly associated with viral hepatitis or cirrhosis.

1. AFP

—**is typically not elevated,** unlike with HCC.

2. Treatment

—is with surgical resection.

3. Overall survival

—is generally better than HCC, potentially because of the greater likelihood of resectability of FHCC tumors at the time of diagnosis.

C. Liver metastases

—are the **most common tumors of the liver.**

—occur much more frequently than any of the primary liver tumors.

1. Tumors that frequently spread to the liver include

—colorectal, lung, and breast cancers.

—melanoma.

—neuroendocrine tumors (i.e., carcinoid).

—other visceral malignancies.

—renal cell carcinoma.

2. Diagnosis

a. Serum carcinoembryonic antigen (CEA)

—is a sensitive **indicator** of metastatic colorectal lesions but lacks specificity (it may be elevated with other disease processes).

—is a reliable indicator for disease recurrence in patients with previously treated colorectal cancer.

b. Imaging techniques

—such as CT scan and, more recently, intraoperative ultrasound, reliably identify colorectal metastases to the liver.

3. Liver resection for metastatic lesions

—other than colorectal cancer have shown little survival benefit.

a. Five-year survival

—after partial hepatic resection for limited hepatic metastases from a colorectal primary is 30%–35%.

—with untreated hepatic metastases is $< 5\%$.

b. Operative mortality

—for partial hepatic resection for metastatic disease is approximately 5%.

c. Factors that determine resectability include

—the size, number, and location of metastatic lesions.

—the extent of the primary tumor.

—Resectable lesions represent a small percentage of liver metastases.

d. Unresectable metastatic lesions

—in other regions of the body (i.e., lung, brain) are contraindications to hepatic resection of liver metastases.

4. **Cystic lesions within the liver**

—**may represent malignant neoplasms** such as ovarian and pancreatic cystadenocarcinomas, as well as cystic degeneration of metastatic solid tumors.

D. **Other malignant lesions of the liver**

1. **Hepatoblastomas**

—are primary malignant tumors of the liver seen primarily **in boys younger than 2 years old** (see *BRS Surgical Specialties,* Chapter 3).

—are associated with hemihypertrophy and Beckwith-Wiedeman syndromes (see Table 15-3).

2. **Cholangiocarcinomas**

—are primary malignant tumors of **biliary ductal epithelium** (see Chapter 6).

—can **present as intrahepatic** or extrahepatic lesions.

V. Portal Hypertension

A. **Portal venous system (Figure 15-5)**

—is valveless, unlike most other veins.

—This allows elevated venous pressure in this system to be transmitted to multiple venous beds via an extensive collateral network of veins.

1. **Normal portal venous pressure**

—is generally less than 12 mm Hg.

2. **Elevated portal pressure** can lead to

—reconstitution and dilation of the umbilical vein leading to the characteristic **caput medusa.**

—varicosities around the umbilicus.

3. **The coronary veins**

—act as collaterals between the portal vein and the systemic venous system of the lower esophagus.

B. **Causes of portal hypertension**

—may be presinusoidal, sinusoidal, or postsinusoidal.

1. **Presinusoidal causes**

—**Schistosomiasis** is the most common cause of portal hypertension worldwide.

—**Portal vein thrombosis** accounts for 50% of portal hypertension in **children.**

2. **Sinusoidal causes** include

—**cirrhosis.**

—congenital hepatic fibrosis (rare).

—**Alcoholic cirrhosis** is the most common cause of portal hypertension in the United States.

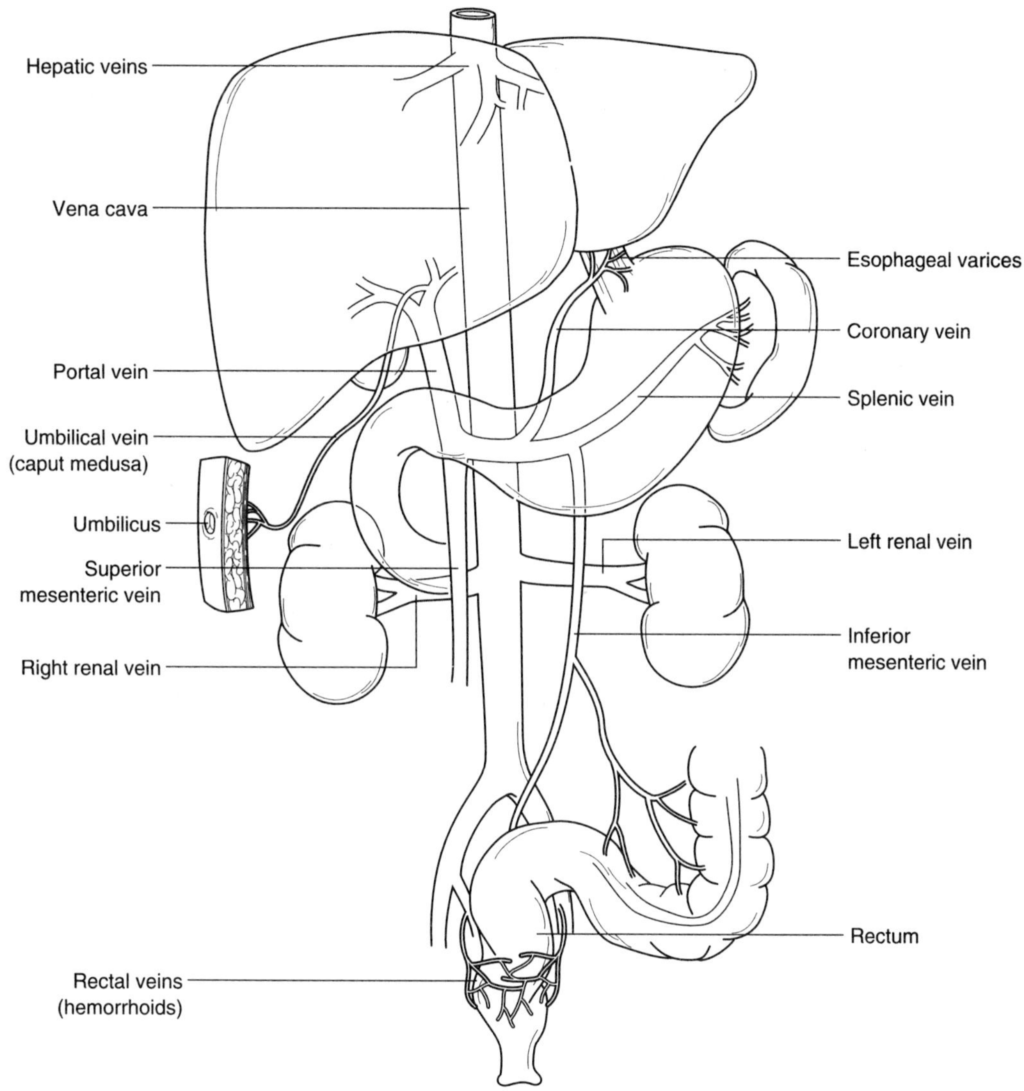

Figure 15-5. Portal venous system. (Adapted from Jarrell BE, Bruce RA, III: *NMS Surgery,* 2nd ed. Baltimore, Williams & Wilkins, 1991, p 216.)

3. **The rare postsinusoidal causes** include
   —**Budd-Chiari syndrome (hepatic vein occlusive disease)**.
   —constrictive pericarditis.
   —chronic heart failure.

C. **The four major consequences of portal hypertension are**
   —ascites.
   —portosystemic venous shunts and varices.
   —congestive splenomegaly.
   —hepatic encephalopathy.

D. Esophageal varices

1. **Approximately 90% of upper gastrointestinal bleeding** in patients with portal hypertension is secondary to bleeding varices.
   —Mortality with acute variceal hemorrhage is approximately 50%.
   —An algorithm for the management of acute variceal hemorrhage is outlined in Figure 15-6.
2. **Endoscopic sclerotherapy**
   —is generally the initial treatment of acute variceal hemorrhage after initial resuscitative measures have been started.
   a. The varices are injected with a **sclerosing agent** that stops the bleeding in over 90% of patients.
   b. **Balloon tamponade** and repeat sclerotherapy may be performed if bleeding recurs or persists.
   c. **Late esophageal stricture** may occur in as many as 25% of patients after sclerotherapy.
      —These strictures are often easily managed with dilation.
3. **Medical treatment of esophageal varices**
   —may also include the use of **vasopressin** and **somatostatin.**
   a. These agents cause **visceral vasoconstriction** but may affect other vascular systems as well.

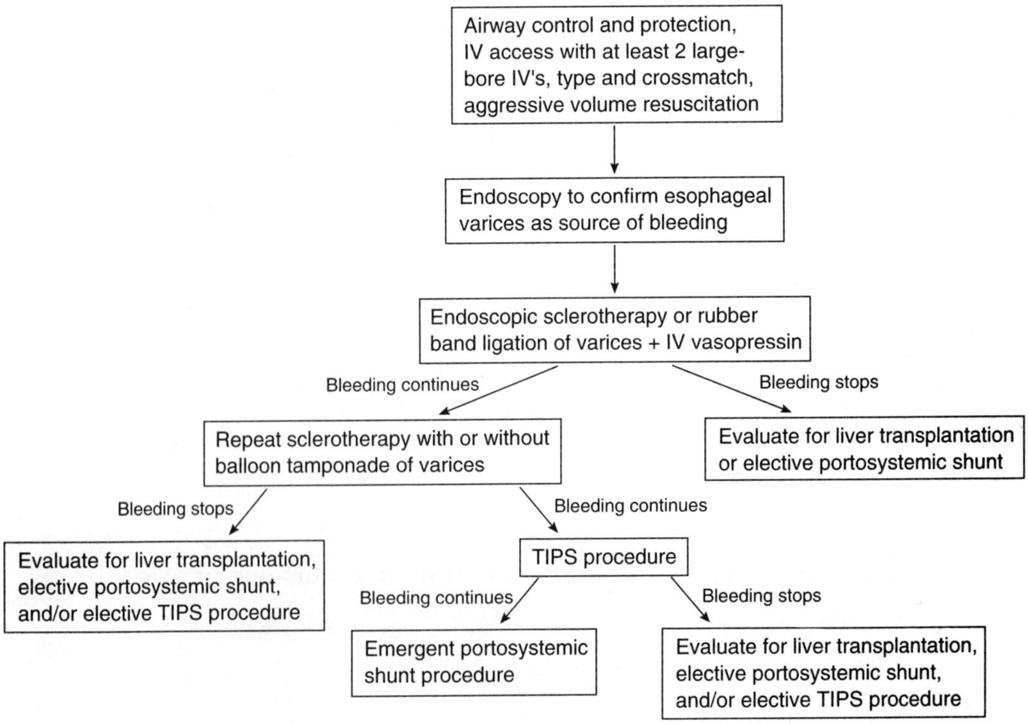

Figure 15-6. Algorithm for the management of acute variceal hemorrhage.

b. Simultaneous **nitroglycerin should be given** when **vasopressin** is administered to patients with coronary artery disease.
   —This will counteract the coronary vasoconstrictive effects of vasopressin.
c. **Propranolol** may decrease portal pressure and prevent recurrent variceal bleeding but has no role in the treatment of acute variceal hemorrhage.
d. **Balloon tamponade** of esophageal varices with a Sengstaken-Blakemore tube may stop acute variceal hemorrhage in 80%–85% of cases.
   —Bleeding recurs in over 50% of patients with balloon deflation.
   —Serious complications such as esophageal rupture may occur in as many as 10% of patients.

4. **Transjugular intrahepatic portocaval shunts (TIPS)**
   —may be inserted percutaneously for refractory variceal bleeding.
   —produces portosystemic shunting of blood using minimally invasive angiographic techniques.
   —often serves as a bridge to hepatic transplantation and as an alternative to surgical shunting procedures.

5. **Surgical portosystemic shunts**
   —are divided into selective and nonselective shunts (**Figure 15-7.**)
   a. **Nonselective shunts**
      —decompress the central portal venous system, thereby decreasing portal pressure.
      —are most effective at decreasing ascites and stopping variceal bleeding.
      —have a **high rate of hepatic encephalopathy** and progressive hepatic failure because portal venous perfusion of the liver is substantially reduced.
      —include end-to-side portocaval shunts, side-to-side portocaval shunts, large mesocaval shunts, and interposition portocaval shunts with an artificial graft.
   b. **Selective shunts**
      —decompress esophageal varices while **preserving some hepatic portal venous flow.**
      —are technically **more difficult to perform;** however, they have a lower risk of producing progressive hepatic failure or hepatic encephalopathy.
      —**The most common selective shunt** is the distal splenorenal shunt, or **Warren shunt.**
      —**Refractory ascites is a contraindication** to the splenorenal shunt because selective shunts tend to precipitate worsening ascites.

6. **Isolated elevation of portal venous pressure**
   —within the gastric portal venous system can be caused by splenic vein thrombosis.
   —can lead to **gastric varices** without altering the rest of the portal venous system.

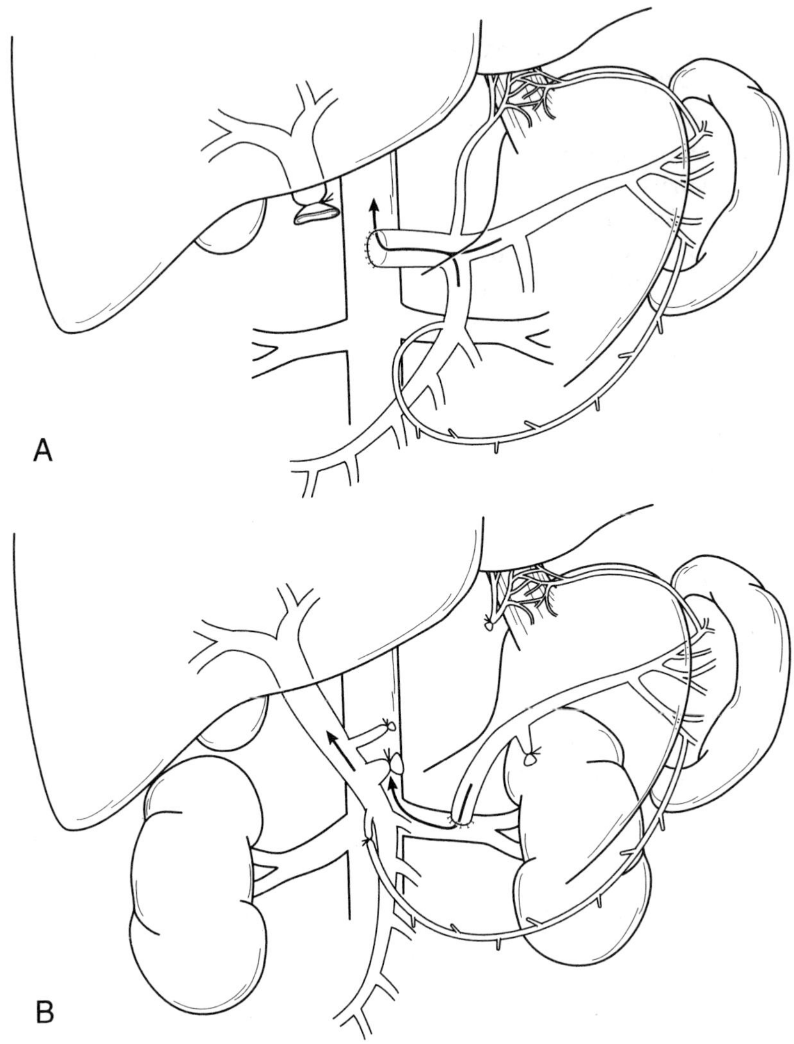

Figure 15-7. Portosystemic shunts. *(A)* Nonselective shunt: end-to-side portal caval shunt. *(B)* Selective shunt: Warren distal splenorenal shunt. (Adapted from Blackbourne LH, Fleischer KJ: *Advanced Surgical Recall.* Baltimore, Williams & Wilkins, 1997, pp 462–463.)

a. **Splenic vein thrombosis**

—is most commonly caused by **pancreatitis.**

—is also noted to occur more frequently in pregnancy.

b. **Recognition is important**

—because adequate **treatment is by splenectomy** alone without the need for portosystemic shunting.

VI. Liver Failure and Ascites

A. The most common cause of liver failure

—is cirrhosis of the liver.

B. Child's Classification

—lists stages of liver failure based on five clinical parameters (**Table 15-4**).

1. **Bilirubin level**
2. **Albumin level**
3. **Severity of ascites**
4. **Severity of encephalopathy**
5. **Nutritional status**

C. Hepatic encephalopathy

—is a **major complication of hepatic failure** and of portosystemic shunts.

—**can lead to neurologic changes,** such as an altered level of consciousness, confusion, intellectual deterioration, and the end-stage characteristic flapping tremor, or asterixis.

1. **The pathogenesis of hepatic encephalopathy is unknown** but is thought to be related to an unidentified cerebral toxin.
2. **Encephalopathy is most often precipitated by**
   —**gastrointestinal bleeding.**
   —dehydration.
   —constipation.
   —sedatives.
   —excessive dietary protein intake.
3. **Treatment is medical with**
   —enteral administration of neomycin and lactulose.
   —protein restriction.
   —treatment of precipitating events.

D. Hepatorenal syndrome

—is renal insufficiency or renal failure associated with hepatic failure.

1. **The etiology**
   —has yet to be identified, although decreased renal perfusion and ischemia are thought to play a major role.
2. **Renal failure**
   —is clinically **difficult to differentiate from prerenal causes of renal failure.**

Table 15-4. Child-Turcot Risk Classification for Liver Failure

	Class A	Class B	Class C
Bilirubin (mg/dL)	<2.0	2.0–3.0	>3.0
Albumin (g/dL)	>3.5	3.0–3.5	<3.0
Ascites	None	Minimal (treatable)	Severe (refractory)
Encephalopathy	None	Minimal	Severe
Nutritional status	Normal	Fair	Poor

3. **Kidney function**

—is restored after liver transplantation in hepatorenal syndrome.

E. **Ascites**

—is a complication of liver failure and portal hypertension.

—can result in a transudate formation within the peritoneal space.

1. **Initial medical management**

—with **diuretics and dietary salt restriction** successfully relieves ascites 95% of the time.

2. **Spironolactone**

—is often a first line diuretic because of the associated hyperaldosterone state often seen with ascites.

3. **Denver and LeVeen shunts**

—are subcutaneous shunts that drain ascitic fluid from the peritoneal cavity to the central venous system.

—Disseminated intravascular coagulation **(DIC)** is a known complication of peritoneovenous shunting of ascitic fluid.

4. **Spontaneous bacterial peritonitis**

—is frequently a fatal complication of persistent ascites.

a. **Risk factors** include

—**nephrotic syndrome.**

—**systemic lupus,** particularly in **children.**

b. Infection is often **monomicrobial.**

—*E. coli* is the most common precipitating agent, followed by *Pneumococcus.*

—Hemolytic streptococci and *Pneumococcus* are the most common organisms in children.

c. **Characteristic findings** include

—fever.

—abdominal pain.

—serum leukocytosis.

d. **Diagnostic findings**

—**Elevated white blood cell count** (> **500/mL**)

—Large numbers of **polymorphonuclear leukocytes within the ascitic fluid** (> 250/mm^3)

—**Blood cultures** and ascitic fluid cultures are often positive, but not always.

e. **Treatment**

—is with broad spectrum antibiotics.

Review Test

Directions: Each of the numbered items or incomplete statements in this section is followed by answers or by completions of the statement. Select the ONE lettered answer or completion that is BEST in each case.

1. A 22-year-old man sustained a gunshot wound to the right upper quadrant (RUQ) and was severely hypotensive on arrival to the emergency room. Intraoperatively, the patient was noted as having a large liver parenchymal injury with severe hemorrhage. A Pringle maneuver was performed to control the hemorrhage for better visualization of the injured parenchyma. After confirmation of appropriate placement of the vascular clamp for the Pringle maneuver, there is persistent bleeding of bright red blood from the liver parenchyma just medial to the falciform ligament. Which of the following structures would mostly likely cause the persistent hemorrhage from the liver parenchyma?

(A) Portal vein
(B) Common hepatic artery from celiac axis
(C) Left hepatic artery arising from left gastric artery
(D) Blood supply to the common bile duct
(E) Blood vessels within the hepatoduodenal ligament

Questions 2–4

A 62-year-old man with a well-known history of alcohol abuse presents to the emergency room with persistent hematemesis and hypotension. Endoscopic examination confirms the presence of diffusely bleeding esophageal and gastric varices.

2. Which of the following are characteristic of the portal venous system and portal hypertension?

(A) Normal portal pressure is generally greater than 12 mm Hg
(B) Esophageal varices arise from dilated branches of coronary veins
(C) The portal vein runs anterior to the common bile duct in the hepatoduodenal ligament
(D) Caput medusa is formed by periumbilical branches of the recanalized ductus arteriosum
(E) Portal pressure > 18 mm Hg may lead to valvular incompetence and subsequent varices

3. Which of the following treatment strategies would be inappropriate in the management of this patient?

(A) Endoscopic sclerotherapy or band ligation
(B) Emergent portosystemic shunt procedure for refractory bleeding
(C) Emergent splenectomy for the gastric varices
(D) Liver transplantation
(E) Placement of a Sengstaken-Blakemore tube

4. Selective portosystemic shunts have which one of the following characteristics?

(A) Ineffective at lowering venous pressure within esophageal varices
(B) Contraindicated for refractory esophageal varices
(C) May cause worsening of ascites
(D) Higher risk of encephalopathy compared with nonselective portosystemic shunts
(E) Large side-to-side portocaval shunt

5. A 45-year-old woman presented to the emergency room with right upper quadrant (RUQ) abdominal pain and fever. The patient states that she had a cholecystectomy 2 years earlier. Computed tomography (CT) scan reveals a 6-cm, fluid-filled mass in the right lobe of the liver that was not noted to be present by ultrasound 2 years ago. Which of the following is the appropriate definitive treatment for the potential cause of this patient's condition?

(A) "Triple" antibiotics alone for a large pyogenic liver abscess
(B) Antibiotics alone for uncomplicated amebic liver abscess
(C) Percutaneous drainage of fluid from echinococcal cyst
(D) Antibiotics alone for a ruptured amebic liver abscess
(E) "Triple" antibiotics alone for a ruptured pyogenic liver abscess

6. A 63-year-old man underwent elective cholecystectomy for chronic biliary colic. Intraoperatively, a 2-cm, irregular mass was identified in the right lobe of the liver. Biopsy revealed a primary hepatocellular carcinoma. Thorough evaluation revealed no evidence of metastatic disease. The patient subsequently underwent resection of this lesion. All of these are potential risk factors for development of hepatocellular carcinoma EXCEPT

(A) Hemochromatosis
(B) Wilson's disease
(C) Hepatic adenoma
(D) Focal nodular hyperplasia
(E) Alcoholic cirrhosis

7. Which of the following would be included in a true functional right hepatic lobectomy?

(A) Hepatic segment IV
(B) All hepatic segments to the right of Cantlies line and segment IV
(C) All hepatic segments to the right of Cantlies line and the entire quadrate lobe
(D) All segments to the right of the falciform ligament
(E) Hepatic segments V–VIII

Questions 8–9

A 57-year-old man with a history of alcohol-induced cirrhosis and chronic hepatic insufficiency presents to the emergency room with complaints of increasing shortness of breath and abdominal bloating worsening over the past 2 weeks. On physical examination, his abdomen is firm but nontender, with notable shifting dullness. In addition, breath sounds are decreased in both lung bases with bibasilar crackles noted. There is no evidence of infiltrate on chest radiograph. His white blood cell count is 9,000 with a normal differential. His prothrombin time is 18, blood urea nitrogen 68, creatinine is 3.5, and albumin is 1.4. Blood and urine cultures are negative.

8. Which of the following is an appropriate statement regarding the management of ascites and its associated complications?

(A) Spontaneous bacterial peritonitis requires prompt surgical drainage
(B) Diuretics should not be used in the initial management of ascites
(C) Peritoneovenous shunts have been shown to improve overall survival in patients with ascites
(D) Disseminated intravascular coagulation is a complication of peritoneovenous shunting
(E) Transjugular intrahepatic portosystemic shunts (TIPS) have no role in the management of refractory ascites

9. The renal failure in this patient has which of the following characteristic findings?

(A) Renal arteriolar vasodilatation
(B) Urine osmolality < 1.010
(C) Many urinary casts on urinalysis
(D) Low urine sodium
(E) Renal function typically does not recover after liver transplantation

Directions: Each set of matching questions in this section consists of a list of four to twenty-six lettered options followed by several numbered items. For each numbered item, select the appropriate lettered option(s). Each lettered option may be selected once, more than once, or not at all.

Questions 10–22

(A) Simple cysts
(B) Cystadenocarcinoma
(C) Hepatic adenoma
(D) Hepatocellular carcinoma
(E) Hemangioendothelioma
(F) Focal nodular hyperplasia
(G) Pyogenic liver abscess
(H) Cavernous hemangioma
(I) Echinococcal cyst
(J) Polycystic disease
(K) Fibrolamellar hepatocellular carcinoma
(L) Hepatoblastoma
(M) Amebic liver abscess

10. A 48-year-old woman with a history of primary ovarian carcinoma 2 months after total abdominal hysterectomy and bilateral salpingo-oophorectomy (TAH BSO) and staging laparotomy presents with a new 2-cm mass in the right lobe of the liver. (SELECT 1 DIAGNOSIS)

11. A 42-year-old woman is found to have a 2-cm, solid mass in the left lobe of the liver during an ultrasound evaluation for biliary colic. Before elective cholecystectomy, a positive red blood cell scan confirms that the lesion is benign. (SELECT 1 DIAGNOSIS)

12. A 34-year-old man presents to the emergency room with a 3-day history of fever and worsening right upper quadrant (RUQ) abdominal pain. Ultrasound reveals a 4-cm, fluid-filled mass in the right lobe of the liver. Attempted percutaneous drainage resulted in a scant amount of thick fluid. Routine bacterial cultures of the aspirated fluid and of the blood were negative. The patient has complete resolution of symptoms with metronidazole therapy. (SELECT 1 DIAGNOSIS)

13. During an elective cholecystectomy, a 43-year-old woman is noted as having a 1-cm, superficial, blue, smooth cystic mass in the right lobe of the liver. (SELECT 1 DIAGNOSIS)

14. During a routine complete blood count, a 43-year-old woman is found to have a platelet count of 53,000. During a thorough evaluation of the thrombocytopenia, an abdominal computed tomography (CT) scan reveals a 5-cm, benign-appearing mass in the right lobe of the liver. Additional laboratory tests are all unremarkable. (SELECT 1 DIAGNOSIS)

15. An 18-month-old healthy boy is noted as having a small palpable mass in the right upper quadrant (RUQ) of the abdomen. Ultrasound reveals a 1-cm, solid, benign-appearing lesion in the periphery of the right lobe of the liver. (SELECT 1 DIAGNOSIS)

16. A 38-year-old woman has been in a motor vehicle accident. During a trauma evaluation, she is found to have a 3-cm, asymptomatic, solid mass in the left lobe of the liver by abdominal computed tomography (CT). The lesion is determined to be benign. However, an elective resection of the lesion is planned given the risk of malignant transformation. (SELECT 1 DIAGNOSIS)

17. A 52-year-old woman has a 2-cm, solid mass within the right lobe of the liver. A computed tomography (CT) scan reveals a lesion with a central stellate scar. (SELECT 1 DIAGNOSIS)

18. During attempted laparoscopic drainage of a benign, 4-cm cystic lesion in the right lobe of the liver, a 38-year-old patient developed rapid onset of hypotension with associated difficulty in ventilation. There was no obvious hemorrhagic source, and emergent chest radiograph was normal. (SELECT 1 DIAGNOSIS)

19. A 63-year-old man with a history of hepatitis B-induced cirrhosis presents with a 20-lb weight loss over the past 3 months. Abdominal computed tomography (CT) scan reveals a 4-cm, irregular, solid mass in the right lobe of the liver. Additional thorough evaluation of the patient is negative. (SELECT 1 DIAGNOSIS)

20. A 34-year-old, thin woman has a large, palpable, irregular liver edge on physical examination. In addition, the left kidney is easily palpable and irregular on physical examination. All liver function tests are within normal limits. Blood urea nitrogen is 45 and creatinine is 3.2. (SELECT 1 DIAGNOSIS)

21. A 33-year-old woman is brought to the emergency room by her husband after she had been complaining of abdominal pain and then suddenly collapsed. Her blood pressure on arrival is 70/40 mm Hg and her abdomen is noted to be tense. Intraoperatively, the patient is found to have a large hemoperitoneum. (SELECT 1 DIAGNOSIS)

22. A 63-year-old man presents to the emergency room with fever and right upper quadrant (RUQ) pain. He is currently being treated as an outpatient for a bout of diverticulitis. Ultrasound reveals a 4-cm, fluid-filled mass in the right lobe of the liver. (SELECT 1 DIAGNOSIS)

Answers and Explanations

1–C. The "Pringle maneuver" is a technique occasionally used in hepatic surgery to control persistent hemorrhage within the liver. It involves compression of the structures within the hepatoduodenal ligament, including the common hepatic artery, the common bile duct, and the portal vein. Typically, the portal vein is posterior to both the common bile duct and the hepatic artery. The hepatic artery is usually medial to the common bile duct. Although there are many anomalies within the hepatic vascular system, one of the most common is the left hepatic artery arising from the left gastric artery. This anomalous artery may not be occluded upon performing the Pringle maneuver and thus may result in persistent parenchymal hemorrhage despite this maneuver. In addition, persistent hemorrhage may also result from back-bleeding arising from injuries to the hepatic veins or to the inferior vena cava, which are not occluded with the Pringle maneuver.

2–E. The portal venous system is a valveless system capable of transmitting elevated portal pressures throughout many collateral venous systems. Portal pressure is generally below 12 mm Hg, although wide variations may exist with and without the development of varices. The coronary veins are a collateral venous system draining blood from the esophagus and cardiac region of the stomach which, when dilated, can produce the characteristic esophageal varices. Increased portal pressure may also lead to dilated periumbilical veins and the characteristic caput medusa.

3–C. Initial management of the patient with actively bleeding varices involves evaluation and control of the airway and initiation of aggressive volume resuscitation. Endoscopy with sclerotherapy with or without band ligation of esophageal varices is an appropriate next step in the management of actively bleeding esophageal varices. In certain situations where endoscopy is not readily available, placing a Sengstaken-Blakemore tube to tamponade the bleeding varices is an acceptable alternative or it may be used as an adjunct to endoscopy. Emergent surgical formation of a portosystemic shunt (i.e., portocaval, mesocaval) to relieve portal pressure is performed less frequently now because of endoscopic therapies but is an appropriate alternative in the treatment of refractory bleeding from esophageal varices. Treatment of isolated gastric varices generally requires splenectomy to allow for selective decompression of the varices. However, performing a splenectomy in this patient with diffuse portal hypertension may worsen the hemorrhage from the esophageal varices and is not indicated. Definitive treatment of esophageal varices is liver transplantation.

4–C. Selective and nonselective portosystemic shunts are both excellent at reducing portal venous pressure and may be used for treatment of esophageal varices. Other less invasive techniques that effectively control bleeding esophageal varices have decreased the need for surgical shunt procedures for the management of bleeding esophageal varices. Nonselective shunts are associated with a higher risk of hepatic encephalopathy when compared with selective shunts because almost all portal venous blood is shunted directly into the systemic venous system with nonselective shunts. Selective shunts are known to cause worsening ascites in patients and these shunts are typically contraindicated in patients with significant ascites. A side-to-side portocaval shunt is a type of nonselective shunt.

5–B. Treatment of most liver abscesses requires adequate drainage, with medical therapy generally serving an adjunctive role. Complicated or large pyogenic liver abscesses such as this one almost always require drainage either percutaneously or surgically. Echinococcal cysts require surgical drainage of cyst fluid followed by instillation of hypertonic saline to kill the remaining organisms. Medical treatment alone is inadequate and drainage, without instillation of hypertonic saline, will not adequately treat the infection. Uncomplicated amebic liver abscesses are an exception in that they may be adequately treated with antibiotic therapy (i.e., metronidazole) alone, although complicated abscesses (i.e., rupture) still generally require surgical management.

6–D. The most common risk factors for the development of hepatocellular carcinoma are cirrhosis secondary to hepatitis B or C infection and alcohol-induced cirrhosis. Other potential risk factors include various disease processes that affect the liver such as hemochromatosis, Wilson's disease, and glycogen storage diseases. There is approximately a 10% risk of malignant transformation of hepatic adenomas to hepatocellular carcinoma. An association between the development of hepatocellular carcinoma and blood-group B has also been demonstrated. Focal nodular hyperplasia is a benign liver lesion that has not been shown to undergo malignant degeneration or transformation.

7–E. A true functional right hepatic lobectomy would include all hepatic segments of the right lobe including segments V–VIII. A right hepatic trisegmentectomy would include hepatic segments IV–VIII. The quadrate lobe includes segments of both the true right and left hepatic lobes, while segment I is the caudate lobe and is not included in a right lobectomy. Cantlies line is an imaginary line to the right of the falciform ligament that divides the true functional right and left hepatic lobes.

8–D. Most cases of ascites can be managed adequately with diuretic therapy. Other techniques for managing refractory ascites include periodic percutaneous drainage, transjugular intrahepatic portosystemic shunts (TIPS), and the surgical placement of peritoneovenous shunts. Peritoneovenous shunts such as the Denver or LeVeen shunts have not been shown to improve survival in patients with liver failure and severe ascites. These shunts are associated with an increased risk of disseminated intravascular coagulation. Spontaneous bacterial peritonitis can often be treated nonsurgically with antibiotic therapy.

9–D. Renal insufficiency secondary to hepatorenal syndrome clinically resembles prerenal causes of renal failure. Characteristics include renal arteriolar vasoconstriction, high urine osmolality, and low urine sodium. Urinary casts typical of acute tubular necrosis are rarely seen in hepatorenal syndrome. Renal function often recovers upon liver transplantation.

10–B. Although cystic hepatic lesions are frequently infectious in nature or otherwise benign, they can include malignant metastatic tumors such as ovarian and pancreatic cystadenocarcinomas. In addition, other solid metastatic tumors may undergo central necrosis and appear as cystic lesions.

11–H. Cavernous hemangiomas are benign tumors of the liver, and are the most common primary lesions of the liver. Hemangiomas may be adequately differentiated from other lesions by computed tomography (CT) examination, although the diagnoses are frequently confirmed by characteristic findings on a red blood cell radionuclide scan.

12–M. An amebic liver abscess caused by *Entamoeba histolytica* can frequently present with fever and right upper quadrant (RUQ) abdominal pain. A fluid-filled mass may be seen on ultrasound or by computed tomography (CT) scan. The fluid within the cyst is often very thick and tenacious and is described as having an "anchovy-paste" consistency. Although most infectious lesions of the liver require drainage, débridement, or both, amebic liver abscesses frequently resolve with metronidazole therapy alone.

13–A. Simple liver cysts are a common incidental finding identified radiographically or at the time of intra-abdominal surgery. These lesions are generally solitary and, upon direct visualization, have a characteristic blue hue. Asymptomatic lesions do not require resection.

14–H. Kasabach-Merritt syndrome is a rare syndrome characterized by sequestration of platelets, potentially leading to a thrombocytopenic coagulopathy. This syndrome is occasionally associated with large cavernous hemangiomas because of platelet sequestration within these lesions. This syndrome may also occur in children with hemangioendotheliomas, although these benign tumors are rare in adults.

15–E. Hemangioendotheliomas are benign vesiculiform tumors seen almost exclusively in children younger than 2 years old. These tumors can easily be differentiated from other tumors, such as hepatoblastomas, with routine radiographic techniques.

16–C. Hepatic adenomas are benign tumors typically presenting as an asymptomatic lesion identified radiographically as an incidental finding. These tumors are almost exclusively found in women of child-bearing age and are associated with oral contraceptive use. Malignant transformation to hepatocellular carcinoma may occur in a small percentage of hepatic adenomas. In addition, there is a risk of spontaneous rupture of these lesions with significant hemorrhage resulting. These factors provide support for the elective resection of medium-sized or large asymptomatic hepatic adenomas.

17–F. Radiographic evidence of a central stellate scar is a characteristic finding of focal nodular hyperplasia. Unfortunately, this finding is not always present and this lesion is often difficult to differentiate from a hepatic adenoma. Unlike a hepatic adenoma, these lesions are not associated with malignant transformation or rupture. Therefore asymptomatic lesions do not require resection. These lesions are composed of hyperplastic Kupffer cells that are easily identified by a sulfur colloid scan.

18–I. Upon drainage of an echinococcal cyst, great emphasis is placed upon avoiding peritoneal spillage of the cyst contents because of the risk of spread of the infection as well as the rare occurrence of anaphylaxis.

19–D. Hepatocellular carcinoma is the most common primary malignant tumor of the liver. Cirrhosis of the liver is the greatest risk factor for development of this tumor. However, metastatic tumors, overall, remain the most common lesions found in the liver.

20–J. Adult polycystic disease is characterized by multiple cystic lesions in both the liver and kidney. It is inherited as an autosomal dominant trait and may present with an enlarged palpable liver or kidneys. Hepatic function (i.e., liver function tests, albumin level, prothrombin time, partial thromboplastin time) is typically unaffected despite extensive cystic involvement of the liver. Morbidity is characteristically associated with renal dysfunction secondary to cystic involvement of the kidneys.

21–C. Spontaneous rupture of a hepatic adenoma with hypotension and a hemoperitoneum is a characteristic complication of these benign tumors. These tumors are associated with oral contraceptive use. There is also an increased risk of rupture of hepatic adenomas with oral contraceptive use. Although other diagnoses may present with hypotension and a hemoperitoneum (i.e., ruptured ectopic pregnancy), a hepatic adenoma should always be considered as a potential source in women of child-bearing age.

22–G. Pyogenic abscesses account for approximately 80% of all infectious lesions of the liver. Pyogenic liver abscesses can often present without an obvious source of infection elsewhere, although intra-abdominal infections such as appendicitis, diverticulitis, and biliary tree infections often serve as a primary source of bacteria.

16

The Biliary Tract

Daniel P. Raymond

I. General

A. Anatomy (Figure 16-1)

1. **The gallbladder is divided** into the **fundus, body, infundibulum,** and **neck.**
   - a. **The neck of the gallbladder**
     —tapers into the **cystic duct,** which joins with the **common hepatic duct** to form the **common bile duct** (CBD).
   - b. **The cystic duct**
     —contains the **spiral valves of Heister,** which have little functional significance.
   - c. **The main blood supply**
     —to the gallbladder is the **cystic artery.**
     - (1) **The cystic artery**
       —arises from the **right hepatic artery** 95% of the time.
       —is usually found within the **triangle of Calot** bounded laterally by the **cystic duct,** medially by the **common hepatic duct,** and superiorly by the **liver.**
     - (2) **Cystic veins**
       —drain directly into the liver and the right portal vein branch.
   - d. **Innervation**
     - (1) The hepatic branch of the left (anterior) vagal trunk provides **parasympathetic innervation.**
     - (2) **Sympathetic fibers,** including sensory fibers that mediate biliary pain, originate from T7–T10 coursing through splanchnic and celiac ganglions.
2. **The biliary ducts**
   - a. **The right and left hepatic ducts** form the **common hepatic duct.**

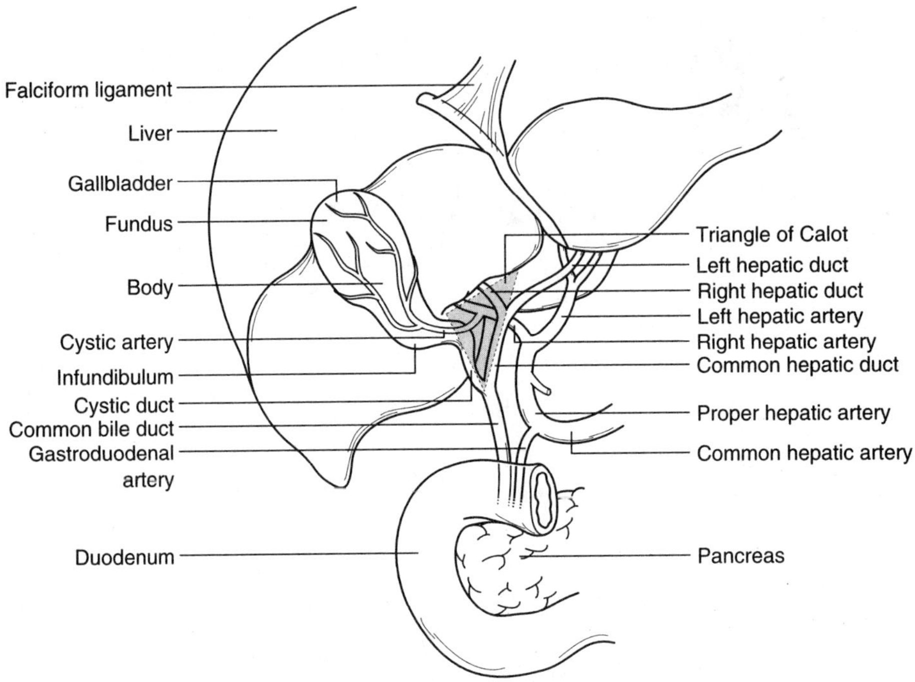

Figure 16-1. Anatomy and arterial supply of the gallbladder. (Adapted with permission from Lippincott Williams & Wilkins. Gray SW, Skandalakis JE: *Atlas of Surgical Anatomy for General Surgeons.* Baltimore, Williams & Wilkins, 1985, p 199.)

—Approximately 25% of the time anterior and posterior portions of the right hepatic duct join the common hepatic duct at different points.

b. **The CBD**

—**begins** in the **hepatoduodenal ligament** as part of the portal triad, and passes posterior to the first portion of the duodenum.

—joins the pancreatic duct to form a common channel leading to the intraduodenal portion called the **ampulla of Vater** in 70% of individuals.

c. **The sphincter of Oddi**

—is a circumferential band of smooth muscle around the ampulla of the CBD and the main pancreatic duct.

d. **The main arterial blood supply**

—comes from branches of the **gastroduodenal** and **right hepatic arteries.** These branches run along the medial and lateral aspects of the bile duct.

3. **Biliary anatomy**

—is highly variable.

a. **The right hepatic artery**

—may arise from the superior mesenteric artery.

b. **An anomalous left hepatic artery**

—may originate from the celiac axis and travel in the medial gastrohepatic ligament.

c. **Accessory hepatic ducts**

—may also be present.

B. Histology

1. **There is no muscularis mucosa or submucosa**

—in the gallbladder wall.

2. **The epithelium**

—is predominately **columnar** with absorptive functions.

—**Rokitansky-Aschoff sinuses** are invaginations of the epithelium seen in the wall of normal gallbladders but are more abundant when inflammation is present.

3. **Ducts of Luschka**

—are microscopic bile ducts that drain directly from the liver into the gallbladder.

—are found in approximately 1% of the population.

C. Radiologic evaluation of the biliary tree

1. **Ultrasound**

a. Ultrasound is the examination of choice for initial evaluation of suspected cholelithiasis or cholecystitis.

b. Drawbacks include operator dependency and limited examination of the CBD.

2. **Radionuclide scan [hepatobiliary iminodiacetic acid (HIDA) scan]**

a. **Intravenous (IV) administered radionuclide is**

—extracted from the bloodstream by the liver.

—excreted into the bile.

—concentrated by the gallbladder.

b. **Opacification of the biliary tree**

—**but not the gallbladder** suggests cystic duct obstruction, and therefore cholecystitis.

c. This scan is also useful for detecting

—a bile leak from a biliary tract injury.

3. **Endoscopic retrograde cholangiopancreatography (ERCP)**

a. **Using upper endoscopy**

—the ampulla of Vater is cannulated.

—contrast is injected to visualize the pancreatic and biliary tree.

b. **ERCP is useful for diagnosing**

—common bile duct stones.

—periampullary disease.

c. **Therapeutic measures may be performed simultaneously,** including

—partial division of the sphincter of Oddi (**sphincterotomy).**

—**stone removal.**

d. Risks include

—bleeding.

—infection.

—perforation.

—**pancreatitis** (5%–10%).

4. Percutaneous transhepatic cholangiography (PTC or THC)

a. A fine needle is passed percutaneously

—through the liver parenchyma with contrast injected into the biliary system.

b. Risks associated with this procedure include

—bleeding.

—infection.

—sepsis.

5. Plain abdominal film

a. Only **10%–15%** of gallstones are radiopaque.

b. Plain films may also demonstrate air in the biliary system associated with a cholecysto-enteric fistula.

6. Oral cholecystography

a. Orally administered contrast

—is secreted in the bile and concentrated in the gallbladder in the absence of biliary tree obstruction.

b. Oral cholecystography is used infrequently because

—the examination takes approximately 10 hours to complete.

—the absorption of contrast is inconsistent.

7. Computed tomography (CT) scan

a. CT scan is useful for

—examining the hepatic parenchyma.

—identifying mass lesions.

—detecting pathologic lymph nodes.

b. CT scans are not used in the routine work-up of gallstones or cholecystitis.

8. Magnetic resonance cholangiopancreatography (MRCP)

—is an emerging technology that may eventually replace invasive cholangiopancreatography.

—Currently, excessive cost is the major limiting factor in the use of MRCP.

II. Physiology

A. Bile is composed predominately of

—bile salts.

—phospholipids (the majority of which is lecithin).

—cholesterol.

1. **Bile salts**
   a. **The liver produces two primary bile salts: cholate** and **chenodeoxycholate.**
   b. **These salts are conjugated**
      —with glycine and taurine to improve water solubility.
2. **After excretion**
   —colonic bacteria can alter these salts to form the **secondary bile salts: deoxycholate** and **lithocholate.**
3. **The primary function of bile is to**
   —transport lipids in micelles and vesicles.
   —aid in digestion and absorption.
4. **Cholesterol solubility in bile is determined**
   —by the relative concentration of the three main components of bile: **cholesterol, bile salts,** and **lecithin.**
   —Alterations in the relative concentration of these components can result in cholesterol crystal formation.

B. Enterohepatic circulation (Figure 16-2)

1. **Ninety-five percent of bile salts are**
   —reabsorbed in the ileum.
   —extracted from portal venous blood by hepatocytes.
2. **Approximately 5% of bile salts**
   —enter the colon where colonic bacteria can convert them to secondary bile salts.

C. Gallbladder function

1. **During fasting**
   —the gallbladder stores and concentrates bile.
2. **During a meal**
   —sphincter of Oddi relaxation and gallbladder contraction are coordinated by neurohumoral mechanisms.
   a. **Cholecystokinin** (CCK)
      —produced by duodenal mucosa in response to a meal is the major stimulus for these functions.
   b. **Vagal stimuli**
      —facilitate the coordinated response to CCK.
      —The **pylorocholecystic reflex** consists of gallbladder contraction and sphincter relaxation in response to antral distension.

D. Bilirubin

1. **Breakdown of red blood cells**
   —leads to production of heme, which is subsequently converted to **biliverdin.**
   a. **Biliverdin** is then reduced to **unconjugated bilirubin.**

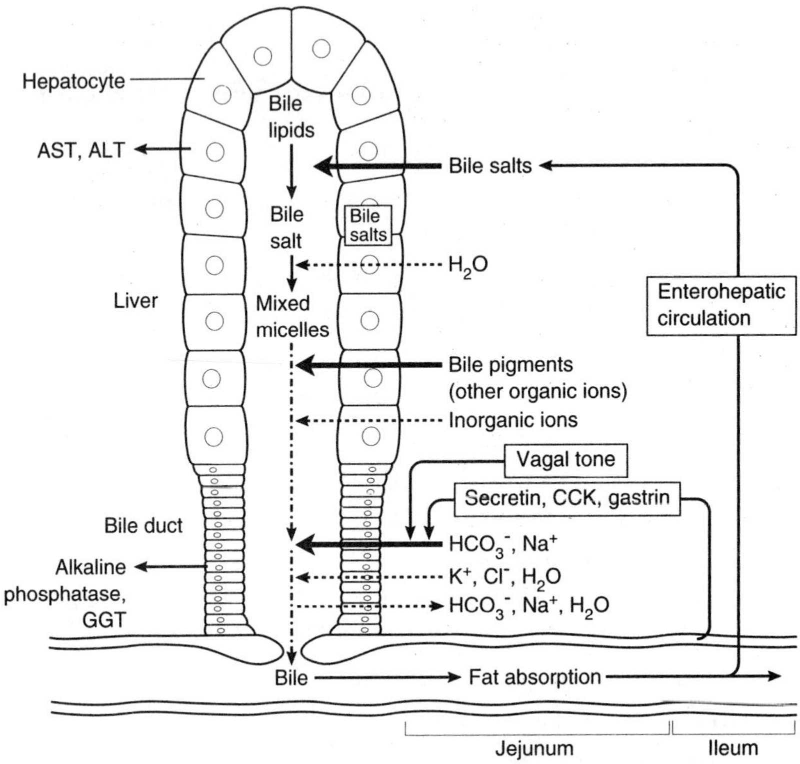

Figure 16-2. The enterohepatic circulation. *AST* = aspartate aminotransferase; *ALT* = alanine aminotransferase; *CCK* = cholecystokinin; *GGT* = gamma-glutamyl transaminase. (Adapted with permission from Way LW: *Current Surgical Diagnosis and Treatment,* 10th ed. Stamford, CT, Appleton & Lange, 1994, p 540.)

b. **Water insoluble unconjugated bilirubin** is bound to albumin in the blood.

2. **Unconjugated bilirubin**

—is converted to **conjugated bilirubin** by hepatocytes in a reaction catalyzed by glucuronyl transferase.

3. **Water soluble conjugated bilirubin**

—is actively secreted into the bile.

4. **Jaundiced patients**

—usually have a total bilirubin ≥ 2.5 mg/dL.

a. Examination of the **sclera of the eye** may demonstrate jaundice in patients with a dark complexion.

b. An algorithm for the work-up of a jaundiced patient is outlined in **Figure 16-3.**

III. Calculous Biliary Disease (Table 16-1)

A. Cholelithiasis

—Approximately 10% of the population have cholelithiasis.

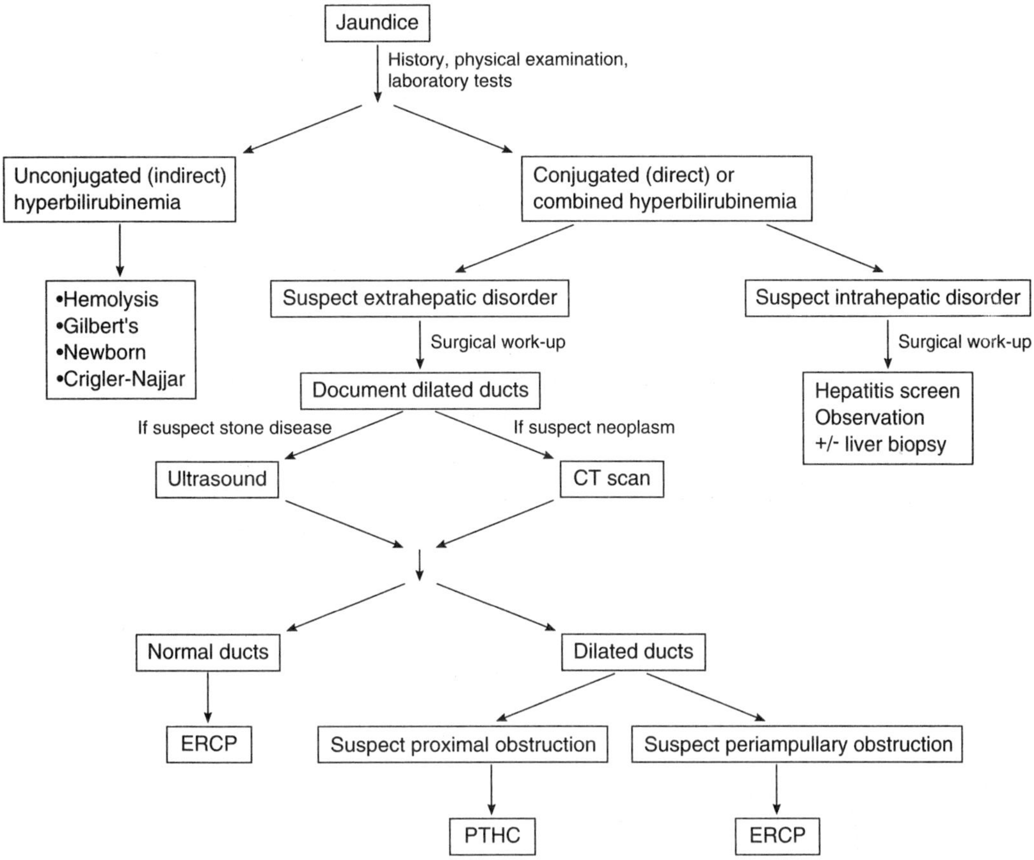

Figure 16-3. Evaluation of the jaundiced patient. *CT* = computed tomography; *ERCP* = endoscopic retrograde cholangiopancreatography; *PTC* = percutaneous transhepatic cholangiography. (Adapted with permission from O'Leary JP: *The Physiologic Basis of Surgery.* Baltimore, Williams & Wilkins, 1996, p 476.)

—The majority of the **gallstones** are asymptomatic.

—Only **30%** of individuals with cholelithiasis eventually have surgery.

B. Cholesterol stones

—account for 75% of all gallstones in the United States.

—form almost exclusively in the gallbladder.

1. Cholesterol supersaturation

—results from alterations in bile components leading to precipitation of cholesterol crystals and subsequent stone formation.

2. Bile stasis

—also contributes to stone formation.

3. **Risk factors for cholesterol stone formation** include

—being female (women are affected 2–4 times more often than men before menopause).

—multiple pregnancies/oral contraceptive use.

Table 16-1. Characteristics of the Various Types of Biliary Calculous Disease

Stone Type	Pathogenesis	Risk Factors	Composition	Presentation
Cholesterol (most common)	Altered bile components, excess cholesterol, bile stasis	Female, obesity, rapid weight loss, prolonged TPN, BCPs	Cholesterol crystals	Biliary colic, cholelithiasis, cholecystitis, secondary ductal stones
Black pigment stone	Altered bilirubin solubilization, bile stasis	Hemolytic disorders, prolonged TPN, cirrhosis, partial ileal resection	Calcium bilirubinate, bile acids, bilirubin polymers	Biliary colic, cholelithiasis, cholecystitis, secondary ductal stones
Brown pigment stone	Bacterial deconjugation of bilirubin, bile stasis	Biliary tract infections	Calcium bilirubinate, bile acids, bilirubin polymers, bacteria	Choledocholithiasis, cholangitis, primary ductal stones
Biliary sludge	Bile stasis	Situations which predispose to bile stasis such as prolonged TPN	Cholesterol crystals, calcium bilirubinate, mucin gel matrix	Biliary colic, incidental ultrasound finding

TPN = total parenteral nutrition; BCPs = birth control pills.

—increasing **age.**

—**obesity.**

—**rapid weight loss.**

—**prolonged total parenteral nutrition (TPN).**

C. Pigment stones

1. Twenty-five percent of gallstones

—in the United States are predominantly pigment stones.

2. Altered solubilization of bilirubin

—results in the precipitation of calcium bilirubinate and other insoluble salts.

3. Black pigment stones are found

—in patients with **hemolytic disorders** and **cirrhosis.**

—almost exclusively in the gallbladder.

a. Other risk factors include

—**chronic TPN** therapy.

—**partial ileal resection.**

b. Important factors in pathogenesis include

—increased bilirubin load.

—impaired hepatic function.

—bile stasis.

4. Brown pigment stones

a. **In Asian populations**
—these are the most common types of stones.

b. **Infection** and bacterial deconjugation
—of bilirubin result in altered solubility.
—are most commonly found in the bile ducts (**primary common duct stones**).

D. **Asymptomatic gallstones**

1. **Approximately 50% of gallstones**
—are truly asymptomatic.
—generally **do not require surgical treatment.**

2. **Relative indications for treatment of asymptomatic gallstones** include
—**large stones** (> 2–3 cm) secondary to increased risk of cholecystitis.
—**calcified (porcelain) gallbladder** due to increased risk of malignancy.
—age over 70 years.
—diabetes.
—immunosuppression.

3. **Care must be taken to recognize**
—atypical complaints suggestive of gallstone disease such as dyspepsia, vague epigastric discomfort, or increased flatulence.

E. **Biliary sludge**
—**is viscous bile** composed of calcium bilirubinate, cholesterol crystals, and mucin gel matrix.
—is generally observed during ultrasound evaluation.
—is most likely a **precursor to gallstone formation.**
—may be associated with **prolonged TPN** use and **fasting.**

IV. Symptomatic Gallstone Disease (Table 16-2)

A. **Biliary colic** is pain caused by
—impaction of a gallstone in the cystic duct.
—transient ductal obstruction.
—possibly, stone passage.

1. **Characteristics of pain**
   a. **Postprandial right upper quadrant (RUQ) pain** often **precipitated by fatty meals** is characteristic, although midepigastric and right lower quadrant (RLQ) pain can occur.
   b. The **onset of pain is** usually rapid, followed by a plateau of discomfort that lasts minutes to hours.
   c. Pain often radiates to the back, inferior to the right scapula.

Table 16-2. Clinical Characteristics of Biliary Tract Disease

Disease	Pathogenesis	Characteristic findings	Treatment
Biliary colic	Transient ductal obstruction, stone passage	Transient postprandial RUQ pain, nausea, vomiting	Elective cholecystectomy
Acute cholecystitis	Cystic duct obstruction with subsequent inflammation	RUQ pain, fever, nausea, vomiting, (+) Murphy's sign, leukocytosis	Urgent cholecystectomy
Choledocholithiasis	Transient or persistent obstruction of biliary duct by a stone	RUQ pain, jaundice, acholic stools, bilirubinuria, elevated alkaline phosphatase, elevated bilirubin. Signs and symptoms tend to fluctuate.	Cholecystectomy plus ERCP with stone removal and sphincterotomy **or** Common bile duct exploration with stone removal
Cholangitis	Bile duct obstruction and infection of bile	Fever, RUQ pain, jaundice, acholic stools, bilirubinuria, signs of sepsis (e.g., mental status changes, hypotension), leukocytosis, elevated alkaline phosphatase, elevated bilirubin, elevated liver transaminases, positive blood cultures	Antibiotics plus ERCP with stone removal and sphincterotomy **or** PTC with stone removal and stenting **or** Biliary bypass (e.g. choledochojejunostomy) plus subsequent cholecystectomy

RUQ = right upper quadrant; ERCP = endoscopic retrograde cholangiopancreatography; PTC = percutaneous transhepatic cholangiography; (+) = positive.

2. **Nausea and vomiting** may also be present.
3. **The clinical manifestations often overlap** with cholecystitis, and the clinical distinction may be difficult.

B. Acute cholecystitis

—occurs in approximately 10% of patients with symptomatic gallstones.

1. **Obstruction of the cystic duct by a gallstone**

   —causes gallbladder distension and subsequent inflammation.

2. **Presentation**

   a. **Seventy-five percent of patients**

   —have had previous attacks of **biliary colic.**

   b. **The pain is**

   —similar to biliary colic.

   —often associated with a meal, but is **unremitting.**

   —associated with increasing abdominal tenderness.

   c. **Patients often complain of**

   —nausea.

   —vomiting.

—anorexia.

d. **Physical findings** include
—RUQ tenderness.
—guarding.
—a palpable gallbladder (30%).
—a positive **Murphy's sign** (inspiratory arrest during deep palpation in the RUQ).

e. **Mild fever and leukocytosis**
—may be present.

f. **Alkaline phosphatase and bilirubin**
—may also be mildly elevated although such findings may also suggest the presence of CBD obstruction.

3. **Radiologic evaluation**

a. **An RUQ ultrasound (Figure 16-4) may demonstrate suggestive findings,** including
—**gallstones.**
—**gallbladder wall thickening.**
—sludge.
—**pericholecystic fluid.**
—CBD dilation suggestive of CBD obstruction.

b. **Murphy's sign**
—induced by the ultrasound probe with maximal tenderness over the gallbladder is suggestive of cholecystitis.

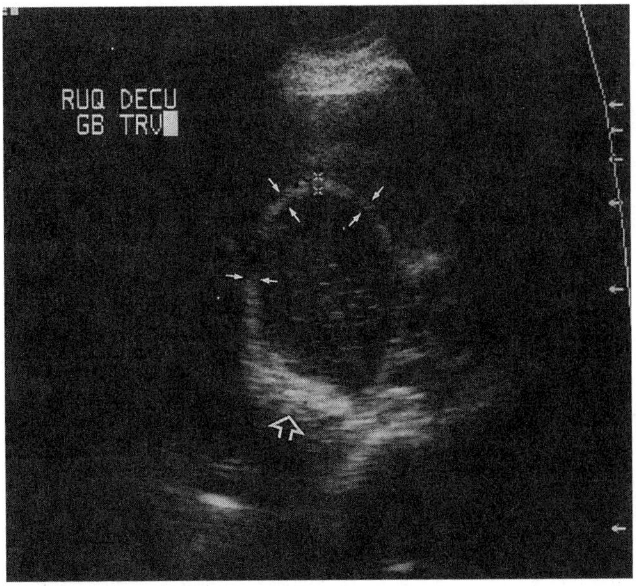

Figure 16-4. Note thickening of the gallbladder wall (small arrows) and multiple small stones (large arrow) in this ultrasound. (Reprinted with permission from Daffner RH: *Clinical Radiology: The Essentials,* 2nd ed. Baltimore, Williams & Wilkins, 1999, p 329.)

c. **Ultrasound is often**

—the only test needed in the work-up of this disease.

d. **A radionuclide scan**

—may be useful when ultrasound findings are equivocal.

—Normal visualization of the biliary tree without visualization of the gallbladder is diagnostic of cystic duct obstruction and acute cholecystitis.

4. Treatment

a. **Laparoscopic cholecystectomy**

—is the procedure of choice for managing uncomplicated acute cholecystitis.

(1) Contraindications include **hemodynamic instability.**

(2) Extensive previous abdominal surgery is a relative contraindication because of adhesions.

b. **Open cholecystectomy**

—through an RUQ incision is the preferred alternative when the laparoscopic approach cannot be performed.

—is associated with a longer hospital stay and a longer convalescence.

c. **Percutaneous transhepatic placement of a cholecystostomy tube**

—using CT or ultrasound guidance may be performed in patients who cannot tolerate surgery.

—When patients are able to tolerate surgery, a cholecystectomy should subsequently be performed.

d. **Fluid resuscitation and perioperative antibiotics**

—are other important components of therapy.

—Organisms may include *Escherichia coli, Klebsiella, Enterococcus,* and *Enterobacter* species.

5. **Complications of acute cholecystitis**

a. **Suppurative cholecystitis**

—with frank purulence in the gallbladder may be associated with sepsis and shock and requires emergent cholecystectomy.

b. **Perforation**

—occurs in 3%–10% of cases.

—can result in peritonitis, abscess formation, or fistula formation.

c. **Gallstone ileus**

—is actually a bowel obstruction, often at the level of the ileum, caused by a gallstone that has passed through a cholecystenteric fistula.

—Obstructive symptoms with **air in the biliary tree** may be suggestive.

d. **Emphysematous cholecystitis (gas in the gallbladder wall)**

—may be produced by certain bacteria such as *Clostridium perfringens.*

—is seen more frequently in **diabetic patients.**

—Sepsis can develop rapidly and **emergent cholecystectomy is required.**

e. **Choledocholithiasis**

—is found in 15% of patients with acute cholecystitis.

C. Acalculous cholecystitis

1. Twenty percent of cases of **acute cholecystitis** occur **in the absence of stones.**
2. **Causative factors** may include
   —bile stasis and altered bile composition.
3. **Acalculous cholecystitis is most commonly associated**
   —with trauma and burn injuries.
   —with prolonged TPN use.
   —in **critically ill patients.**
4. **Complications** include
   —**rapid progression** to **gangrenous cholecystitis.** Surgical treatment with cholecystectomy is required.

V. Choledocholithiasis

A. Primary common duct stones

—are stones that form primarily in the bile ducts.

—are almost exclusively **brown pigment stones** related to stasis and infection.

B. Secondary common duct stones

—are stones that form in the gallbladder and pass into the CBD.

1. Fifteen percent of patients with stones in the gallbladder also have common duct stones.
2. One to 2% of postcholecystectomy patients need further intervention secondary to common duct stones.

C. Presentation

1. **Affected patients**
   —may be asymptomatic.
   —However, jaundice, biliary colic, and suppurative cholangitis may be present.
2. **Incomplete obstruction**
   —**produces the classic picture of** choledocholithiasis with **fluctuating** symptoms of **biliary colic, jaundice,** and **pruritus.**
3. **Complete obstruction**
   —produces a rapidly developing biliary colic.
   —can progress to **cholangitis.**
4. **Other symptoms** include
   —clay-colored stools (acholic stools).
   —dark urine (bilirubinuria).

—possibly, symptoms associated with pancreatitis.

5. **Physical findings** include

   —RUQ tenderness.

   —jaundice.

   —fever.

   —hepatomegaly.

6. **Elevated serum alkaline phosphatase** may be present.

7. **Elevated serum bilirubin** with predominant elevation in direct bilirubin may be present.

   —Transaminases are often normal in uncomplicated choledocholithiasis.

D. Radiologic evaluation

1. **Ultrasound**

   —finding of gallstones with biliary duct dilatation can be diagnostic.

   —The normal CBD is ~8 mm.

2. **Subsequent cholangiography**

   —can characterize biliary anatomy and obstruction.

   —**ERCP** is usually preferred over **PTC** because of its potential therapeutic benefit (e.g., stone removal, sphincterotomy).

E. The goals of treatment include

—stone removal.

—prevention of recurrent disease.

1. **Primary common duct stones**
   - a. **ERCP with stone removal**

     —and sphincterotomy is appropriate treatment.
   - b. **Surgical exploration**

     —of the bile duct with stone removal and sphincterotomy or choledochojejunostomy may be necessary if ERCP is unsuccessful.

2. **Secondary common duct stones**
   - a. **Laparoscopic cholecystectomy**

     —is performed to prevent further disease.
   - b. **Stone removal can be achieved by**

     —**intraoperative choledochoscopy** (fiberoptic camera-guided exploration).

     —formal **common bile duct exploration.**

     —**postoperative ERCP,** if necessary.

F. Complications

1. **Acute pancreatitis**

   —Biliary stones account for approximately 45% of all cases of pancreatitis.

2. **Hepatic abscess** and biliary cirrhosis can be associated with chronic obstruction.

3. **Biliary strictures**

4. **Hemobilia and gallstone ileus** are rare complications.

VI. Cholangitis

—is an **acute bacterial infection** of the biliary tract.
—is associated with **bacterial contamination of bile and biliary obstruction.**

A. **The most common cause** of biliary obstruction

—associated with cholangitis is **choledocholithiasis.**

B. **Other potential causes of obstruction** associated with cholangitis include

—biliary strictures (e.g., iatrogenic).

—neoplasms (rare).

—chronic pancreatitis.

—congenital cysts.

—duodenal diverticula.

C. **Bile is normally sterile, but common organisms in cholangitis** include

—E. coli.

—Klebsiella.

—Enterococcus.

—Pseudomonas.

—Enterobacter.

D. **Presentation**

1. **Classically, patients present with**

—fever.

—RUQ pain.

—jaundice.

—These three signs make up **Charcot's triad.**

2. **Charcot's triad**

—plus hypotension and mental status changes (**Reynolds pentad**) suggests **suppurative cholangitis** (see Chapter 9).

3. **Other symptoms** that may occur include

—bilirubinuria.

—pale acholic stools.

—tender hepatomegaly.

4. **Laboratory findings** include

—leukocytosis.

—elevations in **alkaline phosphatase, transaminases,** and **bilirubin,** with predominant elevation of the direct fraction.

—**Blood cultures** may be positive in 40%–50% of patients.

E. Radiologic evaluation

1. Ultrasound

—will often characterize the obstruction, although cholangiogram may also be useful in some situations.

2. CT scan

—may be helpful, especially when a neoplasm or pancreatitis is suspected.

F. Treatment

1. Initial treatment requires

—**fluid resuscitation.**

—appropriate **antibiotic** administration.

2. Subsequent definitive treatment requires

—**urgent relief of the biliary obstruction.**

a. ERCP with sphincterotomy or PTC

—may be used for stone removal or stent placement across an obstruction and/or biliary tree decompression.

b. Choledochojejunostomy

—may be indicated in cases of neoplasm or stricture.

c. Emergent biliary decompression

—is required in 10% of patients due to sepsis.

G. Complications include

—**sepsis.**

—**stricture formation.**

—**hepatic abscess** formation.

VII. Benign Biliary Strictures

—are most commonly caused by **iatrogenic injuries** and **primary sclerosing cholangitis (PSC).**

A. Iatrogenic injuries

1. Causes of injury include

—laparoscopic cholecystectomy (80%).

—excessive retraction.

—devascularization.

—fibrosis secondary to adjacent inflammatory processes (e.g., abscess).

2. Early presentation of such injuries

—is often secondary to adjacent processes (e.g., bile leak, abscess).

—may occur **days to weeks after surgery.**

—Laboratory evaluation often reveals elevated serum bilirubin and alkaline phosphatase.

3. **Late presentation (years after surgery)**

—is due to stricture formation with signs of biliary obstruction including **recurrent cholangitis, jaundice,** and cirrhosis.

4. **Radiologic evaluation**

a. **PTC** is generally more useful than **ERCP** because it more accurately delineates the biliary tree proximal to the site of obstruction.

b. **Radionuclide studies** (e.g., HIDA scan) can also diagnose a bile leak.

5. **Treatment**

a. **The initial step**

—often involves placement of a catheter into the proximal biliary tree using **PTC** to allow for **decompression proximal to the stricture.**

b. **Appropriate drainage**

—of bile collections or abscesses is also necessary.

c. **If obstruction does not resolve**

—with these treatment measures, surgical treatment may be needed (i.e., **choledochojejunostomy or hepaticojejunostomy**).

d. **Balloon dilation and stenting**

—are being used with increasing frequency in the management of such strictures.

B. Primary sclerosing cholangitis (PSC)

—is an **idiopathic disease** characterized by **inflammatory strictures** of the intrahepatic and extrahepatic bile ducts.

1. **Ulcerative colitis**

—is present in approximately 60% of patients with PSC.

2. **Other less commonly associated conditions** include

—retroperitoneal fibrosis.

—Riedel's thyroiditis.

—pancreatitis.

—diabetes mellitus.

3. **Presentation**

a. **Insidious onset of jaundice and pruritus** often occurs in the fourth to fifth decade.

b. **RUQ pain,** weight loss, fever, and fatigue may also occur with exacerbation of disease with gradual progression to liver failure.

c. **Acute cholangitis is rare** unless biliary tract manipulation has occurred.

4. **ERCP** is often diagnostic

—demonstrating the characteristic **beaded appearance** of multiple intrahepatic and extrahepatic strictures.

5. **Treatment**

a. Percutaneous or endoscopic **balloon dilation**

—of dominant strictures may be useful for **symptomatic relief** of obstruction.

b. **Ursodeoxycholic acid and cholestyramine**

—may relieve symptoms, including pruritus.

c. **An aggressive surgical approach**

—is often advocated because of the insidious **progression to secondary biliary cirrhosis** and eventual liver failure.

(1) **Liver transplantation** is indicated for severe intrahepatic involvement or advanced disease.

(2) **Biliary bypass** (e.g., choledochojejunostomy or hepaticojejunostomy) may be used for isolated extrahepatic bile duct involvement.

6. **Potential complications** include

—cirrhosis.

—gallstone formation.

—**cholangiocarcinoma,** most frequently associated with **ulcerative colitis.**

C. **Other causes of biliary stricture formation** include

—chronic pancreatitis.

—postoperative stricturing of a biliary-enteric anastomosis.

VIII. Malignant Neoplasms of the Biliary Tract

A. Gallbladder cancer

1. **Epidemiology**

a. **Primary gallbladder cancer is rare,** although it is the most common malignant lesion of the biliary tract.

b. The **mean age** at diagnosis is 65

—with a **3:1 female to male ratio.**

c. **Seventy to 90% of cases** are associated with gallstones.

—However, only 0.4% of patients with gallstones develop gallbladder cancer.

d. **Calcification of the gallbladder wall (porcelain gallbladder)**

—is associated with a 25%–60% risk of carcinoma.

—is an indication for cholecystectomy.

2. **Pathology**

a. **Eighty to 90% of gallbladder cancers**

—are well-differentiated **adenocarcinomas.**

b. **The most common site of metastases**

—and **direct tumor spread is the liver.**

c. **Lymphatic spread occurs sequentially**

—to the cystic duct nodes, periportal nodes, and finally to the celiac and superior mesenteric nodes.

3. **Presentation**

a. **The diagnosis**

—**is most commonly made incidentally** at the time of cholecystectomy or laparotomy (90%).

b. **Ninety percent of patients**

—present with **metastatic disease.**

c. **Laboratory findings**

—are related to the extent and location of the tumor.

4. **CT and magnetic resonance imaging (MRI)**

—are useful for characterizing the extent of disease.

5. **Tumor staging**

—is outlined in **Table 16-3.**

6. **Treatment**

a. **Stage I**

—**Cholecystectomy** alone is potentially curative.

b. **Stages II–IV**

—**Radical cholecystectomy** is indicated. This includes cholecystectomy, wedge resection of the liver with 2–3 cm margins around the gallbladder bed, and regional lymphadenectomy.

c. **Stage V**

—Palliative procedures to relieve obstruction such as biliary-enteric bypass procedures are performed.

d. **If the cancer is discovered after laparoscopy,**

—the **trocar sites must be excised** because of a high likelihood of tumor implantation at these sites.

7. **Overall 5-year survival**

—is **< 5%** due to the preponderance of late presentation.

—Average survival currently is **6 months after diagnosis.**

B. **Cholangiocarcinoma**

—is defined as cancer of the bile ducts.

1. **Epidemiology**

a. **Cholangiocarcinoma most commonly occurs**

—between **50–70 years.**

Table 16-3. Staging and Treatment of Gallbladder Adenocarcinoma

Stage	Description	Surgical Treatment
Stage I	Mucosal involvement only	Cholecystectomy
Stage II	Involvement of muscularis layer of the gallbladder	Radical cholecystectomy-cholecystectomy + wedge resection of the liver around the bed of the gallbladder + regional lymphadenectomy
Stage III	All layers of wall involved	
Stage IV	Cystic node involvement	
Stage V	Distant spread including adjacent organs and periportal nodes	Palliative procedures (e.g., choledochojejunostomy)

—with a higher incidence in **males** and people of **southeast Asian origin.**

b. **Other risk factors** include
   —**sclerosing cholangitis.**
   —ulcerative colitis.
   —choledochal cysts.
   —chronic liver infections.
   —congenital hepatic fibrosis.

2. **Pathology**

a. **Tumors may be classified**
   —based on location by dividing the biliary tract into thirds (Figure 16-5).
   —Tumors of the upper third are called **Klatskin tumors.**

b. **Cholangiocarcinomas**
   —are primarily adenocarcinomas.
   —tend to spread by direct extension, frequently involving the portal vein and hepatic artery.

3. **Presentation**

a. **The classic clinical presentation**
   —is **painless jaundice.**
   —Jaundice occurs in 90% of patients and is often associated with pruritus.

b. **Bilirubinuria and acholic stools**
   —may also be present.

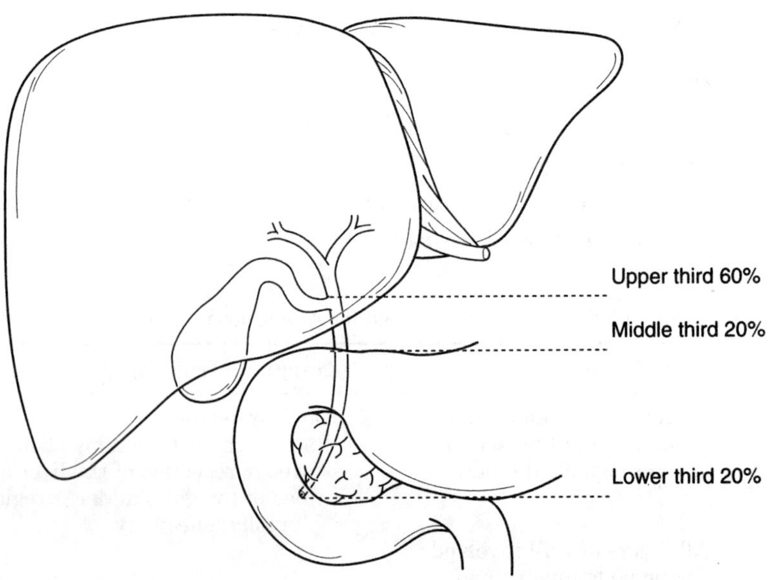

Figure 16-5. Distribution of cholangiocarcinomas. (Adapted with permission from Greenfield LJ, Mulholland MW, Oldham KT, et al: *Surgery: Scientific Principles and Practices,* 2nd ed. Philadelphia, Lippincott-Raven, 1997, p 1061.)

—**Anorexia and weight loss** are markers of advanced disease.

c. **Signs** include
—icterus.
—hepatomegaly.
—possibly, a **palpable gallbladder (Courvoisier's sign).**
—possibly stigmata of cirrhosis (with advanced disease).

d. **Symptoms and signs**
—**do not tend to fluctuate,** as with choledocholithiasis.

e. **Characteristic laboratory findings** include
—persistent elevations of bilirubin and alkaline phosphatase.

4. **Radiologic evaluation**

a. **Cholangiography**
—with PTC or ERCP is the gold standard for diagnosis.

b. **A CT scan**
—may further define a mass lesion and be used in staging.

c. **The discovery of a focal bile duct stenosis**
—in a patient without a history of biliary duct surgery is highly suggestive of a malignant process.

5. **The staging of cholangiocarcinoma**
—is outlined in Table 16-4.

6. **Treatment**

a. **Tumors in the lower third of the bile duct**
—may require radical pancreatoduodenectomy (**Whipple's operation**).

b. **Tumors in the middle third**
—may require **wide resection** and construction of a biliary-enteric anastomosis (e.g., hepaticojejunostomy).

c. **Upper third lesions** (Klatskin tumors)
—are often unresectable.
—If possible, a **wide resection** of the mass **including adjacent liver** parenchyma with subsequent hepaticojejunostomy may be performed.

d. **For unresectable disease**
—palliative stenting is performed either percutaneously, endoscopically, or surgically.

7. **Prognosis**

Table 16-4. Staging of Cholangiocarcinoma

Stage I	Tumor invading but not through the bile duct wall
Stage II	Tumor invading through the wall and involving perimuscular connective tissue
Stage III	Stage II plus local lymph node involvement
Stage IV	Tumor invading adjacent organs including liver, pancreas, duodenum, or vascular structures
Stage V	Distant metastatic spread

a. **The average patient survives**
—less than 1 year after the diagnosis.

b. **Overall 5-year survival**
—is approximately 30%–40% after radical surgery for resectable lesions.

c. **Klatskin tumors have the worst prognosis**
—with an 80%–90% 5-year mortality rate owing to predominant unresectable nature at presentation.

IX. Miscellaneous Biliary Pathologies

A. Congenital abnormalities

1. **Biliary atresia** (see *BRS Surgical Specialties,* Chapter 3)

—is the **most common cause of persistent jaundice in the newborn.**

a. Approximately 90% of people have **complete obliteration** of the biliary tree.

b. Therapeutic interventions include
—**hepatic portoenterostomy** (Kasai procedure), which is not possible with complete obliteration.
—**hepatic transplantation.**

2. **Choledochal cyst**

—is characterized by **congenital segmental dilation** of the extrahepatic biliary duct.

—may be related to **ductal malformation** that causes inappropriate mixing of biliary and pancreatic juices, thus producing ductal wall damage.

—is more commonly seen in females.

—is associated with **intrahepatic cysts** (30%).

a. The classification of choledochal cysts (Types I–V) is outlined in Figure 16-6.

b. **Presentation is variable.**

(1) **Patients may present** in **childhood or adulthood.**

(2) **Characteristics** may include
—epigastric pain.
—fever.
—jaundice.
—cholangitis.

c. **There is a significant risk of**
—cholangiocarcinoma.

d. **Treatment involves** excision of the cyst, followed by biliary bypass.

3. **Caroli's disease** (Type V choledochal cyst)

—is characterized by **congenital intrahepatic ductal dilation** often associated with stone formation and cholangitis.

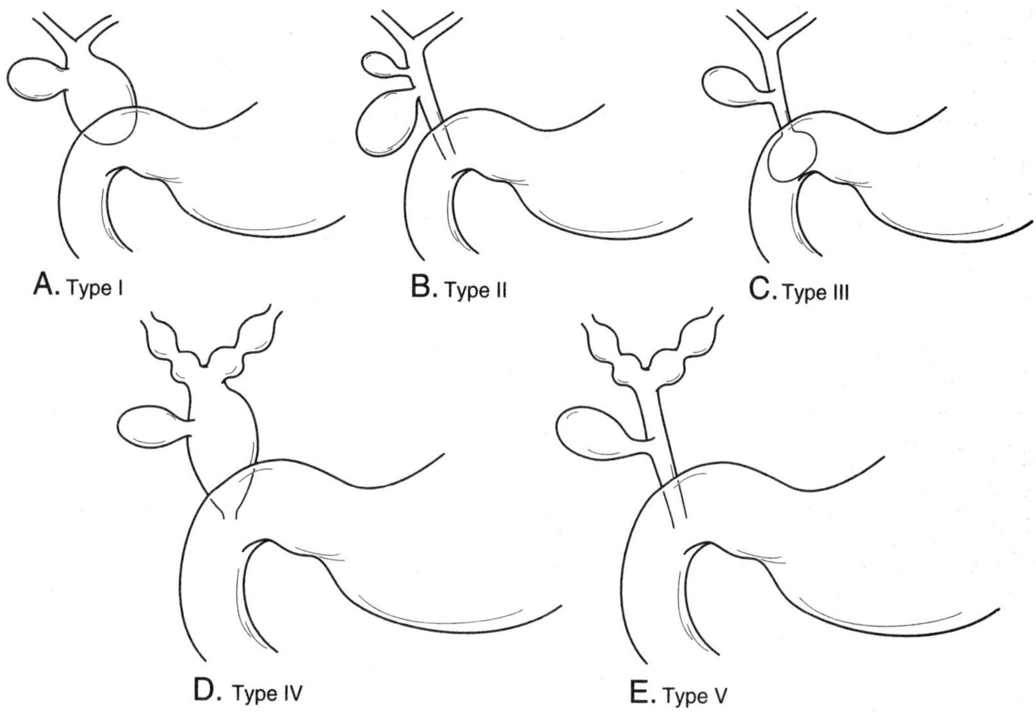

Figure 16-6. Anatomical classification of choledochal cysts. *(A)* Dilation of common hepatic and common bile duct, with cystic duct entering the cyst; most common type. *(B)* Lateral saccular cystic dilation. *(C)* Choledochocele represented by an intraduodenal cyst. *(D)* Multiple extrahepatic cysts, intrahepatic cysts, or both. *(E)* Single or multiple intrahepatic cysts; Caroli's disease. (Adapted with permission from Blackbourne LH: *Surgical Recall.* Baltimore, Williams & Wilkins, 1994, p 219.)

—may be associated with a familial syndrome characterized by **congenital hepatic fibrosis** and **medullary sponge kidney.**

B. Hemobilia

—is defined as bleeding into the biliary tree.

1. **Most cases in the United States**

   —are due to **trauma** or **iatrogenic injury.**

2. **The classic presentation** includes

   —biliary colic.

   —jaundice.

   —guaiac-positive stools.

3. **Diagnosis**

   —often requires **arteriography.**

4. **Treatment of persistent hemobilia** may include

   —embolization.

   —surgical ligation.

C. Ascariasis

—is a parasitic infection that can produce ductal obstruction.

D. Mirizzi syndrome

—**is a rare cause of biliary duct obstruction** due to gallbladder pathology without common duct stone involvement.

1. **A large stone within the gallbladder** may compress the CBD because of anatomic proximity.
2. **Local spread of inflammation** from the gallbladder to the bile duct may also result in ductal narrowing.

Review Test

Directions: Each of the numbered items or incomplete statements in this section is followed by answers or by completions of the statement. Select the ONE lettered answer or completion that is BEST in each case.

1. A 37-year-old woman presents 1 week after a laparoscopic cholecystectomy with complaints of fever, abdominal pain, back pain, and vomiting. Vital signs include: temperature, 38.7° C; blood pressure, 110/80 mm Hg; pulse, 120/min; respiration, 18/min. There is some tenderness in the right upper quadrant (RUQ) with voluntary guarding but no rebound tenderness or distension. Laboratory results include: white blood cells = 18,000; hematocrit = 34; platelets = 572; Na^+ 130; K^+ = 3.3; Cl^- = 95; CO_2 = 29; blood urea nitrogen = 31; creatinine = 0.9; total bilirubin = 8.1; conjugated bilirubin = 6.8; alkaline phosphatase = 700; aspartate aminotransferase (AST) = 150; alanine aminotransferase (ALT) = 209; and lipase = 40. RUQ ultrasound was performed and revealed a dilated common bile duct, no gallbladder, and no significant fluid collections. Which of the following is the most appropriate next step in the management of this patient?

(A) Antibiotics, fluid resuscitation, and observation
(B) Radionuclide hepatobiliary iminodiacetic acid (HIDA) scan
(C) Plain radiograph of the abdomen
(D) Take the patient to the operating room
(E) Endoscopic retrograde cholangiopancreatography (ERCP)

2. A 54-year-old, African-American man with a history of hypertension and sickle cell trait presents with a 24-hour history of nausea, vomiting, and abdominal pain. The patient describes the pain as crampy in nature and worse after eating. His temperature is 38.4° C, blood pressure is 150/96 mm Hg, pulse 105/min, and respiration 6/min. His abdomen is tender in the right upper quadrant (RUQ) and the patient cannot take a deep breath when the examiner is palpating the RUQ. Laboratory results include: white blood cells = 15,000; hematocrit = 39; platelets = 112; total bilirubin = 1.0; conjugated bilirubin = 0.1; and alkaline phosphatase = 62. Which of the following is the most appropriate diagnostic study in the initial evaluation of this patient?

(A) Radionuclide hepatobiliary iminodiacetic acid (HIDA) scan
(B) Plain films of the abdomen
(C) RUQ ultrasound
(D) Computed tomography (CT) scan of the abdomen
(E) Magnetic resonance cholangiopancreatography (MRCP)

3. A 62-year-old, white woman with a history of hypertension, hypercholesterolemia, and peptic ulcer disease presents to the clinic after a routine laparoscopic cholecystectomy. Surgical pathology reveals a 3 mm × 3 mm × 4 mm adenocarcinoma in the wall of the gallbladder that extends into but not through the muscularis layer. A chest radiograph and abdominal computed tomography (CT) scan show no evidence of metastases. Which of the following is the appropriate treatment for this patient's disease?

(A) The patient has been treated appropriately and no further surgery is necessary
(B) Perform a choledochojejunostomy as a palliative measure for relief of potential obstructive symptoms
(C) Perform a wedge resection of the liver around the gallbladder and a regional lymphadenectomy
(D) Perform a pancreaticoduodenectomy to obtain wide margins around the gallbladder
(E) Perform a wedge resection of the liver around the gallbladder, a regional lymphadenectomy, and excision of all trocar sites

4. A 68-year-old, Vietnamese man with a history of hypertension, asthma, and arthritis presents with complaints of pruritus that has gradually worsened over the past 3 weeks. Most recently he also reports some nausea and vomiting. He reports having lost approximately 15 pounds in the past month and attributes this to his nausea and vomiting. On physical examination his temperature is 37.6° C, blood pressure is 160/90 mm Hg, pulse is 87/min, and respirations are 13/min. He is a thin male in no acute distress. Laboratory results include: white blood cells = 8.2; hematocrit = 42; platelets = 208; Na^+ = 132; K^+ = 4.0; blood urea nitrogen = 32; creatinine = 0.7; total bilirubin = 12.0; conjugated bilirubin = 10.8; alkaline phosphatase = 812; amylase = 35; lipase = 60; aspartate aminotransferase (AST) = 212; and alanine aminotransferase (ALT) = 230. A right upper quadrant (RUQ) ultrasound was performed before the patient's referral and reveals no gallstones, gallbladder wall thickening, or common duct dilation. There is, however, intrahepatic ductal dilation. Which of the following is the most likely diagnosis?

(A) Cholangitis
(B) Cholangiocarcinoma
(C) Pancreatitis
(D) Pancreatic cancer
(E) Choledocholithiasis

5. A 42-year-old man with a history of diabetes mellitus and inflammatory bowel disease presents because of a 3-day history of worsening itching. The patient denies any fever, chills, or abdominal pain but does report two episodes of vomiting. The patient also claims to have lost 12 pounds in the last 2 months. After further questioning, the patient reports having had several similar episodes in the past that resolved spontaneously. On physical examination he is jaundiced. Rectal examination is trace positive for blood. Laboratory results include: white blood cell count = 10.0; hematocrit = 33; platelets = 256; blood urea nitrogen = 28; creatinine = 1.1; total bilirubin = 9.0; conjugated bilirubin = 7.6; alkaline phosphatase = 1000; aspartate aminotransferase (AST) = 78; alanine aminotransferase (ALT) = 152; prothrombin time (PT) = 12.2; and partial thromboplastin time (PTT) = 21.8. Which of the following is the most likely diagnosis?

(A) Primary sclerosing cholangitis (PSC)
(B) Choledocholithiasis
(C) Biliary colic
(D) Cholangiocarcinoma
(E) Cholangitis

6. A 75-year-old woman has been in the intensive care unit for the past 3 weeks because of a 20% burn to her back and left arm. Her course has been complicated by adult respiratory distress syndrome (ARDS) and a non-Q wave myocardial infarction. Her cardiovascular status is currently tenuous. Over the past week the patient's white blood cell count has been rising and she grimaces with palpation of the abdomen. Her current white blood cell count is 18,000 with a left shift. Her other laboratory results are unremarkable except for a hematocrit of 29. Current vital signs include: temperature, 38.4° C; blood pressure, 88/48 mm Hg; pulse, 120/min; and respiration, 26/min. Abdominal films are unremarkable. A right upper quadrant (RUQ) ultrasound was performed and revealed a distended gallbladder, thickened gallbladder wall, pericholecystic fluid, no gallstones, and normal common bile ducts. Which of the following is most appropriate in the initial management of this patient?

(A) Endoscopic retrograde cholangiopancreatography (ERCP) with stone removal
(B) Emergent open cholecystectomy
(C) Cholecystostomy
(D) Laparoscopic cholecystectomy
(E) Intravenous (IV) antibiotics and observation

7. A 56-year-old woman with a history of hypertension and gout presents with a 3-day history of worsening abdominal pain, back pain, nausea, and vomiting. The patient claims she has had a history of crampy abdominal pain after eating for almost 1 year but most recently she has been suffering from constant pain. Her temperature is 36.7° C, blood pressure is 168/85 mm Hg, and pulse is 92/min. She is tender to palpation in the midepigastric region and right upper quadrant (RUQ). Laboratory results include: white blood cell count = 10,000; hematocrit = 42; platelets = 210; Na^+ = 138; K^+ = 3.4; Cl^- = 96; CO_2 = 29; blood urea nitrogen = 34; creatinine = 1.3; total bilirubin = 1.2; conjugated bilirubin = 0.3; aspartate aminotransferase (AST) = 50; alanine aminotransferase (ALT) = 80; alkaline phosphatase = 210; amylase = 400; and lipase = 566. Abdominal films are consistent with an ileus. RUQ ultrasound reveals sludge, no wall thickening, no pericholecystic fluid, and a normal bile duct. Which of the following is the most likely cause of this patient's pathology?

(A) Obstruction of the cystic duct by a gallstone
(B) A malignancy obstructing the common hepatic duct
(C) Idiopathic inflammatory strictures of the bile ducts
(D) Passage of a gallstone through the ampulla of Vater
(E) Obstruction and bacterial infection of the biliary tree

8. A 54-year-old, white woman presents with a 48-hour history of worsening crampy abdominal pain. Her pain is exacerbated by eating and is associated with nausea and vomiting. Her temperature is 38.7° C, pulse is 101/min, blood pressure is 130/82 mm Hg, and respiration is 19/min. Her abdomen is tender in the right upper quadrant (RUQ) and she cannot take a deep breath when the examiner palpates in the RUQ. She has no peritoneal signs. Laboratory results include: white blood cells = 16,000; hematocrit = 38; platelets = 316; Na^+ = 134; K^+ = 3.6; Cl^- = 101; CO_2 = 22; blood urea nitrogen = 21; creatinine = 1.0; total bilirubin = 2.0; conjugated bilirubin = 0.8; alkaline phosphatase = 67; aspartate aminotransferase (AST) = 62; alanine aminotransferase (ALT) = 61; and amylase < 30. RUQ ultrasound reveals a distended gallbladder with pericholecystic fluid and multiple echogenic foci in the gallbladder. The common duct appears normal. Which of the following is the most appropriate next step in the management of this patient?

(A) Exploratory laparotomy
(B) Computed tomography (CT) scan of the abdomen
(C) Laparoscopic cholecystectomy
(D) Cholangiopancreatography
(E) Hepatobiliary iminodiacetic acid (HIDA) scan

9. A 68-year-old, diabetic, hypertensive, African-American man was found to have gallstones on an abdominal computed tomography (CT) scan performed as part of a metastatic work-up. The man denies any symptoms except for occasional heartburn, which is treated medically. His vitals signs include: temperature, 37.1° C; blood pressure, 160/90 mm Hg; pulse, 87/min; and respiration, 12/min. His abdomen is soft, nontender, and nondistended. He has normoactive bowel sounds. Which of the following is an appropriate statement regarding the management of this patient?

(A) The patient must have a cholecystectomy
(B) This patient is at no increased risk of developing cholecystitis, versus a diabetic patient without gallstones
(C) If the patient had vague abdominal pain, a laparoscopic cholecystectomy may be helpful
(D) If the patient develops symptoms suggestive of cholecystitis, a CT scan should be repeated
(E) A laparoscopic cholecystectomy for acute cholecystitis is contraindicated in this patient because of the diabetes

10. A 4-year-old boy was in his usual state of good health until approximately 1 month ago when he developed cholangitis. As part of the work-up an endoscopic retrograde cholangiopancreatography (ERCP) was performed and revealed segmental dilation of the common bile duct. A computed tomography (CT) scan was also performed and revealed several intrahepatic cysts, the segmental dilation of the common duct, and no masses. Which of the following is the most appropriate recommendation for this patient?

(A) This is a normal anatomic variant and no surgery is indicated
(B) The patient should have a repeat ERCP to perform a sphincterotomy
(C) The patient should have a cholecystectomy to prevent gallbladder involvement
(D) The patient should have the region of segmental dilation removed followed by biliary reconstruction
(E) The patient should have the dilated region excised, the head of the pancreas removed, and then a biliary bypass

11. A 49-year-old, obese man presents to the emergency room with a 24-hour history of fever, chills, and abdominal pain. He describes crampy pain in the midepigastric region with radiation to the right shoulder. He also reports some associated nausea and vomiting. His vital signs include: temperature, 38.9° C; blood pressure, 156/96 mm Hg; pulse, 99/min; and respiration, 16/min. His sclera are anicteric, his heart is regular, and his lungs are clear to auscultation except for occasional wheezes. Laboratory results include: white blood cells = 14,000; hematocrit = 42; platelets = 221; Na^+ = 132; K^+ = 3.3; Cl = 100; CO_2 = 21; blood urea nitrogen = 20; creatinine = 1.5; glucose = 266; total bilirubin = 1.2; conjugated bilirubin = 0.1; alkaline phosphatase = 242; and amylase = 30. A right upper quadrant (RUQ) ultrasound was attempted but because of the patient's size the gallbladder could not be adequately visualized. Which of the following is the most appropriate next step in the management of this patient?

(A) Endoscopic retrograde cholangiopancreatography (ERCP)
(B) Hepatobiliary iminodiacetic acid (HIDA) scan
(C) Oral cholecystogram
(D) Percutaneous transhepatic cholangiography
(E) The patient should be taken to the operating room

12. A 71-year-old, white man with a history of diabetes mellitus, coronary artery bypass surgery, and a 80 pack-year smoking history presents to the office complaining of severe itching that is not improved with home remedies. He denies fever, chills, or abdominal pain. On physical examination he is a thin, jaundiced, elderly man in no acute distress. Vital signs include: temperature, 36.8° C; pulse, 67/min; blood pressure, 145/67 mm Hg; respiration, 13/min. Laboratory results include: white blood cells = 8000; hematocrit = 32; platelets = 201; Na^+ = 134; K^+ = 3.6; Cl^- = 101; CO_2 = 24; blood urea nitrogen = 31; creatinine = 1.6; glucose = 278; total bilirubin = 11.1; conjugated bilirubin = 8.9; alkaline phosphatase = 1002; and amylase = 100. A computed tomography (CT) scan is performed and reveals dilated intrahepatic ducts but no visualization of the extrahepatic ducts because of a 2 cm × 2 cm × 3 cm mass that appears to involve the common hepatic duct and cystic duct. There is no obvious lymphadenopathy. Which of the following is the most appropriate next step in the management of this patient?

(A) Computed tomography (CT) scan of the chest and a bone scan
(B) Percutaneous transhepatic cholangiography (PTC)
(C) Exploratory laparotomy
(D) Biliary ultrasound
(E) Radical pancreaticoduodenectomy

Directions: Each set of matching questions in this section consists of a list of four to twenty-six lettered options followed by several numbered items. For each numbered item, select the appropriate lettered option(s). Each lettered option may be selected once, more than once, or not at all.

Questions 13–15

(A) Distended gallbladder with thickened wall and pericholecystic fluid. Multiple echogenic foci in the gallbladder. Normal common bile duct and liver.
(B) Normal gallbladder except for a single echogenic foci. Common bile duct distended. Normal liver.
(C) Normal gallbladder. Extrahepatic bile ducts not visualized. Intrahepatic ducts distended.
(D) Normal gallbladder. Normal liver and bile ducts.
(E) Focal stricture of the distal common bile duct with proximal dilation.

Match the right upper quadrant (RUQ) ultrasound result most consistent with the clinical presentation.

13. A 56-year-old, white man with a history of tobacco abuse, hypertension, recent unintentional 80-lb weight loss, and squamous cell cancer of the lung presents with a 24-hour history of right upper quadrant (RUQ) abdominal pain, nausea, and vomiting. He has had similar pains over the past 2 weeks, mostly after eating, but they had resolved spontaneously. The patient denies fever and chills. His temperature is 36.7° C. Physical examination findings are significant for scleral icterus and RUQ tenderness to palpation. Significant laboratory findings include white blood cells = 7800, total bilirubin = 6.8, conjugated bilirubin = 5.6, and alkaline phosphatase = 670. (SELECT 1 RESULT)

14. A 53-year-old, morbidly obese, white woman with a history of diabetes presents with a 36-hour history of worsening crampy midepigastric and right upper quadrant (RUQ) abdominal pain. She claims the pain was initially bad only after meals but has since become constant. She also complains of nausea, vomiting, and fever. Her temperature is 38.5° C. Her physical examination is significant for anicteric sclera, RUQ pain, and inspiratory arrest with deep palpation in the RUQ. Significant laboratory findings include white blood cells = 14,000, K^+ = 3.3, Cl^- = 96, CO_2 = 30, total bilirubin = 1.1, and alkaline phosphatase = 64. (SELECT 1 RESULT)

15. A 58-year-old, diabetic, African-American man with a history of hypertension and hypercholesterolemia presents with a 48-hour history of progressively worsening constant right upper quadrant (RUQ) pain, fever, nausea and vomiting. Vital signs include: temperature, 39.1° C; pulse, 120/min; blood pressure, 100/59 mm Hg; respiration, 21/min. Physical examination is significant for icteric sclera and RUQ tenderness. Significant laboratory findings include white blood cells = 17,000; alkaline phosphatase = 670; total bilirubin = 7.8; conjugated bilirubin = 6.5; aspartate aminotransferase (AST) = 350; alanine aminotransferase (ALT) = 390; and amylase = 45. (SELECT 1 RESULT)

Answers and Explanations

1–E. In addition to iatrogenic biliary tree injury, another complication of laparoscopic cholecystectomy is retained common duct stones, which can lead to obstruction and eventually cholangitis. Endoscopic retrograde cholangiopancreatography (ERCP) would be the examination of choice for evaluation. Not only can the common duct obstruction be identified, but therapeutic measures can be undertaken (e.g., sphincterotomy and stone extraction). If these measures are unsuccessful, surgery may be indicated but would not generally be the initial therapy. Fluid resuscitation and antibiotics are important but the key to initial therapy is to relieve the obstruction. A HIDA scan would help to identify the lesion but ERCP provides better visualization in addition to the potential therapeutic role.

2–C. This clinical picture is consistent with acute cholecystitis. Right upper quadrant (RUQ) ultrasound is the examination of choice for initial evaluation of a patient with possible cholecystitis. Plain films of the abdomen are rarely useful in this situation because only 5% of gallstones appear on such radiographs. A HIDA scan may be used when ultrasound findings are inconclusive; however, it should not be performed as an initial study. Magnetic resonance cholangiopancreatography (MRCP) provides excellent visualization of the biliary tree but it is still limited by cost and inconvenience. Computed tomography (CT) scans are generally not useful in the straightforward evaluation of cholecystitis.

3–E. The appropriate treatment for this gallbladder cancer is a radical cholecystectomy. The patient has already had her gallbladder removed and therefore needs to have the procedure completed with a liver resection with 2–3 cm margins around the gallbladder and a regional lymphadenectomy. In addition, the laparoscopic trocar sites must also be excised to prevent tumor seeding. Wider resections such as a Whipple's operation or palliative procedures are not indicated at this time.

4–B. The presentation of a patient with painless jaundice and no history of abdominal surgery is consistent with either pancreatic cancer or cholangiocarcinoma. The finding of intrahepatic ductal dilation suggests obstruction of the biliary system above the common duct and therefore makes pancreatic cancer less likely. Cholangiocarcinoma and more specifically, tumors involving the upper third of the biliary tree (Klatskin tumors), is the most likely etiology of these findings. Cholangitis often produces a fever and this patient is not febrile.

5–A. This is a characteristic presentation of primary sclerosing cholangitis (PSC). The patient is relatively young and therefore malignancy is less likely. Furthermore, he describes a history of fluctuating symptoms, which is characteristic of PSC and not of cholangiocarcinoma. The lack of pain makes the diagnosis of biliary colic and choledocholithiasis less likely. Of concern is the patient's anemia, guaiac-positive stools, and weight loss. This may be due to colon cancer, which is an increased risk in patients with PSC and ulcerative colitis.

6–C. Acalculous cholecystitis characteristically affects critically ill patients. An appropriate management strategy in an unstable patient with cholecystitis is cholecystostomy that involves percutaneous placement of a catheter in the gallbladder to provide for drainage until the patient is stable enough to tolerate formal cholecystectomy. With simple antibiotics and observation serious morbidity and mortality can affect up to 60% of these patients. On the other hand, the patient is not well enough to tolerate the stress of surgery, so a temporizing measure is needed. Endoscopic retrograde cholangiopancreatography (ERCP) is not indicated in the setting of cholecystitis.

7–D. The most common cause of pancreatitis in the United States is gallstone disease, including passage of a gallstone. Evidence for this includes the long history of biliary colic, which suggests calculous biliary disease. Furthermore, the elevation in alkaline phosphatase suggests recent irritation to the bile ducts, such as that caused by stone passage. In addition, the right upper quadrant (RUQ) ultrasound findings include the precursor to gallstones in the gallbladder as well as a normal duct, which weighs against other diagnoses, including primary sclerosing cholangitis (PSC), cholangitis, and cholangiocarcinoma. There was also no evidence on ultrasound of active biliary tree obstruction.

8–C. The history of colicky pain worsened by eating is classic for cholecystitis. On physical examination the patient has a positive Murphy's sign. Her laboratory tests show evidence of infection but her normal bilirubin and alkaline phosphatase suggest no common duct involvement. The right upper quadrant (RUQ) ultrasound visualizes stones in the gallbladder. The next step for this patient is a cholecystectomy to remove her gallbladder. Further diagnostic tests, such as a HIDA or computed tomography (CT) scan, are not necessary because of the clear evidence of cholecystitis. Endoscopic retrograde cholangiopancreatography (ERCP) is not necessary because there is no suggestion of common duct pathology.

9–C. Surgery for asymptomatic gallstones is not absolutely indicated. The patient's age and diabetes may lead many surgeons to perform a cholecystectomy, but these are relative indications. On the other hand, a cholecystectomy could help this patient, especially if there is a history of vague complaints. A right upper quadrant (RUQ) ultrasound would be the test of choice for initial evaluation if symptoms suggestive of cholecystitis were to develop, not a computed tomography (CT) scan. A laparoscopic approach is not contraindicated because of diabetes. The presence of gallstones in any population is associated with an increased risk of cholecystitis versus those without stones.

10–D. The most likely diagnosis in this case is a choledochal cyst. There is an increased risk of cholangiocarcinoma associated with this congenital abnormality, therefore the recommendation is to have the cyst excised and the biliary tree reconstructed, often with a Roux-en-Y choledochojejunostomy or hepaticojejunostomy. There is no pathology in the pancreas, thus the head of the pancreas should not be removed with the cyst. Additionally, a sphincterotomy would not relieve the obstruction in this patient.

11–B. This patient has a presentation that is highly suggestive of acute cholecystitis. When a right upper quadrant (RUQ) ultrasound is equivocal, the next test of choice is nuclear imaging of the biliary tree, such as a HIDA scan. An oral cholecystogram can give the same information as the HIDA scan but it is much more time-consuming and the reliability is lower owing to the patient's vomiting. Cholangiography is not indicated before the HIDA scan but may be necessary if common duct obstruction is diagnosed. Surgery may be necessary, but not before confirming the diagnosis in this setting.

12–B. This patient is presenting with obstructive jaundice from a mass involving the common hepatic duct and the cystic duct. This is most likely due to gallbladder cancer with extension down the cystic duct but may also be due to cholangiocarcinoma. The next step in evaluation would be cholangiography. Percutaneous transhepatic cholangiography (PTC) is preferred because it can characterize the extent of involvement of the proximal biliary tree, which is important for surgical planning. In addition, a drain may be left in the intrahepatic bile ducts or a stent may be placed to decompress the dilated biliary system. After this has been performed clinical staging and surgical planning can be accomplished. Although computed tomography (CT) may further define a mass lesion and be used in staging, it is not as effective as PTC at outlining the degree of biliary tree involvement. Exploratory laparotomy is not indicated in this setting.

13–B. This patient is presenting with choledocholithiasis most likely related to cholesterol stones formed in the gallbladder caused by his rapid weight loss. Therefore one would expect to see common duct distension caused by the cholesterol stone. In addition, one might expect to find evidence of stone formation in the gallbladder, such as another stone or sludge.

14–A. This patient is presenting with classic acute cholecystitis. Characteristic findings of acute cholecystitis on right upper quadrant (RUQ) ultrasound could reveal gallstones, a distended gallbladder, pericholecystic fluid, and thickening of the gallbladder wall.

15–B. This patient is presenting with cholangitis. Characteristic findings include fever; right upper quadrant (RUQ) pain; icteric sclera (Charcot's triad); and elevated bilirubin, alkaline phosphatase, and transaminases. The RUQ ultrasound should show evidence of biliary obstruction, the dilated ducts. The ultrasound picture of cholangitis and choledocholithiasis are very similar but the clinical picture can easily separate the two. The most likely cause of cholangitis in this setting is choledocholithiasis.

17

Pancreas and Spleen

Thomas G. Gleason

I. Pancreas

A. Embryology

1. The **pancreas develops from**

   —the **dorsal pouch** (the endodermal lining of the duodenum) and the **ventral pouch** (the hepatic diverticulum).

   a. The **ventral pouch**

      —migrates posteriorly and clockwise to fuse with the dorsal pouch.

   b. **Failure of normal clockwise rotation**

      —results in an **annular pancreas.**

2. The **ventral duct normally fuses**

   —with the distal dorsal duct to form the main pancreatic duct, the **duct of Wirsung.**

   a. **Pancreas divisum (Figure 17-1)**

      —occurs when these ducts do not fuse (in 25% of people).

   b. The **unfused proximal dorsal duct**

      —forms the accessory **duct of Santorini.**

B. Anatomy

1. The **pancreas consists of** the

   —head (with uncinate process).

   —neck.

   —body.

   —tail.

2. **Blood supply** (**Figure 17-2**)

   a. The **head**

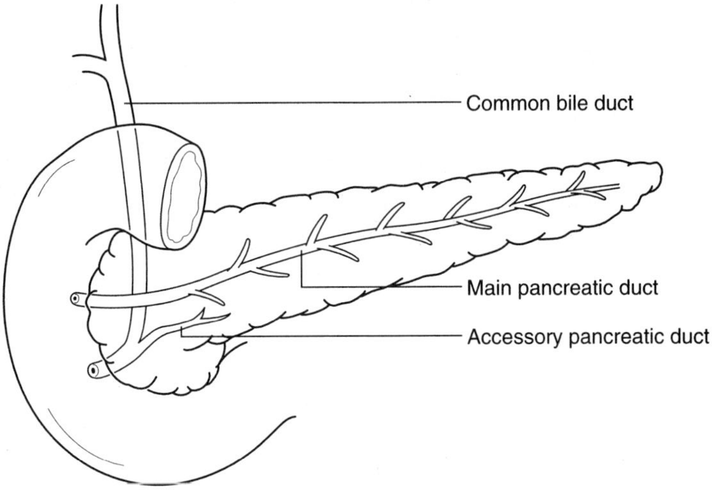

Figure 17-1. Pancreatic divisum. No connection between the main pancreatic and accessory pancreatic ducts. (Reprinted with permission from Howard JM, Jordan, Jr GL, Reeber HA: *Surgical Diseases of the Pancreas.* Baltimore, Williams & Wilkins, 1987, p 22.)

—is supplied by the anterior and posterior **pancreaticoduodenal** arteries and veins.

b. The **proximal body**

—is supplied by the superior and inferior **pancreatic** arteries and veins originating from the celiac or splenic arteries.

c. The **distal body and tail**

—are supplied by the short branches of the **splenic** and **gastroepiploic** arteries and veins and the dorsal pancreatic artery.

3. **Nodal groups**

a. The **pancreatic head**

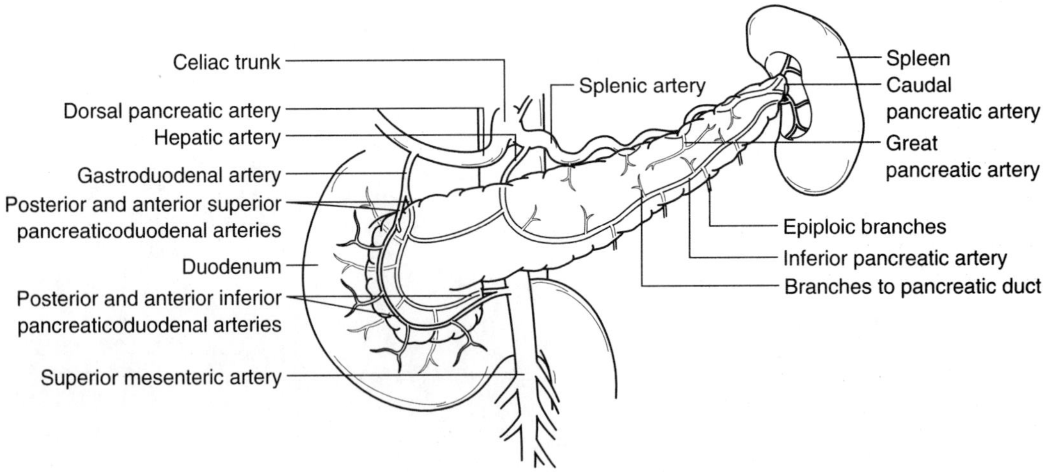

Figure 17-2. Arterial supply of the pancreas. (Reprinted with permission from Howard JM, Jordan, Jr GL, Reeber HA: *Surgical Diseases of the Pancreas.* Baltimore, Williams & Wilkins, 1987, p 26.)

—drains into the subpyloric, portal, mesocolic, and aortocaval nodes.

b. The **body and tail**

—drain into the retroperitoneal celiac, mesocolic, mesenteric, and aortocaval nodes.

C. Histology and physiology

1. Exocrine cells

a. **Acinar cells**

—contain digestive enzymes (e.g., amylase, lipase, phospholipase A_2, trypsin, chymotrypsin, elastase).

b. **Ductal cells**

—secrete an electrolyte **solution high in bicarbonate** (HCO_3^-).

2. Pancreatic secretions

a. **Cholecystokinin** and **acetylcholine**

—stimulate enzyme secretion.

(1) Most **peptidases** are secreted in inactive forms: trypsin, chymotrypsin, elastase, kallikrein, carboxypeptidase A and B.

(2) The peptidases are activated intraluminally by **enterokinase.**

(3) Nucleases, lipase, and amylase are secreted in their active forms.

b. **Secretin** and vagal efferents

—stimulate HCO_3^- secretion—the substrate is a clear, isotonic, basic solution (pH 8), with 30–120 mEq/L HCO_3^-.

3. Endocrine cells: islets of Langerhans

a. **Alpha cells** produce **glucagon.**

b. **Beta cells** produce **insulin.**

c. **Delta cells** produce **somatostatin.**

d. **F cells** produce **pancreatic polypeptide.**

e. **Islets also produce**

—vasoactive intestinal peptide (VIP).

—serotonin.

—pancreastatin.

—calcitonin gene related peptide (CGRP).

—neuropeptide Y.

—gastrin-releasing peptide.

II. Pancreatitis

A. Acute pancreatitis

1. Etiology

a. The most **common causes** of pancreatitis are **alcohol abuse and gallstones.**

b. **Other causes** include

—endoscopic retrograde cholangiopancreatography (ERCP).

—trauma.

—hyperlipidemia.

—medications (e.g., azathioprine, furosemide, glucocorticoids, cimetidine).
—*Ascaris lumbricoides* and *Opisthorchis sinensis*.
—viruses (e.g., coxsackie, mumps)
—hypercalcemia.
—scorpion bite.

2. **Enzymes contributing** to saponification, hemorrhage, and necrosis include
—trypsin.
—lipase.
—phospholipase A_2.
—elastase.

3. **Signs and symptoms**
a. **Patients typically present with**
—**abdominal pain.**
—nausea.
—**vomiting.**
—**anorexia.**
b. **Signs of complex disease** include
—retroperitoneal hemorrhage of the flank (**Grey Turner sign**).
—umbilicus (**Cullen sign**).
—inguinal ligament (**Fox sign**).

4. Diagnosis
—Work-up should focus on identifying the cause and severity of illness.
a. **Laboratory studies** should include
—amylase.
—lipase.
—values needed for establishing **Ranson's criteria (Table 17-1)**.
b. **Ranson's criteria**
—are used as a prognostic indicator in pancreatitis.
(1) Patients with **more than 3 Ranson's criteria** are at high risk for developing **complicated pancreatitis** (abscess or necrosis).
(2) **Mortality** sharply rises with more than 3 Ranson's criteria (see Table 17-1)
c. **Abdominal imaging** (i.e., computed tomography [CT] scan with intravenous [IV] contrast) may show
—a sentinel loop.
—edematous pancreas.
—nonenhancement of the pancreas (necrotic pancreatic tissue).
d. **Ultrasound**
—is used to identify gallstone disease and biliary ductal dilation.
e. **ERCP**
—helps evaluate pancreatic ductal anatomy and pathology.

Table 17-1. Ranson's Criteria and Predicted Mortality

Less than 24 Hours		
Age		> 55
White blood cells (WBC)		$> 16 \times 10^3/\mu L$
Lactate dehydrogenase (LDH)		> 350 IU/L
Asparate aminotransferase (AST)		> 250 IU/L
Glucose		> 200 mg/dL
Less than 48 Hours		
Fluid sequestration		> 6 L
Base deficit		> 4
Po_2		< 60 mm Hg
Hematocrit (Hct) decrease		$> 10\%$
Ca^{2+}		< 8 mg/dL
Blood urea nitrogen (BUN) increase		> 5 mg/dL
Predicted Mortality		
Number of Criteria	***Percent Mortality***	
3–4 signs	28%	
5–6 signs	40%	
> 7 signs	100%	

5. Treatment

—is **nonoperative** unless complications develop (i.e., necrosis or infection).

a. Aggressive fluid resuscitation

—is an essential part of treatment.

b. Intubation and mechanical ventilation

—should be instituted if significant pulmonary dysfunction occurs (e.g., partial pressure of oxygen [pO_2] less than 60 mm Hg).

c. Nasogastric decompression

—is used to relieve vomiting.

d. Nutritional support

—is an important adjunct, but controversy exists about which form is ideal.

(1) Most agree that early in a course of complicated acute pancreatitis total parenteral nutrition (**TPN**) is indicated.

(2) If patients tolerate enteral feeding, it should initially occur distal to the ampulla of Vater via a nasoenteric tube or jejunostomy.

e. ERCP with **endoscopic sphincterotomy** (ES)

—is indicated in patients with gallstone pancreatitis and biliary obstruction.

f. The use of **prophylactic antibiotics** (i.e., imipenem-cilastatin)

—lowers the infection rate.

—may lower the mortality rate in **necrotizing pancreatitis** (see II C 2).

B. Gallstone pancreatitis

—is characterized by pancreatitis identified in the setting of cholelithiasis.

1. **Blockage of the pancreatic duct**
   —appears to play an important role.
2. **Uncomplicated pancreatitis with concomitant biliary obstruction**
   —should be treated by **preoperative ERCP with ES** and stone extraction.
   a. **Laparoscopic cholecystectomy**
      —should then be performed, once the acute pancreatitis resolves.
   b. **Intraoperative cholangiography** (IOC)
      —should be performed to confirm the absence of common bile duct obstruction.
3. **Gallstone pancreatitis without biliary obstruction**
   —should initially be treated medically, followed by laparoscopic cholecystectomy before discharge.

C. **Complicated acute pancreatitis**

1. **Pancreatic abscesses**
   —are typically polymicrobial.
   a. **Well-circumscribed abscesses**
      —should be **drained percutaneously.**
   b. **Operative drainage** should be reserved
      —for failed attempts at percutaneous drainage.
      —with infected pancreatic necrosis or multiloculated, poorly defined fluid collections.
2. **Necrotizing pancreatitis**
   a. **Sterile (uninfected) necrosis**
      (1) These patients should be **treated nonoperatively** during the first several weeks to better delineate viable and nonviable pancreatic tissue.
      (2) Necrotic tissue or **fluid collections** should be **sampled percutaneously** with CT-guidance if the patient develops bacteremia, sepsis, or deterioration.
      (3) Administering **antibiotics** with imipenem-cilastatin **decreases the infection rate** in patients with sterile pancreatic necrosis.
   b. **Infected necrosis**
      (1) If CT-guided aspirates demonstrate **infection,** débridement of necrotic pancreatic tissue (**necrosectomy**) and operative drainage (open or closed) are indicated.
      (2) Many patients require reoperation for further débridement.
      (3) **IV antibiotics** directed at the organisms cultured from the pancreatic bed are indicated.
   c. **Peritoneal lavage**
      —has been proposed as an adjunctive therapy for necrotizing pancreatitis.
3. **Enterocutaneous or enteroperitoneal fistulae**

—develop in over 20% of patients with pancreatic necrosis.

—Over **50%** of enterocutaneous fistulae will **resolve spontaneously** after adequate drainage is established (see Chapter 13).

D. Pancreas divisum (see **Figure 17-1**)

1. The majority of patients with **pancreas divisum**

   —have no clinical manifestations.

2. A minority of patients with **accessory duct (duct of Santorini) stenosis**

   —develop recurrent acute pancreatitis.

3. These patients can be **treated**

   —endoscopically or surgically.

   a. **Endoscopic treatment** includes

      —dilation.

      —sphincterotomy, stent placement, or both.

   b. **Surgical therapy**

      —entails a **transduodenal sphincteroplasty.**

E. Chronic pancreatitis

—corresponds with **irreversible parenchymal fibrosis.**

1. **Manifestations** of chronic pancreatitis may include

   —recurrent bouts of acute pancreatitis.

   —chronic abdominal pain.

   —anorexia and weight loss.

   —malabsorption and steatorrhea.

   —diabetes.

2. The **majority of cases** in the United States are caused by **alcohol abuse.**

3. The **diagnosis** is based on clinical and radiographic findings.

   —**CT findings** typically demonstrate an **atrophied gland,** areas of dilated pancreatic duct, and **calcifications.**

4. Primary **treatment**

   a. **Abstinence from alcohol**

      —will help prevent acute exacerbations.

   b. **Supportive care**

      —will include pain control and **nutritional support.**

5. Relative **indications for surgery** include

   —refractory, disabling pain.

   —concern of concomitant malignancy.

   —biliary obstruction.

   —complications of pseudocysts (e.g., bowel obstruction, splenic artery pseudoaneurysm, splenic vein thrombosis).

6. **Operative techniques** used for chronic pancreatitis
   a. Drainage procedures
      (1) The **Duval procedure** is a retrograde drainage with distal resection and end-to-end pancreaticojejunostomy.
      (2) The modified **Peustow procedure** is a side-to-side pancreaticojejunostomy.
      (3) The **Frey procedure** is a longitudinal pancreaticojejunostomy with partial pancreatic head resection.
   b. Resection procedures
      (1) **Distal pancreatectomy** is useful in chronic pancreatitis secondary to distal pancreatic trauma.
      (2) A modified **Whipple procedure (Figure 17-3)** may be appropriate for an inflammatory mass of the pancreatic head.
      (3) **Total pancreatectomy** is rarely indicated for diffuse chronic pancreatitis with a nondilated pancreatic duct.
   c. **Splanchnicectomy**
      —or celiac ganglionectomy or ganglion ablation may be useful for pain control.

F. Pancreatic pseudocysts

—are **nonepithelialized, encapsulated** pancreatic fluid collections.

1. Typically, **pseudocysts mature**
   —from pancreatic fluid collections **several weeks after bouts of acute pancreatitis.**

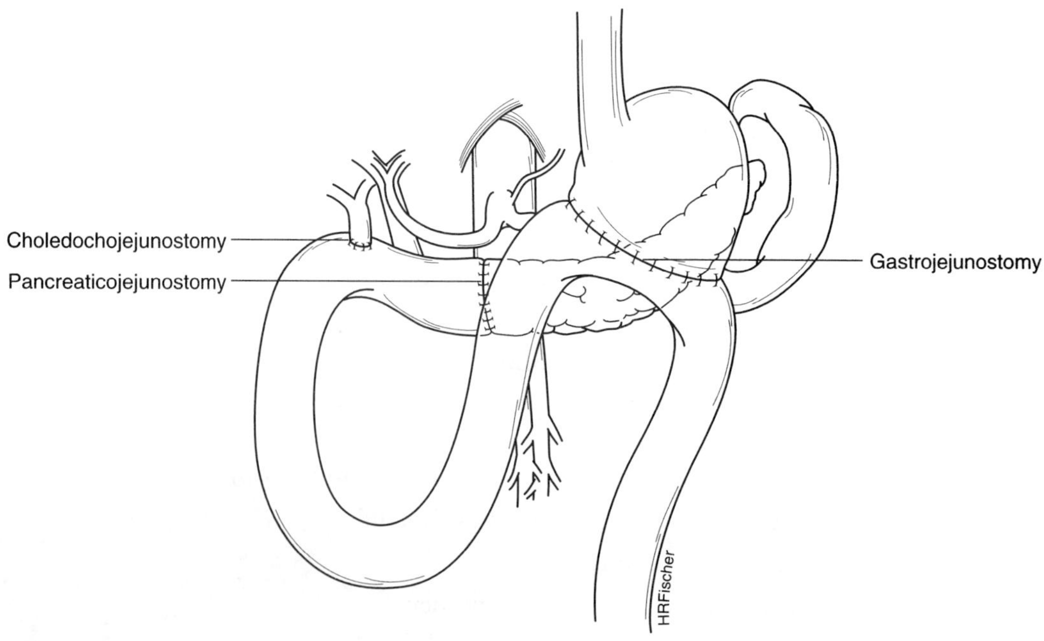

Figure 17-3. Anastomoses of a standard pancreaticoduodenectomy (Whipple procedure). (Reprinted with permission from Bell RH, Rikkers LF, Mulholland MW: *Digestive Tract Surgery.* Philadelphia, Lippincott-Raven, 1995, p 866.)

2. **Symptoms** include pain, fever, weight loss, and bowel obstruction by external compression.
3. A **CT scan** is often diagnostic (Figure 17-4).
4. **Small cysts** (< 5 cm)

   —will usually resolve spontaneously.
5. **Large cysts** (> 6 cm)

   —are more likely (75%) to require **drainage,** but they should be allowed to mature a capsule for at least **6 weeks** before attempted drainage.

   a. **Image-guided percutaneous drainage**

      —has a failure or reaccumulation rate of at least 30%–40%.

   b. **Operative drainage techniques** (e.g., **cystgastrostomy)**

      —have significantly lower recurrence rates than percutaneous techniques.

   c. **Endoscopic cystgastrostomy or cystenterostomy**

      —are newer techniques that may be used for draining these cysts, but recurrence rates are not yet defined.

G. **Pancreatic fistulae**

1. Pancreatitis-associated **pleural effusions**

   —may require ERCP with pancreatic stent placement to control pancreatic drainage.
2. **Pancreatic ascites**

   —When persistent, these should similarly be treated by pancreatic **ductal stenting.**
3. **Low-output (< 200 mL/day) pancreaticocutaneous fistulae**

   —typically **resolve spontaneously.**

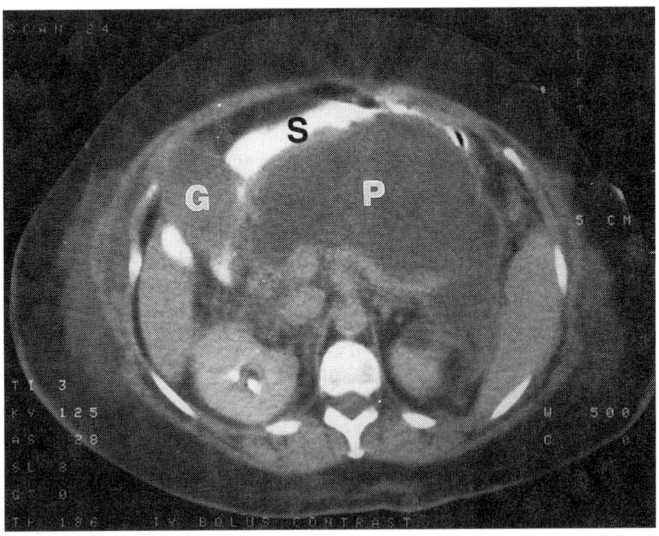

Figure 17-4. CT scan of a pancreatic pseudocyst. G = gallbladder; P = pseudocyst; S = stomach compressed by pseudocyst. (Reprinted with permission from Daffner RH: *Clinical Radiology: The Essentials,* 2nd ed. Baltimore, Williams & Wilkins, 1999, p 333.)

a. **Treatment**

—is similar to treatment of small bowel fistulae (see Chapter 13).

b. **Octreotide**

—may help decrease the volume of a fistula and convert a high-output (> 200 mL/day) into a low-output fistula.

H. **Pancreatic insufficiency**

—**generally refers to** pancreatic **exocrine insufficiency,** but often occurs with endocrine insufficiency.

1. It **generally occurs in the setting of**

—long-standing chronic pancreatitis.

—after total pancreatectomy (over **90% of exocrine function must be lost**).

2. **Symptoms**

—include **malabsorption and steatorrhea.**

3. **Diagnosis**

—**To confirm diagnosis, fecal fat testing** and the **secretin** or cholecystokinin **test** are used most frequently.

4. **Treatment**

—includes a high-carbohydrate, high-protein diet with **pancreatic enzyme replacement.**

III. Pancreatic Carcinoma

A. **Epidemiology and pathology**

1. The **incidence**

a. Pancreatic carcinoma

—occurs in approximately **1/10,000 people.**

—is twice as common in African Americans and 1.5 times as common in men versus women.

b. This carcinoma typically develops in the seventh decade of life.

c. **Tobacco use** appears to be a risk factor for its development.

2. Ninety percent of **pancreatic carcinomas** are of **ductal cell origin.**

a. **Sixty to seventy percent of adenocarcinomas** arise in the **head** of the pancreas.

b. The majority (60%–65%) of **periampullary cancers** are pancreatic.

3. **Pancreatic adenocarcinomas** typically metastasize to the lymph nodes, liver, and peritoneal surfaces.

4. **Five-year survival rates** range from **0%–10%** in the United States. Most patients die within one year.

5. **Other neoplasms** of the **exocrine pancreas** have a more favorable prognosis than adenocarcinomas.

a. **Papillary-cystic neoplasms**

—of the pancreas are usually cured by resection.

b. Serous cystadenomas

—are generally **benign** and are treated with resection to exclude malignancy.

c. Mucinous cystadenomas

—often contain **malignant** cells and, like cystadenocarcinomas, have a 60% 5-year survival rate after surgery.

d. Pancreatic lymphomas

—are rare (1%–2% of pancreatic cancers) and are treated with chemotherapy.

e. Metastatic tumors

—of the pancreas are rare but can arise from renal cell carcinomas or other non-Hodgkin's lymphomas.

B. The tumor-node-metastasis (TNM) staging system

—for pancreatic cancers is outlined in **Table 17-2.**

C. Presentation and diagnosis

1. **Most patients present** with **weight loss, jaundice,** or both.
2. **Other manifestations** include
   —abdominal pain.
   —nausea and anorexia.
   —jaundice.
   —hepatomegaly.
   —vomiting secondary to duodenal obstruction.
3. **Laboratory signs** include
   —elevated conjugated bilirubin.

Table 17-2. Tumor-Node-Metastasis (TNM) Staging System of Pancreatic Carcinoma

Stage	Primary Tumor	Nodal Disease	Distant Metastases
I	T1 or T2	N0	M0
II	T3	N0	M0
III	T1, T2 or T3	N1	M0
IV	T1, T2 or T3	N0 or N1	M1

Primary tumor

T1	No extension beyond the pancreas
T2	Limited direct extension (e.g., to duodenum, bile ducts, or stomach)
T3	Extension incompatible with resection

Nodal disease

N0	None
N1	Regional nodal disease

Distant metastases

M0	None
M1	Distant metastatic disease

—elevated alkaline phosphatase.

—mild elevations of amylase.

4. **Nonspecific tumor markers** include

—mucin-associated carbohydrate antigens (e.g., **CA 19–9**).

—carcinoembryonic antigen (**CEA**).

—mutated **c-K-*ras***.

5. **Important imaging modalities** include

—contrast-enhanced dynamic CT.

—magnetic resonance cholangiopancreatography (MRCP).

—ERCP.

—percutaneous transhepatic cholangiography (PTHC).

—radiolabeled octreotide scanning.

—endoscopic ultrasound.

6. **Radiographic studies**

—may reveal a classic "**double duct sign**" (**Figure 17-5**) when both the pancreatic and common bile ducts are dilated.

7. **Fine-needle aspiration (FNA)** remains somewhat controversial.

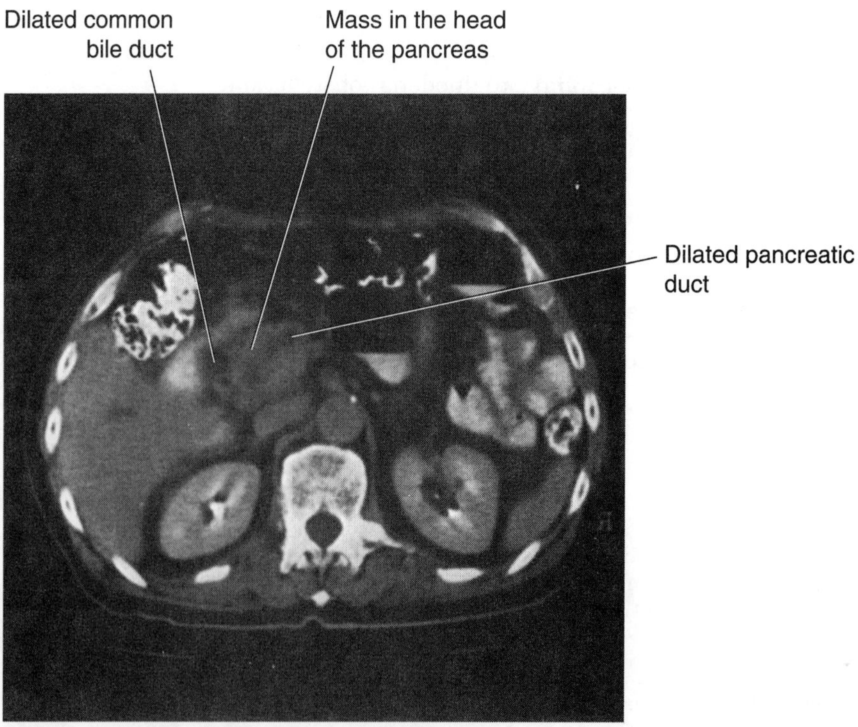

Figure 17-5. Carcinoma of the head of the pancreas near the ampulla of Vater. CT scan demonstrates dilation of both the pancreatic and bile ducts ("double duct sign"). (Reprinted with permission from Howard JM, Idezuki Y, Ihse I, Prinz RA: *Surgical Diseases of the Pancreas,* 3rd ed. Baltimore, Williams & Wilkins, 1987, p 141.)

—It does, however, appear to have reasonable sensitivity (≈70%) and excellent specificity (100%).

D. Treatment of pancreatic adenocarcinoma

1. **Cure** can only be achieved with **surgical resection.**
2. **Resectability** is definitively determined intraoperatively, although spiral CT and MRI can predict vascular involvement.
   a. **Laparotomy allows palpation of the**
      —pancreatic head.
      —superior mesenteric artery.
      —superior mesenteric vein.
      —portal veins.
      —nodal beds.
   b. **Laparoscopy is less invasive**
      —but requires the use of ultrasound to evaluate for vascular invasion and nonvisible nodal beds.
   c. **Contraindications** to curative resection include
      —**liver metastases.**
      —**peritoneal metastases.**
      —**nodal metastases beyond the zone of resection** (e.g., periaortic).
      —**tumor invasion** of the superior mesenteric artery.
3. The **type of resection depends** on tumor location.
   a. **Tumors of the head**
      —require a **Whipple procedure** [see II E 6 b (2)].
   b. **Tumors of the tail and body**
      —are treated by distal or extended **distal** (near-total) **pancreatectomy.**
   c. **Total pancreatectomy**
      —for pancreatic cancer is generally avoided.
4. Pre- or postoperative **adjuvant chemoradiotherapy**
   —(**5-fluorouracil** and external beam radiation) may increase 2-year survival rates.
5. **Complications of pancreaticoduodenectomy** include
   —delayed gastric emptying.
   —**pancreatic fistula** (10%–20%).
   —infection.
   —bile leak.
   —pancreatitis.
6. **Postoperative prognosis may be affected by**
   —lymph node involvement.
   —vascular invasion.
   —a clear margin of resection.
   —the need for blood transfusions.

7. **Patients with unresectable tumors**

—may require palliative surgery to treat intractable jaundice or duodenal obstruction.

a. **Jaundice**

—can be palliated by internal or external biliary stents or a biliary bypass (choledochojejunostomy).

b. **Duodenal obstruction**

—can be treated by gastrojejunostomy.

IV. Endocrine Pancreatic Neoplasms

—are **rare,** occurring at a rate of 5 cases per million people per year.

A. Endocrine pancreatic tumors

—arise from neural crest cells called amine precursor uptake and decarboxylation (APUD) cells.

—may be **functional** or **nonfunctional,** presenting as a space-occupying lesion (**Table 17-3**).

1. **Functional tumors**

a. **Insulinomas**

—are the most common endocrine tumor of the pancreas.

—Most (90%) insulinomas are **benign.**

Table 17-3. Endocrine Tumors of the Pancreas

Tumor	Features	Usual Site	Diagnosis	% Malignant	Treatment
Insulinoma	**Whipple's triad**	Pancreas, evenly distributed	Fasting glucose and insulin levels	**10%**	Enucleation or resection
Gastrinoma	**Peptic ulcers, diarrhea**	**Gastronoma triangle**	Secretin stimulation test	**50%**	Resection, omeprazole
VIPoma	**Watery diarrhea, hypokalemia, achlorhydria**	Distal pancreas	Elevated PP and VIP in setting of diarrhea	**> 50%**	Resection, distal pancreatectomy, octreotide
Glucagonoma	**Diabetes, necrolytic migratory erythema**	Body and tail of pancreas	Skin biopsy, fasting glucagon level	**> 80%**	Resection, distal or extended-distal pancreatectomy
Somatostatinoma	Diabetes, steatorrhea, gallstones	Periampullary head of pancreas	Fasting somatostatin level	**> 90%**	Resection of bulky disease, cholecystectomy
Nonfunctional	Large mass: **pain, weight loss, jaundice**	Throughout pancreas	Abdominal imaging: CT/MRI	**50%–90%**	Resection, chemotherapy

VIPoma = vasoactive intestinal peptide tumor; PP = pancreatic polypeptide; CT = computed tomography; MRI = magnetic resonance imaging.

(1) Symptoms

(a) Most patients present with **catecholamine surge**–related symptoms, such as palpitations, diaphoresis, and tachycardia induced by hypoglycemia and relieved by carbohydrates.

(b) Whipple's triad is typically documented:

—symptomatic hypoglycemia during fasting.

—serum glucose measurements of less than 50 mg/dL.

—relief of symptoms when administered glucose.

(2) Diagnosis

(a) Insulinomas are diagnosed by concomitantly measuring **insulin** and **glucose** levels during a monitored fasting period of 12–18 hours.

(b) Measuring **proinsulin** or **C-peptide levels** can exclude the possibility of surreptitious insulin.

(3) Fewer than 10% of patients with insulinoma

—have the multiple endocrine neoplasia (MEN) I syndrome, but those that do often have multiple insulinomas (see Chapter 20).

b. Gastrinomas typically present with

—abdominal pain.

—intractable peptic ulcer disease (PUD).

(1) Of patients with **recurrent PUD,** 2% have gastrinomas.

(2) Occurrence

—Seventy-five percent of gastrinomas occur **sporadically.**

—Twenty-five percent occur in patients with MEN type 1 (see Chapter 20).

(3) Gastrinomas are associated with

—amplification of the ***HER-2/neu*** proto-oncogene.

(4) Initial diagnosis

—is confirmed with the **secretin stimulation test.**

(5) Gastrinomas typically (90%) **are found**

—within the **gastrinoma triangle (Figure 17-6)**.

(6) Half of these tumors are **malignant.**

c. Vasoactive intestinal peptide tumors (VIPomas)

—present with the **Verner-Morrison** or **WDHA syndrome** (watery diarrhea, hypokalemia, and achlorhydria.)

(1) Diagnosis

—of these tumors is typically made by excluding other causes of diarrhea and documenting elevated VIP levels.

(2) Ten percent of VIPomas are extrapancreatic (i.e., retroperitoneum, thorax).

(3) Over 50% of VIPomas present with **metastatic** disease to lymph nodes or liver.

d. Glucagonomas present with

—severe dermatitis.

—diabetes.

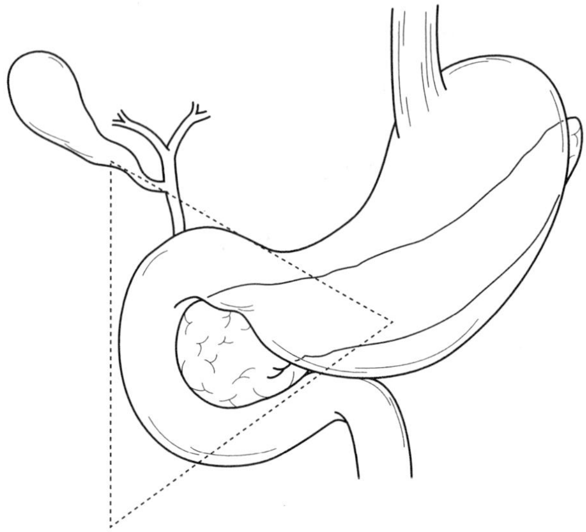

Figure 17-6. Gastrinoma triangle. (Reprinted with permission from Greenfield LJ, Mulholland MW, Oldham KT, Zelenock GB: *Surgery: Scientific Principles and Practice,* 2nd ed. Philadelphia, Lippincott-Raven, 1997, p 839.)

—stomatitis.

—weight loss.

(1) The **dermatitis**

—is called **necrolytic migratory erythema.**

—tends to wax and wane in severity, spreading in a serpentine-like fashion.

(2) Skin biopsy aids in diagnosis

—but elevated fasting **glucagon levels** are more conclusive.

(3) These **tumors tend to be**

—fairly large.

—easily seen by contrast-enhanced CT.

e. Somatostatinomas

—have less distinguishable symptomatology often including steatorrhea, diabetes, hypochlorhydria, and gallstones.

—These tumors are **very rare,** occurring in fewer than 1 in 40 million people per year.

2. Nonfunctional tumors

a. These tumors present

—with symptoms of pain, weight loss, and jaundice because they are large and **space-occupying.**

b. Nonfunctional endocrine tumors

—tend to have a protracted, indolent course relative to pancreatic carcinomas.

c. Pancreatic polypeptide levels

—may be elevated in these patients, but this is not specific for these tumors.

B. Treatment

1. **All pancreatic endocrine tumors**

—are primarily treated by resection.

a. **Metastatic disease** precludes curative resection.

b. The **type of resection indicated**

—depends on the tumor **histology** and **location** (see **Table 17-3**).

(1) **Insulinomas** can usually be **enucleated** although some may require formal resection.

(2) **Gastrinomas** and **somatostatinomas** typically require pancreaticoduodenectomy.

(3) **VIPomas** and **glucagonomas** usually require distal pancreatectomy.

(4) **Nonfunctional tumors** may require either a Whipple procedure or a distal pancreatectomy.

2. **Octreotide**

—(or omeprazole for gastrinoma) may be helpful in ameliorating symptoms in patients with VIPomas and glucagonomas.

3. **Chemotherapy**

—(e.g., streptozocin and doxorubicin) may be helpful with nonfunctional pancreatic endocrine tumors and insulinomas.

4. **Radiotherapy** has not improved survival.

C. Survival rates

1. **Insulomas**

—Over 90% are **curable** with resection.

2. **Gastrinomas**

—Sixty to seventy percent are curable with resection.

3. **Somatostatinomas**

—Most are **incurable.**

4. **Nonfunctional tumors**

—After resection, the **5-year survival rate** is 50%.

V. Spleen

A. Embryology

1. **The spleen arises** from **mesenchymal cells** in the dorsal mesogastrium.

2. **Accessory spleens** occur in **20%** of people and are most frequently found within the splenic hilum or the splenic ligaments.

B. Anatomy

1. The **arterial blood supply** is primarily via the **splenic artery,** which does not branch until it enters the hilum.

a. **Short gastric vessels**

—emanate from the left gastroepiploic artery supplying some arterial blood.

b. The **venous drainage vessels**

—parallel the arterial supply with the splenic vein abutting the posteroinferior aspect of the pancreas.

2. The **splenic parenchyma consists of**

—**red pulp** (erythrocytes).

—**white pulp** (lymphocytes and monocytes).

3. **Blood either passes** through capillaries directly into venous **sinusoids** (closed circulation), or into the red pulp (open circulation).

C. **Physiology of the spleen**

1. The **red pulp** of the spleen acts as a **filter** to remove damaged or aged erythrocytes.

2. The **white pulp** of the spleen harbors leukocytes that serve to mount both nonspecific and specific **immune responses.**

a. **Within the spleen macrophages phagocytose**

—cellular, particulate debris and poorly **opsonized bacteria.**

b. The **lymphocyte population**

—produces a large percentage of nonspecific **opsonins** including **tuftsin, properdin,** and fibronectin.

c. **Antigen processing**

—occurs in the spleen upon interaction between macrophages and helper T cells.

VI. Diseases Treated by Splenectomy (Table 17-4)

A. **Splenic trauma**

—is the **primary indication** for splenectomy.

1. **Splenic injuries**

—are **graded** by severity (**Table 17-5**).

2. **Indications for operative intervention** associated with splenic trauma include

—**hemodynamic instability.**

—**arterial "blushing" or "pooling of contrast" on abdominal CT.**

—**active bleeding** confirmed by falling blood counts and the need for blood transfusions (> 2 units packed red blood cells [PRBC]).

3. **Patients with grade IV or V injuries**

—generally require splenectomy.

4. **Primary repair of the spleen (splenorrhaphy)**

—should be attempted only in hemodynamically stable patients.

B. **Hereditary spherocytosis (HS)**

1. HS is a **hereditary disease**

Table 17-4. Indications for Splenectomy

Disease	Description and Caveats
Trauma	**Resection with hilar involvement, significant parenchymal disruption, active bleeding**
ITP	Steroid therapy; IV gamma globulin and plasmapheresis are primary therapies; **resection reserved for refractory disease**
TTP	Resection as last resort after failed medical therapy
Myeloproliferative diseases	Resection for symptomatic splenomegaly—may reduce transfusion requirements
Lymphoma	Resection occasionally indicated for **symptomatic splenomegaly**
Hereditary spherocytosis	**Resection is curative**
Felty's syndrome	Resection improves responses to infection and treats symptomatic splenomegaly
Splenic abscess	CT-guided percutaneous drainage occasionally successful, otherwise resection
Parasitic cysts	Resection indicated
Sarcoidosis, Gaucher's disease	Resection for **symptomatic splenomegaly** may improve symptoms
Splenic vein thrombosis	Resection cures the sinistral portal hypertension

ITP = idiopathic thrombocytopenic purpura; IV = intravenous; TTP = thrombotic thrombocytopenic purpura; CT = computed tomography.

—transmitted by an **autosomal dominant** trait.

—characterized by the formation of **poorly deformable erythrocyte membranes.**

2. **Red blood cells**

—are **sequestered** and destroyed by the spleen.

3. **Patients**

—become anemic.

—become jaundiced.

—develop splenomegaly.

4. **Splenectomy** is **curative** and should be delayed until age 4.

C. Idiopathic thrombocytopenic purpura (ITP)

—occurs as a result of the development of **anti-platelet antibodies** (immunoglobulin [Ig]G) that direct platelet destruction and sequestration in the spleen.

Table 17-5. Grading System for Classification of Splenic Injuries

Grade	Description of Injury
I	**Subcapsular hematoma < 10% surface area, capsular tear < 1 cm**
II	Subcapsular/intraparenchymal hematoma 10%–50% surface area/< 5 cm diameter, laceration 1 cm–3 cm depth
III	Large (> 50% surface area, > 5 cm diameter) subcapsular/intraperitoneal hematoma, expanding or ruptured hematoma, > 3 cm laceration involving trabecular vessel
IV	Laceration involving hilar or segmental vessel
V	**Hilar avulsion or shattered spleen**

1. The **clinical manifestations**
   —occur as a result of **thrombocytopenia:** purpura, ecchymoses, bleeding from mucosal surfaces, and hematuria.
   —The spleen is **not** enlarged.
2. **Treatment**
   a. **Initial treatment** should include
      —**corticosteroids** and IV **gamma globulin** directed at binding and neutralizing the antiplatelet antibodies.
   b. For **refractory cases**
      —that do not respond to steroids, Vinca alkaloids, cyclophosphamide, danazol, and plasmapheresis have been used.
   c. **Splenectomy**
      —is frequently effective.
      —is reserved for patients who fail medical therapy or require continued steroid therapy to maintain adequate platelet counts.
   d. **Platelet transfusions**
      —should **not** be given **preoperatively.**
      —**should** be given after the splenic blood supply is ligated.

D. **Thrombotic thrombocytopenic purpura (TTP)**
   —is characterized by **diffuse aggregation of platelets.**
   —Hyaline membrane deposits throughout capillary systems, causing profound thrombocytopenia.
   1. A **pentad syndrome**
      —of **fever, purpura, hemolytic anemia, hematuria, and neurologic changes** is typical.
   2. **Hemolytic uremic syndrome (HUS)**
      —of children has a similar presentation and disease course.
   3. **Treatment**
      a. **Plasmapheresis** is the mainstay of treatment.
      b. **Splenectomy** is reserved for patients with disease refractory to plasmapheresis and is frequently unsuccessful at effectively treating TTP.

E. **Splenic abscesses**
   —are typically caused by hematogenous spread of a bacterial infection (**endocarditis** and **IV drug abuse** most common).
   —may be amenable to CT-guided percutaneous drainage but may require splenectomy.

VII. Hypersplerism

—refers to a **condition associated with splenomegaly,** decreased and/or **dysfunctional circulating platelets,** and responsive **bone marrow hypertrophy.**

A. **Types**
   1. **Primary hypersplenism**

—is very rare and is a diagnosis of exclusion.

2. **Secondary hypersplenism** is more common and is associated with several diseases, such as
   —myeloproliferative diseases.
   —infections (e.g., mononucleosis).
   —portal hypertension.
   —congestive heart failure.
   —Felty's syndrome (arthritis, splenomegaly, neutropenia).
   —amyloidosis.
   —sarcoidosis.
   —malignancies (e.g., lymphomas).
   —acquired immunodeficiency syndrome (AIDS).
   —Gaucher's disease.
   —polycythemia vera.
   —systemic lupus erythematosus.

B. **Splenectomy** is generally indicated

—in patients with **primary hypersplenism.**

—in symptomatic splenomegaly associated with secondary hypersplenism (see Table 17-4).

VIII. Overwhelming Postsplenectomy Infection (OPSI)

A. **After splenectomy**

—patients are at risk for developing a life-threatening bacterial infection (0.5%).

B. **Mortality**

—from OPSI can be as high as **80%–90%.**

C. **Causes of OPSI**

—are most often related to **encapsulated organisms,** particularly *pneumococcal* species (*Streptococcus pneumoniae*).

D. **Prophylaxis**

—should include **vaccination** against *Pneumococcal species, Meningococcal species, and Haemophilus influenza B.*

—**Vaccinations** should ideally be given 10 days before splenectomy.

—After splenectomy **children** should also receive prophylactic **penicillin** through adolescence.

E. **Infections**

—in postsplenectomy patients should be aggressively diagnosed and treated.

Review Test

Directions: Each of the numbered items or incomplete statements in this section is followed by answers or by completions of the statement. Select the ONE lettered answer or completion that is BEST in each case.

1. A 52-year-old man presented to his primary care physician 3 months ago with severe epigastric pain after an episode of hematemesis. Esophagogastroduodenoscopy (EGD) at that time revealed two large peptic ulcers in the first portion of the duodenum. He was placed on omeprazole after *Helicobacter pylori* titers were negative. After 6 weeks he returned to his physician with improved but continued pain. Repeat EGD revealed that the original ulcers were significantly smaller but there were several new ulcers both in the duodenum and in the antrum of the stomach. What is the next most appropriate step in the management of this patient?

(A) Repeat EGD in 6 weeks
(B) Abdominal ultrasound
(C) Highly selective vagotomy
(D) Vagotomy and pyloroplasty
(E) Secretin stimulation test

2. A patient with a suspected gastrinoma has a markedly elevated serum gastrin level and the level failed to drop appropriately after secretin administration. Abdominopelvic computed tomography (CT) scan failed to reveal any pancreatic mass. Endoscopic ultrasound was also unrevealing. Which of the following would be the most appropriate next step in managing this patient?

(A) Distal pancreatectomy
(B) Vagotomy and pyloroplasty
(C) Mobilization of the duodenum and intraoperative ultrasound
(D) Whipple procedure (pancreaticoduodenectomy)
(E) Metronidazole, omeprazole, and clarithromycin therapy

3. A 45-year-old man presents to the emergency room complaining of severe epigastric pain that radiates to his back and left scapula. He has had severe nausea and vomiting associated with the pain for 3 days. Nothing seems to relieve his pain. He drinks about a fifth of bourbon a day. He has not had a bowel movement in several days. He also complains of a very dry mouth. He is afebrile and normotensive with a heart rate of 110 beats/min. He is mildly tender on abdominal examination. His serum amylase level is 650 IU/L. Which of the following is the most appropriate initial step in the management of this patient?

(A) Exploratory laparotomy and pancreatic débridement
(B) Discharge and close follow up as outpatient
(C) Obtain an abdominopelvic computed tomography (CT) scan
(D) Perform esophagogastroduodenoscopy (EGD)
(E) Admit for intravenous (IV) hydration and withhold oral feeding

4. A 57-year-old man with a history of biliary colic presents with a 2-day history of severe epigastric and left upper quadrant (LUQ) pain, intractable nausea, and vomiting. He was admitted to an outside hospital for intravenous (IV) hydration, but over the first 24 hours of his hospital course he became progressively more ill. Abdominopelvic computed tomography (CT) scan demonstrated an enlarged common bile duct, a markedly edematous pancreas with portions of the pancreas which do not enhance, and several liters of ascites. His left flank became markedly ecchymotic, and his abdomen became progressively more distended. He was then transferred to the intensive care unit at your tertiary care hospital. Despite infusion of 10 L of crystalloid over the last 12 hours, he remains hypotensive. Laboratory studies reveal a white blood cell count of 24,000, a Po_2 of 55 mm Hg, a blood glucose of 280 mg/dL, bilirubin of 4.3, and a lactate dehydrogenase of 495 IU/L. Based on Ranson's criteria, which of the following indicates this patient's mortality risk upon entering the intensive care unit?

(A) 0%
(B) 20%
(C) 40%
(D) 80%
(E) 100%

5. A patient with necrotizing pancreatitis would benefit most from which of the following therapeutic measures?

(A) Placement of a pulmonary artery catheter
(B) Blood transfusion
(C) Endoscopic pancreatic stent placement
(D) Emergent surgical exploration
(E) Initiation of broad spectrum antibiotic therapy with imipenem/cilastatin

6. A patient with a high-output pancreatic fistula is most likely to suffer from which one of the following metabolic derangements?

(A) Hyponatremia
(B) Hyperkalemia
(C) Respiratory alkalosis
(D) Metabolic acidosis
(E) Metabolic alkalosis

7. A 39-year-old woman presents with severe epigastric pain, nausea and vomiting. She states she has been anorexic for 2 days. She weighs 240 lb and gave birth to her fourth child 2 years ago. Examination reveals mild tachycardia and abdominal tenderness in the epigastrium and the left upper quadrant (LUQ). Ultrasound examination demonstrates multiple large gallstones in the gallbladder and a dilated common bile duct. The pancreas was poorly visualized secondary to her body habitus. Her serum bilirubin is measured at 3.8 mg/dL, amylase at 1,200 IU/L, lipase at > 6,000 IU/L, and white blood cell count at 17,500. In addition to intravenous (IV) hydration, which of the following is the most appropriate approach to managing this patient?

(A) Antibiotics and endoscopic retrograde cholangiopancreatography (ERCP) with endoscopic sphincterotomy
(B) Antibiotics and exploratory laparotomy
(C) Observation
(D) Antibiotics and observation
(E) Antibiotics and laparoscopic cholecystectomy

8. A 73-year-old man is brought to your clinic by his wife because of her concerns of his "wasting away." He describes having lost 60 lb over the last 6 months. He appears cachectic with a scaphoid abdomen. You note a fullness to his epigastrium. Abdominopelvic computed tomography (CT) reveals a mass in the head of the pancreas and a 3-cm hypodense lesion in the liver. Which of the following is appropriate in the management of this patient?

(A) Pancreaticoduodenectomy (Whipple procedure)
(B) Image-guided percutaneous biopsy of the liver lesion
(C) Radiotherapy
(D) Choledochojejunostomy
(E) Total pancreatectomy

9. A 41-year-old woman with human immunodeficiency virus (HIV) presents to her physician with complaints of bleeding gums and easy bruising throughout her extremities. Examination reveals a palpable spleen below the left costal margin, multiple soft tissue ecchymoses of her extremities, and multiple petechiae on her hands and feet. Blood counts reveal a platelet count of 27,000/μL. Evaluation of the plasma reveals antiplatelet antibodies. Which of the following is the most appropriate initial therapy?

(A) Glucocorticoids
(B) Platelet infusions
(C) Splenectomy
(D) Methotrexate
(E) Danazol

10. A 54-year-old woman presents with complaints of intermittent episodes of marked diaphoresis and palpitations. She describes feeling like her heart is racing during these episodes, and it makes her feel quite anxious. She has learned that eating food will relieve her symptoms. Screening laboratory tests reveal a blood glucose level of 55 mg/dL. The woman weighs 122 lb and appears otherwise healthy. A fasting glucose level performed the next day was 50 mg/dL and her serum insulin level was markedly above fasting norms. Abdominopelvic computed tomography (CT) demonstrated a discrete, 1-cm tumor in the body of the pancreas. Which of the following is the most appropriate therapy for this patient?

(A) Oral propranolol therapy
(B) Wide local excision of the tumor
(C) Distal pancreatectomy
(D) Enucleation of the tumor
(E) Pancreaticoduodenectomy

11. A 38-year-old woman with no history of alcohol use or cholelithiasis has suffered from intermittent epigastric abdominal pain, nausea, and vomiting for most of her adult life. She takes no medicines. Recently, evaluations have included esophagogastroduodenoscopy, an upper gastrointestinal barium study, and an abdominal ultrasound that have all been unrevealing. She now presents with the same constellation of symptoms. Examination is unremarkable, however laboratory studies reveal an amylase of 1200 IU/L and a lipase of 4400 IU/L. Repeat abdominopelvic computed tomography (CT) scan reveals only an edematous pancreatic head. Which of the following is the next most reasonable diagnostic or therapeutic modality?

(A) Endoscopic ultrasound
(B) Percutaneous transhepatic cholangiography (PTHC)
(C) Enteroclysis
(D) Hepatobiliary scintigraphy (HIDA scan)
(E) Endoscopic retrograde cholangiography (ERCP)

12. A 22-year-old woman presents to the emergency room after having fallen off a galloping horse. She complains of left lower chest wall pain and is mildly short of breath. She is hemodynamically stable. There is a large bruise over her left flank. Chest radiograph demonstrates several fractured ribs on the lower left side. Abdominopelvic computed tomography (CT) scan reveals a 1 x 3 cm^2 subcapsular splenic hematoma and some fluid adjacent to the spleen. Which of the following is the most appropriate next step in the management of this patient?

(A) Emergent splenectomy
(B) Splenorrhaphy
(C) Pneumococcal vaccine administration
(D) Chest wall splinting
(E) Bedrest and observation

13. A 26-year-old man presents to his primary physician with complaints of intermittent, crampy epigastric pain, nausea, and vomiting shortly after eating. He usually vomits undigested food and this relieves the pain and nausea. He has preferred to eat soft foods his whole life, and he often relies on liquids. He is otherwise healthy and well-developed. Upper gastrointestinal barium study reveals a markedly narrowed second portion of the duodenum. Laboratory studies are unremarkable. Which of the following is the most likely diagnosis for this patient?

(A) Gallstone pancreatitis
(B) Pancreatic carcinoma
(C) Pancreas divisum
(D) Annular pancreas
(E) Cholelithiasis

14. A 44-year-old woman was hospitalized 3 weeks earlier with acute pancreatitis believed to be secondary to the azathioprine therapy, which was used as maintenance immunosuppressive for her transplanted kidney. The azathioprine therapy was discontinued, and she gradually recovered. She presents to clinic today with a new complaint of early satiety, intermittent nausea, and one episode of postprandial vomiting. Abdominopelvic computed tomography (CT) reveals a 5-cm, round, fluid collection within the lesser sac. Which of the following is the most appropriate therapy for the management of this patient?

(A) Observation and follow-up CT in 3–6 weeks
(B) Laparotomy and cystgastrostomy
(C) Gastroscopy and endoscopic cystgastrostomy
(D) Percutaneous drainage
(E) Restart azathioprine therapy

15. Patients having undergone splenectomy are at increased risk of developing overwhelming sepsis from which of the following organisms?

(A) *Helicobacter pylori*
(B) *Klebsiella pneumoniae*
(C) *Bacteroides fragilis*
(D) *Staphylococcus aureus*
(E) *Enterococcus faecium*

16. A 48-year-old, alcoholic male has been hospitalized over the last 20 years more than 30 times for episodes of acute pancreatitis. He now presents to the emergency department complaining of mid-back pain and horribly malodorous and frequent soft stools. He describes that the stools float in the toilet. He also explains that he has lost 30 lb over the last 6 months. Which of the following therapeutic measures is the best option to improve this patient's health maintenance?

(A) Total pancreatectomy
(B) Oral pancreatic enzyme replacement
(C) Total parenteral nutrition
(D) Octreotide therapy
(E) High-fat diet

17. A 57-year-old, male alcoholic with chronic pancreatitis has had several episodes of acute pancreatitis in the last year. Today he presents to the emergency department with hematemesis. After admission to the intensive care unit and resuscitation, esophagogastroduodenoscopy (EGD) reveals large gastric varices, one of which is actively bleeding. The bleeding varix is successfully banded, but over the next 12 hours the patient's hematocrit continues to fall despite blood transfusions, and fresh blood continues to drain from a nasogastric tube. Upon review of an abdominal computed tomography (CT) scan performed 1 month ago you note a markedly calcified pancreas, large gastric varices, and no enhancement of the splenic vein. Which of the following is the most appropriate next step in the management of this patient?

(A) Emergent splenectomy
(B) Repeat EGD and sclerotherapy
(C) Sengstaken-Blakemore tube placement
(D) Excision of the gastric varices
(E) Intravenous (IV) vasopressin

18. A 33-year-old woman presents with complaints of frequent paroxysms of profuse diaphoresis and a "racing heart." She has seen several physicians about these concerns, but none have "helped her." Occasionally, these episodes result in her fainting. She generally feels better if she eats right after the onset of symptoms. A portable glucometer demonstrates that she has a normal blood glucose level in your clinic. Reports from other physicians demonstrate that she has had several low blood glucose levels and elevated insulin levels documented. She explains that her symptoms do not occur every day. Which of the following laboratory tests may aid in establishing her diagnosis?

(A) Glucagon level
(B) Lactate dehydrogenase level
(C) Erythrocyte sedimentation rate
(D) C-peptide level
(E) Somatostatin stimulation test

Answers and Explanations

1–E. This patient may have Zollinger-Ellison syndrome (gastrinoma with intractable peptic ulcer disease), although this must be initially confirmed. A secretin stimulation test is often diagnostic. In patients with ZE syndrome, secretin administration increases serum gastrin levels, in contrast to the normal physiologic inhibition of gastrin secretion by secretin. Repeating the esophagogastroduodenoscopy (EGD) is unnecessary at this time because the patient does not seem to be actively bleeding. Abdominal ultrasound would not be particularly helpful, but once diagnosed, a gastrinoma can at times be localized by endoscopic ultrasound. Neither ulcer operation (vagotomy or pyloroplasty) is indicated before ruling out a gastrinoma.

2–C. Gastrinomas are located in the gastrinoma triangle in the majority of cases. They can often be seen by abdominal computed tomography (CT), magnetic resonance imaging (MRI), or endoscopic ultrasound. Other localizing modalities include selective portal venous gastrin sampling or radiolabeled octreotide scanning. Alternatively, as in this question, it is reasonable to explore the abdomen, initially focusing on the gastrinoma triangle by exposing and examining the duodenum and pancreatic head using intraoperative ultrasound. Neither distal pancreatectomy nor a Whipple procedure should be performed before more aggressive attempts are made at localizing the tumor. Ulcer operations are not indicated in patients with Zollinger-Ellison syndrome; even those with unresectable or metastatic tumors should be treated with omeprazole. This patient does not have *Helicobacter pylori,* thus antibiotic therapy would not be appropriate.

3–E. This patient has acute pancreatis most likely secondary to alcoholism. He does not appear to have peritonitis nor is he in extremis. He has signs of intestinal ileus and is assuredly dehydrated. The initial management of a patient with acute pancreatitis should be fluid resuscitation and restriction of oral intake. Surgery for acute pancreatitis is reserved for patients with complications of pancreatitis or infected pancreatic necrosis. Discharging a severely dehydrated patient with acute pancreatitis would not be safe. Esophagogastroduodenoscopy would not be helpful in the initial management of this patient and would not be well tolerated. An abdominopelvic computed tomography (CT) scan is useful in evaluating patients with severe, acute pancreatitis, to help in identifying signs of pancreatic necrosis and fluid collections, but it is not indicated initially in patients with uncomplicated pancreatitis.

4–C. This patient has hemorrhagic necrotizing pancreatitis which is made evident by his Grey Turner sign (left flank ecchymosis) and the computed tomographic findings. With a history of biliary colic, the pancreatitis is likely secondary to gallstones. He has at least six of Ranson's criteria, notably (1) age over 55, (2) fluid sequestration > 10 L, (3) white blood cell count > 16,000, (4) $Po_2 < 60$, (5) glucose > 200, (6) lactase dehydrogenase > 350. His mortality risk is at least 40%.

5–E. While placement of a pulmonary artery catheter may help manage the fluid resuscitation of this patient, its use has not been shown to significantly improve patient outcome. Blood transfusion may be appropriate to improve oxygen-carrying capacity in the setting of retroperitoneal hemorrhage, but without blood loss or hemolysis there is no benefit to transfusion. Placement of an endoscopically placed pancreatic stent in the setting of necrotizing pancreatitis would likely worsen the pancreatitis. Emergent surgical exploration is not recommended in the initial treatment of patients with sterile necrotizing pancreatitis because patient survival has not been improved by this approach. The patient with necrotizing pancreatitis should be assumed to have sterile necrosis until proven otherwise. Those patients who have culture-proven bacterial sepsis or signs of deterioration despite aggressive supportive care should undergo a fine-needle aspiration of pancreatic fluid collections or necrotic debris for Gram stain and culture to prove the presence of infected necrosis. The presence of infected necrosis then dictates surgical débridement. The use of imipenem/cilastatin in patients with necrotizing pancreatitis has been shown to decrease infection-related complications and, therefore, would benefit the patient.

6–D. Patients with high-output pancreatic fistulae can develop a profound metabolic acidosis secondary to loss of bicarbonate in the pancreatic secretions. These patients may partially compensate by increasing their minute ventilation, however this compensation is not enough to cause an alkalosis. Octreotide therapy is often helpful in decreasing the volume of output from the fistula, and thus decreasing the amount of lost bicarbonate. These patients generally do not develop significant hyponatremia or hyperkalemia.

7–A. This patient has gallstone pancreatitis with both laboratory and ultrasound evidence suggesting an impacted gallstone at the ampulla of Vater. The most appropriate care would involve fluid resuscitation followed by endoscopic stone extraction, cholangiopancreatography, and sphincterotomy. Any time endoscopic retrograde cholangiopancreatography (ERCP) is performed, the patient should be given prophylactic antibiotics because of the associated risk of cholangitis. Based on the information given, neither exploratory laparotomy nor cholecystectomy is indicated at this time. The patient's gallbladder should be removed electively after resolution of her gallstone pancreatitis to prevent recurrence. Observation in the setting of an impacted gallstone is likely to worsen the severity of pancreatitis and lead to cholangitis.

8–B. This patient likely has pancreatic carcinoma with a metastasis to the liver. First, the liver lesion should be biopsied before embarking on resection of the primary tumor. This could be achieved either percutaneously, laparoscopically, or by laparotomy. If feasible, percutaneous needle biopsy is the least invasive and the most desirable as a first step in planning the care of this patient. A Whipple procedure is generally not indicated in patients with stage IV pancreatic carcinoma. Total pancreatectomy is no longer recommended for pancreatic carcinoma. Biliary bypass (choledochojejunostomy) is not indicated in patients with metastatic pancreatic carcinoma who do not have biliary obstruction. Radiotherapy for end-stage pancreatic carcinoma is ineffective.

9–A. Patients with human immunodeficiency virus (HIV) are at increased risk of developing idiopathic thrombocytopenic purpura (ITP), which is what this patient has. Patients typically develop antiplatelet antibodies that appear to facilitate platelet sequestration and destruction in the spleen. Initial therapy includes using steroids and intravenous (IV) immunoglobulin (Ig)G therapy to induce a remission. Patients will typically respond to the steroids by an increase in their platelet counts. If the platelet counts begin to fall upon steroid withdrawal, splenectomy is indicated. Refractory cases that do not respond to steroids may respond to other agents like cyclophosphamide and danazol. Platelet infusions should generally not be given to patients with ITP before splenectomy because these platelets will quickly be sequestered in the spleen and will not function. Immediately after splenectomy, platelets may be given. Life-threatening hemorrhage should be treated with emergent IgG therapy. Methotrexate is an antineoplastic agent and therefore not appropriate in this case.

10–D. This woman has an insulinoma. She is experiencing catecholamine surges at times of profound hypoglycemia as a compensatory mechanism to promote glycogenolysis and release of glucose stores. Propranolol may help ameliorate the palpitations and anxiety, but it will not address the underlying problem. Over 90% of insulinomas are benign, and most can be successfully enucleated. The lesion described is small and enucleation should be curative. Distal pancreatectomy is possible, but is more resection than is necessary, and pancreaticoduodenectomy would not address her tumor.

11–E. This patient has signs of acute pancreatitis based on her clinical presentation, laboratory, and radiologic evaluation. With no history of alcohol consumption or gallstones other causes must be ruled out. Pancreas divisum is often a cause of intermittent acute pancreatitis in patients in whom other causes have been ruled out. The best way to identify an anatomical cause of this patient's acute pancreatitis is by endoscopic retrograde cholangiography (ERCP). Moreover, ERCP has the advantage over other imaging techniques by allowing treatment options at the time of the investigation (i.e., endoscopic sphincterotomy or pancreatic duct stent placement). Repeat ultrasound would offer no additional information. Percutaneous transhepatic cholangiography (PTHC) is more difficult in the absence of a dilated biliary tree and does not often provide good detail of the pancreatic ductal anatomy. Enteroclysis will not address the question of etiology of pancreatitis. Hepatobiliary scintigraphy does not provide any image of the pancreatic ducts.

12–E. This patient has a grade II splenic injury and is hemodynamically stable. This warrants a conservative management with close observation and bedrest for a defined period of time (3–7 days). Emergent splenectomy would be premature and likely subject this patient to the risks of laparotomy and splenectomy unnecessarily. Splenorrhaphy would be an appropriate option (as would splenectomy) if this patient did not tolerate conservative management (i.e., she continued to bleed and required blood transfusions while being observed). The pneumococcal vaccine should only be given if the patient undergoes splenectomy. Chest wall splinting is unnecessary, would further restrict her chest wall motion, and would not address her splenic injury.

13–D. This patient has symptoms of gastric outlet obstruction or, as in this case, duodenal obstruction. Several of these diseases could result in duodenal obstruction. However, the fact that he is young, otherwise healthy, and has avoided solid foods all his life suggests he has a congenital problem. He does not describe symptoms of biliary colic nor does he have signs of cancer. Episodic pain is not typical during bouts of acute pancreatitis, and pancreas divisum does not cause duodenal obstruction. Annular pancreas fits best with his history, his constellation of present symptoms, and his upper gastrointestinal study.

14–A. This patient, who recovered from an episode of acute pancreatitis 3 weeks ago, appears to have an evolving pancreatic pseudocyst. The majority of small pseudocysts (< 5 cm) will resolve spontaneously. Those larger are likely to require intervention. Pseudocysts should not be drained until they have a mature capsule, which generally takes 6–8 weeks from the time of the acute pancreatitis. Therefore, none of the drainage procedures (laparotomy and cystgastrostomy; gastroscopy and endoscopic cystgastrostomy; percutaneous drainage) are appropriate only 3 weeks after the resolution of the acute pancreatitis. The inciting agent—azathioprine—should not be restarted this early. It can be substituted with other agents if necessary.

15–B. Overwhelming postsplenectomy infection (OPSI) is an uncommon event, occurring at a rate of 0.3%–1.8% among adults over an 8-year follow-up. The mortality rate of postsplenectomy sepsis is approximately 50%, and thus it must be taken very seriously. Encapsulated organisms are the usual causes. Among the organisms listed only *Klebsiella pneumoniae* is encapsulated.

16–B. This patient has chronic pancreatitis and signs of pancreatic insufficiency with steatorrhea and weight loss secondary to malabsorption. Total pancreatectomy is not likely to improve the patient's health. Oral pancreatic enzyme replacement will treat both this patient's fatty stools and his malabsorption. He should also initiate a high-carbohydrate, high-protein diet to stabilize his weight. Although total parenteral nutrition may help this patient's malnourishment acutely, it is not a good option as it would restrict his activities, require a central venous catheter, carry a significant risk of morbidity, not provide optimal nutrition, and be quite costly. Octreotide therapy would likely make this patient's symptoms worse, as it would inhibit any remaining pancreatic exocrine function. A high-fat diet would worsen this patient's steatorrhea.

17–A. This patient developed splenic vein thrombosis secondary to pancreatitis. He has since developed sinistral portal hypertension with massive gastric varices formed from the enlarged short gastric veins, which now drain the splenic blood supply completely. Splenectomy will cure this patient's left-sided portal hypertension. It should be understood that emergent laparotomy in the setting of variceal bleeding carries a high mortality rate. Repeat esophagogastroduodenoscopy (EGD) in a patient with actively bleeding, large gastric varices that have failed one attempt at banding is not likely to be successful, will delay definitive therapy, and will increase his mortality risk. Sengstaken-Blakemore tubes are useful as a temporizing measure in patients with intractable esophageal varices, however they do not work well with gastric varices. Excision of the varices is not curative and risks inappropriate gastric devascularization. Intravenous (IV)) vasopressin may be temporizing, but does not address the underlying pathology and has not been shown to reduce mortality in this setting.

18–D. This patient may be feigning illness by administering insulin surreptitiously. This possibility can be excluded by measuring either proinsulin or C-peptide (an insulin precursor) levels. None of the other tests would be likely to aid in the diagnosis. Somatostatin is an inhibitory enzyme, not a stimulating one.

18

Breast

Laurence H. Brinckerhoff and Craig L. Slingluff Jr.

I. Overview of Breast Development and Function

A. Embryology

1. **Normal female breast development**

   —depends on **estrogen** and **progesterone.**

2. **Milk line regression**

   a. **Failure of regression** results in **accessory breast tissue.**
      —This is most commonly found in the axilla.
      —The most common congenital breast anomaly is accessory nipple(s), or **polythelia.**

   b. **Abnormal regression** may lead to underdevelopment of the breast, or **amastia.**
      —The **Poland syndrome** is amastia associated with hypoplasia of the chest wall and pectoralis muscles.

B. Anatomy

1. The **normal breast**

   —has a "teardrop" shape resulting from the extension of the breast tissue into the axilla, the "**axillary tail,**" or the "**tail of Spence.**"

2. **Breast asymmetry**

   —is common.

   —usually represents a normal variation.

3. **Vascular supply**

   a. **The medial and central portions are supplied by**
      —perforating branches from the **internal mammary artery.**

   b. **Laterally, the breast is supplied by**
      —the lateral thoracic.

—the thoracodorsal and suprascapular and perforating branches of the intercostal arteries.

4. **The venous drainage**

—runs in parallel to the arterial supply.

—includes a venous plexus in the subareolar region.

5. **The lymphatic drainage**

—plays an important role in the **spread of breast cancer.**

a. Of the entire **breast lymphatic drainage,** 97% flows into the axilla. The remainder flows to the internal mammary nodes.

b. **Any quadrant of the breast can drain to the internal mammary nodes.**

6. **Regional breast nodes**

—are important in the evaluation of breast cancer.

a. The **three different levels of axillary nodes**

—are defined by their relation to the **pectoralis minor muscle (Figure 18-1).**

(1) **Level I nodes** are lateral to the pectoralis muscle, within the axillary fat pad.

(2) **Level II nodes** are beneath or inferior to the pectoralis minor muscle.

(3) **Level III nodes** are medial to the pectoralis muscle.

b. **Rotter's nodes** (see Figure 18-1)

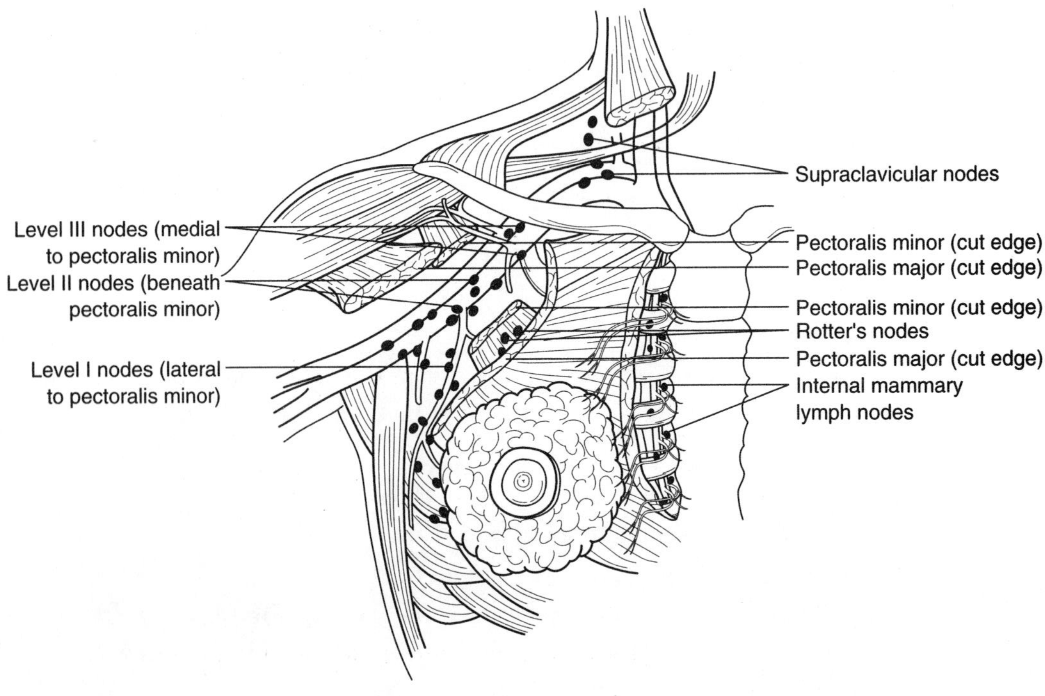

Figure 18-1. Lymphatic drainage of the breast. (Adapted with permission from Lawrence P. *Essentials of General Surgery,* 2nd ed. Baltimore, Williams & Wilkins, 1994, p 275.)

—are usually too small to be visualized.

—are located between the pectoralis major and pectoralis minor muscles.

c. **Internal mammary lymph nodes**

—directly drain a small portion of breast tissue.

d. **Supraclavicular nodes**

—also need to be assessed in patients with breast cancer.

7. **Fascial elements of the breast**

—There are two distinct but connected fascial elements of the breast.

a. **The fascial envelope**

—surrounds the breast tissue.

—extends to the pectoralis major and serratus anterior muscle fascia.

b. **Suspensory ligaments of Cooper**

—are fascial strands extending from the facial envelope through the breast tissue to the skin (**Figure 18-2).**

(1) These subdivide the breast into segments.

(2) Breast cancers involving these strands may cause **skin dimpling.**

C. **Histology**

1. **Breast tissue**

—has two histologically distinct tissues: **lobular** and **ductal.**

a. **Both tissues have associated stroma comprised of**

—connective tissue.

—nerves.

—blood vessels.

—lymphatics (see Figure 18-2).

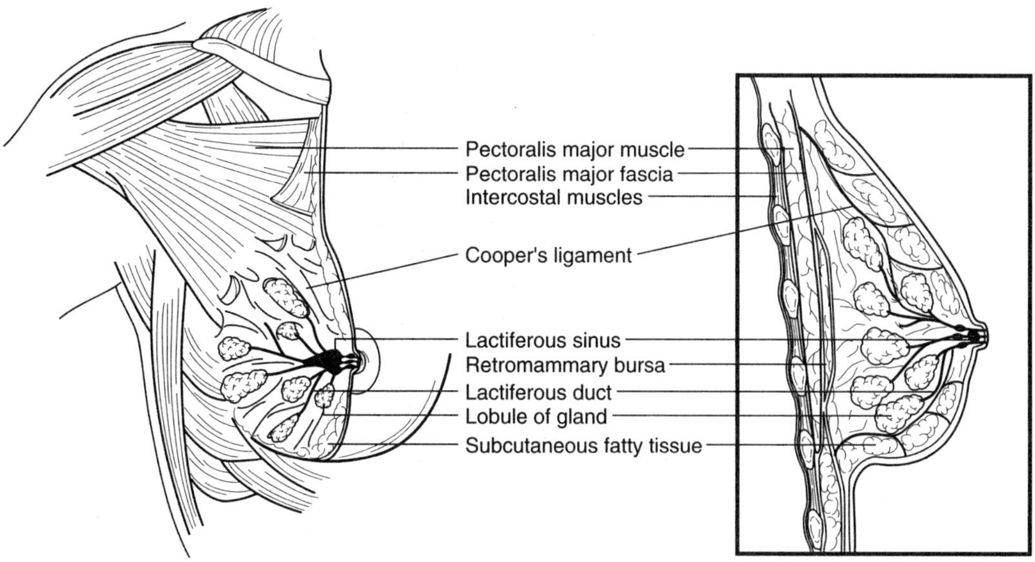

Figure 18-2. A tangential and sagittal view of the breast. (Adapted with permission from O'Leary P. *The Physiologic Basis of Surgery,* 2nd ed. Baltimore, Williams & Wilkins, 1996, p 287.)

b. The **lobule**

—is the functional unit of the breast.

(1) **Alveoli** are terminal elongated tubular ducts.
(2) Around 10–100 alveoli coalesce to form larger lobular ductal units.
(3) Twenty to 40 coalesce to form an excretory duct.

c. The **ductal tissue**

—is a double layer of cuboidal and columnar cells.

(1) These ducts form the channels for milk flow during **lactation.**
(2) These ducts define the lobes of the breast.

D. Physiology

1. **Estrogen**

—stimulates epithelial proliferation and blood flow to the breast.

2. **Progesterone**

—induces the cellular differentiation of alveolar cells into secretory cells.

3. **Prolactin**

—is produced from the **anterior pituitary.**

—stimulates alveolar milk secretion.

a. **Nipple stimulation**

—during breast feeding promotes secretion of prolactin.

b. **Cortisol and insulin**

—play a permissive role for prolactin function.

4. **Oxytocin**

—is produced from the **posterior pituitary.**

—stimulates contraction of breast myoepithelia.

—Nipple stimulation during breast feeding induces milk ejection.

5. **At menopause** the lack of estrogen and progesterone results in atrophy of the breast glandular tissue.

II. Basic Surgical Terminology

A. A lumpectomy

—refers to the removal of a lesion with a small rim of normal tissue.

B. Axillary lymph node dissection

—is the removal of the level I and level II axillary lymph nodes for **staging purposes.**

—current data shows no survival advantage to axillary node dissection versus observation for clinically palpable nodes.

C. Subcutaneous mastectomy

—is the removal of the bulk of the breast tissue, with preservation of the nipple-areolar complex.

D. A total mastectomy

—is the removal of all the breast tissue, including the nipple-areolar complex.

E. **Radical mastectomy** is the en bloc excision of

—the breast.

—the overlying skin.

—pectoralis major and minor muscles.

—level I, II, and III lymph nodes.

F. **Modified radical mastectomy**

—is a **total mastectomy** combined with **an axillary node dissection.**

III. Evaluation of Breast Abnormalities

A. **Breast imaging**

1. **Mammography**

—can detect a large proportion of nonpalpable breast cancers.

a. **Palpation**

—detects 10%–20% of bilateral mammogram (MMG)-negative cancers.

b. **The sensitivity of an MMG increases with age**

—due to replacement of dense parenchymal tissues by fatty tissues.

c. Of **MMG-positive, nonpalpable lesions**

—only 15%–25% are cancerous.

d. A **spiculated, dense lesion**

—with ill-defined margins is likely to be cancer (**Figure 18-3A**)

e. **Other lesions** suggestive of cancer on MMG include

—clusters of microcalcifications (Fig 18-3B).

—asymmetric densities.

—ductal asymmetry.

—distortion of normal breast architecture.

—skin or nipple distortion.

2. **The American Cancer Society's recommendations for a screening MMG**

a. **Age 35–39:** a baseline MMG.

b. **Age 40–49:** an MMG every 1–2 years.

c. **Over age 50:** an MMG yearly.

d. **All women undergoing breast biopsy**

—should have an MMG for evaluation of synchronous ipsilateral or contralateral disease.

e. An MMG should be considered for **all symptomatic women.**

f. **If there is a family history of breast cancer**

—screening should start 5 years before the age of the youngest affected relative.

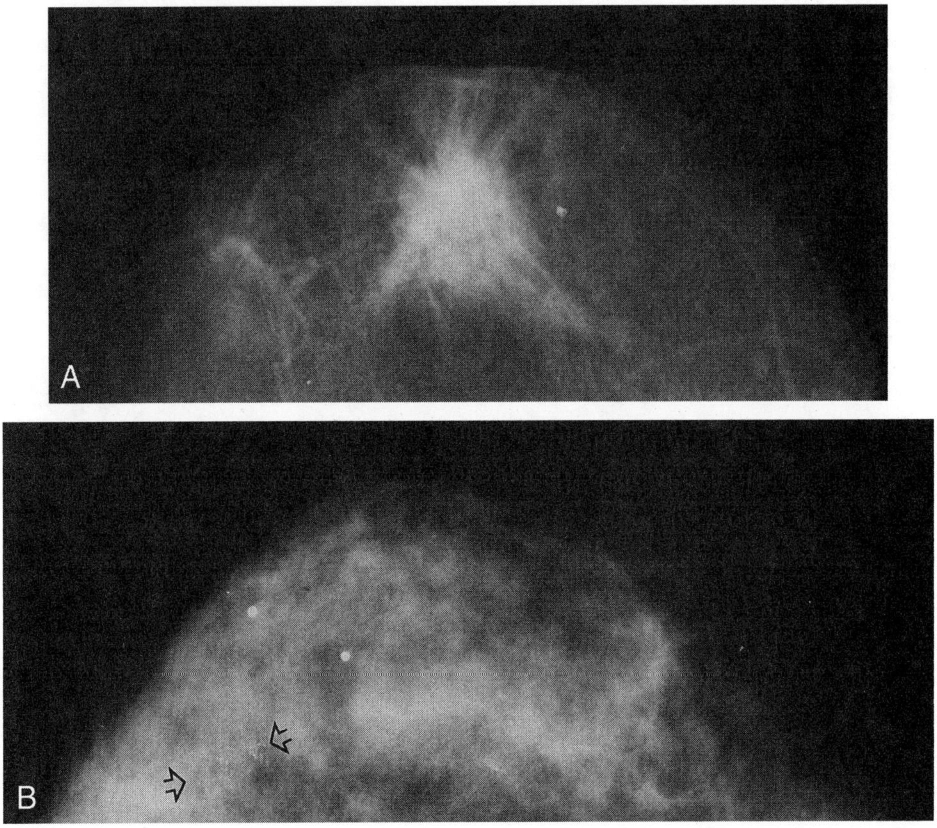

Figure 18-3. Mammograms demonstrating characteristic findings of breast carcinoma. (*A*) Note spiculated irregular margins of breast lesion. (*B*) Note clustered microcalcifications. (Reprinted with permission from Daffner RH: *Clinical Radiology: The Essentials,* 2nd ed. Baltimore, Williams & Wilkins, 1999, pp 245 and 247.)

B. General approach to suspicious nonpalpable mammographic lesions

1. Only about 15%–25% of these lesions will be **malignant.**
2. Independent of a woman's age these lesions require a **tissue biopsy.**

C. General approach to the palpable breast mass (Figure 18-4).

1. Many breast cancers present as a **palpable mass.** Thus self breast examination is a primary method for diagnosis.
2. **Women over age 30 and postmenopausal women**
   a. **Obtain an MMG**
      —to screen for occult concurrent disease.
   b. **Regardless of the MMG results**
      —**biopsy** of any and all suspicious lesions is mandatory.
      (1) Fine needle aspiration (FNA)
         —for palpable lesions provides cells for analysis.
         —provides a rapid, minimally invasive cellular diagnosis.
         —The accuracy of FNA depends on the cytologist.

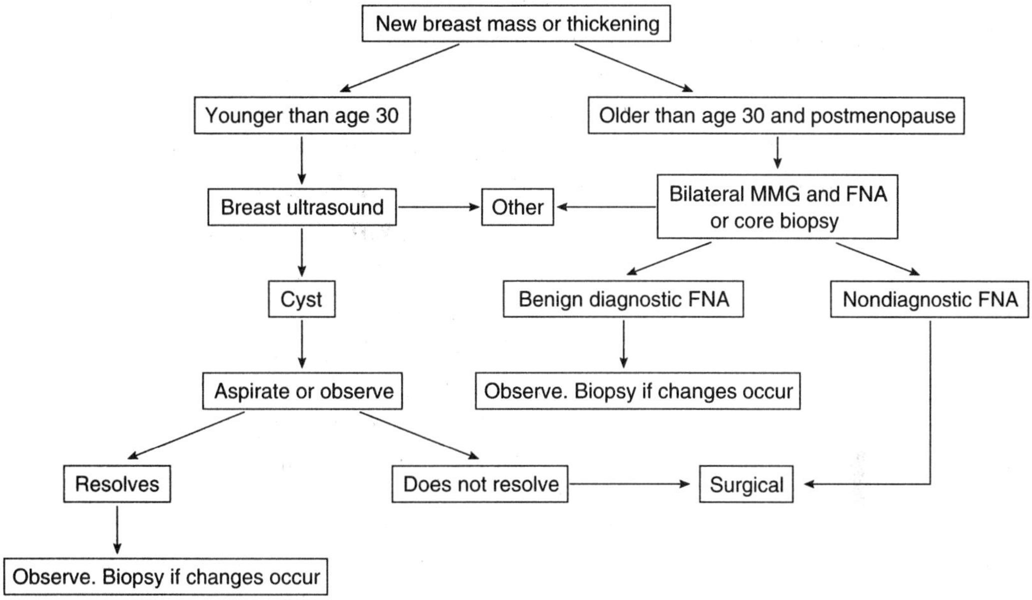

Figure 18-4. Approach to a new breast mass or thickening. MMG = mammogram; FNA = fine needle aspiration.

(2) Needle localized excisional biopsy

—provides intact tissue sections for analysis.

(a) Incisional biopsy is indicated for masses larger than 3 cm.

(b) Excisional biopsy is the gold standard for lesions smaller than 3 cm.

(3) Core needle biopsy

—may be substituted for needle localization because it also provides intact tissue sections for analysis.

—may be comparable to surgical excisional biopsy in accuracy.

—is considered to be a minimally invasive procedure.

—There have been reports of a higher level of false-negatives.

—This procedure is considered better than FNA because it allows for **histologic analysis.**

3. Women under the age of 30

a. Most of these patients have a low risk of cancer, unless there is a family history of breast cancer at a young age.

b. Fibroadenomas (see IV B)

—**Ultrasound** may be used to help diagnose fibroadenomas.

(1) For a **presumptive diagnosis** of fibroadenoma, it is reasonable to follow the breast mass over several months.

(2) A **definitive diagnosis** can be obtained using FNA.

(3) If a presumed **fibroadenoma enlarges,** surgical **excision** is indicated.

c. Cysts

—**Ultrasound** may also be used to help diagnose cysts.

(1) Cysts may be aspirated and followed with serial ultrasounds.

(2) If the cyst is **complex** or returns after aspiration, surgical excision is indicated.
(3) If it becomes **symptomatic** or painful, it may be appropriate to remove the cyst.

IV. Benign Breast Disorders (Table 18-1)

A. Fibrocystic changes or fibrocystic disease

—refer to a continuum of a disease state in response to cyclical hormones.

1. **Both** are **characterized** by nodular, lumpy breast tissue, which **varies with the hormone cycle.**
2. **Neither diagnosis carries an increased risk of cancer.**

Table 18-1. Benign Breast Disease

Breast Pathology	Histology	Presentation	Radiographic	Treatment
Fibrocystic disease	Microscopic and macroscopic **cyst**	Mastodynia, breast masses, or nipple discharge	Clustered **microcalcifications** on MMG	Reassurance
Sclerosing adenosis	**Fibrosis, adenosis** with lymphocytic infiltratio	Mastodynia, breast masses, or nipple discharge	Clustered **microcalcifications** on MMG	Reassurance
Fibroadenoma	Lobular stromal tissue; epithelium-lined duct-like structures	Painless, slow growing **mass; firm rubbery texture**	Solid mass on ultrasound	Observation; surgical excision when symptomatic or uncertain diagnosis
Radial scar	Fibroelastic tissue with radiating ducts and epithelial hyperplasia	Abnormality on MMG	MMG showing a stellate, irregular, spiculated mass	Reassurance
Intraductal papilloma	Diagnosis is made by ductography	**Bloody nipple discharge;** serous nipple discharge	**Ductography** Showing lesions close to nipple, on a long stalk	**Subareolar excision**
Mastodynia				
Cyclic	Fibrocystic disease	Pain before menses	Microcalcifications	Reassurance, NSAIDs, acetaminophen, danazol BCPs, elimination of caffeine
Continuous	Single fluid filled cyst	Pain not related to menses	Fluid filled mass	Reassurance, NSAIDs, acetaminophen, danazol BCPs, elimination of caffeine

MMG = mammogram; NSAIDs = nonsteroidal anti-inflammatory drugs; BCPs = birth control pills.

3. **Fibrocystic change**

—refers to patients without significant symptoms.

4. **Fibrocystic disease**

—refers to women with severely symptomatic breasts.

a. **Signs and symptoms include**

—mastodynia (i.e., breast pain) (see IV C 9).

—breast masses.

—nipple discharge (see IV C 8).

b. Care must be taken to **rule out** other causes of pain such as infection and cancer.

5. Some of the **risk factors** differ from those of breast cancer, and include

—early menarche.

—late menopause.

—irregular menses.

—small breast size.

—normal or low body weight.

—history of cyclic breast mass.

—history of spontaneous abortions.

6. The classic **histologic changes** are **microscopic** and **macroscopic cysts.**

a. **Fibrosis and adenosis** with lymphocytic infiltration is characteristic.

b. **Mild to moderate ductal or lobular hyperplasia** may be present with no atypia.

c. **Many of these findings** can be found in normal breast tissue.

d. **Sclerosing adenosis** is a **histologic subtype** of fibrocystic change.

(1) Most commonly it **presents as** a cluster of microcalcifications on MMG without an associated palpable mass or pain

(2) It is **easily confused with breast cancer** histologically and radiographically.

(3) **Wire localization** and **surgical excision** may be required for diagnosis.

(4) It is **distinguished from cancer** by the regularity of nuclei and absence of mitoses.

7. **Primary treatments are reassurance** and symptomatic relief.

B. **Fibroadenoma** (see Table 18-1)

1. **Overview**

—It is the **most common breast tumor** in **adolescents** and **young women.**

—Patients will have **multiple fibroadenomas** in 10%–15% of cases.

2. **Characteristics of a fibroadenoma** include

—a **painless, slow growing mass** found on self-breast examination.

—growth to several centimeters in size, and then no further progression.

—changes in size and symptoms with menstrual cycle.

—**well-circumscribed,** oval or round, mobile masses.

—firm **rubbery texture** (may become rock hard with degeneration).

—Fibroadenomas may enlarge quickly during pregnancy.

3. **Diagnosis**

   a. **On MMG** fibroadenomas **rarely have a characteristic nature.**

      —However, with degeneration, they will appear as classic "popcorn calcifications."

   b. **Ultrasound evaluation** is seldom definitive, but may substantiate the diagnosis.

4. **Treatment**

   —is based on the probability of missing a primary breast cancer.

   a. **Women under age 30** with a confirmed diagnosis may be observed and followed up.

      —Removal is indicated only if the mass enlarges or changes in character.

   b. **Women 30 and over** require an FNA for a definitive diagnosis.

      —If FNA is nondiagnostic, or if any changes occur, surgery is indicated.

5. **Giant fibroadenomas** (larger than 5 cm)

   —are a subclass of the simple adenoma.

   —usually occur immediately after menarche or menopause.

   —Recurrence is rare if excision is complete.

C. **Other benign breast diseases**

1. **Radial scar** (radial sclerosing lesions) (see Table 18-1)

   a. The **classic MMG shows** a **stellate, irregular, spiculated mass lesion**.

   b. Though **hard to differentiate from cancer** there is no increased risk.

      —A **tissue diagnosis** is required to differentiate from cancer.

2. **Fat necrosis**

   a. **Pathophysiology and presentation**

      —The pathophysiology is thought to be **inflammatory necrosis** frequently related to **trauma.** Only about 50% of cases, however, are associated with known trauma.

      —The **attendant fibrosis** may cause skin dimpling and a mass effect.

   c. **Diagnosis**

      —Microscopically, **macrophages** laden with fat lobules, or foreign body giant cells are diagnostic.

   d. **Treatment**

      —involves reassurance without excision.

3. **Periductal mastitis**

—(i.e, mammary duct ectasia, plasma cell mastitis) is an uncommon disease.

a. **Pathological characteristics**

—are dilated mammary ducts with inspissated secretions and marked periductal inflammation.

b. **Signs and symptoms**

—include noncyclical mastodynia; nipple retraction; thick, white creamy nipple discharge; and sterile subareolar abscesses.

c. **History**

—Most patients will give a history of difficulty with **breast-feeding.**

d. **Diagnosis and treatment**

—depend on the involved symptoms.

(1) If there is the typical **discharge,** then only reassurance is indicated.

(2) If an **abscess** has formed, surgical incision and drainage is indicated.

4. **Infectious mastitis**

a. When a **primary infection of the breast is suspected clinically,** care must be taken to rule out inflammatory breast cancer.

b. Although uncommon, **80% of infections** are associated with **breast-feeding.**

c. The **most common pathogen** is ***Staphylococcus aureus.***

d. In **nonlactating women,** mastitis may also be caused by

—**chronic infections** (e.g., actinomycosis, tuberculosis, syphilis).

—**autoimmune diseases** (e.g., lupus erythematosus).

e. **Most infections**

—begin as skin cellulitis.

—may be treated with antibiotics safe for feeding the infant.

5. **Galactoceles**

—are breast cysts that are filled with milk.

a. It is **almost exclusively seen** after breast-feeding and represents dilated obstructed breast ducts.

b. **Treatment**

—ranges from simple aspiration to surgical incision and drainage.

6. **Mondor's disease**

—is **thrombophlebitis** of superficial veins of the breast.

a. This **inflammation typically**

—**affects** the lower outer quadrant.

—**presents as** a **palpable, cord-**like mass with associated burning pain.

b. The **etiology is unknown**

—but it is associated with trauma and strenuous exercise.

c. **Treatment**

—with nonsteroidal anti-inflammatory drugs (NSAIDs) is indicated if pain is severe.

7. **Intraductal papilloma** (see Table 18-1)

—is the most common cause of **bloody nipple discharge,** although half the time the discharge is serous.

a. **These lesions are usually**

—small.

—nonpalpable.

—close to the nipple.

b. **Diagnosis**

—can be made by ductography.

c. **Treatment**

—with subareolar excision is generally curative.

d. **Diffuse papillomatosis**

—affects multiple ducts and both breasts.

(1) The papillomas are larger than when papillomas occur as a single lesion.
(2) The discharge is serous, not bloody.
(3) There is an **increased risk of breast cancer** (40% develop breast cancer).

8. **Nipple discharge**

a. **Most causes** of nipple discharge are benign.

b. **Intraductal papillomas and breast cancer** can produce a bloody or blood-tinged serous discharge.

c. **Subareolar infections**

—produce purulent discharge with tender areola.

d. **Galactorrhea**

—is defined as a milky white discharge.

—is usually bilateral, and not related to lactation or breast stimulation.

(1) It may signify an increase in **prolactin secretion.**
  (a) The most common cause is **pituitary microadenoma.**
  (b) **Drugs** have also been shown to increase prolactin levels, including phenothiazines, metoclopramide, birth control pills (BCPs), α-methyldopa, reserpine, and tricyclic antidepressants (TCAs).
(2) Hypothyroidism as well as hyperthyroidism has also been associated.
(3) It is usually associated with amenorrhea.

e. **Fibrocystic disease**

—uncommonly produces green/yellow or brown discharges.

9. **Mastodynia** (i.e., breast pain) (see Table 18-1)

a. **Malignancy** is rarely associated with mastodynia.

b. It needs to be distinguished from **Tietze syndrome,** which is costochondritis of the upper ribs with referred pain to the breast.

c. There are **two distinct types** of mastodynia: **cyclic and continuous.**
   (1) **Cyclic mastodynia**
   —is characterized by pain before the menstrual period.
      (a) The pain may be referred to the axilla or to the underside of upper arm.
      (b) It is most commonly associated with **fibrocystic** disease.
   (2) **Continuous mastodynia**
   —is characterized by continual pain unrelated to the menstrual cycle.
   —often represents an acute or subacute infection.
   —most commonly presents as a **single large cyst.**

d. **Treatment**
   (1) Progressing from cyclic to continuous, mastodynia is usually **refractory** to treatment.
   (2) Most patients can be treated with **reassurance.**
   (3) Treatment for **persistent pain** includes using NSAIDs or acetaminophen, eliminating methylxanthines and caffeine, smoking cessation, danazol (a weak androgen), BCPs, vitamin E, and tamoxifen.

V. Noninvasive Breast Cancer/Premalignant Breast Cancer (Table 18-2)

A. Ductal carcinoma in situ (DCIS)

1. This **lesion contains malignant cells**

   —from the ductal epithelium **without microinvasion** (invasion through the basement membrane).

2. The **median age of diagnosis**

   —is between **50–60,** but it is also found in **young women.**

3. Based on histologic findings, there are four major **distinct forms of DCIS:**

   a. **Comedo DCIS**
   —is the most aggressive form, with the highest microinvasion rate.
   —can display multicentricity (simultaneous occurrence in **different breast quadrants).**

   b. **Solid DCIS**
   —is identified by malignant cells completely filling the ducts.

   c. **Cribriform DCIS**
   —has small, uniform cells in a fenestrated pattern.

   d. **Micropapillary DCIS**
   —tends to be multicentric.

4. **Microinvasion is rare**

   —in lesions smaller than 2.5 cm.

5. **Classic MMG findings**

Table 18-2. Premalignant and Malignant Breast Cancer

Breast Pathology	Histology	Presentation	Treatment	Comments
Premalignant Breast Cancer				
Ductal carcinoma in situ (DCIS)	Noninvasive adeno-carcinoma cells (five subtypes)	Clustered **micro-calcifications** on **MMG**	Segmental mastectomy or **lumpectomy** with **post-operative radiation;** axillary node dissection for lesion > 3 cm	**Comedo** is the most **aggressive** subtype
Lobular carcinoma in situ (LCIS)	**Multicentric** and **multi-focal** lesions are **common**	Pathologic examination	Close observation	Risk factor for **ductal carcinoma**
Invasive Breast Cancer				
Infiltrating ductal carcinoma Medullary Tubular Mucinous (colloid) Secretory (juvenile)	Invasive adenocarcinoma cells in a fibrous stroma	**Mass on self-breast exam**	Lumpectomy + axillary node dissection + radiation therapy or modified radical mastectomy	Juvenile carcinoma may present before age 30
Infiltrating lobular carcinoma	Multicentric and multi-focal	Pathologic examination; mass effect on MMG	Lumpectomy + axillary node dissection + radiation therapy or modified radical mastectomy	

MMG = mammogram.

—are **clustered microcalcifications** (see Figure 18-3B).

a. Between **25%–35%** of untreated DCIS will develop into **invasive cancer.**

b. Approximately **10%** of women will develop DCIS in the **contralateral breast.**

6. **Treatment options** for DCIS may include

a. **Total mastectomy,** with or without reconstruction.

—This option is usually considered too aggressive for DCIS lesions.

—It may be indicated if the majority of the breast has DCIS changes.

b. **Segmental mastectomy (lumpectomy),** with or without **postoperative radiation.**

—Postoperative radiation therapy may reduce the local recurrence rate to 10%.

—Patients with a small, low grade DCIS may not need postoperative therapy.

c. An **axillary node dissection** or **sentinel node biopsy**

—may be considered for a DCIS lesion larger than 3 cm.

7. **Close follow-up**

—with physical examination and MMG is essential.

B. **Lobular carcinoma in situ (LCIS)**

1. **Lesions** are

—defined histologically by terminal lobule intra-epithelial proliferation.

—generally **nonpalpable** and diagnosed by pathologic evaluation.

—primarily found in **premenopausal women.**

2. **LCIS is a risk factor** for developing **bilateral breast cancer.**

—Bilateral disease occurs in 30%–50% of patients.

3. **A diagnosis of LCIS** confers a 5% chance of having a synchronous invasive lesion.

—Sixty to seventy percent of invasive lesions associated with LCIS are **ductal** carcinomas.

4. **Multifocal disease**

—(i.e., simultaneously occurring lesions within the **same breast quadrant**) and **multicentric** disease is common.

5. Although controversial, **treatment options** for LCIS may include close **observation** or bilateral prophylactic mastectomy without axillary node dissection.

VI. Invasive Breast Cancer (see Table 18-2)

A. **Overview**

1. **Incidence**

—There are approximately 150,000 new cases of female breast cancer and 44,000 deaths per year secondary to breast cancer.

—The incidence of breast cancer has increased **150% since 1970.**

2. It has been estimated that 7% (1/14) of women who reach age 70 will develop breast cancer.

B. **Risks factors for breast cancer** are covered in **Table 18-3.**

C. **Adenocarcinoma of the breast**

1. **Invasive ductal carcinoma/infiltrating ductal carcinoma**

—represents **70%–80%** of all breast cancer.

a. **Invasive adenocarcinoma cells** in a fibrous stroma, sometimes with associated microcalcifications, are typically observed microscopically.

b. **Ductal cancers typically metastasize** to axillary lymph nodes and may spread to bone, lung, liver, and brain.

Table 18-3. Risk Factors for Developing Breast Cancer

Greatly Increased Risk	Moderately Increased Risk
Increasing age	Nulliparity or first birth after age of 30
Female gender	Menarche before age 12, menopause after age 55
Strong family history: two or more first degree relatives with bilateral, premenopausal breast cancer	Moderate family history: one or more relatives with breast cancer, not bilateral or premenopausal
DCIS, LCIS, atypical ductal or lobular hyperplasia	Low-dose ionizing radiation in childhood or adolescence
History of contralateral breast cancer	Other cancers: colon, endometrial
BRCA-1, BRCA-2 (genetic tumor markers)	Diet: high-fat or high-calorie diets

Oral contraceptives and the use of postmenopausal conjugated estrogens have not been shown to increase the long-term risk of breast cancer. **Many women diagnosed with breast cancer do not have a risk factor other than gender.**
DCIS = ductal carcinoma in situ; LCIS = lobular carcinoma in situ.

c. When **mixed in histology** the clinical behavior is like that of ductal cancer.

2. **Variants of invasive ductal carcinoma**

a. **Medullary carcinoma**

—represents about 6% of all the breast cancers.

—tumors are typically larger than ductal carcinomas.

(1) Typically, marked lymphocytic infiltration and large pleomorphic nuclei are observed microscopically.
(2) Ninety plus percent are estrogen- and progesterone-positive.
(3) This variant carries a **better prognosis** than other invasive ductal carcinomas.

b. **Tubular carcinoma**

—represents about 2% of all the breast cancers.

(1) These tumors are typically smaller, being identified on screening MMG.
(2) Small tubule formation of over 75% of the tumor with stroma and elastic tissue is observed microscopically.
(3) This variant carries a **better prognosis** than other invasive ductal carcinoma.

c. **Mucinous (colloid) carcinoma**

—represents about 2% of breast cancers.

(1) Microscopically, there is an abundance of extracellular mucin.
(2) This variant may confer a better prognosis.

d. **Secretory carcinoma (juvenile carcinoma)**

—is a very rare variant.

(1) The mean age of diagnosis is 25, but ranges from 11–75.
(2) These slow growing, mobile tumors are commonly mistaken for fibroadenomas.
(3) Small, secretion filled, glandular cells in a lobulated pattern can be seen microscopically.

3. Invasive lobular carcinoma/infiltrating lobular carcinoma

—represents about 5%–10% of invasive breast cancers.

a. These tumors **differ from ductal cancer.**

—Microcalcifications are rarely seen on MMG.

—They are usually **extensively infiltrating,** often with no distinct tumor mass.

—Multicentricity and multifocality are much more common.

b. A **single-file arrangement** of adenocarcinoma cells is observed microscopically.

—If larger **signet-ring cells** can be seen, there is a **poorer prognosis.**

c. These tumors metastasize to axillary lymph nodes, bone, lung, liver and brain. They may also metastasize to the **meninges and serosal surfaces.**

4. Treatment guidelines

—for infiltrating ductal or lobular carcinoma are covered in Table 18-2.

D. Other histologic types of breast cancer

1. Metaplastic adenocarcinoma

—takes the appearance of nonglandular tumors.

a. The **most common types of metaplasia** are squamous and pseudosarcomatous.

b. The **prognosis** is the same as that of the tumor from which it was derived.

—Although uncommon, **squamous carcinoma** has a **worse prognosis** than ductal cancer.

2. Adenoid cystic carcinomas

—are large, well circumscribed lesions.

—have a **better prognosis** than ductal cancers.

—can be thought of as a large cyst containing DCIS.

E. Factors that influence prognosis

1. The most important **prognostic factor**

—for patients without clinically advanced disease is the number of **lymph nodes positive** for cancer.

2. Other factors, in order of importance, include

—tumor size.

—histologic grade.

—estrogen receptor and progesterone receptor status.

—the histologic type.

VII. Management of Breast Cancer

A. Assessment of breast cancer

1. Diagnose all evident local and systemic disease (Table 18-4).

2. Assess for the **extent** of regional and systemic disease.

Table 18-4. Indications and Staging Studies After the Diagnosis of Breast Cancer

Study	Indication
Complete blood count, liver function tests	Routine
Chest radiograph	Routine
Bilateral mammogram	Routine
Computed tomography scan of the liver	Symptoms, abnormal liver function test
Bone scan	Suggestive symptoms, locally advanced primary, abnormal alkaline phosphatase

—If there is evidence of lymphatic microinvasion, there is a 30% chance of either regional or systemic disease.

B. Treatment for breast cancer

1. **Treatment** is based on the **stage of the disease.**

   —The American Joint Committee on Cancer tumor-node-metastasis (TNM) staging is outlined in **Table 18-5.**

2. The **approach for breast cancer management** is based on disease location.

   a. **Local control:** lumpectomy with irradiation or mastectomy.

   b. **Regional control:** axillary lymph node dissection, irradiation to localized disease.

   c. **Systemic disease:** chemotherapy.

   d. **Micrometastatic disease:** hormonal therapy, chemotherapy, or both.

3. **Adjuvant therapy** includes chemotherapy and hormonal therapy.

   —**Decisions** about adjuvant therapies are affected by factors such as age and receptor status **(Table 18-6).**

4. Even women **without** evidence of **lymphatic microinvasive breast cancer** may benefit from antiestrogen therapies and/or chemotherapy.

C. Microinvasive breast cancer

—is DCIS with a focus (<10%) of microinvasion in biopsy.

1. The **incidence**

   —of axillary node metastasis is 0%–10%.

2. **Axillary node dissection**

   —is not felt to be warranted in these patients.

3. **Treatment**

   —is similar to the treatment for DCIS: lumpectomy with postoperative radiation therapy.

D. Early-stage breast cancer (T1–T2, N0–N1)

—represents 75% of patients who present with breast cancer.

1. There are **three standard treatment options** with equivalent survival rates:

   a. Lumpectomy, axillary node dissection, followed by postoperative radiation.

Table 18-5. The American Joint Committee on Cancer Tumor-Node-Metastasis (TNM) Staging

Tumor (T)
Tx —Primary tumor cannot be assessed
T0 —No evidence of primary tumor
Tis —Carcinoma in situ: intraductal or loblar carcinoma in situ, or Paget's disease of the nipple with no tumor
T1 —Tumor mass < 2 cm in diameter
T2 —Tumor > 2 cm and < 5 cm in diameter
T3 —Tumor > 5 cm in diameter
T4 —Tumor of any size with direct extension to chest wall or skin

Nodes (N)
Nx —Regional nodes cannot be assessed—previously removed
N0 —No regional lymph node metastasis
N1 —Metastasis to movable ipsilateral axillary lymph nodes
N2 —Metastasis to ipsilateral axillary nodes that are fixed, nonmobile
N3 —Metastasis to ipsilateral internal mammary lymph nodes

Distant Metastasis (M)
Mx —Presence of disease cannot be assessed
M0 —No evidence of distant metastasis
M1 —Distant metastasis

Stage	T	N	M
Stage 0	Tis	N0	M0
Stage I	T1	N0	M0
Stage IIA	T0	N1	M0
	T1	N1	M0
	T2	N0	M0
Stage IIB	T2	N1	M0
	T3	N0	M0
Stage IIIA	T0	N2	M0
	T1	N2	M0
	T2	N2	M0
	T3	N1	M0
	T3	N2	M0
Stage IIIB	T4	Any N	M0
	Any T	N3	M0
Stage IV	any T	Any N	M1

b. Modified radical mastectomy alone.
c. Modified radical mastectomy with reconstruction.

2. **Determining which treatment option** to use depends on multiple variables:
   a. If the **breast is small,** then lumpectomy may yield a poor cosmetic result.
   b. If there is **aggressive histology,** a more aggressive treatment may be advocated.
   c. Patient's desires, age, and reliability for follow-up are all considered.
3. **Axillary node dissection** is important for **staging,** even with nonpalpable nodes.
   a. **Axillary node status is a major predictor of 5-year survival.**
      (1) **No positive axillary nodes:** confers a 75% five-year survival.

Table 18-6. Indications for Adjuvant Chemotherapy

Tumor Size	ER/PR Status	Nodal Status	Recommendations: Premenopausal	Recommendations: Postmenopausal
< 1 cm	+	–	No adjuvant therapy	No adjuvant therapy
> 1 cm	+	–	Chemotherapy plus tamoxifen	Tamoxifen
	–	–	Chemotherapy	Chemotherapy
Any size	+	+	Chemotherapy plus tamoxifen	Chemotherapy plus tamoxifen
	–	+	Chemotherapy	Chemotherapy

ER = estrogen receptor; PR = progesterone receptor.

(2) With **1–3 nodes positive:** 60%.

(3) With **4–10 nodes positive:** 40%.

b. Among early breast cancers with **nonpalpable axillary nodes,** 20%–30% will have nodal disease identified with surgery.

c. The **nodal status**

—also helps to direct adjuvant chemotherapy (see VII B 3).

d. Minimally invasive techniques

—like sentinel node biopsy may allow for an accurate assessment of the nodal status of patients with little pain and risk.

E. Locally advanced breast cancer

1. This cancer is comprised of **large (T3) tumors** or extensive regional disease without distant metastasis.

a. About 10%–20% of patients present with this stage of breast cancer.

—**About 75%** will have clinically palpable axillary or supraclavicular nodes.

b. About 20% of patients who appear to be stage III on examination will be stage IV after complete staging.

2. Inflammatory breast cancer

—is a rare, virulent form of breast cancer.

a. It usually **presents** as an **erythematous, warm breast, with edema and pain (peau d'orange).**

b. Tumor emboli in dermal lymphatics can be seen in skin biopsies for diagnosis.

3. Locally recurrent breast cancer

—is usually only focal disease.

—may be controlled with a salvage mastectomy.

—Postmastectomy recurrence typically occurs within 2 years and is associated with distant disease and a median survival of 2–3 years.

4. Paget's disease of the nipple

—is a sometimes weeping, eczematous lesion of the nipple.

—may be associated with edema and inflammation.

—usually represents **malignant cells within the milk ducts.**

5. **Metastatic breast cancer**

   —generally cannot be cured.

   a. The median survival is about 2 years.

   b. **Treatment** with surgery and chemotherapy is generally palliative.

VIII. Atypical Breast Cancer

A. Cystosarcoma phylloides

—are rare tumors, representing about 0.5%–1.0% of breast tumors.

1. The **median age** at presentation is **50.**
2. Microscopically there are stromal and epithelial elements.
3. These are usually **larger tumors,** and can be benign or malignant.
4. These tumors **rarely metastasize.**

   —If they do, they can metastasize to the lung, bone and mediastinum (note **not** axilla).

5. **Treatment** is **local excision** without axillary node dissection.

B. Occult breast cancer

—is breast cancer presenting as **axillary metastases** with an **unknown primary.**

1. Fifty-five to seventy-five percent of these patients are found to have cancer after mastectomy.
2. **Radiation therapy** may be an option for patients who desire breast conservation.
3. **Treatment** is usually modified radical mastectomy.

C. Male breast cancer

1. **Overview**

   a. There are approximately 900 new cases of male breast cancer per year, about 1% of breast cancer cases.

   b. Mean age of presentation is 60–65.

2. **Risk factors** include

   —previous radiation.

   —family history.

   —Klinefelter's syndrome.

   —protracted hyperestrogenemic state.

3. **These tumors are**

   —ductal in origin, and 80% are estrogen receptor-positive.

   —tend to **metastasize** early in the course of the disease.

3. **Treatment** is a **modified radical mastectomy.**

Review Test

Directions: Each of the numbered items or incomplete statements in this section is followed by answers or by completions of the statement. Select the ONE lettered answer or completion that is BEST in each case.

1. A newborn is found to have an additional nipple in the right axilla. Which of the following characteristics are most likely to be associated with this condition?

(A) Amastia
(B) Hypoplasia of the ipsilateral chest
(C) Hypoplasia of the ipsilateral breast
(D) Normal development
(E) Bilateral breast hyperplasia

2. A newborn is examined immediately after birth and is found to have bilateral breast hyperplasia with an associated creamy-white discharge. What is the most appropriate evaluation for this patient?

(A) Immediate computed tomography (CT) scan of the brain to evaluate for a microadenoma and possible surgery
(B) Observation with reassurance to the parents that this is a known normal phenomenon
(C) Bilateral ductography and simple mastectomy to remove diffuse papillomas
(D) Close observation of the newborn and thyroid supplementation
(E) Close observation and a toxin scan of both mother and infant

3. A 45-year-old, premenopausal woman presents to her doctor with a new breast mass discovered on self-breast examination. It is a small, firm, mobile mass in the left lower outer quadrant of her breast. There are no skin changes or dimpling and no lymph nodes palpable in her axilla. Which of the following histories would confer the greatest concern that this mass represents an invasive ductal carcinoma?

(A) Her sister had postmenopausal breast cancer
(B) She had her menarche before age 12
(C) She had never been pregnant
(D) She had a history of atypical lobular hyperplasia
(E) She had been on birth control pills (BCPs) for 5 years when in her 20s

4. A 48-year-old, premenopausal woman presents to her doctor for routine health maintenance. She is found to have a small, firm palpable breast mass in her left breast. The patient undergoes a bilateral mammogram (MMG) to evaluate for concurrent disease, subclinical breast disease presenting simultaneously with the mass. The MMG shows no abnormalities, including no microcalcifications or mass effect near the area of the palpable breast mass. Which of the following is the most appropriate next step in the evaluation of this patient?

(A) Close observation to evaluate for increases in size or decreased mobility
(B) Ultrasound evaluation in 1 year
(C) Fine needle aspiration (FNA) for cellular evaluation
(D) Excisional biopsy and axillary node dissection
(E) Core needle biopsy and axillary node dissection

5. A 54-year-old woman presents with a clinically node-positive, 3-cm infiltrating ductal carcinoma in her left breast. She has no other symptoms. Which of the following would be appropriate for the initial evaluation of this patient?

(A) Chest radiograph, bone scan, complete blood count with liver function tests, bilateral mammogram (MMG), and a computed tomography (CT) scan of the liver
(B) Chest radiograph, bone scan, bilateral MMG, and a CT scan of the liver
(C) Chest radiograph, complete blood count with liver function tests, and a bilateral MMG
(D) Chest radiograph, bone scan, and a complete blood count with liver function tests
(E) Chest radiograph, bone scan, bilateral MMG, and a CT scan of the liver

6. A 34-year-old woman underwent a wide local excision, axillary node dissection, and postoperative radiation to her left breast for a node-positive, 2-cm, infiltrating ductal carcinoma 3 years ago. She received adjuvant chemotherapy at that time. She now presents with a new 2-cm mass in the same breast, and it shows infiltrating ductal carcinoma. She has no other symptoms and has no palpable lymph nodes. Which of the following is the most appropriate treatment for this patient?

(A) Re-excision to free margins, second axillary node dissection, and radiation therapy
(B) Combination chemotherapy alone
(C) Left total mastectomy
(D) Left modified mastectomy
(E) Combination chemotherapy and radiation therapy

Questions 7–8

7. A 43-year-old professional woman presents to your office with questions about breast cancer screening. She has never had a mammogram previously, but does monthly self-breast examinations and has not noted any masses. Her mother was diagnosed with breast cancer at age 65, but she has no other relatives with cancer. She has had 3 children and her menarche was at age 13. The best screening routine for this patient is to obtain a baseline mammogram

(A) At age 45, then every 2 years after age 50
(B) Now, then every 2 years thereafter
(C) Now, then every 2 years until age 50, then yearly thereafter
(D) Now, and then every 6 months thereafter
(E) Now, and then every 5 years thereafter

8. This patient undergoes a bilateral mammogram (MMG) and is discovered to have an area of microcalcifications in her right breast. She then undergoes a needle localized excisional biopsy that demonstrates a cellular, monomorphic pattern, with poorly cohesive intact cells, nuclear crowding, and a variation in nuclear size, prominent nucleoli, and clumping of the chromatin. There is no evidence of microinvasion and the largest diameter is 1 cm. The margins are negative. Which of the following management options is most appropriate?

(A) Modified radical mastectomy
(B) Reassuring the patient that the process is benign
(C) Axillary node dissection with postoperative breast radiation therapy
(D) Breast radiation therapy alone
(E) Axillary node dissection alone

9. A 55-year-old woman status post-breast conservation therapy for ductal carcinoma in situ (DCIS) develops a large, fixed node in her right axilla. There are no breast masses on physical examination, and a bilateral mammogram (MMG) demonstrates no abnormalities. You obtain a fine needle aspiration (FNA) from the axillary mass, which shows adenocarcinoma cells. Which of the following is the most appropriate next step in the management of this patient?

(A) Axillary node dissection for staging, and radiation therapy to the breast
(B) Axillary node dissection for staging alone
(C) Radical mastectomy
(D) Modified radical mastectomy
(E) Radiation to the axillary mass without surgery

10. A 28-year-old woman presents to your office with painful breasts. She states that she used to suffer from pain in her breasts only before her period, but the pain now never goes away and she can no longer function normally. She does take birth control pills (BCPs), but does not smoke and does not drink coffee. On physical examination, you find no dominant masses and no nodes positive in her axilla. No nipple discharge is expressible. Over the next few months you try to treat her pain conservatively, but without success. Which of the following is the best approach to the treatment of this patient?

(A) Continue with observation alone because the process is self-limiting
(B) Prescribe more potent pain relieving drugs such as narcotics
(C) Launch an extensive work-up for invasive ductal carcinoma
(D) Prescribe danazol, with follow-up to evaluate for side effects
(E) Obtain bilateral ultrasounds to localize the fibroadenomatous disease

11. A 37-year-old woman presents to the clinic with a history of left-sided bloody nipple discharge. She denies any pain or any changes on self-breast examination. She has no other complaints. She is very concerned because her sister died at the age of 42 of breast cancer. On physical examination, you cannot appreciate any dominant masses. There is a small amount of blood-tinged nipple discharge. On mammogram (MMG), there are no abnormalities seen. Which of the following is the most appropriate next step in the evaluation and treatment of this patient?

(A) Observation with strict instructions to return when and if the bloody discharge occurs again
(B) Ultrasound to evaluate for any cystic masses
(C) Re-examination in 6 months with bilateral mammogram (MMG)
(D) Simple mastectomy and close follow-up
(E) Ductography and potential subareolar excision

12. A 66-year-old woman returns to your office 10 years after being treated for advanced left breast cancer. At that time, she had a radical mastectomy and radiation therapy to her axilla for regional control. She states that for the last 4 years, she has noticed swelling in her left hand and now is somewhat distressed because there seems to be a rash progressing up her arm. On physical examination, she does have 4+ pitting edema in her hand as well as multiple painless purplish red nodules that seem to be spreading up her arm. Which of the following is the most likely diagnosis for this mass?

(A) Bacterial cellulitis
(B) Paraneoplastic coagulopathy
(C) Post-traumatic hematoma
(D) Lymphangiosarcoma
(E) Lymphoma

Directions: Each set of matching questions in this section consists of a list of four to twenty-six lettered options followed by several numbered items. For each numbered item, select the appropriate lettered option(s). Each lettered option may be selected once, more than once, or not at all.

Questions 13–17

(A) Infiltrating ductal carcinoma
(B) Comedo intraductal carcinoma
(C) Lobular carcinoma in situ
(D) Medullary carcinoma
(E) Inflammatory carcinoma

Match each histologic type of breast cancer with the most likely associated description.

13. Associated with lymphocytic infiltration and a good prognosis. (SELECT 1 TYPE)

14. Significant likelihood of multicentric ipsilateral disease. (SELECT 2 TYPES)

15. Highest likelihood of bilateral disease. (SELECT 1 TYPE)

16. Dermal lymphatic invasion. (SELECT 1 TYPE)

17. Most common carcinoma presenting as a breast mass. (SELECT 1 TYPE)

Answers and Explanations

1–D. The failure of the regression of the milk line results in accessory breast tissue. The most common congenital breast anomaly is accessory nipple(s), or polythelia, and is associated with normal breast development. Accessory breast tissue, separate from the main breast mound, is most commonly found in the axilla. A complete accessory breast, possessing both breast tissue and nipple, is rare. Abnormal or total regression of the milk line may lead to underdevelopment of the breast, or amastia, and is usually associated with hypoplasia of the ipsilateral chest wall and pectoralis muscles, or Poland syndrome.

2–B. The epithelial bud differentiates from the retained thoracic portion of the milk line, developing from the seventh week of gestation to birth. This bud forms into the nipple and functional breast tissues. Thus, these tissues may respond to in utero maternal hormone stimulation by hypertrophy and the postbirth production of colostrum. Therefore, although a microadenoma causing an increase in prolactin levels is the most common cause of bilateral nipple discharge in adults, in the newborn population this is a known normal phenomenon and requires only observation and reassurance of the parents. Diffuse papillomatosis is primarily seen in an older population and produces a serous discharge. Both hyperthyroidism and hypothyroidism have been associated with a bilateral discharge, but this is rare and is usually seen in adults. There are a few toxins that can cause developmental abnormalities in the newborn, however these usually cause extensive global abnormalities.

3–D. The risk of breast cancer increases with age, and the majority of invasive ductal carcinomas present as a new mass on physical examination. All of the histories described are considered risk factors for the development of breast cancer. However, having never been pregnant, having an early menarche before age 12, or having a sister who had postmenopausal breast cancer all confer a lower risk than having the premalignant changes of atypical lobular hyperplasia, **estimated to be four to five times the risk.** In addition, both lobular carcinoma in situ (LCIS) and lobular hyperplasia are strong risk factors for the development of **invasive ductal carcinoma.** Birth control pills (BCPs) have not been shown to confer an increased long-term risk for breast cancer.

4–C. There are a large number of women without risk factors who develop breast cancer each year. The most common presentation for breast cancer is a new mass on physical examination. Therefore, great care must be taken to rule out breast cancer in any women who present with a new breast mass; observation is inadequate in this patient. Even though the sensitivity of a mammogram (MMG) increases with age due to replacement of dense parenchymal tissues by fatty tissues, palpation detects 10%–20% of MMG-negative cancers. Most women over the age of 30 presenting with a new mass on physical examination require a definitive, cell-based, diagnosis. If a cyst was found on an ultrasound study, suggesting a benign process, close follow-up and serial exams may be indicated rather than immediate biopsy. A fine needle aspiration (FNA) would be the most appropriate next step in this patient owing to the pretest's likelihood that this lesion is malignant. However, if the FNA was nondiagnostic, excisional biopsy or a core needle biopsy would be indicated. Axillary node dissection would be premature at this point.

5–C. This patient is presenting with a locally advanced tumor and therefore has a relatively high risk for metastatic disease. Infiltrating ductal carcinoma usually spreads to regional lymph nodes first, then can metastasize to the lungs, liver, and bone. Therefore, a chest radiograph and liver function tests are indicated. Bone metastases will either be painful or cause an increase in alkaline phosphatase. If the patient does not have either of these, then a bone scan is not indicated. A bilateral mammogram (MMG) is indicated in all patients presenting with recurrent disease to evaluate for concurrent disease. A computed tomography (CT) scan of the liver is not as sensitive for small liver metastases, and therefore would only be obtained if the liver function tests were abnormal.

6–C. Local recurrence in the breast occurs in approximately 10% of patients who are treated with wide local excision, axillary node dissection, and radiation therapy. "Salvage" total mastectomy is usually required and survival rates approach those obtained when a modified radical mastectomy is performed originally. In the absence of palpable lymph nodes, a second lymph node dissection is unnecessary. The effect of radiation on tissues is cumulative and does not diminish with time. Therefore, use of more radiation therapy in this patient increases the risk of toxicity to normal tissues and thus is usually not considered appropriate. Chemotherapy alone would be inappropriate because of a lower long-term survival with this approach.

7–C. This woman has only one risk factor for developing breast cancer; her mother was diagnosed with postmenopausal disease. All women, however, should obtain a baseline mammogram (MMG) between the ages of 35 and 39. Then, if there are no abnormalities, a screen MMG should be obtained every 1–2 years between the ages of 40 and 49, and yearly thereafter. An MMG should be obtained in all women over the age of 30 that present with breast symptoms even when there are no palpable lesions. Mammography can detect 90% of nonpalpable breast lesions.

8–D. This patient's lesion is most consistent with ductal carcinoma in situ (DCIS), therefore simple reassurance is inappropriate. Other findings on mammogram (MMG) that are suggestive of DCIS include asymmetric densities, ductal asymmetry, and distortion of normal breast architecture and skin or nipple distortion. Once a diagnosis of DCIS has been made, there are multiple factors that help determine the most appropriate treatment. Patient's preference and reliability for close follow-up, breast size, and family history are all taken into account. In this patient, local control of her DCIS was obtained with the lumpectomy. If this lesion had been observed, there would be approximately a 30% chance that it would develop into an invasive carcinoma. Because the lesion was small (< 3 cm in diameter) and there was no evidence of microinvasion, an axillary node dissection is not indicated. Although some may advocate the use of a modified radical mastectomy for such lesions, most people would agree that this is too aggressive for DCIS. Postoperative radiation therapy has been shown to be beneficial in reducing the local recurrence rate for small DCIS lesions.

9–D. In any patient with ductal carcinoma in situ (DCIS), close follow-up with breast examination and mammogram is essential. This patient now has evidence of regional metastatic disease with an unknown primary. In this case, axillary node dissection is not only used for staging, but is also considered therapeutic because of the overall reduction in tumor mass. However, axillary node dissection alone does not adequately treat the unknown primary, and thus a mastectomy is indicated. Radiation of the axilla may also treat the regional disease, but this is inadequate and does not address the unknown primary breast lesion. Most people would agree that a radical mastectomy is too aggressive for such a patient. A modified radical mastectomy, the removal of all the breast tissue combined with an axillary node dissection, is the most appropriate therapy for this patient because it provides treatment for the regional disease as well as for the unknown primary. Approximately 55%–75% of patients with occult breast cancer are found to have lesion on mastectomy.

10–D. The patient is suffering from mastodynia, which is rarely associated with malignancy, or fibroadenomas. She has progressed from cyclic to continuous mastodynia and thus represents a population of patients who are usually refractory to conservative therapy. However, in this situation, treatment with reassurance alone is inappropriate because of the disabling nature of her disease. Narcotics do not provide good pain relief for such a disease. Danazol has been shown to be very effective for such patients, as well as low-dose tamoxifen. Danazol is usually well tolerated, but may cause amenorrhea, body fat redistribution, hirsutism, acne, weight gain, and deepening of the voice. Long-term use has been associated with liver function abnormalities.

11–E. Most causes of nipple discharge are benign, however, spontaneous nipple discharge that is bloody tinged may represent cancer. Therefore, in low risk patients, observation combined with serial examinations is probably sufficient. However, in the high-risk patient, great care is required to confirm the diagnosis of an intraductal papilloma and observation is inadequate. Intraductal papillomas are the most common cause of bloody nipple discharge, although half the time the discharge is serous. These are usually small, nonpalpable lesions close to the nipple that are usually not seen on mammogram (MMG) or ultrasound, so evaluation in 6 months with MMG or ultrasound would usually miss the papilloma. Diagnosis is generally made by ductography and curative treatment consists of subareolar excision. There is no increased risk of cancer, so simple mastectomy may be too aggressive for the treatment of this disease. Diffuse papillomatosis affects multiple ducts and both breasts. The papillomas are larger and the discharge is serous, not bloody. With this diagnosis, there is an increased risk of breast cancer (40%), therefore simple mastectomy may be indicated.

12–D. Long-standing lymphedema of any kind predisposes to the development of lymphangiosarcoma. Most of these tumors develop in patients with massive lymphedema, usually as a result of the combination of a complete axillary node dissection (including the level III nodes) and axillary radiation. A single discrete tumor is rarely encountered. Rather, purplish red nodules are usually seen and are easily mistaken for bacterial cellulitis. These tumors are almost always high-grade and spread rapidly to involve most of the arm as well as the shoulder and chest wall. Pulmonary metastases are also commonly found at the time of diagnosis. Most patients die within 2 years of presentation. If these lesions represented a post-traumatic hematoma or the manifestations of a paraneoplastic coagulopathy, they would probably be painful. Lymphomas are typically solitary masses.

13–D. Medullary carcinoma usually presents as a palpable mass with smooth borders on mammogram (MMG) that mimic a benign condition. However, histologic examination reveals its malignant nature and typically has marked lymphocytic infiltration. Overall, it carries a relatively good prognosis.

14–B, C. The comedo form of ductal carcinoma in situ (DCIS) has the highest microinvasive rate and multicentric rate of these lesions. It is best treated with lumpectomy and postoperative radiation therapy. Lobular carcinoma in situ (LCIS) is also characterized by a high rate of multicentricity.

15–C. Lobular carcinoma in situ (LCIS) is usually considered a major risk factor for ductal carcinoma and usually presents as an incidental finding on breast biopsy of another lesion in postmenopausal women. Approximately 20%–25% of women who are found to have LCIS will develop breast cancer within 15 years of the diagnosis, with both breasts being at equal risk.

16–E. Inflammatory carcinoma, a variant of infiltrating ductal carcinoma, is characterized by the clinical appearance of inflammation (peau d'orange, warmth, edema, and pain) secondary to dermal lymphatic invasion. Its prognosis is poor.

17–A. Although there are variants of infiltrating ductal carcinoma, overall this lesion is the most common malignancy presenting as a breast mass.

19

Thyroid and Parathyroid

James J. Gangemi

I. Functional Anatomy

A. The thyroid gland

—develops from **endoderm of the first and second pharyngeal pouches.**

1. **Altered migration may result in**

   —**thyroglossal remnants** (cysts).

   —ectopic thyroid tissue (**lingual thyroid**).

2. **Lingual thyroid tissue**

   —may persist in the region of the **foramen cecum at the base of the tongue.**

   —that causes dysphagia, dyspnea, or dysphonia may be treated via suppression with thyroid hormone or ablation with radioactive iodine.

3. The **pyramidal lobe**

   —extending upward from the isthmus is a **remnant** of this migration.

   —is present in 80% of patients.

B. The **small parathyroid glands**

—are characteristically located **adjacent and posterior to the thyroid gland.**

1. **Most individuals (80%–90%)**

   —have **4 parathyroid glands,** 2 on each side.

2. The paired **superior parathyroid glands**

   —arise from the **fourth branchial pouch** in close proximity to the origin of the thyroid gland (floor of foregut).

3. The paired **inferior parathyroid glands**

—arise from the **third branchial pouch** along with the thymus.

—migrate farther and thus are more likely to be found in **ectopic locations** such as the **anterior mediastinum.**

4. **Other potential ectopic sites include**

—intrathyroid, posterior mediastinum, or near the tracheoesophageal groove.

C. **Arterial supply and venous drainage**

—of the thyroid and parathyroid **(Figure 19-1)**

1. **Arterial supply**

—is via the **inferior and superior thyroid arteries.**

2. **Venous drainage**

—is via the **superior, middle, and inferior thyroid veins.**

3. The **middle thyroid veins**

—drain directly into the internal jugular veins.

—are present in 50% of individuals.

D. The **recurrent laryngeal nerve**

—runs in the tracheoesophageal groove lateral to the ligament of Berry (a posteromedial suspensory ligament of the thyroid) before entering the larynx.

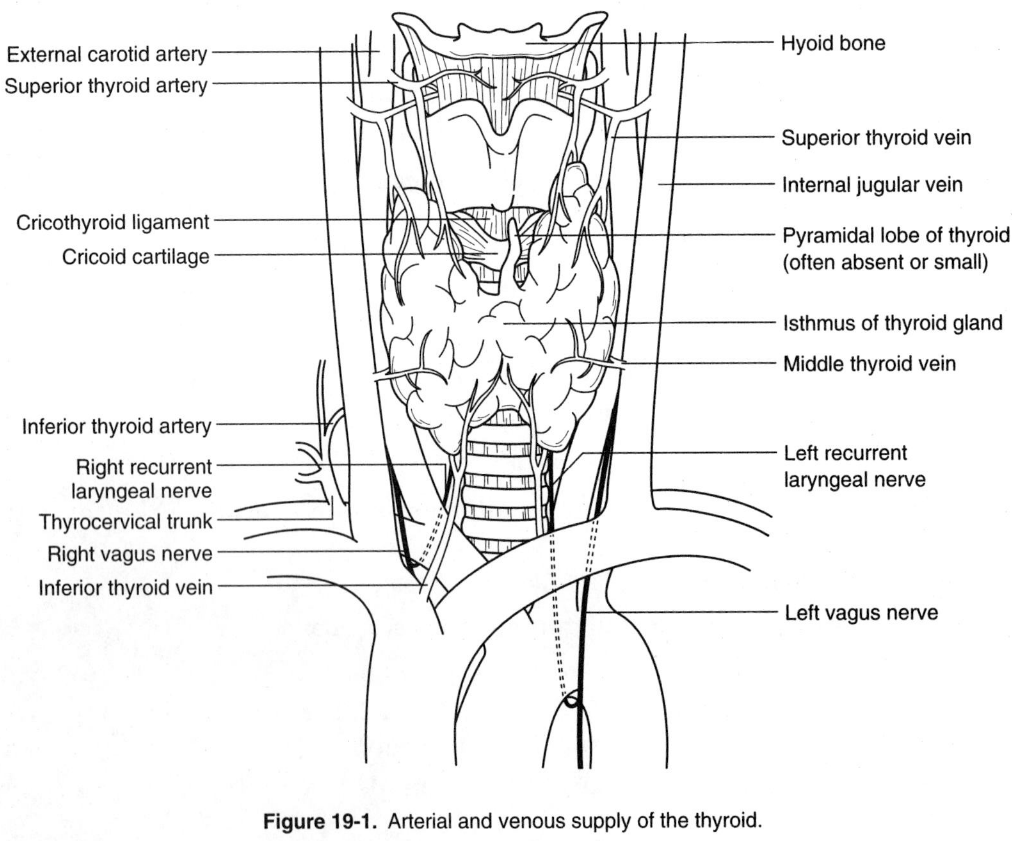

Figure 19-1. Arterial and venous supply of the thyroid.

1. **Unilateral injury to the nerve**

—causes ipsilateral **paralysis of the vocal cord** and failure of cord abduction, which may result in **hoarseness.**

2. **Bilateral cord injuries**

—may result in either complete loss of voice or **airway obstruction,** requiring immediate intubation or tracheostomy.

E. Superior laryngeal nerve

—runs adjacent to the superior pole of the thyroid to innervate the cricothyroid muscle.

—injury may result in an inability to attain high tones.

II. Physiology

A. Thyroxine (T_4) and triiodothyronine (T_3)

—are the principal hormones secreted by the thyroid.

1. **T_4 and $T_3$are stored**

—**in the colloid** via linkages with thyroglobulin.

2. **T_4 and T_3 become instantly bound**

—to albumin and thyroxine-binding globulin.

3. Most **T_3 in euthyroid patients**

—is produced by peripheral conversion of T_4 to T_3.

B. Thyroid hormone secretion

—**is regulated by feedback mechanism** involving the hypothalamus and pituitary gland.

1. **Thyrotropin-releasing factor** (TRF)

—is formed in the **hypothalamus.**

—stimulates the release of thyrotropin (**thyroid stimulating factor [TSH]**) from the **pituitary.**

2. **TSH secretion** is controlled in feedback manner by serum thyroid hormone levels.

3. **TSH** binds to specific receptors on the thyroid plasma membrane, stimulating increased cyclic adenosine monophosphate (cAMP) production and thyroid cellular function.

III. The Thyroid Nodule

A. Overview

1. **Eighty-five percent of thyroid nodules are benign.**

2. **Nodules are four times more common in women**

—although there is an equal distribution of thyroid cancer.

B. Risk factors for malignancy

—are outlined in **Table 19-1.**

C. Evaluation

1. Aspiration cytology

—is the single most helpful procedure for evaluation of a thyroid nodule.

2. Fine needle aspiration (FNA)

—is very accurate in colloid nodules and papillary cancer.

—can be used to **diagnose and treat cystic lesions,** which are **rarely malignant.**

3. "Follicular cytology"

—on fine needle aspirates **can represent a benign follicular nodule or a follicular cancer.**

—In this setting of an indeterminate diagnosis, excision is recommended.

4. Ultrasound

—may be used to characterize very small nodules (as small as 1 mm).

—can delineate cystic from solid lesions.

5. Thyroid nuclear medicine scan

—uses ^{99m}technetium to identify hyperfunctional ("hot") or hypofunctional ("cold") nodules within the thyroid.

—is used less frequently today because both cold and hot nodules may harbor a malignancy (Table 19-1).

6. Thyroid function tests

—are **not** very useful as a diagnostic test, because most thyroid cancers are euthyroid.

7. Excision

—is required for any nodule, cystic or solid, that **persists for 3 months.**

Table 19-1. Characteristics Associated with a Relatively Higher Probability of Malignancy in Thyroid Nodules

Age < 30 or age > 60
Solid lesions > cystic lesions
Cold nodules > hot nodules on thyroid scan (20%–25% of cold nodules are malignant versus < 1% of hot nodules)
History of radiation to head/neck (30% develop nodules; 30% are malignant)
Multiple endocrine neoplasias
Single nodules > multiple nodules
Enlarging nodules on thyroid hormone suppression
Nodules associated with dysphasia, dyspnea, hoarseness, vocal cord paralysis, Horner syndrome, or adenopathy

IV. Benign Diseases of the Thyroid

A. Causes of hyperthyroidism (thyrotoxicosis)

1. Graves' disease or toxic diffuse goiter

—accounts for 80% of all cases of hyperthyroidism.

a. This is an **autoimmune disease** resulting from **thyroid-stimulating immunoglobulin.**

b. **Incidence**

—is **six to seven times higher in females.**

c. **Manifestations include**

—**thyrotoxicosis** symptoms, which include heat intolerance, thirst, increased appetite, weight loss, sweating, and palpitations (e.g., atrial fibrillation).

—**diffuse goiter.**

—**exophthalmos.**

—**vitiligo.**

d. **Diffuse, increased uptake of radioiodine** (^{131}I) within a symmetrically enlarged gland is diagnostic and differentiates Graves' disease from other causes of thyrotoxicosis.

e. **Medical treatment**

(1) **Antithyroid drugs**

—Medical management with antithyroid drugs may be used as definitive treatment or in preparation for surgery or radioiodine treatment.

—**Propylthiouracil (PTU) or methimazole** inhibits function of the gland without destroying tissue.

—The **recurrence rate is high** (43% 1-year), and there is a risk of **agranulocytosis** with these agents.

(2) **Radioactive ^{131}I thyroid ablation**

—is effective treatment associated with **low recurrence,** although **70% develop hypothyroidism** within 10 years.

—is **contraindicated in children, women of childbearing years, patients with concomitant thyroid nodules,** or those with extremely large glands.

f. **Surgery**

—is rarely required.

(1) **Indications for surgery** include

—noncompliant patients.

—recurrence after medical therapy.

—children and women of childbearing age.

—presence of a very large gland or concomitant thyroid nodules.

(2) **Bilateral subtotal thyroidectomy or total thyroidectomy** may be performed.

—**β-Adrenergic blockers** (propranolol) are initiated 1 week before surgery to control symptoms.

—**Potassium iodide or Lugol's solution** is initiated 2 weeks before surgery to **decrease the vascularity of the gland.**

2. **Toxic multinodular goiter (Plummer disease)**
   a. This **disease typically affects women older than 50 years.**
   b. **Treatment** involves thyroidectomy after adequate medical therapy.
   c. **Bilateral subtotal thyroidectomy** is most commonly used.
      —**^{131}I does not reduce goiter size and may cause acute enlargement.**

3. **Solitary toxic nodule**
   a. These nodules are **most commonly found** in **women in the fifth decade** of life.
   b. **Functional nodules causing hyperthyroidism** are usually larger than 3 cm in diameter.
   c. The **nodules** eventually develop central necrosis and become cold.
   d. **Evaluation and treatment**
      —is similar to that described for a thyroid nodule (see III C).

B. Thyroiditis

—Causes and treatments are characterized in **Table 19-2.**

1. **Hashimoto's thyroiditis**
   —or **chronic lymphocytic thyroiditis,** is the **most common form** of chronic thyroiditis.

2. **Subacute thyroiditis (de Quervain thyroiditis)**
   —typically occurs in younger females with a **recent viral infection.**

3. **Acute suppurative thyroiditis** and **Reidel thyroiditis**
   —are rare.

C. Thyroid storm

—represents a massive uncontrolled release of thyroid hormone.

1. **Precipitating events** may include
   —**surgery.**
   —**anxiety.**
   —**excessive palpation of gland.**
   —**adrenergic stimulants.**
   —This typically occurs in patients with undiagnosed hyperthyroidism who are undergoing major stress.

2. **Symptoms include**
   —tachycardia.
   —fever.
   —numbness.
   —irritability.

Table 19-2. Causes and Treatment of Thyroiditis

Cause	Pathology	Clinical Findings	Treatment
Hashimoto's thyroiditis (chronic lymphocytic thyroiditis)	Autoimmune: antimicrosomal and antithyroglobulin antibodies in serum; diffuse lymphocytic infiltrate with germinal centers on histology	Most common cause of spontaneous hypothyroidism; middle-age women; diffuse, slowly progressive goiter with firm, rubbery, lobulated gland; may mimic a neoplasm	Treat with thyroid hormone replacement (levothyroxine)
Subacute thyroiditis (de Quervain thyroiditis)	Etiology unknown	Young females with recent viral infection; tender to palpation, weakness, fatigue, referred pain to jaw	Often self-limited for a few weeks with aspirin and steroids helpful; surgery only for refractory disease
Acute suppurative thyroiditis (rare)	Acute bacterial infection caused by *Streptococcus* or *Staphylococcus* species, pneumococci, coliforms	Typically follow URI: severe neck pain, dysphagia, fever, chills	Surgical drainage and débridement
Reidel's struma (rare)	"Woody" and fibrous thyroid involving adjacent strap muscles and carotid sheath; etiology unknown	Localized pain and compression of adjacent structures may occur: retroperitoneal fibrosis, fibrosing mediastinitis, sclerosing cholangitis	Often self-limited; steroids may be beneficial

URI = upper respiratory tract infection.

—vomiting.

—diarrhea.

3. **High output cardiac failure**

—may occur and is the usual cause of death.

4. **Preventative measures** include

—administration of PTU and beta-blocking agents (e.g., propranolol) for 3–4 weeks before surgery.

5. **Treatment of thyroid storm** includes

—mechanical **cooling,** and administering **oxygen and fluids.**

—preventing adrenal failure: **steroid therapy.**

—administering **β blockers** to relieve symptoms.

—administering **PTU** along with **iodine** (potassium iodide), which decreases serum thyroid hormone levels by inhibiting release of hormone from the thyroid gland.

—emergent subtotal thyroidectomy, although rarely required.

V. Thyroid Cancer (Table 19-3)

A. Overview

1. **Thyroid cancer** is the **most common endocrine malignancy** in the United States.
2. These cancers are an **uncommon cause of death** because the majority of these lesion are well differentiated and relatively nonaggressive.

B. Papillary carcinomas represent the majority of thyroid tumors.

—Mixed papillary/follicular carcinoma acts like very aggressive papillary carcinomas.

C. Follicular carcinomas are generally more aggressive than papillary carcinomas.

1. **Follicular carcinomas are** occasionally **difficult to differentiate** from follicular adenomas on FNA.

   —**Microvascular or local invasion on FNA** is characteristic of carcinoma, although indeterminate lesions may require resection.
2. **Hürthle cell tumors are variants of follicular carcinoma** that generally present at an older age.
   (1) **Unlike most follicular carcinomas,** these tumors are **generally resistant to ^{131}I radioablation.**
   (2) **Treatment**

   —**Large** (> 2 cm) or locally invasive Hürthle cell tumors are treated with **total thyroidectomy** with local lymph node biopsy.

   —With **positive nodes, modified lymph node dissection** of the neck is indicated, unlike with follicular lesions.

   —For **smaller,** less aggressive lesions, **lobectomy** may be appropriate.

D. Medullary carcinoma

—arise from **parafollicular, or C, cells** of the thyroid that secrete **calcitonin.**

1. **Sporadic cases** are usually unilateral.
2. **Familial cases,** associated with multiple endocrine neoplasia (MEN) II (see Chapter 20), are **often bilateral.**

E. Anaplastic carcinoma

—is the **most aggressive tumor** of the thyroid.

—may present with airway compromise.

—is often fatal despite surgery.

F. Treatment options for each tumor

—are outlined in **Table 19-3.**

1. For **metastatic papillary** or **follicular carcinoma** diagnosed preoperatively, **total thyroidectomy is performed to facilitate uptake of ^{131}I** into the metastases for ablation.

Table 19-3. Characteristics of Thyroid Cancer

Tumor	Epidemiology	Pathology	Prognosis	Treatment
Papillary (80%)	Affects young adults and children, women >men; most common tumor following neck irradiation	Slow-growing, often multicentric; psammona bodies on histology are characteristic; spread is via lymph nodes	Tumors <1.5 cm rarely metastasize; 5%–15% have lung metastases at diagnosis; 90% 5-year survival	Small tumors (<1.5 cm) may be treated with lobectomy and isthmusectomy; large tumors and metastases treated with total thyroidectomy and ^{131}I ablation
Follicular (10%)	Peaks at age 50–60, women>men	May be confused with adenoma on FNA; capsular or vascular invasion is diagnostic. Spread is characteristically hematogenous (bone, lung, brain, and liver)	85% 5-year survival without angioinvasion; 45%–50% with angioinvasion	Subtotal or total thyroidectomy depending on lesion size and location; postoperative ^{131}I ablation reduces recurrence rate and effectively treats metastases
Medullary (5%)	Sporadic cases peak at age 50–60; familial cases (10%–15%) associated with MEN II peak at 20–40	Secretes calcitonin; arises from parafollicular C-cells (neural crest tissue); presence of amyloid on histology is characteristic	Lymph node metastases frequently present at diagnosis; 30% will have microscopic disease in uninvolved lobe	Total thyroidectomy with lymph node dissection (bilateral if tumor bilateral)
Anaplastic (1%–2%)*	Peaks at age >70; seen in patients with longstanding nodular goiter	Poorly differentiated rapidly growing carcinoma	Often associated with lymph node metastases at diagnosis, most aggressive thyroid cancer with <2% 1–2 year survival	Total thyroidectomy for rare resectable lesions; palliative chemoradiation therapy, palliative resection

*Lymphoma and squamous cell carcinoma account for the rest of thyroid tumors.
^{131}I = iodine 131; FNA = fine needle aspiration; MEN = multiple endocrine neoplasia.

2. Thyroid hormones are also administered to suppress TSH stimulation of tumor growth.

G. Operative and postoperative complications

1. Recurrent laryngeal nerve injury

—The overall risk is 0.2%–3% at primary operation, but increases to 6% for re-operations.

2. Hypoparathyroidism with resultant hypocalcemia

—may result from bilateral dissection via **devascularization** of the parathyroid glands.

3. **Excessive postoperative hemorrhage**

—may lead to airway compromise and requires immediate re-exploration and possible drain placement.

4. **Injury to the superior laryngeal nerve**

—may result in a weak voice, which frequently goes unnoticed except in singers.

VI. Parathyroid

A. Functions of parathyroid hormone (PTH) include

—increasing mobilization of calcium and phosphate from bone.

—promoting active calcium reabsorption in distal nephron.

—inhibiting phosphate reabsorption in the proximal tubule.

—stimulating 1,25-dihydroxyvitamin D_3 and increasing gut absorption of calcium and phosphorous.

B. Primary hyperparathyroidism

—is characterized by excessive, abnormally regulated secretion of **PTH,** which results in **hypercalcemia.**

1. **Overview**
   a. A small percentage of patients have a history of **radiation exposure** as a child.
   b. Primary hyperparathyroidism peaks between the ages of 50–60, with a female:male ratio of 3:1.
2. **Etiology and pathology**
   a. **Adenomas**
   —There is **single adenoma** in **80%–85%** of patients.
   —There is a 2%–4% incidence of multiple adenomas.
   —Histologically, there is proliferation of chief cells in a single focus with a compressed rim of surrounding normal tissue.
   b. **Diffuse hyperplasia of all 4 glands**
   —occurs in 15% of patients.
   —may be associated with MEN I in 25%–35% of patients (see Chapter 20).
   —Histologically, diffuse chief cell hyperplasia is seen with cords or sheets of chief cells.
   c. **Parathyroid carcinoma**
   —occurs in 0.5–1.0% of patients.
3. The **causes of hypercalcemia** are outlined in **Table 19-4.**
   a. **Humoral hypercalcemia of malignancy**

Table 19-4. Causes of Hypercalcemia

Cause	Pathogenesis	PTH
Malignancy*	Hematologic: 25% (myeloma, leukemia) Nonhematologic: 75% (lung, breast, head and neck tumors)	Decreased or normal
Primary hyperparathyroidism*	Adenoma (80%–85%), diffuse hyperplasia (15%), parathyroid carcinoma (rare)	Increased
Familial hypocalciuric hypercalcemia	Autosomal dominant mutation in calcium sensing receptor	Decreased or normal
Immobilization	Associated with bone demineralization	Decreased or normal
Granulomatous disease	Sarcoidosis, tuberculosis	Decreased or normal
Vitamin D and vitamin A excess	Increased absorption	Decreased or normal
Other drugs	Thiazide diuretics, lithium	Decreased or normal
Other endocrine disorders	Addison disease, hyperthyroidism	Decreased or normal
Tertiary hyperparathyroidism	Hypercalcemia associated with chronic renal failure persisting after correction of renal failure (e.g., kidney transplant)	Increased
Milk-alkali syndrome	Excessive intake of calcium supplements in addition to milk	Decreased or normal

*Malignancy and primary hyperparathyroidism are the two most common causes of hypercalcemia. PTH = parathyroid hormone.

—(50% of cancer hypercalcemia) leads to increased bone resorption and suppressed bone formation.

—is characterized by **elevated calcium and urinary cAMP with low serum phosphate** and normal or low PTH.

—is **caused by a PTH-related protein** secreted by the tumor.

b. Hematologic malignancies

—(e.g., multiple myeloma, lymphoma) may be associated with **elevated phosphates and low urinary cAMP.**

—Lytic bone lesions may be caused by interleukin (IL)-β and tumor necrosis factor (TNF)-β that cause increased osteoclastic bone resorption.

4. Clinical manifestations

—of hypercalcemia are characterized in **Table 19-5.**

a. Mild chronic hypercalcemia

—Most patients are **asymptomatic.**

b. Hypercalcemic symptoms

—are related to the **magnitude and the rate of rise.**

—Hypercalcemia related to **malignancy** is often associated with a rapid rise and is frequently symptomatic.

Table 19-5. Clinical Manifestations of Hypercalcemia

Neuromuscular	Mental confusion, obtundation, coma, fatigue, lethargy, malaise, muscle weakness, depression, apathy, inability to concentrate
Renal	Nephrolithiasis (most frequent complication of primary hyperparathyroidism developing in 15%–20% of patients) Nephrocalcinosis (calcification of renal parenchyma): severe cases may not improve with parathyroidectomy
Cardiovascular	Hypertension that correlates with degree of renal impairment Shortened QT interval on electrocardiogram Heart block
Skeletal	Bone pain Radiographic evidence (uncommon, 1%–2%) Pathologic fractures Subperiosteal cortical resorption on radial aspect of middle phalanx of second/third finger Salt-and-pepper pattern of skull on radiograph "Brown tumor": localized proliferation of osteoclasts typically involving long bones Osteitis fibrosa cystica (rare)
Gastrointestinal	Nausea and vomiting, anorexia, constipation, peptic ulcer disease, pancreatitis: rare, cholelithiasis: elevated calcium in bile

5. **Diagnosis**

   a. **Hypercalcemia and elevated levels of PTH**

   —(> 60 mEq/mL) are hallmarks of primary hyperparathyroidism.

   b. **Because of extensive calcium binding by albumin**

   —**total serum calcium levels vary based upon albumin levels.**

   —For every 1 mg/dL fall in serum albumin, total serum calcium levels drop 0.8 mg/dL even in the setting of normal calcium balance.

   —**True hypocalcemia** is characterized by decreased **ionized calcium levels,** which accurately reflect functional extracellular calcium levels despite hypoalbuminemia.

   c. **Hypophosphatemia**

   —will occur in 35% of patients.

   d. **Elevated urinary cAMP and urinary calcium**

   —may be present (35%–40%).

   e. **Bone densitometry**

   —is very sensitive and determines the extent of cortical bone loss.

   f. **Preoperative localization of lesions**

   —with ultrasound or nuclear medicine scan is **rarely** indicated for primary disease.

   —Localization is frequently indicated for reoperative procedures.

6. **Treatment of primary hyperparathyroidism**

   a. **Symptomatic disease**

   —**Surgery** is the **only definitive therapy** for treatment of symptomatic disease.

   b. **Asymptomatic or mild disease**

   —at the time of diagnosis seldom progresses clinically, biochemically, or radiologically.

c. The **cure rate**
—for initial operation is 90%–95%.

7. **Principles of surgical correction**
a. **Location and number of glands**
—**may be highly variable.**
b. **To rule out lesions in multiple glands**
—bilateral neck dissection with **identification of all 4 glands** may be necessary.
c. **To confirm the presence or absence of parathyroid tissue**
—frozen sections should be performed.
(1) This is not helpful in differentiating diseased tissue from normal tissue.
(2) Intraoperative measurement of local venous PTH may also be used to confirm removal of a functional parathyroid lesion.
d. **Treatment of adenomas**
(1) **Single or multiple enlarged glands**
—**should be resected,** leaving normal or atrophic glands.
(2) If **only 3 normal glands are identified**
—after thorough exploration, ipsilateral thyroidectomy is often performed on the side where only 1 gland was found.
(a) In this setting, 96% of the remaining glands are intrathyroidal.
(b) Videoscopic parathyroid resection is also being used for the surgical treatment of benign parathyroid disease.

8. **Multiglandular hyperplasia**
—may be treated with subtotal or total parathyroidectomy.
a. **Subtotal parathyroidectomy**
—involves removing 3.5 glands, while leaving the remaining tissue with the native blood supply.
b. **Total parathyroidectomy**
—is **followed by autotransplantation** of gland fragments to the nondominant forearm or sternocleidomastoid muscle.
(1) Autotransplantation makes reoperation for recurrence easier.
(2) This is the preferred procedure for familial disease.
c. **Permanent hypoparathyroidism**
—occurs in 5% of patients.

C. **Persistent or recurrent disease**
1. **Persistent hyperparathyroidism**
—after surgical exploration occurs in less than 5% of patients.
—is often related to a single diseased gland remaining in the neck.
2. **Recurrent disease**
—often develops after a period of hypocalcemia.
—is often related to **regrowth of diseased tissue.**

—may occur because of inadvertent microscopic implantation during resection.

—Recurrent parathyroid carcinoma should be considered in this setting.

3. **Preoperative localization**

—is **recommended for recurrent disease.**

a. **Adhesions** make reoperation more difficult.

b. **Ectopic location**

—of glands is also more likely in this setting.

c. **Localization methods**

(1) **Ultrasonography** is most useful for lesions close to or within the thyroid.

(2) **Computed tomography (CT) or magnetic resonance imaging (MRI)** offers superior visualization of **deeper structures and ectopic adenomas,** especially in the mediastinum.

(3) A **technetium-99m-Sestamibi** scan may also help localize diseased tissue.

d. **Invasive localization**

—is reserved for unsuccessful noninvasive localization

(1) Selective angiography.

(2) Venous sampling with measurement of PTH can be combined with angiography for complete identification.

4. **Surgical reexploration**

—has 60%–80% success rate.

a. There is an **increased incidence of complications** such as **unilateral recurrent nerve injury (5%–10%)** and **permanent hypoparathyroidism (10%–20%).**

b. **Median sternotomy** and **mediastinal exploration** is necessary in 1%–2% of patients.

c. The **superior parathyroids** may be posterior to the esophagus and as superior as the pharynx.

D. **Secondary hyperparathyroidism**

—is a consequence of **chronic renal failure.**

1. **These patients are unable** to synthesize the active form of vitamin D, which results in **hypocalcemia and compensatory elevation of PTH.**

2. **Untreated patients become symptomatic with**

—**bone demineralization.**

—**calcification of soft tissues.**

—**accelerated vascular calcification.**

—pruritus.

—painful skin ulcerations from subcutaneous calcium deposition.

3. **Treatment** is generally **medical** with

—**dialysis** with high-calcium bath.

—phosphate-binding antacids.

—**calcium supplements.**

4. **Surgical treatment**

—is rarely indicated except for refractory cases.

E. Tertiary hyperparathyroidism

1. **This type of hyperparathyroidism**

—is characterized by **persistent disease in patients with secondary hyperparathyroidism despite renal transplantation** secondary to dysregulated parathyroid function.

—is associated with **hypercalcemia and elevated PTH levels.**

2. **Treatment** often requires surgical resection with subtotal thyroidectomy.

F. Parathyroid carcinoma

1. **Compared with adenomas** patients with **parathyroid carcinomas are younger,** with an equal male:female ratio.
2. **Patients are more frequently symptomatic** with elevated levels of calcium, PTH, and alkaline phosphatase.
3. **Histologically, characteristics include**

—a trabecular pattern.

—mitotic figures.

—**capsular invasion.**

—**angioinvasion.**

4. The **affected glands** are often adherent to surrounding tissue.
5. **Treatment** is with **radical resection of** the involved gland, the ipsilateral thyroid gland, and regional lymph nodes.

—**Chemotherapy** and **radiation therapy** provide no additional benefit.

—The **recurrence rate** is ~50%.

—Long-term **prognosis** is poor.

—**Survival** depends on complete resection at the initial operation.

Review Test

Directions: Each of the numbered items or incomplete statements in this section is followed by answers or by completions of the statement. Select the ONE lettered answer or completion that is BEST in each case.

1. During a routine check-up, an otherwise healthy 38-year-old woman is found to have hypercalcemia on a routine chemistry panel. Additional work-up reveals an elevated parathyroid hormone (PTH) levels as well. At the time of operation, which of the following histopathologic findings would suggest the presence of parathyroid carcinoma in this patient?

(A) Diffuse proliferation of chief cells in all 4 glands
(B) Sheets of chief cells in all 4 glands
(C) Focal chief cell hyperplasia extending through the capsule
(D) Focal chief cell hyperplasia compressing a normal rim of tissue
(E) Focal chief cell hyperplasia in 2 different glands

2. A 35-year-old woman presents with flank pain and hematuria, and during evaluation is found to have calcium phosphate stones in her urine along with hypercalciuria and hypercalcemia. Subsequent work-up reveals an elevated parathyroid (PTH) level. After resolution of this episode of renal colic, she undergoes elective neck exploration. Initial exploration of the right neck posterior to the right lobe of the thyroid reveals 2 diffusely enlarged parathyroid glands, which are successfully removed. Which of the following is the most appropriate statement regarding the subsequent management of this patient?

(A) No additional exploration if an adenoma is identified on frozen section
(B) Exploration of the left side only if hyperplasia is identified
(C) Exploration of the left side only if an adenoma is identified
(D) Resection of 3.5 parathyroid glands if an adenoma is seen on frozen section
(E) Performance of frozen sections and exploration of the left side

3. A 42-year-old woman presents for elective total thyroidectomy for a follicular carcinoma of the thyroid gland diagnosed by fine needle aspiration (FNA). Intraoperatively, ligation of which of the following vessels is necessary to obtain complete vascular control of the thyroid gland in this patient?

(A) Inferior and superior thyroid arteries; and inferior, middle, and superior thyroid veins
(B) Inferior, middle, and superior thyroid arteries; and inferior and superior thyroid veins
(C) Inferior and superior thyroid arteries and veins; and thyroid ima artery
(D) Inferior, superior, and middle thyroid veins; and superior, middle, and thyroid ima arteries
(E) Inferior, middle, and superior thyroid arteries and veins; and thyroid ima vein

4. A 56-year-old woman presents to the office with a 2-cm neck mass just left and lateral to the trachea in the inferior lobe of the left thyroid gland. Fine needle aspiration (FNA) reveals a moderately differentiated tumor that stains strongly for amyloid. In addition, her calcitonin is elevated. Which of the following is the most appropriate therapy for this patient?

(A) Total thyroidectomy with radioiodine (^{131}I) ablation therapy
(B) Total thyroidectomy with bilateral lymph node dissection
(C) Total thyroidectomy with left-sided lymph node dissection
(D) Left lobectomy and isthmusectomy with left-sided lymph node dissection
(E) Left lobectomy and isthmusectomy alone

5. A 47-year-old woman presents to the office with complaints of a 4-month history of worsening fatigue and weight gain. Palpation of the thyroid gland reveals an irregular lobulated gland bilaterally. Laboratory evaluation demonstrates serum antimicrosomal antibodies. Which of the following best describes the histologic findings that are likely to be identified upon biopsy of this patient's thyroid?

(A) Diffuse sheets and cords of chief cells
(B) Proliferation of parafollicular cells with amyloid
(C) Well differentiated tumor with psammoma bodies
(D) Diffuse lymphocytic infiltrate with germinal centers
(E) Follicular cell proliferation with vascular invasion

6. A 41-year-old woman presents to the office with a 3-cm nodule in the right lobe of the thyroid gland involving part of the isthmus. Fine needle aspiration (FNA) of the lesion reveals a well differentiated lesion with lamellar mineral deposits surrounding necrotic cells (psammoma body). Which of the following is the most appropriate treatment for this patient?

(A) Right lobectomy with isthmusectomy and radioiodine (^{131}I) therapy
(B) Total thyroidectomy and postoperative ^{131}I therapy
(C) Total thyroidectomy alone
(D) Right lobectomy with isthmusectomy alone
(E) Total thyroidectomy with right-sided lymph node dissection

7. A 54-year-old woman undergoes an elective total thyroidectomy for follicular cell carcinoma. The dissection was noted to be somewhat difficult but the patient tolerated the procedure well. Twelve hours postoperatively the patient is noted to be very anxious. On physical examination she is noted to have facial fasiculations and facial muscle twitching to palpation. Which of the following is the most appropriate therapy for this patient?

(A) Administration of calcium supplements
(B) Direct laryngoscopy to identify paralyzed vocal cord
(C) Re-exploration and evacuation of hematoma
(D) Immediate reintubation
(E) Immediate forearm implantation of inadvertently resected parathyroid tissue

8. A 35-year-old man with a 5-year history of end-stage renal disease requiring hemodialysis presents to the emergency room with complaints of right leg pain after minor trauma to the area. Plain radiographs reveal a fracture line along the tibia with notable bone demineralization and soft tissue calcification. Further work-up reveals elevation of parathyroid hormone (PTH) and a decreased ionized calcium level. Which of the following is the most appropriate treatment measure for this patient's underlying condition?

(A) Resection of 3.5 parathyroid glands
(B) Resection of all parathyroid glands with autotransplantation
(C) Radiation therapy to the parathyroid glands
(D) Calcium supplements, vitamin D, and alteration of dialysis fluid
(E) Calcium restriction and alteration of dialysis fluid

9. A 75-year-old man presents to the office for a routine check-up. The patient states that he has been doing well except for some mild low-back pain, which he attributes to working too much in the yard. A chemistry panel reveals an elevated calcium level but no other significant abnormalities. Plain radiographs reveal multiple lytic lesions within the vertebral bodies of L4 and L5. After a thorough physical examination, which of the following tests is most appropriate in the subsequent evaluation of this patient?

(A) Serum parathyroid hormone (PTH) levels and neck ultrasound
(B) Serum PTH levels and measurement of creatinine clearance
(C) Neck exploration and resection of 3.5 parathyroid glands
(D) Transrectal ultrasound of the prostate and prostate-specific antigen levels
(E) Serum PTH and computed tomography (CT) scan of the neck

10. A 46-year-old woman presents to the office with a 3-cm mass in the right lobe of the thyroid. On physical examination, the mass is noted to be cystic in nature. Fine needle aspiration (FNA) of the cyst reveals colloid. Which of the following is the most appropriate management strategy for this patient?

(A) No further therapy and continued observation
(B) Total thyroidectomy alone
(C) Right lobectomy and isthmusectomy
(D) Total thyroidectomy and radioiodine (^{131}I) therapy
(E) Total thyroidectomy and right-sided lymph node dissection

Answers and Explanations

1–C. Differentiating a parathyroid adenoma from a carcinoma may sometimes be difficult. Adenomas are characterized by focal chief cell hyperplasia compressing a normal rim of parathyroid tissue. Characteristic histologic findings of a carcinoma include microvascular invasion and invasion of the surrounding capsule. Focal hyperplasia in 2 glands is suggestive of multiple adenomas. Diffuse proliferation of chief cells, or sheets or cords of chief cells in all 4 glands is suggestive of diffuse parathyroid hyperplasia.

2–E. As many as 15%–20% of patients will have multiple adenomas at the time of surgery. During a neck exploration for parathyroid disease, identification of all glands is important if diffuse hyperplasia is a concern. In the patient described, frozen sections of the initial 2 glands should be performed to confirm the presence of parathyroid tissue in the resected specimens. Despite the findings, exploration of the left side should be performed for the reasons mentioned above.

3–A. A general understanding of the arterial and venous supply to the thyroid gland is essential for adequate vascular control during resection. The thyroid gland is generally supplied by 2 major arteries: the inferior and superior thyroid arteries. A small percentage of patients (10%–15%) will have an accessory thyroid ima artery arising directly from the aortic arch. There are 3 major veins draining the thyroid gland: the superior, inferior, and middle thyroid veins. Variations of both the arterial and venous systems may exist.

4–C. The presence of amyloid on histologic examination is a classic finding for medullary carcinoma of the thyroid. These tumors arise from parafollicular, or C, cells and may secrete calcitonin, which is also a characteristic diagnostic finding. Treatment involves total thyroidectomy and central lymph node dissection on the side of the lesion. If bilateral tumors are identified, then bilateral lymph node dissection may be required. A lobectomy and isthmusectomy would be inadequate therapy for this tumor. These tumors are insensitive to radioiodine (^{131}I) ablation therapy, although external beam radiation therapy to the neck is considered in some patients with this disease.

5–D. The presence of antimicrosomal or antithyroglobulin antibodies in the serum is suggestive of Hashimoto's thyroiditis, which is a frequent cause of hypothyroidism. This disease can present with a diffusely enlarged gland although a firm, rubbery, multilobulated gland may also be present and may mimic thyroid tumors. The characteristic histopathologic finding of Hashimoto's thyroiditis is diffuse lymphocytic infiltrate with normal germinal centers. Diffuse sheets and cords of chief cells suggests diffuse parathyroid hyperplasia. Parafollicular, or C, cell proliferation with the presence of amyloid is suggestive of medullary thyroid carcinoma. Psammoma bodies are characteristic of papillary tumors. Extensive follicular cell proliferation with vascular invasion is suggestive of a follicular carcinoma.

6–B. Psammoma bodies are a classic histologic finding of papillary carcinoma of the thyroid gland. Appropriate surgical treatment of large papillary carcinomas near the isthmus includes total or near total thyroidectomy with postoperative radioiodine (^{131}I) ablation therapy because these lesions are sensitive to ^{131}I. A lymph node dissection is generally not required in these patients. For some small papillary carcinomas (< 1.5 cm) involving 1 lobe only, some advocate lobectomy and isthmusectomy alone; however, in this setting this would be considered inadequate treatment.

7–A. Postoperative hypoparathyroidism with resultant hypocalcemia is most commonly caused by devascularization of the parathyroid glands rather than removal of all the glands. After thyroid surgery, permanent hypoparathyroidism is quite rare, although temporary hypocalcemia may be present. Signs and symptoms of the resultant hypocalcemia in the postoperative period include paresthesias, tetany, seizures, mental status changes, Chvostek sign (facial twitching with tapping of the facial nerve), and Trousseau sign. Treatment involves administration of calcium supplements (e.g., intravenous calcium gluconate). Recurrent laryngeal nerve injury is unlikely to cause these signs and symptoms; thus, laryngoscopy or reintubation is not necessary. A hematoma is also unlikely to present in this manner. Delayed forearm transplantation, hours after removal of the specimen would not be helpful acutely and is unlikely to be successful.

8–D. This patient has characteristic findings of secondary hyperparathyroidism in a patient on chronic hemodialysis. The presence of a pathologic fracture precipitated by minor trauma with bone demineralization and soft tissue calcification in association with an elevated parathyroid hormone (PTH) and hypocalcemia is characteristic of this disease. Treatment involves administering calcium supplements, vitamin D, and adding calcium to dialysate fluid. Calcium restriction and altering dialysis fluid are contraindicated in this setting. Parathyroid resection is not indicated in the treatment of secondary hyperparathyroidism. Radiation therapy plays no role in the treatment of hyperparathyroidism.

9–D. Malignancy is a frequent cause of hypercalcemia. In the setting described, metastatic disease to the lumbar vertebrate should be suspected as the cause of hypercalcemia rather than a primary disorder of the parathyroid gland. Adenocarcinoma of the prostate gland frequently metastasizes to the vertebral bodies and produces characteristic osteoblastic lesions, as described. Transrectal ultrasound of the prostate and measurement of prostate-specific antigen levels would be appropriate in the evaluation of this patient before any work-up of parathyroid disease. Multiple myeloma may also cause osteoblastic lesions; this is seen most commonly in men 50–60 years old. Other tumors that should be considered in this setting include lung, colon, and breast (women > men) cancers. Measurement of PTH or neck exploration would not be useful in the evaluation or management of this patient's primary disease process.

10–A. Most cystic masses are benign in nature and represent simple colloid-filled cysts. Simple needle-guided drainage of these lesions is adequate therapy. Recurring lesions or cystic lesions that persist for longer than 3 months may require resection. It should be noted that some carcinomas of the thyroid may undergo central necrosis and appear cystic, although cytology will generally identify these lesions. Formal resection in the setting of a simple colloid nodule is not indicated. Formal resection or ablation therapy is not required for simple cystic lesions that respond to needle-guided drainage.

20

Adrenal Gland

P. James Renz, III

I. Functional Anatomy

A. Adrenal glands

1. The adrenal glands are retroperitoneal organs located near the superior pole of each kidney (Figure 20-1).
2. Each gland is composed of two functionally distinct regions, the cortex and medulla.
   a. The **cortex** arises from primitive **mesoderm.**
   b. The **medulla** arises from **ectodermal neural crest cells** that migrate to the adrenal cortex.
      —Extra-adrenal rests of **neural crest tissue** along the aorta may persist in the retroperitoneum. The **organ of Zuckerkandl** is the most notable example, located at the aorta at the level of the inferior mesenteric artery.

B. Arterial supply and venous drainage

1. The **arterial supply**
   —is derived from the **inferior phrenic artery, aorta, and the renal artery,** which form the superior, middle, and inferior suprarenal arteries, respectively.
2. The **adrenal veins**
   a. The **short right adrenal vein** drains into the **inferior vena cava.**
   b. The **left adrenal vein** drains into the **left renal vein.**

C. Lymphatic drainage and innervation

1. **Lymphatics**
   —**parallel** the vascular supply.
   —**drain** into para-aortic, subdiaphragmatic, and renal lymph nodes.
2. There is **no innervation to the cortex**

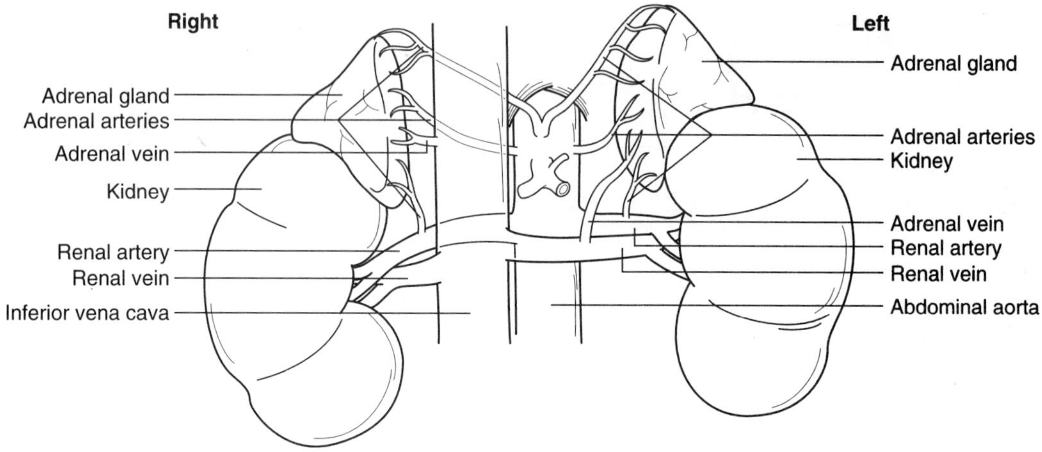

Figure 20-1. Adrenal anatomy. (Adapted with permission from O'Leary JP: *The Physiologic Basis of Surgery.* Baltimore, Williams & Wilkins, 1996, p 332.)

—although the **medulla** receives **preganglionic sympathetic innervation** via the splanchnic nerves.

II. Physiology of the Adrenal Cortex

A. Overview

1. The **cortex is subdivided** into 3 zones that are characterized by distinct steroid secretory patterns.
   - a. **Outer zona glomerulosa: aldosterone** secretion.
   - b. **Middle zona fasciculata:** predominantly **cortisol** secretion.
   - c. **Inner zona reticularis:** predominantly **androgen** secretion.
2. The **various pathways involved in steroid synthesis** within the adrenal cortex are outlined in **Figure 20-2.**
3. The **adrenal steroids** exist in unbound and bound (active) forms.
   —Binding is mainly by **corticosteroid binding globulin** and **albumin.**

B. Secretory products

1. **Glucocorticoids**
   - a. **Cortisol**
     —is the principal glucocorticoid in humans.
     —is released in episodic bursts with a **diurnal peak around 4–6 AM.**
   - b. **Secretion** is stimulated and regulated by the episodic secretion of adrenocorticotropic hormone (ACTH), sympathetic activation, and feedback inhibition of cortisol.
2. **Aldosterone**
   - a. Aldosterone

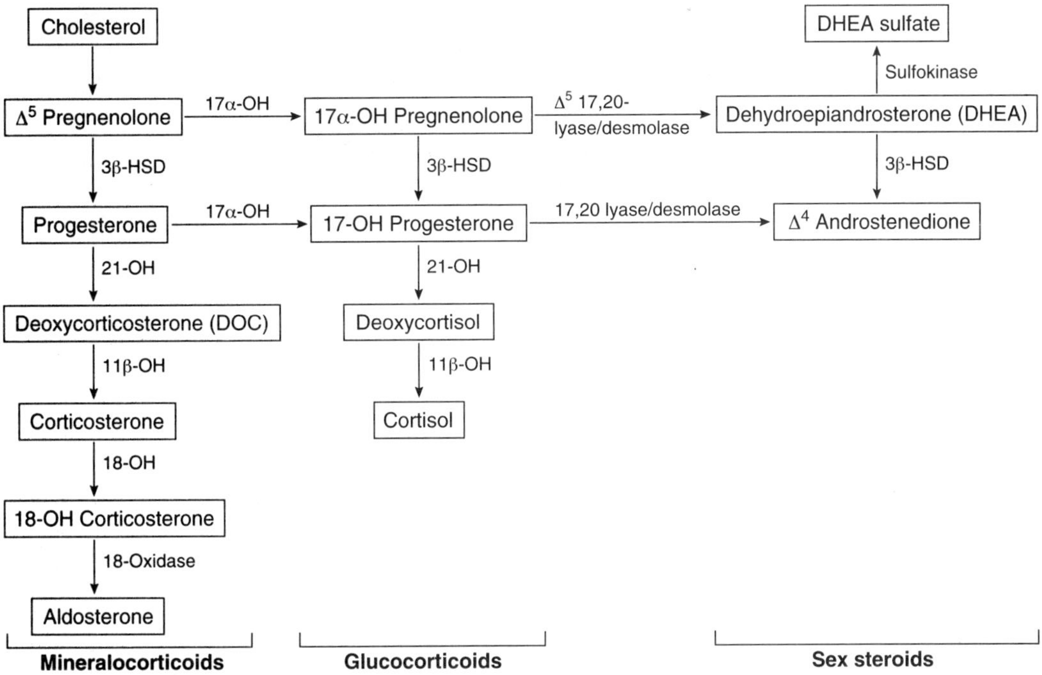

Figure 20-2. Steroid biosynthetic pathway. (Adapted with permission from O'Leary JP: *The Physiologic Basis of Surgery.* Baltimore, Williams & Wilkins, 1996, p 333.)

—**stimulates renal sodium reabsorption** and the **secretion of potassium,** hydrogen, and ammonia.

b. Secretion is stimulated by the activation of the renin-angiotensin system, hyperkalemia, and ACTH.

3. Sex steroids

a. Dehydroepiandrosterone (DHEA)

—is the major sex steroid produced by the adrenal cortex.

b. Secretion is stimulated and regulated by ACTH, not gonadotropins.

c. Actions of sex steroids

(1) DHEA influences male external genitalia and ductal structures.

—Its absence prompts development of female genitalia in the fetus.

(2) This steroid also promotes development of **male secondary sexual characteristics.**

III. Diseases of the Adrenal Cortex

A. Hyperadrenocorticism (i.e., Cushing's syndrome)

—is caused by chronically **elevated levels of cortisol and corticosterone.**

1. Causes of Cushing's syndrome

a. The **most common cause of Cushing's syndrome** is chronic **exogenous administration of corticosteroids.**

b. Other endogenous causes of Cushing's syndrome are outlined in **Table 20-1.**

2. **Clinical manifestations** include

—truncal obesity.

—moon facies.

—purple striae.

—hirsutism.

—hypertension.

—menstrual disorders.

—Buffalo hump.

—muscle wasting.

—easy bruising.

—diabetes mellitus.

—amenorrhea.

—impotence.

—edema.

—osteoporosis.

—emotional lability.

3. **Evaluation of Cushing's syndrome**

—includes appropriate laboratory and radiologic assessment (**Figure 20-3**).

a. **Screening tests**

—document hyperadrenocorticism.

—include 24-hour **urinary free cortisol** and the low-dose dexamethasone suppression test.

b. **Diagnostic tests**

(1) These tests differentiate causes of Cushing's syndrome.

Table 20-1. Causes of Endogenous Cushing's Syndrome*

Etiology	Pathogenesis	Laboratory Findings
Cushing's disease (70%) **Ecotopic ACTH syndrome** (e.g., lung cancer)	**ACTH-dependent**	Suppression of cortisol with **low-dose and high-dose** dexamethasone, high ACTH, and increased skin pigmentation
Adrenal adenoma **Adrenal carcinoma** **Adrenal hyperplasia**	**ACTH-independent**	No suppression of cortisol with low-dose or high-dose dexamethasone, and low ACTH
Major depression **Alcoholism**	PseudoCushing's syndrome	Suppression of cortisol with low-dose dexamethasone

*Exogenous administration of corticosteroids remains the leading cause of Cushing's syndrome.
ACTH = adrenocorticotropic hormone.

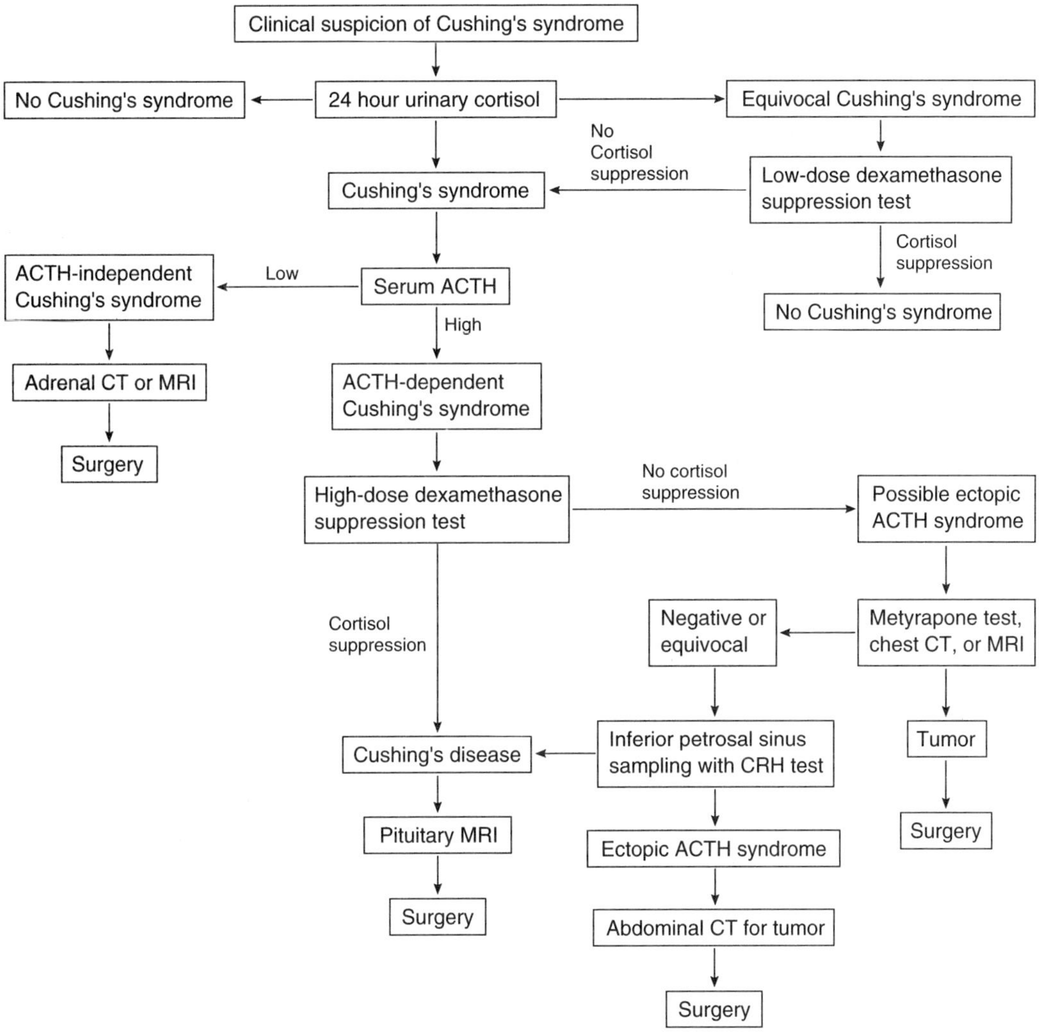

Figure 20-3. Algorithm for evaluation of Cushing's syndrome. (Adapted with permission from Sabiston DC: *Scientific Principles of Surgery.* Saunders, 1997, p 681.) *ACTH* = adrenocorticotropic hormone; *CT* = computed tomography; *MRI* = magnetic resonance imaging; *CRH* = corticotropin releasing hormone.

(2) Tests include

—serum ACTH levels.

—high-dose dexamethasone suppression test.

—metyrapone stimulation test.

—inferior petrosal sinus sampling.

c. Radiologic assessment

(1) A **magnetic resonance imaging (MRI)** scan should be performed if a **pituitary lesion** is suspected.

(2) An **abdominal computed tomography (CT)** scan is performed if an **adrenal source** is suspected.

(3) A **chest and abdominal CT** may identify an **ectopic** source.

(4) An **NP-59 radionuclide imaging** study may differentiate

adrenal adenoma or hyperplasia (positive uptake) from an adrenal carcinoma (negative uptake).

4. **Treatment**
   a. **Cushing's disease**
      —is treated with **transsphenoidal resection** of the pituitary lesion in adults.
      —is treated with irradiation in children.
   b. An **adrenal adenoma**
      —is treated with **unilateral adrenalectomy.**
   c. **Nodular hyperplasia**
      —is treated with **bilateral adrenalectomy** with or without reimplantation.
   d. **Adrenal carcinoma** (see III E)
   e. **Ectopic ACTH syndrome**
      (1) **Treatment**
         —involves either **resection of the primary lesion** or debulking of unresectable lesions and metastases.
      (2) **Pharmacological adrenalectomy**
         —with agents that **block adrenal steroid production** (e.g., **metyrapone, aminoglutethimide, ketoconazole, or mitotane**) may be performed for **inoperable lesions.**
      (3) **Bilateral adrenalectomy**
         —may be performed if one is unable to localize the source or if uncontrollable hypercortisolism is present.

B. Hyperaldosteronism (i.e., Conn's syndrome)

1. **Overview**
   —This syndrome is caused by hypersecretion of aldosterone, which is **more common in females** (2:1).
   —It usually presents in the third to fourth decade.

2. **Etiologies**
   a. **Primary causes** (decreased plasma renin) include
      —aldosterone-producing adenoma (65%–85%).
      —bilateral adrenal hyperplasia (25%).
      —unilateral adrenal hyperplasia.
   b. **Secondary causes** (increased plasma renin) include
      —renal artery stenosis.
      —congestive heart failure.
      —cirrhosis.
      —pregnancy.
      —diuretic therapy.
      —Bartter's syndrome (renin-secreting tumor).

3. **Clinical manifestations** include
   —**hypertension secondary to sodium retention without edema.**

—weakness and fatigue.

—polyuria and polydipsia.

—tetany secondary to hypokalemia.

—menorrhagia.

4. Evaluation of Conn's syndrome

a. Initial laboratory studies include

—serum potassium.

—24-hour urine aldosterone.

—plasma renin activity.

b. The **saline infusion test**

—can be used to confirm the diagnosis because **saline infusion** causes a decrease in **plasma aldosterone** levels in normal patients, but is **unaffected in hyperaldosteronism.**

c. Studies differentiating hyperplasia from an adenoma

—include postural studies and 18-hydroxycorticosterone levels.

(1) Postural studies

—Because of persistent renin suppression associated with **adenomas,** morning **plasma aldosterone levels remain unchanged or decreased** in the upright position versus initial supine measurements.

—In **hyperplasia,** the postural renin response is not suppressed, thus the **aldosterone level increases** in the **upright position.**

(2) 18-hydroxycorticosterone levels

—are greater than 100 ng/dL with **adenomas.**

—are less than 100 ng/dL with **hyperplasia.**

d. Radiographic assessment

—is often used to localize and differentiate lesions.

(1) CT and MRI localize lesions in approximately 90% of cases.

(2) Adrenal venous sampling and NP-59 scintigraphy help differentiate adenomas from hyperplasia.

5. Treatment

—is **surgical** for **adrenal adenomas.**

—is **medical** for **adrenal hyperplasia.**

a. Both **adenomas and hyperplasia**

—are treated with potassium supplementation, calcium channel blockers, and diuresis.

b. Adrenalectomy

—**Unilateral adrenalectomy** is performed for **adenomas.**

—**Subtotal adrenalectomy** may be performed for **hyperplasia associated with symptomatic hypokalemia refractory to medical therapy.**

C. Adrenogenital syndromes

—**are caused by** congenital adrenal hyperplasia (90%) or adrenal neoplasms (10%).

1. **Congenital adrenal hyperplasia (CAH)**

—represents inherited defects of enzymes necessary for cortisol synthesis, which shunts cortisol precursors into androgen pathways (**Table 20-2**).

a. **21-Hydroxylase deficiency**

—is the most common enzymatic defect that causes CAH (90%).

—**occurs** in 1 in 10,000 live births.

—**causes** deficits of aldosterone and cortisol and **increased production of testosterone.**

(1) **Clinical manifestations** include

—diarrhea.

—hypovolemia.

—hyponatremia.

—hyperkalemia.

—hyperpigmentation.

—virilization.

(2) **Diagnosis**

—**Increased 17-hydroxyprogesterone and testosterone** levels are often diagnostic.

(3) **Treatment**

—is with glucocorticoid and mineralocorticoid replacement, and in females with ambiguous genitalia, surgical correction as well.

b. **11-B-hydroxylase deficiency**

—is the second most common enzymatic defect causing CAH (5%).

2. **Adrenal neoplasms**

—that cause adrenogenital syndromes are usually adrenal carcinomas or adenomas.

a. **Virilizing adrenal tumors** are **more common in women.**

Table 20-2. Syndromes of Congenital Adrenogenital Hyperplasia

Deficiency	Characteristics	Salt Metabolism
21-Hydroxylase	Genotypic females present with ambiguous external genitalia and postnatal virilization	Salt wasting
11-B-hydroxylase	Genotypic females present with ambiguous external genitalia and postnatal virilization	Hypertension
17-Hydroxylase	Genotypic males present with ambiguous external genitalia	Hypertension
3β-Dehydroxylase	Genotypic males and females may present with ambiguous external genitalia and postnatal virilization in females	With or without salt wasting

(1) **Clinical manifestations** include
—premature hirsutism.
—macrogenitosomia praecox.
—small testes and infertility in boys.
—clitoral enlargement and premature pubic hair in girls.

(2) **Symptoms**
—**Men** are often **asymptomatic.**
—**Women** display **hirsutism** and **masculinization.**

(3) **Diagnosis**
(a) **Elevated levels of plasma DHEA,** testosterone, and urine 17-ketosteroids are frequently present.
(b) **CT scanning** may be useful for localization of lesions.
(c) The **ACTH stimulation test** may also help to confirm such tumors.

(4) **Treatment**
—involves **surgical resection and the administration of mitotane** for recurrent disease.

b. Feminizing adrenal tumors

(1) **Clinical manifestations** include
—impotence.
—amenorrhea.
—gynecomastia.
—testicular atrophy in men.
—precocious puberty.
—breast enlargement.
—early menses.

(2) **Diagnosis**
—Elevated **urinary 17-ketosteroids** and estrogens are often diagnostic.

(3) **Treatment**
—is again surgical, while mitotane may be administered for recurrent disease.

D. Adrenal insufficiency (i.e., Addison's disease)

1. Overview

—This disease occurs in 1 in 5000 hospitalized patients, usually during the third to fifth decades.

2. Etiologies

a. Primary causes (adrenal source) include
—autoimmune disorders (65%–85%).
—infectious sources (30%).
—adrenal hemorrhage.

b. Secondary causes include
—withdrawal of exogenous steroids.
—pituitary disease.

—surgical resection or injury to the glands.

—adrenal metastases.

3. **Clinical manifestations**
   a. These **result from glucocorticoid** and mineralocorticoid **deficiencies.**
   b. **Signs and symptoms** include

—fever.

—nausea and vomiting.

—lethargy and fatigue.

—abdominal pain.

—weight loss.

—hypotension.

—anorexia.

—diarrhea.

—hyperpigmentation.

4. **Diagnosis**
   a. An **ACTH stimulation test**

—often confirms the diagnosis (**Table 20-3**).

   b. Other **laboratory abnormalities** include

—**hyponatremia.**

—**hyperkalemia.**

—**azotemia.**

—**hypoglycemia.**

—low plasma.

—urinary cortisol.

5. **Treatment** includes

—**saline and glucose administration**

—**glucocorticoid replacement.**

—mineralocorticoid replacement for chronic disease.

E. **Adrenocortical carcinoma**

1. **Overview**
   a. These are rare tumors occurring with a bimodal age distribution (**before age 5 and during the fifth decade**).

Table 20-3. Characteristics of Adrenal Insufficiency

	Primary Adrenal Insufficiency	Secondary Adrenal Insufficieny
ACTH levels	Increased	Decreased
Aldosterone levels	Increased	Decreased
ACTH stimulation test	Increased ACTH levels Decreased cortisol levels	Decreased ACTH levels Decreased cortisol levels
Skin pigmentation	Hyperpigmentation	Normal pigmentation
Headaches, vision loss	Rare	Frequent

ACTH = adrenocorticotropic hormone.

b. Sixty percent secrete hormones.

c. Fifty percent present as a large mass, and approximately 50% have metastases.

2. Clinical manifestations

a. Presenting symptoms in adults typically include

—abdominal pain.

—increased abdominal girth.

—weight loss.

—weakness.

—anorexia.

—nausea.

b. Children display

—virilization over 90% of the time.

3. Evaluation and staging

—should include CT, MRI, and a bone scan.

4. Treatment involves

—**attempted complete resection,** in addition to medical therapy for control of symptoms.

a. **Recurrences** may be treated with reoperation.

b. Debulking and chemotherapy, involving mitotane, are beneficial in **controlling symptoms** and **prolonging survival.**

IV. Physiology of the Adrenal Medulla

A. Cells of the adrenal medulla

—produce biologically active catecholamines including **epinephrine (80%), norepinephrine (20%),** and dopamine.

B. Catecholamine secretion

1. **Secretion is stimulated** by

—sympathetic activation.

—anorexia.

—endotoxins.

—body temperature changes.

2. **Secretion is inhibited** by prostaglandins.

V. Diseases of the Adrenal Medulla

A. Pheochromocytoma

1. Overview

a. These tumors

—are **slow-growing, catecholamine-secreting** tumors.

—arise from chromaffin cells of the **adrenal medulla** (85%) or **sympathetic ganglia.**

—**usually present** in the fourth to fifth decades.

—are **rare** with fewer than 0.1% per year, but there is an increased frequency in association with multiple endocrine neoplasia **(MEN) II syndromes** (see VI C).

b. The **"Rule of Tens"** associated with pheochromocytomas include:

—**10% are malignant.**

—**10% are familial** (associated with MEN syndrome).

—**10% are found in children.**

—**10% are bilateral** (50% in children and 100% in familial forms).

—**10% are extra-adrenal.**

c. Malignancy

—is more common in women (3:1), children, and extra-adrenal locations.

2. Clinical manifestations include

—**hypertension** (95%) that is frequently episodic.

—**headache** (80%).

—**diaphoresis** (70%).

—**palpitations** (60%).

3. The **differential diagnoses** include

—essential hypertension.

—migraines.

—tachycardia.

—endocrine abnormalities.

—central nervous system (CNS) disorders.

—tumors.

—pregnancy.

—renal artery stenosis.

4. Evaluation of pheochromocytoma

—involves confirmation of catecholamine excess and tumor localization.

a. Laboratory evaluation

(1) Urinary vanillylmandelic acid (VMA) **and metanephrine levels** may be elevated.

(2) Urinary free or serum catecholamine levels may be useful markers in equivocal cases.

(3) The **clonidine suppression test** may be useful if urinary catecholamines are equivocal and the diagnosis is strongly suspected because clonidine will not suppress norepinephrine levels in affected patients.

b. Radiologic assessment

(1) CT or **MRI** may help to localize tumors.

(2) **Metaiodobenzylguanidine (MIBG) radionuclide scanning** is particularly helpful in identifying extra-adrenal tumors.
(3) **Arteriography or fine needle aspiration (FNA) is not indicated.**

5. Treatment

—involves both medical and surgical therapy.

a. Medical treatment

—**should precede surgical resection.**

(1) **Reversal of vasoconstriction** with **α-blockade** (e.g., phenoxybenzamine, prazosin) is essential.
  (a) α-Blockade should be administered 1 week preoperatively to **prevent vascular instability.**
  (b) Phenoxybenzamine is also indicated if blood pressure is over 200/130 mm Hg, there are uncontrolled hypertensive attacks, hematocrit is over 50%, or with anticipated use of β blockers.
(2) Administer fluids and restore blood volume.
(3) Following appropriate α-blockade, **administration of β-blockers** is often indicated (e.g., propranolol).
  (a) This is indicated for heart rate over 130, for arrhythmias, or if the tumor secretes large amounts of epinephrine.
  (b) **β Blockers should never be administered before α blockade** because unopposed α activity may result, causing vasoconstriction and cardiac failure.
  (c) **Metyrosine** inhibits tyrosine hydroxylase, causing decreased synthesis of catecholamines; this may also be beneficial.
(4) **Morphine** and **meperidine** should be avoided preoperatively because they may stimulate catecholamine release or cause hypotension.

b. Surgical treatment

—involves **resection or debulking** to control symptoms.

—Negative localization still warrants exploratory laparotomy.

6. Complications include

—hypertension.

—hypotension.

—intracranial bleeding.

—arrhythmias.

—congestive heart failure.

—myocardial infarction.

B. A neuroblastoma

—is an embryonal tumor of neural crest origin that arises in the sympathetic chain (see *BRS Surgical Specialties,* Chapter 3).

C. A ganglioneuroma

—is a rare, benign, often asymptomatic tumor of neural crest origin involving the adrenal gland or sympathetic trunk.

V. Incidental Finding of an Adrenal Mass (Incidentaloma)

A. Incidentalomas

—are unsuspected adrenal masses identified during evaluation of other processes (Figure 20-4).

—are **frequently benign** (e.g., adenomas), but a portion of incidentalomas may be metastatic disease or **adrenal carcinomas** (5%).

B. Evaluation of incidentalomas

—is necessary to identify a hormonally active lesion or an adrenocortical carcinoma.

1. **Laboratory studies** include

—**serum potassium.**

—**24-hour urinary free cortisol.**

—**urine 17-hydroxycorticosteroids, VMA, and metanephrines.**

—**plasma aldosterone and renin levels,** if hypertensive or hypokalemic.

2. **Radiologic assessment**

—includes a chest radiograph and abdominal CT scan.

—may also include an **MRI** or **MIBG scan** for suspicious or symptomatic lesions.

C. Surgical resection

—is indicated for lesions with significant malignant potential.

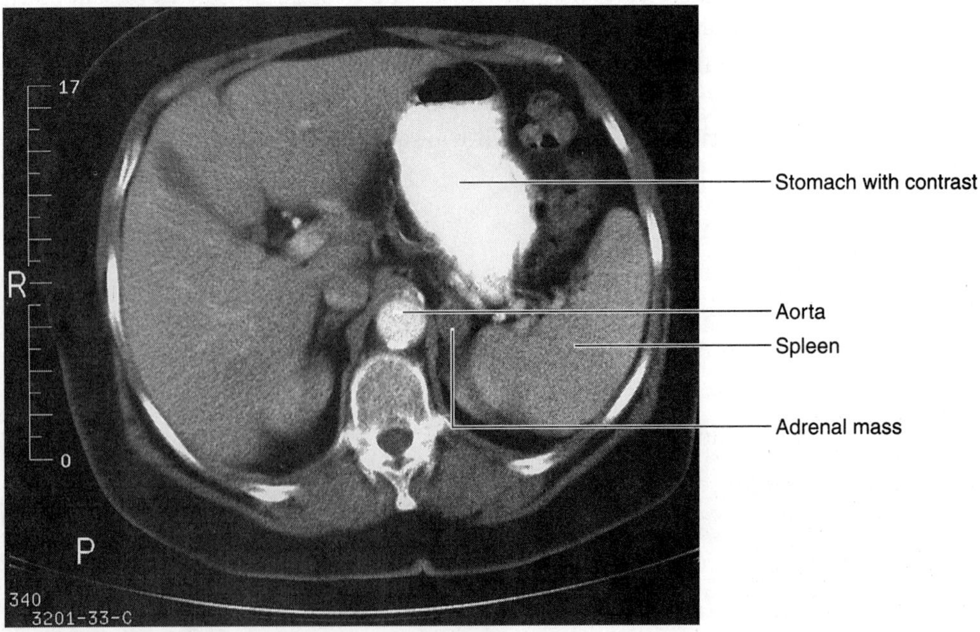

Figure 20-4. Incidental finding of an adrenal mass on an abdominal computed tomography (CT) scan performed for trauma evaluation.

1. **Tumors** with a **higher potential for malignancy** include
   —**functional tumors** (e.g., hormone-producing tumors).
   —**tumors that are enlarging over time.**
   —**tumors larger than 5 cm.**
   —**Tumors that meet these criteria** generally require **surgical resection.**
2. Nonfunctional, stable **tumors smaller than 3 cm**
   —**have a lower potential for malignancy.**
   —may be managed with close follow-up and serial CT scans.
3. **Tumors 3–6 cm**
   —may require additional diagnostic work-up.
   —should be treated individually.

VI. Multiple Endocrine Neoplasia (MEN) Syndromes (Table 20-4)

A. Overview

1. MEN syndromes are a group of **familial disorders**

characterized by the development of neoplasms in multiple endocrine glands.

2. They are **derived from APUD** (*a*mine *p*recursor *u*ptake *d*ecarboxylation) **cells.**
3. The **neoplasms may develop** synchronously or metachronously.
4. These **syndromes are inherited** in an **autosomal dominant fashion** with **100% penetrance** but variable expressivity.

B. MEN I syndrome (i.e., Wermer's syndrome)

—is caused by a defect in chromosome 11, which involves a tumor suppressor gene.

1. **Common components of MEN I syndrome** include
   —primary **hyperparathyroidism** (see Chapter 19 VI B).

Table 20-4. Multiple Endocrine Neoplasia (MEN) Syndromes

Syndrome	Components
MEN I (Wermer's)	Parathyroid hyperplasia (90%) Pancreatic islet tumors (80%) Pituitary tumors (65%)
MEN IIA (Sipple's)	Medullary thyroid carcinoma (100%) Pheochromocytoma (50%) Parathyroid hyperplasia (40%)
MEN IIB	Medullary thyroid carcinoma (100%) Pheochromocytoma (50%–90%) Mucosal neuromas (100%) Marfanoid habitus (70%)

—**pancreatic islet cell tumors** (see Chapter 17 IV B).

—**pituitary tumors.**

2. **Most patients present** with **pancreatic hypersecretion.**
   a. The **most common tumors**
      —include **gastrinomas** (60%) and **insulinomas** (30%). These present with symptoms of **peptic ulcer disease or hypoglycemia,** respectively.
   b. **Neoplasms**
      —are usually malignant, multicentric, and microadenomas.
3. **Hyperparathyroidism**
   —**presents similarly** to sporadic hyperparathyroidism with hypercalcemia (see Chapter 19 VI B, C).
   —usually presents in the third to fourth decade of life, but rarely before age 10.
4. **Pituitary neoplasm**
   a. Pituitary tumors are **associated with**
      —headaches.
      —visual field defects.
      —galactorrhea and amenorrhea in women.
      —hypogonadism in males.
   b. Neoplasms are usually **prolactinomas** (40%).
5. **Diagnosis**
   —begins with biochemical confirmation of hypersecretory states.
6. **Treatment**
   —involves attention to all neoplastic changes.
   a. **If hypercalcemia is present, total parathyroidectomy with autotransplantation**
      —is recommended over subtotal parathyroidectomy because of a high incidence of recurrence.
   b. **Resection of pancreatic tumors**
      —depends on the type of tumor present.
   c. **Bromocriptine**
      —is often used to decrease the size and inhibit hormone production of prolactinomas, and is followed by surgical ablation, irradiation, or both.
   d. Cabergoline or pergolide may also be used to decrease the size of pituitary prolactinomas.
7. **Differences exist**
   —between the neoplastic disorders in familial (MEN) forms and sporadic forms.
   a. **Gastrinomas**
      —are usually malignant with MEN I, but benign with sporadic forms.
   b. **Insulinomas**

—are **multiple with MEN I,** but generally solitary with sporadic forms.

C. MEN II syndrome

1. These **disorders can be divided** into **MEN IIA** (Sipple's syndrome) and **MEN IIB.**

—Both **MEN IIA and IIB are highly associated with medullary thyroid carcinoma and pheochromocytomas.**

—Additional associations are listed in Table 20-4.

2. Clinical manifestations

a. Medullary thyroid carcinoma

(1) These **tumors arise** from **C-cells that secrete calcitonin,** which **inhibits bone resorption and decreases calcium** levels.
(2) These tumors usually **present** in the **second to third decade,** as opposed to the fifth to sixth decade in sporadic forms.
(3) This is often the **earliest expressed defect** in MEN II syndromes.
(4) Diarrhea is the **most common symptom.**
(5) Tumors are often **bilateral.**

b. Pheochromocytoma

(1) These **tumors usually present** in the second to third decades.
(2) Sixty to eighty percent are bilateral (only 10% of sporadic forms are bilateral).
(3) These tumors are nearly always benign (90%), unless they are extra-adrenal (50%).

c. Hyperparathyroidism (see Chapter 19 VI).

3. Evaluation

a. Evaluation begins with confirmation of a hypersecretory state and tumor localization.

b. Laboratory findings may include

—elevated calcium levels.

—elevated calcitonin levels (> 300 pg/mL).

—increased calcitonin with pentagastrin challenge.

—elevated urinary catecholamines and metabolites.

—presence of the *ret* oncogene

4. Treatment

a. Unilateral or bilateral adrenalectomy

—should be performed for unilateral and bilateral pheochromocytomas, respectively.

b. Thyroidectomy and parathyroidectomy

—can be performed simultaneously 1–2 weeks after adrenalectomy.

c. A **total thyroidectomy with central lymph node dissection**

—is generally performed for medullary thyroid tumors.

—Many surgeons advocate total thyroidectomy with a radical neck dissection for MTC associated with MEN II.

d. A **total parathyroidectomy with autotransplantation**

—is generally performed for hypercalcemia or an enlarged parathyroid gland.

5. **Differences between familial (MEN) and sporadic forms**
   a. **Medullary thyroid carcinoma**
      —is **usually bilateral with MEN.**
      —is often more aggressive when associated with MEN.
      —is unilateral with sporadic forms.
   b. **Pheochromocytomas**
      —are **usually bilateral (60%–80%) with MEN.**
      —are unilateral (90%) with sporadic forms.

Review Test

Directions: Each of the numbered items or incomplete statements in this section is followed by answers or by completions of the statement. Select the ONE lettered answer or completion that is BEST in each case.

1. A 26-year-old woman presents with anxiety and hypertension, and is diagnosed with a presumed pheochromocytoma based on preliminary laboratory studies. Which of the following diagnostic tests is contraindicated for pheochromocytoma?

(A) Computed tomography (CT)
(B) Magnetic resonance imaging (MRI)
(C) Metaiodobenzylguanidine (MIBG) radionuclide scanning
(D) Selective arteriography
(E) Ultrasound

2. Which of the following adrenal masses could be treated with observation and follow-up after a complete metabolic work-up?

(A) Nonfunctioning, 3-cm, solid adrenal mass in a 38-year-old man
(B) Nonfunctioning, 7-cm, cystic adrenal mass in a 25-year-old woman
(C) Functioning, 2-cm, cystic mass in a 45-year-old woman
(D) Nonfunctioning, solid mass that has doubled in size in 1 year in a 67-year-old man
(E) A 10-cm, solid adrenal mass in a 56-year-old man

3. A 45-year-old man presents with a 4-cm adrenal mass that has been diagnosed as a pheochromocytoma by preoperative testing. Preoperative preparation in this patient should initially include which of the following?

(A) Administration of phenoxybenzamine
(B) Administration of propranolol, followed by phenoxybenzamine
(C) Administration of furosemide
(D) Fluid restriction
(E) Administration of propranolol

4. A 40-year-old woman who has been treated with prednisone for 2 years for rheumatoid arthritis undergoes emergent splenectomy after a motor vehicle accident. Postoperatively, the patient develops fever, abdominal pain, nausea, and vomiting. Laboratory data reveal hyperkalemia, hypoglycemia, and hyponatremia. Immediate measures should include which of the following?

(A) Rapid correction of hyponatremia
(B) Administration of saline, glucose, and dexamethasone
(C) Saline infusion and fludrocortisone
(D) Intravenous hydrocortisone alone
(E) Plasma adrenocorticotropic hormone (ACTH) and cortisol levels after initiation of therapy

5. A 45-year-old man presents to the emergency room after having fallen from a height of 12 feet. He complains only of abdominal pain, and a computed tomography (CT) scan is eventually performed to evaluate his abdomen. No injuries are noted but a 5-cm solid adrenal mass is detected. Which of the following studies is inappropriate in the work-up of this lesion?

(A) Serum potassium
(B) Serum aldosterone
(C) Fine needle aspiration (FNA)
(D) Chest radiograph
(E) Urine metanephrines

6. A 62-year-old man presents with an 8-cm, nonfunctioning adrenal tumor. Which of the following statements is true regarding the surgical approach in this patient?

(A) The anterior approach is usually used for patients with potential bilateral disease
(B) The posterior approach is used for lesions larger than 5 cm because of greater exposure of the retroperitoneum
(C) The lateral approach is the preferred method for patients with bilateral adrenal disease
(D) Laparoscopic adrenalectomy is contraindicated in right-sided lesions because of the short adrenal vein
(E) Laparoscopic adrenalectomy is contraindicated in lesions larger than 4 cm

Directions: Each set of matching questions in this section consists of four to twenty-six lettered options followed by several numbered items. For each numbered item, select the appropriate lettered option(s). Each lettered option may be selected once, more than once, or not at all.

Questions 7–11

(A) Cushing's disease
(B) Ectopic adrenocorticotropic hormone (ACTH) syndrome
(C) Adrenal carcinoma/adenoma
(D) Hyperaldosteronism
(E) Adrenogenital syndrome
(F) Pheochromocytoma
(G) Primary hyperparathyroidism
(H) Multiple endocrine neoplasia (MEN) II syndrome

Match the following surgical causes of hypertension with their respective clinical scenarios.

7. A 30-year-old man presents with truncal obesity, hypertension, and weakness. Work-up reveals increased urine cortisol and decreased plasma ACTH. (SELECT 1 CAUSE)

8. A 65-year-old man presents with truncal obesity, hypertension, and weight loss. Work-up reveals increased urinary cortisol and ACTH. (SELECT 2 CAUSES)

9. A 30-year-old man presents with hypertension and weakness. Work-up reveals the following laboratory values: $Na^+ = 153$, $K^+ = 1.9$, blood pressure = 150/98, central venous pressure = 15. (SELECT 1 CAUSE)

10. A 26-year-old man presents with episodic hypertension and anxiety. Work-up reveals increased urinary vanillylmandelic acid (VMA) and metanephrines. (SELECT 1 CAUSE)

11. A 30-year-old woman presents with a 4-month history of hypertension and a thyroid mass. Work-up reveals hypercalcemia. (SELECT 1 CAUSE)

Answers and Explanations

1–D. Computed tomography (CT), magnetic resonance imaging (MRI), metaiodobenzylguanidine (MIBG) scans, and ultrasound can all be used in the work-up of a suspected adrenal mass. Ultrasound is the least useful of these tests owing to limited resolution and limited visualization of surrounding anatomy. In addition, ultrasound can only visualize tumors larger than 2 cm. CT scan provides more information about surrounding anatomical structures and is useful for detecting tumors as small as 1 cm. MIBG selectively accumulates in chromaffin tissue and will do so more rapidly in a pheochromocytoma than in normal tissue. Selective angiography is contraindicated because a sudden increase in intraglandular pressure can cause a massive release of catecholamines and precipitate a hypertensive crisis.

2–A. General criteria that are considered indications for surgical intervention for an adrenal mass include functional tumors of any size, tumors that increase in size during follow-up, and nonfunctional tumors that are 6 cm or larger. These tumors are at greatest risk for harboring malignancy. Nonfunctioning adrenal tumors smaller than 6 cm are unlikely to harbor malignancy and some surgeons advocate simple observation and follow-up computed tomography (CT) scans in 3 to 6 months. Some surgeons use 3–4 cm as the upper limit instead of 6 cm.

3–A. The physiologic effects seen in a patient with a pheochromocytoma are a result of α- and β-adrenergic stimulation. α-Receptor blockade (e.g., phenoxybenzamine, phentolamine) should be instituted before surgery to counteract the diffuse vasoconstriction seen in patients with an active pheochromocytoma. The vasodilation that ensues after α blockade will result in a functional hypovolemia, making diuretic therapy (e.g., furosemide) and fluid restriction contraindicated before surgery. β-antagonist therapy (e.g., propranolol) is often needed after α antagonist therapy is instituted to counteract the reflex tachycardia that may result. However, β-antagonist therapy should never be started before α blockade, as it can result in unopposed α stimulation from the pheochromocytoma, causing malignant hypertension and congestive heart failure.

4–B. Emergency measures in the treatment of acute adrenal insufficiency include establishment of intravenous (IV) access, immediate assessment of serum electrolyte, glucose, and adrenocorticotropic hormone (ACTH) levels, and subsequent infusion of 2–3 liters of isotonic saline. Treatment with IV dexamethasone should also be instituted. Initiation of therapy before measuring plasma ACTH and cortisol may interfere with assessment of these hormones. Rapid correction of hyponatremia is rarely indicated, as central pontine myelinolysis can result. Fludrocortisone has no role in the acute management of acute adrenal insufficiency, although it is used in the treatment of chronic insufficiency. Hydrocortisone alone without adequate administration of fluids is inadequate therapy.

5–C. The work-up of adrenal incidentalomas should include serum and urine testing to assess the possibility of a functional tumor. A chest radiograph should also be obtained to rule out the possibility of a metastatic lesion from the chest. Fine needle aspiration (FNA) has no place in the work-up of a new adrenal lesion because the information obtained is rarely helpful unless the lesion is metastatic. In addition, FNA may be dangerous because of the risk of precipitating a hypertensive crisis in a patient with a pheochromocytoma.

6–A. Adrenal tumors can be removed by a variety of surgical approaches. An anterior approach is preferred for suspected bilateral tumors because it allows for inspection of both glands through a single incision. The posterior approach is generally better tolerated postoperatively but gives only limited exposure. The lateral approach is used for large, unilateral tumors or for bilateral tumors in obese or high-risk patients, although it is not generally the preferred method because of the postoperative pain and morbidity associated with bilateral subcostal flank incisions. Laparoscopic adrenalectomy is more difficult in right-sided and large lesions, but is not contraindicated in either scenario.

7–C. This patient exhibits the signs and symptoms of plasma cortisol excess. Possible causes include Cushing's disease, ectopic adrenocorticotropic hormone (ACTH) syndrome, adrenal cancer, adrenal adenoma, and iatrogenic causes. However, the fact that this patient's plasma ACTH is decreased rules out Cushing's disease (primary pituitary source). Although not one of the choices listed, it should be noted that ACTH may be decreased in the presence of signs and symptoms of Cushing's syndrome with exogenous administration of corticosteroids.

8–A, B. There are numerous potential causes of Cushing's syndrome. Both ectopic adrenocorticotropic hormone (ACTH) production and Cushing's disease would produce elevated cortisol and ACTH. These two possible causes can usually be differentiated from one another with the aid of a dexamethasone suppression test.

9–D. Elevated serum sodium, decreased serum potassium, and hypertension are the classic signs of hyperaldosteronism (i.e., Conn's syndrome). Work-up of this patient would include 24-hour urine aldosterone as well as plasma renin activity. Diagnostic studies are needed to differentiate adrenal hyperplasia from an adenoma because the treatments differ for these two possible causes (medical therapy for hyperplasia versus surgical treatment for an adenoma).

10–F. Complaints of episodic hypertension should raise suspicion for a pheochromocytoma, especially in young patients. Increased levels of catecholamine breakdown products (vanillylmandelic acid and metanephrines) in the urine essentially confirms the diagnosis. Further localization studies include abdominal computed tomography (CT), magnetic resonance imaging (MRI), or metaiodobenzylguanidine (MIBG) scan.

11–H. The diagnosis of pheochromocytoma should be considered in any young patient who presents with hypertension. Furthermore, the additional finding of a thyroid mass should raise suspicion for the multiple endocrine neoplasia (MEN) II syndrome (pheochromocytoma, medullary thyroid cancer, and hyperparathyroidism). Preoperative work-up should include serum calcium levels in patients with suspected MEN II syndrome because any parathyroid dysfunction can be addressed at the same time as the thyroid mass. Should a pheochromocytoma also be present, it should be addressed first at a separate procedure.

21

Skin Cancer and Soft Tissue Sarcomas

Lee W. Thompson

I. Melanoma

A. Etiology and epidemiology

1. **Melanocytes** originate from **neural crest cells.** Therefore, melanoma can occur anywhere that neural crest cells migrate in the embryo.
2. **Melanoma occurs**

   —**primarily in the skin.**

   —rarely in the **eye and mucous membranes** (e.g., oral mucosa, anorectum, female genital tract).
3. **Melanomas represent**

   —a minority of skin cancers (3%–5%), but can cause at least 65% of the deaths from skin cancer.
4. The **characteristic melanoma patient**

   —has a **fair complexion** (i.e., Celtic complexion).

   —has a history of **sunburning easily.**

   —may be younger than other patients with skin cancer (80% of melanoma patients are from ages 25–65).
5. A **significant risk factor**

   —for the development of melanoma is **intermittent, unaccustomed sun exposure** (e.g., sunburns).
6. Other **risk factors** and **associated conditions** include

   —**sporadic dysplastic nevi** (20-fold increase over the general population).

—**familial dysplastic nevi syndrome** (B-K mole syndrome, atypical mole syndrome) associated with 100% lifetime risk of melanoma.

—**large congenital nevi** (larger than 20 cm) have a 5%–20% lifetime risk of melanoma.

—**familial predisposition**.

—**xeroderma pigmentosum**.

—**previous skin cancer** (10-fold increase risk with previous melanoma).

B. The **clinical appearance** and **symptoms**

—of melanoma are outlined in **Table 21-1**.

C. The **four main pathologic types** of melanoma

—are outlined in **Table 21-2**.

D. Prognostic factors

1. The **depth of invasion**

—**is an important prognostic indicator for melanoma.**

—Two **classification systems** are used to describe the depth of invasion of the tumor: **Clark's level of invasion (Table 21-3)** and **Breslow thickness (Table 21-4)**.

2. **Nodal status**

—also correlates with prognosis.

—With 1–2 positive nodes, 5-year survival is 30%–55%.

3. **Distant metastasis**

—is associated with a very poor survival.

4. **Other factors associated** with a relatively **poor prognosis**

a. **Location:** posterior neck, scalp, upper back > trunk > hands and feet, listed from worse to better prognosis.

b. **Men** have a worse prognosis than do women.

c. **Ulcerated lesions** have a worse prognosis than nonulcerated lesions.

Table 21-1. Important Factors in the Evaluation of a Skin Lesion

***A**symmetry*	Irregular elevations	Any nodular area, indentation, or nonuniformity in elevation should raise the suspicion of a melanoma.
***B**orders*	Irregular borders	More likely **melanoma:** borders that blend, are difficult to see, and are nondiscrete More likely **benign:** smooth, discrete, uniform borders
***C**olor*	Variation in color	The variation in color across a lesion is more worrisome than any particular color in a uniform lesion.
***D**egeneration*	Ulceration, itching, bleeding, or rapid changes	Worrisome symptoms for melanoma

Table 21-2. Pathologic Classification of Malignant Melanomas

Type	Epidemiology	Common Site	Metastatic Potential
Superficial spreading (70%)	Equally common among men and women; median age 50	Sun-exposed areas	Intermediate aggressiveness
Nodular (15%–30%)	More common in men; peaks in the 5th decade	Sun-exposed areas; may occur in normal skin without pre-existing nevi	Most aggressive form
Lentigo maligna melanoma (10%–15%)	More common in women; median age 70	Sun-exposed areas (head, neck, and dorsum of the hand); frequently arises at site of Hutchinson freckle (benign, brown, macular lesion)	Least aggressive
Acral lentiginous (rare)	Uncommon except in dark-skinned people; median age 60	Occurs on the palms, soles, and subungual regions; more than 75% involve large toe or thumb	Intermediate aggressiveness

d. **Vertical growth characteristics** have a worse prognosis than radial growth characteristics.

e. **Ocular** and **mucosal melanomas** are more aggressive than cutaneous lesions.

E. Evaluation

1. Biopsy of suspected melanoma

—**must include the full depth** of the lesion to evaluate tumor thickness.

2. Total excisional biopsy

—should be attempted for small lesions.

Table 21-3. Clark's Level Classification System for Melanoma

Clark's Level*	Definition
I	All tumor cells confined to the epidermis with no invasion through the basement membrane (melanoma in situ)
II	Tumor cells penetrate through basement membrane into the papillary dermis, but not to the reticular dermis
III	Tumor cells fill the papillary dermis and abut the reticular dermis but do not invade it
IV	Tumor invades reticular dermis
V	Tumor cells invade the subcutaneous tissue

*For staging purposes, the Breslow thickness has largely replaced Clark's levels for characterization of primary lesion (see Table 21-4).

Table 21-4. Breslow Classification System and Staging of Melanoma

Staging Factors	Breslow Tumor Thickness (mm)	Melanoma Stage	Overall Mortality*
Tumor	≤ 0.75	IA	0%
	0.76–1.49	1B	33%
	1.50–2.49	IIA	32%
	2.50–3.99	IIA	69%
	≥ 4.00	IIB	84%
Lymph node involvement	Any	III	~50%†
Distant metastases	Any	IV	> 95%

*Mortality rates vary widely depending on the study and have generally improved significantly over the past several years.
†Mortality increases with increasing number of involved lymph nodes.

3. **Physical examination**

   —of all possible draining lymph nodes should be performed.

4. Although **not routine, other tests** can be used during evaluation.
   a. A **chest radiograph** may identify lung metastasis.
   b. **Lactate dehydrogenase** and alkaline phosphatase may be measured to screen for hepatic metastasis.
   c. Recently, **lymphoscintigraphy** has been used to identify the "sentinel lymph node" (see I F 3 a).

F. **Treatment**

1. With **all stages** of **melanoma**

   —**the primary lesion is treated with wide local excision.**

   a. The **size of the margin** generally depends on the depth of invasion (**Table 21-5**).
   b. The **lesion site,** such as on the head and neck, may influence margin size.

2. Most patients with **stage I disease**

   —**will be cured by resection alone**.

3. **Stage IIA and IIB melanomas**

   —(based on depth of invasion) are also treated with **wide local excision of the primary lesion**.

   a. **Cutaneous areas** usually drain first to a single or small group of lymph nodes known as the **sentinel lymph node.**

Table 21-5. Recommended Margin of Resection for Wide Local Excision of Melanoma

Depth of Melanoma	Recommendation for Margins
Melanoma in-situ	0.5 cm
≤ 1 mm thick	1 cm
1 mm to 4 mm thick	2 cm
> 4 mm thick	3 cm

b. Some **surgeons currently recommend** performing a **sentinel lymph node biopsy** at the time of initial resection.

c. If the **sentinel lymph node does not have melanoma then the other lymph nodes are unlikely to be positive** (98% sensitivity).

4. Patients with **stage III tumors**

—in addition to wide local excision, **should also undergo full lymph node dissection** of the affected lymph node group.

a. **Five-year survival** with resected positive nodes is 30%–50%.

b. Postoperatively, some high-risk patients receive **interferon-α.**

c. Other types of immunotherapy and chemotherapy are currently being evaluated.

5. **Resection of metastasis (Stage IV)**

—is warranted for **palliation of symptoms.**

a. For some patients, **resection of metastasis** has provided long disease-free intervals.

b. In eligible patients, **resection of single lesions** (e.g., lung) that will require a relatively low-risk procedure remains **the best chance for cure** and long-term survival.

c. Melanoma may **rarely metastasize** to the **gastrointestinal tract.**

—This causes obstruction or bleeding, which may require resection of the affected bowel.

6. **Other therapies**

a. **Interleukin-2 therapy** has a significant response rate in patients with advanced disease.

b. **Chemotherapeutic agents** have generally **not** been shown to provide benefit in the treatment of melanoma.

c. **Tumor vaccine therapy** and other types of immunotherapy are currently being investigated.

II. Nonmelanoma Skin Cancer

A. Etiology and epidemiology

1. **Skin cancer**

—is the most common malignancy in the United States.

—is **70 times less likely to develop in African Americans.**

2. **Basal cell** and **squamous cell carcinomas**

—make up the vast majority of nonmelanoma skin cancers.

3. **Basal cell cancers occur**

—**3–4 times more frequently than squamous cell cancers.**

4. **Basal cell** and **especially squamous cell cancers**

—are related directly to **chronic sun exposure.**

—occur most commonly on areas of the body that receive chronic sun exposure.

5. **Patients who develop a skin cancer**
   —have a 36%–50% chance of developing a second primary skin cancer in the 5 years following the original diagnosis.

B. **Overall risk factors** include

—**fair skin, red or blonde hair, blue eyes.**

—**Celtic origin.**

—**immunosuppression** (e.g., transplant patient).

—**exposure to ultraviolet (UV) light** (especially UVB).

—**exposure to ionizing radiation.**

—**chemical exposure** (polycyclic aromatic hydrocarbons, e.g., coal tar; chlorophenols; arsenic; psoralen).

—**precursor skin lesions** (e.g., **actinic keratosis, Bowen's disease**).

C. The **differential diagnoses of a skin lesion** may include, in addition to malignant skin lesions, these **benign conditions:**

—actinic keratoses.

—keratoacanthoma.

—warts.

—acneform papules.

—eczema.

—chalazia.

—seborrheic keratoses.

D. **Squamous cell carcinoma** (cutaneous)

1. **Specific risk factors** include
   —**human papillomavirus.**
   —**immunosuppression.**
   —**old scars and burns (Marjolin's ulcer** is a squamous cell carcinoma that develops at the site of an old scar or burn).
   —sinus tracts.
   —venous stasis ulcers.
   —tobacco use, which is a significant risk factor for mucosal squamous cell carcinomas (i.e., lip, gums).
2. **Precursor lesions** include
   —actinic keratosis.
   —Bowen's disease.
   —Queyrat erythroplasia.
3. **Appearance**
   a. Lesions are usually red to reddish brown, but may be pearly.

b. The surface may be crusted, scaly, or hyperkeratotic with erosions and ulcers.

c. These lesions are **typically painless and have poorly defined borders** and develop over a period of weeks to 2–3 months.

4. **Metastasis**

a. **Squamous cell cancers metastasize**

—more frequently than basal cell cancers but much less frequently than melanomas.

b. **Factors predictive of metastasis** include

—**degree of differentiation** (grade).

—**depth of penetration and size.**

—**location of lesion** (lip and ear have highest risk).

—**recurrent lesions** (25%–45% rate of metastasis).

—**age.**

—**immune status of patient.**

E. **Basal cell carcinoma**

1. **These carcinomas**

—are slow-growing.

—are locally destructive malignancies.

—have an **extremely low incidence of metastasis.**

2. **Incidence is related to total sun exposure**

—however, basal cell cancer appears to be related more to **irregular sun exposure** than to persistent sun exposure.

—More than **80%** of **basal cell cancers** are found on the **head and neck,** with the nose as the most common site.

3. **Genetic alterations**

—that are known to be caused by UV light are common in basal cell cancer cells.

4. **Subtypes** of **basal cell cancer**

a. **Nodular:** pearly translucent nodule often with central ulceration (rodent ulcer).

b. **Micronodular:** group of small, nodular lesions.

c. **Superficial:** flat, scaly, eczema-like lesion.

—Tumor often extends beyond the clinically positive border.

d. **Infiltrative:** lesions are often difficult to see because they blend with the skin.

e. **Morpheaform:** flat, firm, yellow-to-tan lesion that often extends well beyond the clinically positive borders.

f. **Mixed:** composed of more than one of the above tumor elements.

g. **Basosquamous cell carcinoma:** separate foci and components of both basal cell and squamous cell tumors.

F. **Treatment**

1. **Wide local excision**

—of lesions with negative margins is associated with a **95%–99% cure rate.**

a. **Margins of 5 mm are acceptable for most lesions** although some complex lesions may require 10 mm margins.

b. **Recurrent basal cell cancers** should be treated aggressively because the rate of re-recurrence is high.

2. **Mohs' micrographic technique**

a. **Lesions are removed** with what is thought to be a 2–3 mm margin.

b. The **excision is continued until the margins are free** of microscopic disease.

—Therefore the procedure has theoretically 100% margin control.

c. This **technique is designed** to provide adequate resection of lesions with sparing of normal tissue (i.e., face lesions).

d. This method is **contraindicated if a melanoma is suspected.**

3. **Other procedures** used for treating **small lesions** include

—curettage and electrodesiccation.

—cryosurgery.

—CO_2 or neodymium laser.

—topical 5-fluorouracil.

—topical or oral retinoids.

—intralesional interferon-α_{2b}.

4. **Systemic chemotherapy**

—is reserved for tumors that are inoperable or metastatic.

5. **Radiation therapy**

—is generally reserved for inoperable lesions.

6. Although rare, **lymph node metastasis**

—can be treated with lymph node dissection or possibly radiation therapy.

III. Soft Tissue Sarcomas

A. Introduction and epidemiology

1. **Most sarcomas arise** from tissues that developed from **embryonic mesoderm.**

a. Because of their origin, soft tissue sarcomas can arise anywhere in the body.

b. Approximately **50% arise in the extremities.**

2. **Half of all sarcomas occur in children.**

3. When these **lesions metastasize, spread is almost uniformly by hematogenous route.**

4. **Lymph node involvement is uncommon.**

B. Risk factors

1. **Radiation exposure**

   —A 7–20 year latency period is generally present for radiation-induced sarcomas.

2. **Thorotrast**

   —is associated with angiosarcoma of the liver 18–36 years later.

   —was once used as a contrast medium, but is no longer available.

3. **Chemical exposures** include

   —phenoxyacetic acids (herbicides).

   —chlorophenols.

   —vinyl chloride.

   —arsenic.

4. **Chronic lymphedema**

   —Stewart-Treves syndrome is the classic **lymphangiosarcoma** in post-mastectomy, postirradiated patients with a lymphadenomatous arm after breast cancer treatment.

   —The lymphangiosarcomas occur outside the irradiated field.

5. **Genetic syndromes**

   —associated with sarcoma development are listed in **Table 21-6**.

C. **Diagnosis**

1. **Most sarcomas** are large (larger than 5 cm), grow rapidly, and are painless.

2. **Patients may wrongly associate these lesions** with trauma, thus delaying consultation with a physician.

3. **Presenting signs** of a **visceral or retroperitoneal sarcoma** include

   —asymptomatic abdominal mass (most common presentation).

   —gastrointestinal bleeding.

   —bowel obstruction.

   —neurologic deficits.

4. The ratio of benign to malignant tumors is greater than 100 to 1.

Table 21-6. Familial Syndromes Associated with the Development of Sarcomas

Syndrome	Tumor Types
Neurofibromatosis	Benign or malignant central nervous system tumor; malignant peripheral nerve sheath tumor; pheochromocytoma
Li-Fraumeni cancer syndrome	Childhood rhabdomyosarcoma, as well as many other tumors later in life including sarcomas
Hereditary retinoblastoma	Retinoblastoma, as well as many other tumors later in life including sarcomas
Tuberous sclerosis	Angiomyolipoma
Gardner's syndrome	Familial adenomatous polyposis and multiple intra-abdominal desmoid tumors

5. Most sarcomas present as a **soft tissue mass that must be differentiated from**
   - —reactive processes.
   - —benign tumors.
   - —calcified post-traumatic muscle masses (myositis ossificans).
   - —metastatic carcinomas.
   - —melanoma.
   - —lymphoma.
6. **Indications for biopsy** of soft tissue masses include
   - —symptomatic lesions.
   - —enlarging lesions.
   - —lesions larger than or equal to 5 cm.
   - —new masses that persist for longer than 5 weeks.

D. Prognosis and staging

1. **The histologic grade of the primary tumor**
   - —**is the predominant factor in predicting metastatic recurrence and mortality.**
2. **Factors used to establish tumor grade** include
   - —cellularity.
   - —differentiation.
   - —pleomorphism.
   - —necrosis.
   - —number of mitoses.
3. **Tumors larger than or equal to 5 cm**
   - —are more likely to metastasize.
   - —are associated with a higher mortality.
4. **Overall morbidity and mortality**
   - —may also be related to the site of the primary lesion and its resectability.
5. A **summary of sarcoma staging** based on tumor grade and size is outlined in **Table 21-7.**
6. The **risk of recurrence** remains significant after 5 years without disease.
   - —Factors associated with recurrence and disease specific mortality are included in **Table 21-8.**

E. Diagnosis and treatment of site-specific sarcomas

1. **Sarcomas of the extremities**
   - a. **A chest radiograph**
     - —is essential because **88% of metastases from extremity lesions are to the lung.**

Table 21-7 Staging System for Sarcomas

Stage	Grade	Size	Metastasis
IA	Low	< 5 cm	No
IB	Low	> 5 cm	No
IIA	Moderate	< 5 cm	No
IIB	Moderate	> 5 cm	No
IIIA	High	< 5 cm	No
IIIB	High	> 5 cm	No
IVA	Any	Any	Lymph nodes only
IVB	Any	Any	Distant

b. Computed tomography (CT) or magnetic resonance imaging (MRI) scans

—are frequently useful for operative planning and for identifying metastasis.

c. Biopsy of the lesion

(1) Three **methods** most commonly used to obtain biopsy material include

—excisional biopsy.

—incisional biopsy (preferred in most situations).

—Tru-cut needle biopsy.

(2) The biopsy is performed so that the biopsy incision can be included in the definitive sarcoma resection.

(3) Meticulous hemostasis must be maintained because the hematoma can disseminate and assist spread of tumor cells.

d. Treatment of sarcomas smaller than 5 cm

—is via **wide en bloc surgical resection** with 2–4 cm wide tumor-free margins.

(1) **Limb-sparing procedures should be performed** with amputation reserved for situations when no other option exists.

(2) Radiation therapy should be combined with surgery if the tumor margins are of concern.

Table 21-8. Factors Associated with Increased Recurrence Rates and Mortality in Sarcomas

Increased Local Recurrence	Increased Distant Recurrence	Increased Disease-Specific Mortality
Age > 50 years Positive primary margins Histologic subtypes (e.g., peripheral nerve tumors)	Lesions ≥ 5 cm High grade lesions Deep location of tumor Histologic subtypes (e.g., leiomyosarcoma > liposarcoma)	Large tumor size High grade lesions Deep location of tumor Treatment of recurrent disease Positive primary margins Lower extremity tumors Histologic subtypes (e.g., leiomyosarcomas and peripheral nerve tumors)

e. **Treatment of extremity sarcomas larger than 5 cm**
   (1) **Limb sparing surgery combined with adjunctive radiation therapy** is the treatment of choice.
   (2) Although a group of these patients will have local recurrences that require further resection and treatment, long-term survival is not affected.

f. Patients with **tumors larger than 10 cm**

   —are usually good candidates for preoperative or neoadjuvant radiation therapy.

g. **Chemotherapy does not** currently

   —play a significant role in the treatment of soft tissue sarcomas.

2. **Visceral or retroperitoneal sarcoma**
   a. A **CT or MRI scan** of the abdomen and pelvis allows for assessment of the primary lesion and metastatic disease.
   b. A **chest radiograph** to identify metastasis is essential.
   c. The **predominant lesions identified** are **leiomyosarcoma and liposarcoma.**
   d. **Surgical resection** is the mainstay of treatment for these sarcomas.
      (1) Tumors are usually very large at the time of diagnosis.
      (2) Resection of adjacent organs is routine, although the impact on long-term survival is limited.
      (3) **The ability to completely resect the primary tumor is the most important prognostic factor**.
      (4) Incomplete resections do not improve long-term survival.
      (5) **Unresectability** is usually related to **peritoneal implants or extensive vascular involvement**.
      (6) The incidence of local recurrence is high, although many recurrences can be re-resected.

3. **Head and neck sarcomas**
   a. **Many of the head and neck sarcomas** occur in the **pediatric population**.

      —**Rhabdomyosarcoma** is the most common.

   b. Even for **small lesions** tumor-free margins are difficult to obtain owing to the close proximity of vital structures.
   c. **Postoperative radiation therapy** is a very important part of local control because adequate margins are often difficult to obtain.

4. **Sarcoma of the breast**

   —accounts for fewer than 1% of all breast tumors.

   a. These lesions **rarely metastasize** to the lymph nodes, unlike breast carcinoma.
   b. **Treatment** involves **en bloc resection** with wide margins, as in other parts of the body.

      —Lymph node dissection is not routinely performed, unlike in carcinoma of the breast.

F. **Treatment of local recurrence**

1. **If complete resection can be accomplished then the recurrence should be resected.**

2. **Re-irradiation** combined with resection of the recurrence has been shown to decrease local recurrence rates in certain patient populations.

G. **Metastatic sarcoma**

1. **Overall, 20% of patients** with sarcoma present with distant metastasis.
2. **Palliative resection of symptomatic lesions and radiation therapy are used on an individual basis.**
3. **Resection of locally advanced disease** and metastatic lesions can offer longer disease-free survival, but the risk of the procedure must be weighed against that potential benefit.
4. **Resection of isolated pulmonary metastasis may be associated with a 20%–30% increase in the 5-year survival rate.**
5. The role of **chemotherapy** in the treatment of metastatic disease is still being investigated.

H. **Kaposi's sarcoma**

—is a rare, aggressive sarcoma seen most commonly in **severely immunosuppressed patients** (e.g., acquired immunodeficiency syndrome [AIDS]).

1. **These lesions involve** the skin or mucous membranes and occasionally the intestinal tract.
2. **Surgery is indicated** with intestinal perforation or hemorrhage, although overall survival is very low.

I. **Desmoid tumors**

—may be **considered low-grade sarcomas** or a reactive process.

1. **When resected,** desmoids **frequently recur locally but rarely metastasize.**
2. **Trauma or surgery** commonly precedes the development of desmoids.
3. These **lesions are divided into three subgroups.**
   a. **Extra-abdominal desmoids**
      —tend to occur on the muscles of the back, shoulders, chest wall, and thigh.
   b. **Abdominal desmoids**
      —arise in the musculoaponeurotic structures of the anterior abdominal wall.
      —classically occur during or following **pregnancy**.
   c. **Intra-abdominal desmoids**
      —are associated with **Gardner's syndrome.**
      —may be associated with **diffuse retroperitoneal fibrosis**.

Review Test

Directions: Each of the numbered items or incomplete statements in this section is followed by answers or by completions of the statement. Select the ONE lettered answer or completion that is BEST in each case.

1. A 54-year-old man presents to the office with a complaint of a mass in his left thigh increasing in size over the past several months. On examination, the patient is noted to have a firm 6-cm mass on his left anterior thigh with no other significant findings. An incisional biopsy reveals a soft tissue sarcoma. Which of the following is the most appropriate statement regarding the initial evaluation and management of this patient?

(A) A sentinel lymph node biopsy should be performed because sarcomas spread almost uniformly through lymphatics to lymph nodes
(B) A chest radiograph should be obtained because sarcomas spread almost uniformly by a hematogenous route with a majority going to the lung
(C) Resection alone is the next step because growth is so slow that where it spreads is not a concern
(D) Multiple local skin biopsies should be performed because sarcomas usually spread superficially through the skin
(E) Immediate amputation should be performed because of the aggressive nature of sarcomas occurring in the extremities

2. A 66-year-old, diabetic woman underwent a lumpectomy/axillary node dissection with postoperative radiation therapy 17 years ago for breast adenocarcinoma. The patient gives a history of a severe skin "reaction" to the radiation and a history of chronic swelling of the affected arm. She now presents with a mass in the upper portion of the affected extremity, recently diagnosed as a lymphangiosarcoma. Which of the following factors in this patient is thought to be most important in the source of this sarcoma?

(A) History of previous breast malignancy
(B) Chronic lymphedema
(C) History of radiation exposure
(D) Advanced age
(E) History of chronic diabetes

3. A 54-year-old construction worker presents to the office for a routine check-up. He is noted to have a 6-mm, dark lesion under the fingernail of a finger on his left hand. He denies any trauma to the area. The area is nontender with no evidence of infection. Which of the following is an appropriate statement regarding the lesion identified in this patient?

(A) This is the most common form of melanoma
(B) This lesion occurs most commonly in white males
(C) This lesion developed from a subungual hematoma
(D) This is the most aggressive form of melanoma
(E) This lesion can also develop on the soles of the feet

4. Three years ago, a 55-year-old man had a sarcoma resected from his anterior superior thigh that had positive margins on the pathology specimen. He was treated with postoperative radiation therapy to salvage his leg. Unfortunately he developed a recurrent lesion that appears to be 4–5 cm medial to the femoral neurovascular bundle. Which of the following is the most appropriate treatment measure for this patient?

(A) Surgical resection
(B) Doxorubicin and ifosfamide combination
(C) Immunotherapy combined with interferon-α
(D) Observation until lesion becomes symptomatic
(E) Radiation therapy alone

5. A 63-year-old woman presents to the office for a routine check-up. She states that she recently read an article that discussed the different types of skin cancer and that a friend of hers recently had a basal cell cancer removed. She is inquiring about her risk for the development of skin cancer. In describing the risk factors for development of nonmelanoma skin cancers to this patient, which of the following is accurate regarding the relative risks?

(A) Pre-existing keratoacanthoma is a greater risk than pre-existing Bowen's disease
(B) Immunocompetence is a greater risk than immunosuppression
(C) Brown eyes is a greater risk than blue eyes
(D) Brunette hair is a greater risk than blonde hair
(E) Ultraviolet (UV)B exposure is a greater risk than UVA exposure

6. During routine chest radiography, a 63-year-old man is found to have an isolated 1-cm mass in the upper lobe of his right lung. Biopsy of the lesion reveals a melanoma. In addition to examining all skin and mucous membrane surfaces, which of the following would be most appropriate in the subsequent evaluation of this patient to identify the primary lesion?

(A) Funduscopic examination, proctoscopy, and chest computed tomography (CT).
(B) Funduscopic examination and abdominal CT
(C) Chest CT
(D) Chest and abdominal CT
(E) Funduscopic examination and small bowel contrast study

7. During an abdominal computed tomography (CT) scan performed for complaints of vague abdominal discomfort, a 55-year-old man is found to have a 6-cm mass near the midline in the retroperitoneum suggestive of a sarcoma. Which of the following is an appropriate statement regarding the evaluation and management of this patient?

(A) The presence of multiple peritoneal implants is an appropriate indication for surgical resection of asymptomatic disease
(B) In addition to surgical resection, radiation therapy is a key component of the treatment regimen
(C) Because of the location of this lesion, metastases are more likely found in the liver versus the lung
(D) Given the patient's age and location of the tumor, this lesion is most likely a rhabdomyosarcoma
(E) After initial surgical resection, if the lesion recurs locally, re-resection is appropriate

8. A 45-year-old woman presents to the office with complaints of a hard mass in her abdomen. She is otherwise healthy and has 3 children, 1 recently born by cesarean section. Upon examination, the patient is noted to have a firm, 3-cm, subcutaneous mass, inferior to the umbilicus and just lateral to the midline. Excisional biopsy of the lesion reveals a desmoid tumor. Upon discussion of this lesion with the patient during follow-up, which of the following is an appropriate statement regarding the nature of this lesion?

(A) These lesions rarely recur after resection
(B) These lesions may be a high risk for metastasis
(C) These lesions may behave like low-grade sarcomas
(D) These lesions are frequently associated with retroperitoneal fibrosis
(E) Postoperative chemotherapy is a key component of therapy

Answers and Explanations

1–B. A chest radiograph is essential in the evaluation of patients with sarcomas because the lung is the most common site of metastasis. In contrast, sarcomas rarely metastasize via the lymphatics, and thus biopsy of the sentinel lymph node is not routinely performed. Preoperative evaluation of patients with sarcoma allows for identification of metastatic disease, which occurs frequently with these lesions. Sarcomas preferentially spread via hematogenous routes and rarely spread superficially to the skin. In addition, performing multiple biopsies may increase the likelihood of tumor seeding of the blood and metastasis. Limb-sparing procedures are currently preferred over amputation in the management of most extremity sarcomas.

2–B. The pathogenesis of the development of lymphangiosarcomas in these patients is related to the presence of chronic lymphedema. These lesions often occur outside the irradiated field and are not specifically related to the pre-existing breast cancer. Advanced age and a history of diabetes are also not direct risk factors for the development of these lesions. Lymphangiosarcomas may also arise in association with lymphedema caused by filarial infection (elephantiasis) or other chronic lymphedematous states.

3–E. Although overall these lesions are rare, acral lentiginous melanomas generally occur in regions of the body not exposed to the sun, including the palms, soles, and subungual regions. This form of melanoma most commonly occurs in patients with dark skin. Although these tumors are frequently mistaken for traumatic subungual hematomas, these tumors do not develop specifically from these injuries. Melanomas of the digits frequently require amputation for adequate resection. The most aggressive type of melanoma is the nodular variant, not acral lentiginous lesions.

4–A. Surgical re-resection is still the most appropriate treatment strategy even for recurrent lesions. Radiation therapy may play an adjunctive role but is not the best therapy when used alone. Chemotherapy and immunotherapy play little, if any, role in the local treatment of recurrent disease. Observation alone would be inappropriate.

5–E. Exposure to ultraviolet (UV) light is a risk factor for the development of nonmelanoma skin cancers, although among the different types, UVB light is associated with a greater risk than UVA light. Bowen's disease is a premalignant lesion that predisposes to squamous cell carcinoma, while a keratoacanthoma is a benign lesion. Immunosuppression is also a significant risk factor for skin cancers. Other characteristics that may be associated with a greater risk of skin cancer development include fair skin, blue eyes, and blonde hair. These factors are generally related to the sensitivity of the patient's skin to light exposure.

6–A. By far the most common site of melanoma is on the skin surfaces, therefore, all patients should undergo extensive examination of skin surfaces to identify the primary lesion. If a primary skin lesion is not identified, other potential sites for melanoma development include the mucous membranes (e.g., mouth, nasal passages), on the fundus of the eye, and in the anorectal region. Otoscopy is also essential to identify potential lesions within the ear canal. Therefore, a careful funduscopic examination should be performed, in addition to careful evaluation of the anorectum with proctoscopy if necessary. A chest and abdominal computed tomography (CT) and a small bowel contrast study are not routinely indicated in this setting. Approximately 5% of patients will not have an identifiable primary lesion in the setting of metastatic disease.

7–E. Repeat surgical resection is still the most appropriate treatment strategy for locally recurring sarcomas. The presence of peritoneal implants is generally a contraindication to surgical resection of asymptomatic sarcomas. Preoperative assessment may also include angiography to rule out potential vascular invasion, which is another common contraindication to resection of the lesion. Radiation of the retroperitoneum is associated with significant morbidity and does not play a significant role in the treatment of recurrent retroperitoneal sarcomas. Although visceral sarcomas may frequently metastasize to the liver, retroperitoneal sarcomas rarely do; and the lung is generally the most common location of metastatic disease. The most common lesions in this site in patients in this age group are leiomyosarcomas and liposarcomas.

8–C. Desmoid tumors are soft tissue tumors that can behave like low-grade sarcomas; however, they rarely metastasize. Despite the low frequency of metastasis, these lesions frequently recur locally despite resection. There are 3 subgroups of desmoid tumors and the abdominal wall desmoids frequently occur during or following pregnancy and may be related to previous scars. The intra-abdominal desmoids are associated with Gardner's syndrome and are prone to the development of retroperitoneal fibrosis. The primary treatment is surgical resection, with some lesions responding to radiation therapy. Chemotherapy does not play a significant role in the treatment of these lesions.

Comprehensive Examination

Directions: Each of the numbered items or incomplete statements in this section is followed by answers or by completions of the statement. Select the ONE lettered answer or completion that is BEST in each case.

1. A 65-year-old man is admitted to the surgical intensive care unit following pancreatic débridement for necrotizing pancreatitis. The patient is extubated, although his respiratory status remains guarded. Parenteral nutrition therapy is initiated with 35 kcal/kg/day; 65% is administered as carbohydrates, 30% as lipids, and 5% as protein. The patient also receives vitamin supplements. Over the next 24 hours the patient complains of worsening fatigue and numbness around his lips. He develops a tremor in both hands and becomes more lethargic as the day continues until he must be reintubated. This patient's abnormality would be most adequately treated if he were administered

(A) KPO_4^-
(B) $MgCl_2$
(C) KCl
(D) Thiamine
(E) Insulin

2. A 27-year-old, 80-kg, male athlete sustained deep partial-thickness burns to approximately 60% total body surface area (TBSA). He has been receiving lactated Ringer's in direct accordance with the Parkland formula calculations for volume resuscitation, however, he remains tachycardic with a heart rate of approximately 110 beats/min. Which of the following is true with regard to fluid management in this patient?

(A) A Foley catheter is not necessary in this patient if he is awake
(B) A urine output of 30 mL/hour is not satisfactory in this patient
(C) Tachycardia is the most reliable marker of inadequate resuscitation
(D) One 18-gauge intravenous (IV) catheter is sufficient for treating this patient
(E) If significant peripheral edema is present, IV fluid rates should be decreased

3. A 70-year-old man with an asthma exacerbation suffers a first time episode of atrial fibrillation in the hospital. The ventricular response is 160, but the patient's blood pressure remains stable. The decision is made to cardiovert the rhythm, however, secondary to increasing dyspnea. Ketamine is administered intravenously, the man loses consciousness but continues to spontaneously ventilate, and is successfully converted to sinus rhythm after one 100 J synchronized cardioversion. Upon awakening he complains of intensely frightening illusions. Which of the following premedications could have lessened this unwanted side effect?

(A) Propofol
(B) Fentanyl
(C) Lidocaine
(D) Etomidate
(E) Midazolam

4. A 15-year-old boy is admitted with the chief complaint of right lower quadrant abdominal pain, nausea, vomiting, and anorexia for the past 5 hours. His vital signs are: respiration, 24/min; heart rate, 90 beats/min; blood pressure, 120/70 mm Hg; temperature, 38.3°C. Which of the following findings is most likely to be present in this patient?

(A) Pelvic crepitus
(B) Psoas sign
(C) Murphy's sign
(D) Flank ecchymosis
(E) Periumbilical ecchymosis

5. A 63-year-old man is being treated with a 7-day course of oral antibiotics for an acute episode of diverticulitis. Now, 4 days into the course of antibiotics, the patient presents with persistent fever and worsening pain and advancing erythema in the perineal area. Upon evaluation, he is felt to have worsening necrotizing fasciitis of the perineum extending to and including the scrotum. Which of the following would be an appropriate treatment strategy for this patient?

(A) Aggressive débridement of the affected tissue with orchiectomy and intravenous (IV) antibiotics
(B) Aggressive débridement of the affected tissue with sparing of the testes and IV antibiotics
(C) Sitz baths 4 times a day and broad spectrum oral antibiotics
(D) Sitz baths 4 times a day and broad spectrum IV antibiotics
(E) Aggressive débridement of the affected tissue with orchiectomy and immediate resection of affected colon with primary reanastomosis

6. A 42-year-old man undergoes elective laparoscopic hernia repair for bilateral inguinal hernias. On postoperative day one, the patient develops worsening abdominal pain associated with nausea and vomiting. On physical examination, the patient is noted to have severe abdominal pain with rebound and guarding. Which of the following is the most likely cause of this patient's findings?

(A) Strangulation of bowel
(B) Recurrence of the hernia
(C) Iatrogenic bowel injury
(D) Wound infection
(E) Adhesion formation

7. A 45-year-old woman underwent an uneventful total colectomy for ulcerative colitis. On postoperative day 5, the patient was found to be minimally responsive. Physical examination reveals a temperature of 40.0°C; blood pressure of 70/36 mm Hg; pulse of 130/min; respiration of 32/min; and cold, clammy skin, diaphoresis, and cool extremities. There was 85 mL of urine output overnight. Laboratory studies showed a white blood cell count of 2.2, hematocrit = 44.1, platelets = 700,000, Na^+ = 145, K^+ = 5.9, Cl^- = 111, HCO_3^- = 18, blood urea nitrogen = 64, and creatinine = 3.0. Urinalysis was significant for renal tubular cells. Which of the following statements is true regarding this patient's renal function?

(A) This patient is anuric and must immediately be started on hemodialysis
(B) Treating the initial condition has little effect in allowing renal function to recover
(C) Certain drugs and transfusion reactions are potential etiologies of this condition
(D) Persistent disease will result in severe metabolic alkalosis, hypokalemia, and dehydration
(E) In most patients, this complication is irreversible

8. A 65-year-old woman presents with obstructive jaundice and a history of 20-lb weight loss. She denies any complaints of fever, pain, nausea, or vomiting. Her abdominal examination is unremarkable. An endoscopic retrograde cholangiopancreatography (ERCP) has been performed and reveals a focal common bile duct stenosis with dilation of the common hepatic and intrahepatic ducts. Significant laboratory values include a normal white blood cell count, total bilirubin = 12.0, conjugated bilirubin = 11.2, alkaline phosphatase = 2000, and normal transaminases. Which of the following is the most likely diagnosis?

(A) Primary sclerosing cholangitis
(B) Cholangitis
(C) Choledochal cyst
(D) Mirizzi's syndrome
(E) Cholangiocarcinoma

9. A 30-year-old healthy woman presents to the office 1 year after having an uncomplicated cesarean section. She complains of a persistently large, unsightly scar at the surgical site, which is found to be a hypertrophic scar. Intralesional triamcinolone improves the appearance of the scar. The effect of this drug is best described by which of the following mechanisms?

(A) Enhancement of collagenase activity
(B) Decrease in the number of active fibroblasts
(C) Increase in collagen turnover, making the scar more susceptible to local pressure treatment
(D) Inhibition of intracellular collagen synthesis
(E) Inhibition of extracellular intermolecular collagen cross-linking, increasing collagen solubility

10. A 50-year-old man receives a transfusion of packed red blood cells (PRBCs) for anemia secondary to chronic gastrointestinal bleeding. Fifteen minutes after the infusion begins, the patient develops back pain, chills, fever, and dark urine. His temperature is 38.8°C (102°F), his pulse rate is 124/min, his respiratory rate is 28/min, and his blood pressure is 116/44 mm Hg. Examination reveals moderate respiratory distress and crackles throughout his lung fields. Which of the following is the most likely source of this patient's problem?

(A) Infection secondary to bacterial contamination of donor blood
(B) Donor leukocytes reacting with the recipient's red blood cells (RBCs)
(C) Recipient antibodies reacting to donor RBCs
(D) Volume overload secondary to rapid administration of blood
(E) Hypocalcemia secondary to citrate in the donor blood

11. One month after an orthotopic liver transplant, a 43-year-old woman presents to the office with complaints of fatigue and weakness. On physical examination she is noticeably jaundiced. She denies fever or chills. Her aspartate aminotransferase (AST) and alanine aminotransferase (ALT) are significantly elevated, as is her total bilirubin. Her chest radiograph is clear, and blood and urine cultures are negative. Doppler ultrasound of the right upper quadrant reveals no fluid collections and a patent hepatic artery and portal vein. Liver biopsy reveals portal lymphocytic infiltration and injury to the bile canaliculi. Which of the following is the most appropriate initial therapy for this patient?

(A) Glucocorticoids
(B) Cyclosporine
(C) Cyclophosphamide
(D) Azathioprine
(E) Mycophenolate mofetil

12. A 73-year-old man with chronic obstructive pulmonary disease is hospitalized for recurrent pneumothoraces. He has been critically ill in the surgical intensive care unit with multiple bouts of pneumonia and sepsis for 5 weeks. On reviewing his laboratory data you notice a steady trend downward of his hematocrit from 48% to 21%. Which of the following would be the most appropriate initial step in the management of this patient?

(A) Emergent laparotomy
(B) Observation
(C) Colonoscopy
(D) Nasogastric tube placement and stools for guaiac
(E) Immediate mesenteric angiography

13. An 18-year-old college student presents with 4 hours of severe chest and epigastric pain after a night of binge drinking. She states that she vomited several times upon returning home and that the pain began shortly thereafter. She is currently stable and her chest radiograph reveals pneumomediastinum and a pleural effusion on the left side. Which of the following is true regarding this scenario?

(A) As is the case in more than 75% of cases, this patient can be treated successfully with intravenous (IV) hydration and antibiotics alone
(B) Primary repair of the esophagus is unlikely to be successful in this patient
(C) Boerhaave's syndrome is the most common cause of esophageal perforation
(D) Despite proper intervention, survival is generally less than 50% in this patient
(E) Radical procedures such as esophageal exclusion are usually not necessary in patients who present within 24 hours of the injury

14. A 35-year-old man with hypertension and end-stage renal disease secondary to systemic lupus erythematosus is receiving an axillary block as the anesthetic for an arterioventricular fistula placement. During injection of the local anesthetic (bupivacaine) into the axilla, the patient abruptly seizes. Which of the following agents given intravenously would be most appropriate in the treatment of this patient's seizure?

(A) Fentanyl
(B) Succinylcholine
(C) Midazolam
(D) Etomidate
(E) Lidocaine

15. A 57-year-old man with severe liver disease from alcohol abuse is admitted to the hospital with worsening ascites and encephalopathy. He is placed on the recipient list for a donor liver and managed in the intensive care unit. Because of his encephalopathy, he is unable to eat; therefore, he is started on enteral nutritional support via a nasoduodenal feeding tube. He is receiving 1.3 mg protein/kg/day with a predominance of branched-chain amino acids. Which of the following is an appropriate statement regarding the administration of branched-chain amino acid to patients in this setting?

(A) Branched-chain amino acids include leucine, isoleucine, and alanine
(B) Muscle preferentially metabolizes these amino acids
(C) The liver preferentially metabolizes these amino acids
(D) Branched-chain amino acids act as hepatotoxins in liver failure
(E) Branched-chain amino acids are nonessential amino acids

16. A 72-year-old man is evaluated in the emergency room with a primary complaint of nausea and vomiting for 2–3 days and a 2- to 3-week history of intermittent right upper quadrant pain. His past surgical history is significant for triple coronary artery bypass surgery. Physical examination reveals a distended abdomen with hyperactive bowel sounds. Rectal examination is heme-negative. His temperature is 37.7°C (100°F), his heart rate is 105 beats/min, and his blood pressure is 140/75 mm Hg. His abdominal radiograph shows multiple step-ladder air–fluid levels throughout the abdomen and notable air within the biliary tree. Which of the following is the most likely diagnosis?

(A) Superior mesenteric artery syndrome
(B) Cancer of the colon
(C) Obstruction caused by adhesions
(D) Sigmoid diverticulitis
(E) Gallstone ileus

17. A 64-year-old man presents to your office with right breast hyperplasia. He states that he has only noticed his right breast getting bigger over the last few months, but his wife stated that she thought he had always been a little bigger on the right. He states that he does drink, but no more than a few beers each night. On physical examination, you notice that his right breast is larger than his left, and there is a firm mass just under the nipple. There are no palpable masses in his axilla, but the mass does seem to be fixed to the chest wall. Which of the following is the most appropriate treatment for this patient?

(A) A lumpectomy, axillary node dissection with postoperative radiation therapy
(B) Fine needle aspiration (FNA) and, if malignant disease is discovered, a modified radical mastectomy
(C) FNA and, if malignant disease is discovered, a radical mastectomy
(D) Systemic chemotherapy alone
(E) Observation

18. A 62-year-old man with a history of a previous episode of diverticulitis presents to the emergency room with complaints of fever, nausea, and abdominal pain that is greatest in the left lower quadrant. Computed tomography (CT) scan reveals multiple sigmoid diverticula, a 4-cm abscess in the left lower quadrant, and free air in the peritoneum. Which of the following is the most appropriate course of management for this patient?

(A) Percutaneous drainage of the abscess and administration of intravenous (IV) antibiotics
(B) Emergent resection of the affected colon with end colostomy and abscess drainage
(C) Percutaneous drainage of the abscess, IV antibiotics, and elective resection at a later date
(D) Emergent total colectomy with abscess drainage
(E) Emergent operative drainage of the abscess, IV antibiotics, and elective resection of the colon at a later date

19. Which of the following is characteristic of malignant tumors of the liver?

(A) α-Fetoprotein may be elevated with hepatic metastases or hepatocellular carcinoma
(B) Alcoholic cirrhosis is the most common cause of hepatocellular carcinoma worldwide
(C) Hepatocellular carcinoma is the most common malignant lesion of the liver
(D) Fibrolamellar variant of hepatocellular carcinoma is associated with a worse prognosis compared with hepatocellular carcinoma
(E) Hepatoblastoma is generally insensitive to chemotherapy

20. A 34-year-old man with acquired immunodeficiency syndrome (AIDS) and a recent episode of *Pneumocystis carinii* infection has been suffering from progressive symptoms of early satiety, abdominal bloating, weight loss, and intermittent, dull left upper quadrant abdominal pains. Physical examination reveals a markedly enlarged spleen, the tip of which is palpable in the left lower quadrant. Abdominopelvic computed tomography (CT) scan confirms massive splenomegaly but no other masses are identified. Antiplatelet antibodies are not identified in his blood. Which of the following is the most appropriate therapy for this patient?

(A) Elective splenectomy
(B) Plasmapheresis
(C) Emergent splenectomy
(D) Intravenous (IV) gamma globulin
(E) Splenic artery embolization

21. A 42-year-old woman with a history of Graves' disease currently being treated medically presents with a 3-cm mass in the left lobe of the thyroid. Fine needle aspiration (FNA) reveals follicular cell carcinoma. Before induction, during palpation of the thyroid gland, the patient develops sudden fever and tachycardia intraoperatively. Which of the following is the most appropriate treatment measure in this setting?

(A) Administration of calcium carbonate
(B) β-Blockade, propylthiouracil (PTU), and Lugol's solution
(C) Thyroxine administration
(D) Mechanical cooling and dantrolene
(E) Administration of 4 units of packed red blood cells (PRBCs)

22. A 65-year-old, obese woman underwent a left hemicolectomy with primary re-anastomosis for colon adenocarcinoma. On postoperative day 14, the patient complains of abdominal pain, anorexia, and fever (temperature of 39.1°C). Her physical examination is significant for mild diffuse abdominal tenderness, a mildly distended abdomen with few bowel sounds, and guarding in the left lower quadrant. Laboratory studies show a white blood cell count of 16.9 (91% polys), and are otherwise within normal limits. Computed tomography (CT) scan of the abdomen reveals a fluid collection in the left lower quadrant. An anastomotic leak is diagnosed. Which of the following is true regarding her intestinal anastomoses?

(A) Anastomotic leaks occur more frequently in the colon than in the small bowel because of the increased bowel wall thickness of the colon
(B) Avoidance of gross contamination while making anastomoses has little impact on the incidence of leakage because the abdomen may be easily irrigated before closure
(C) The presence of a leak requires immediate re-operation with exteriorization of the bowel
(D) Ensuring the absence of distal obstruction is important in creating successful intestinal anastomoses
(E) Percutaneous drainage should not be attempted because it carries a high failure rate

23. A 38-year-old, African-American woman with a history of gastroesophageal reflux disease and sickle cell disease presents with a 36-hour history of nausea, vomiting, and right upper quadrant pain. The pain is described as spasmodic in nature and is exacerbated by eating. The patient denies fever, chills, and previous abdominal surgery. Her vital signs are: temperature, 36.9° C; pulse, 101/min; blood pressure, 140/86 mm Hg; and respiration, 13/min. Her abdomen is soft but tender to palpation in the right upper quadrant. Her laboratory results are: white blood cells = 6000; hematocrit = 34; platelets = 212; Na^+ = 132; K^+ = 4.1; Cl^- = 104; CO_2 = 25; blood urea nitrogen = 14; creatinine = 0.8; glucose = 89; total bilirubin = 7.5; conjugated bilirubin = 6.6; alkaline phosphatase = 540; and amylase = 41. A right upper quadrant ultrasound reveals multiple gallstones and a distended common duct but no other abnormalities. Which of the following statements is appropriate regarding this patient's condition?

(A) The patient most likely has a common bile duct obstruction from a stone formed in the gallbladder
(B) The pathogenesis of this patient's condition is related to bile stasis and bacterial deconjugation of bilirubin
(C) Fluctuating symptoms are uncommonly associated with this disease
(D) Pain on palpation is an uncommon finding in this disease
(E) An endoscopic retrograde cholangiopancreatography (ERCP) may be diagnostic but plays no role in the treatment of this disease

24. A 45-year-old woman sustains multiple injuries in a motor vehicle accident, including a splenic laceration requiring emergent splenectomy, a transverse process fracture of the third lumbar vertebrae, and a fracture of the shaft of the left tibia. During placement of a Swan-Ganz catheter via the left subclavian vein, the patient suddenly develops hypotension with a blood pressure of 80/60 mm Hg initially. A chest tube is placed without improvement in her blood pressure. A large quantity of blood is noted to be coming out of the endotracheal tube. Which of the following is the most likely cause of this patient's hypotension?

(A) Tension pneumothorax
(B) Severe hemothorax
(C) Cardiac perforation
(D) Pulmonary artery perforation
(E) Acute pulmonary embolus

25. A 28-year-old woman presents to the surgical clinic with a known history of a thyroid nodule. History reveals that her mother and sister died secondary to thyroid cancer and a hypertensive crisis, respectively. Fine needle aspiration (FNA) of the thyroid mass reveals medullary thyroid carcinoma. Which of the following is correct regarding further treatment of this patient?

(A) Surgical treatment of her thyroid cancer involves lobectomy and isthmusectomy
(B) If a pheochromocytoma is found, a laparoscopic approach is contraindicated in this patient
(C) If a pheochromocytoma is found, the posterior approach should be used
(D) If hyperparathyroidism is found, the patient can generally be managed with parathyroidectomy of the adenoma
(E) Urine tests for catecholamines, metanephrines, vanillylmandelic acid, parathyroid hormone, and calcium should be obtained

26. A 62-year-old woman presents with a 3-cm, dark, elevated mass on her upper back. The report of an incisional biopsy of the lesion performed at another hospital states that the lesion is a melanoma, 0.7 mm thick. Which of the following is the most appropriate therapy for the treatment of the primary lesion?

(A) Wide local excision of the lesion with 1-cm margins
(B) Cryosurgical ablation of the lesion
(C) Wide local excision of the lesion with 5-cm margins
(D) Mohs' microsurgical technique of surgical resection
(E) Wide local excision of the lesion with 2-cm margins

27. A 45-year-old woman presents with a 3-cm neck mass in the right lobe of the thyroid partially involving the isthmus. Fine needle aspiration (FNA) of the lesion reveals a poorly differentiated Hürthle cell variant of follicular carcinoma. Which of the following is the most appropriate treatment for this patient?

(A) Lobectomy and isthmusectomy followed by radioiodine (^{131}I) ablation therapy
(B) Total thyroidectomy followed by ^{131}I ablation therapy
(C) ^{131}I ablation therapy followed by total thyroidectomy
(D) Total thyroidectomy with node dissection for positive nodes
(E) Lobectomy and isthmusectomy

28. After a motor vehicle accident, a 28-year-old woman was found to have a 3-cm, simple liver cyst on computed tomography (CT) scan during her evaluation in the emergency room. The patient was found to have isolated orthopedic injuries and was discharged 2 days later. Which of the following would be a contraindication to surgical management or percutaneous drainage of a simple liver cyst in this patient?

(A) Pain associated with cyst
(B) Fever, chills, and positive cultures from cyst contents
(C) Hemorrhage within cyst
(D) Rupture of cyst
(E) Presence of von Meyenburg complexes (biliary ductal epithelium) within biopsy specimen of cyst wall

29. A 38-year-old man presents with a firm nodule in his neck and hypertension that has been refractory to medical therapy. Subsequent work-up also reveals a pheochromocytoma as the probable source of the patient's hypertension as well as a medullary thyroid cancer consistent with the diagnosis of the multiple endocrine neoplasia (MEN) II syndrome. Which of the following is true regarding the sequence of treatment of this patient?

(A) Immediate resection of the pheochromocytoma should be performed, followed by resection of the medullary cancer at a later date
(B) Control of hypertension and resection of the pheochromocytoma and the medullary cancer during the same procedure
(C) Control of hypertension and resection of the pheochromocytoma, followed by neck exploration and resection of the medullary cancer at a later date
(D) Resection of the cancerous lesion first, followed by resection of the pheochromocytoma
(E) Resection of the pheochromocytoma, followed by neck irradiation

30. A 30-year-old man sustained multiple injuries in a motor vehicle accident. On hospital day two, he remains intubated in the intensive care unit in critical condition and it is decided that enteral nutritional support should be initiated. During placement of a nasogastric feeding tube to 40 cm the patient's blood pressure is noted to drop precipitously to 50/30 mm Hg. During forceful insufflation of air through the feeding tube there are no sounds noted over the epigastric region. Which of the following would be the most appropriate definitive step in the management of this patient?

(A) Removal of the feeding tube and fluid resuscitation
(B) Removal of the feeding tube and chest tube placement
(C) Injection of contrast through the feeding tube to assess placement
(D) Removal of the feeding tube and immediate laparotomy
(E) Removal of the feeding tube and immediate pulmonary angiogram

31. A 59-year-old woman is taken to the operating room and undergoes an exploratory laparotomy for a high-grade small bowel obstruction. During the operation she is found to have a large leiomyoma that is obstructing the distal ileum. A large segment of the terminal ileum is resected with the tumor. Which of the following long-term nutritional risks is associated with this procedure?

(A) Dumping syndrome
(B) Pernicious anemia
(C) Hypercalcemia
(D) Afferent loop syndrome
(E) Iron deficiency anemia

32. A 29-year-old, breast-feeding mother presents to the clinic with the primary complaint of right breast tenderness. She states that the tenderness began suddenly, and was first associated with pain when she began breast-feeding, but now is continuous. She denies fever, chills, or any other associated symptoms. On physical examination, she has a tender right breast with an area of erythema in the lower outer quadrant. There is no expressible discharge and no definitive masses to palpation. Which of the following is the most appropriate treatment for this patient?

(A) Place patient on nonsteroidal anti-inflammatory drugs (NSAIDs)
(B) Antibiotics to cover skin organisms, *Staphylococcus aureus,* and discontinue breast-feeding until pain resolves
(C) Antibiotics to cover skin organisms, *S. aureus,* and continue breast-feeding
(D) Consider placing patient on danazol
(E) Reassure the patient that with continued breast feeding her pain should resolve

33. A patient who has been diagnosed with diverticular disease presents with massive hemorrhage. After the site of bleeding is well localized, the patient continues to bleed and requires 5 units of blood over the next 24 hours. Which of the following therapies will provide the lowest morbidity and least chance of rebleeding?

(A) Surgical resection of the diseased segment
(B) Angiographic embolization of the bleeding vessel
(C) Angiographic vasopressin infusion
(D) Subtotal colectomy
(E) Further observation and transfusion as needed

34. A 16-year-old boy presents to the emergency room 36 hours after being bitten in the hand during an altercation. He is febrile [39.0°C (102.2°F)] and he has purulent drainage from the 2-cm wound over the metacarpophalangeal joint of his ring finger. The finger cannot be actively extended. Which of the following is the most appropriate management strategy?

(A) Topical cleansing followed by oral antibiotics
(B) Débridement and irrigation followed by intravenous (IV) antibiotics
(C) Repair of the affected extensor tendon followed by skin closure
(D) Repair of the affected extensor tendon followed by open packing
(E) Application of a sterile dressing and close observation

35. A 59-year-old man presents to the emergency department with complaints of persistent fever and mild left lower quadrant abdominal pain for the previous 4 days. The patient is otherwise healthy and denies nausea or vomiting. Physical examination reveals localized pain to deep palpation in the left lower quadrant without rebound or guarding. Subsequent computed tomography (CT) scan reveals a localized 8-cm pelvic abscess with multiple diverticula noted throughout the sigmoid colon. Which of the following is the most appropriate next step in the management of this patient?

(A) Percutaneous drainage of the abscess with adjunctive antibiotics
(B) Immediate laparotomy with resection of adjacent bowel
(C) Antibacterial agents alone should be sufficient treatment
(D) Antibiotic therapy directed against principally aerobic bacteria
(E) Antifungal therapy should be initiated because of a significant risk of fungal contamination

36. A 55-year-old man has been experiencing chronic epigastric burning pain for the past 10 years. He initially was able to control his symptoms with over-the-counter medications. However, his pain has persisted despite a 12-month course of ranitidine and most recently a 6-month course of omeprazole. Repeat endoscopy reveals a persistent duodenal ulceration without active bleeding. Multiple biopsies reveal no evidence of malignancy or *Helicobacter pylori.* Which of the following operations is associated with the lowest morbidity, but the highest recurrence in this patient?

(A) Truncal vagotomy
(B) Truncal vagotomy and pyloroplasty
(C) Vagotomy and antrectomy
(D) Parietal cell (highly selective) vagotomy
(E) Total gastric resection

37. A 21-year old woman is brought to the emergency room because she has been experiencing lower abdominal pain for the past 8 hours that has been getting progressively worse. The date of her last menstrual period was 8 weeks ago. The patient was found by paramedics to be pale and lethargic. Examination now reveals a distended abdomen with rigidity and guarding diffusely. Her vital signs are: heart rate, 120 beats/min; blood pressure, 70/30 mm Hg; respiration, 28/min; temperature, 36.0°C. Which of the following is the most likely diagnosis?

(A) Appendicitis
(B) Crohn's disease
(C) Ectopic pregnancy
(D) Perforated duodenal ulcer
(E) Torsed ovary

38. A 24-year-old man is involved in a motor vehicle accident resulting in a severe closed head injury. This injury is believed to be irreversible and evaluation for possible organ donation is undertaken. Which of the following would exclude him as a heart-beating organ donor?

(A) Absence of response to painful stimuli
(B) Intact deep tendon reflexes
(C) Intact gag reflex
(D) Core body temperature of 38.2°C
(E) The requirement of 10 μg/kg/min of dopamine for hemodynamic stability

39. A 55-year-old woman undergoes an excisional biopsy for a palpable breast mass. The biopsy results return indicating invasive ductal adenocarcinoma of less then 1 cm in diameter, and no cancer cells at the margin of the biopsy. Which of the following is the most appropriate next step in the treatment of this patient?

(A) Axillary node dissection or sampling for staging, and radiation therapy to the breast
(B) Axillary node dissection for staging alone
(C) Radiation therapy to the breast alone
(D) Simple mastectomy
(E) Radical mastectomy

40. Work-up of a right-sided colon mass found in a 68-year-old, otherwise healthy woman reveals an incompletely resected adenocarcinoma upon colonoscopic polypectomy. The patient subsequently undergoes an elective segmental colonic resection of the lesion, which confirms adenocarcinoma upon pathologic evaluation. Which of the following adjuvant therapies would be appropriate in the further management of this patient?

(A) Chemotherapy for stage III adenocarcinoma
(B) Chemotherapy for stage I adenocarcinoma
(C) Radiation therapy for stage II adenocarcinoma
(D) Radiation therapy for stage III adenocarcinoma
(E) Chemotherapy and radiation therapy for stage III adenocarcinoma

41. A 180-kg, 21-year-old man with spina bifida and lower extremity paralysis is in the medical intensive care unit with urosepsis. The patient also has a history of a seizure disorder. The patient was extubated after a prolonged period of intubation, however, his respiratory status continues to deteriorate and the decision is made to reintubate. His blood pressure is 78/40 mm Hg, respiration rate exceeds 30/min, and the SaO_2 is 89% on 100% oxygen. The anesthesiologist judges the airway to be difficult because of limited neck motion and inability to visualize the uvula with mouth opening. Which of the following is the most appropriate strategy in the initial airway management of this patient?

(A) Rapid sequence intubation with etomidate and rocuronium
(B) Rapid sequence intubation with thiopental and rocuronium
(C) Rapid sequence intubation with propofol and rocuronium
(D) Topical anesthesia (lidocaine) to the airway
(E) Intubation after administration of ketamine and rocuronium

42. A 79-year-old woman underwent an uneventful abdominal-perineal resection for a rectal cancer. She was slow to recover and on postoperative day 10, she was noted to have an open, excoriated wound near her buttocks and blisters on both heels. Which of the following statements most accurately reflects this condition?

(A) This is a common complication in all populations of postoperative patients
(B) Frequent bathing and skin conditioners frequently cause this complication
(C) Quantitative skin cultures are necessary to ensure proper treatment of the colonizing flora
(D) Early mobilization and frequent position changes have little impact in preventing this complication
(E) Maintaining proper nutritional status is helpful in the prevention and treatment of this condition

43. A 55-year-old, obese woman presents with a painful 4-cm mass just below the umbilicus in the midline. The patient states that she had noticed the mass for several years but presents today because of progressively worsening pain associated with the mass over the past day. On physical examination there is an exquisitely tender mass just under the umbilicus. Although difficult, the mass is eventually reduced with firm pressure and moderate sedation. After reduction of the mass, the patient continues to complain of abdominal pain and is noted to have significant guarding and rebound tenderness. Which of the following is the most appropriate treatment strategy for this patient?

(A) Immediate abdominal exploration
(B) Immediate local wound exploration and hernia repair
(C) Discharge and plan for elective hernia repair
(D) Discharge and elective hernia repair if the hernia recurs
(E) Observation and exploration if the pain worsens

44. A 32-year-old man presents with a history of intermittent dysphagia, most often following a hurried swallow. These episodes generally occur with solids and he reports a history of mild gastroesophageal reflux symptoms. Upper endoscopy reveals the presence of a Schatzki's ring. Which of the following statements is true regarding this patient?

(A) This patient almost certainly has an associated type II esophageal hernia
(B) A Schatzki's ring is covered by columnar epithelium on both the upper and lower surfaces
(C) This is a premalignant lesion, similar to Barrett's esophagus
(D) Symptomatic lesions generally respond to either rigid or pneumatic dilation of the ring
(E) The presence of gastroesophageal reflux symptoms and a Schatzki's ring is an indication for fundoplication without any further preoperative studies

45. A 44-year-old is started on parenteral nutritional therapy for acute necrotizing pancreatitis. He undergoes pancreatic débridement and shows some improvement in the immediate postoperative period. On postoperative day 3, the patient gradually becomes increasingly lethargic and confused. His heart rate is 140 beats/min, blood pressure is 80/40 mm Hg, and respiration is 24/min. His $K^+ = 3.7$, $Na^+ = 145$, $Cl^- = 120$, blood urea nitrogen = 75, and creatinine = 1.7. His hematocrit is 45%. Arterial blood gas is pH 7.24, $PO_2 = 85$ on 2 L nasal cannula, $PCO_2 = 30$, and $HCO_3^- = 19$. He is currently receiving fluids via parenteral nutrition with 35 kcal/kg/day: 60% carbohydrates, 35% kcal as lipids, and the rest as protein. He is also receiving morphine sulfate via a patient-controlled analgesia pump. Which of the following would most likely account for this patient's current status?

(A) Deficiency in thiamine
(B) Hypoglycemia
(C) Hyperglycemia
(D) Dehydration
(E) Morphine overdose

46. A patient presents to the emergency room after sustaining a gunshot injury to the right chest. The entrance wound is approximately 2 inches below the nipple and along the anterior axillary line with an exit wound near the posterior axillary line on the right. Along with the placement of a chest tube, treatment should include which of the following?

(A) Performance of a subxiphoid window
(B) Immediate aortogram
(C) Immediate median sternotomy
(D) Exploratory laparotomy
(E) No further treatment

47. A 52-year-old man with a history of hypertension is referred for biopsy-proven gastric adenocarcinoma. The patient states that the cancer was found when he underwent a routine upper endoscopy for the evaluation of his epigastric pain. The pain has been recent in onset, about 1 month. Otherwise, the patient denies any melanotic stools or weight loss. Extensive evaluation does not demonstrate any metastatic disease. Which of the following would be the best advice to give to this patient?

(A) Undergo chemotherapy and radiation only
(B) Undergo surgical resection
(C) Have a repeat computed tomography scan (CT) in 6 months to evaluate for regression
(D) Undergo a gastric bypass for symptomatic relief
(E) Undergo radiation therapy alone

48. A 57-year-old woman underwent an abdominal hysterectomy for fibroids 8 years ago. She now presents to the emergency room with a 2-day history of worsening nausea and vomiting, as well as complaints of crampy central and lower abdominal pain. On physical examination her temperature is 37.7°C (100°F), her heart rate is 110 beats/min, her respiratory rate is 16/min, and her blood pressure is 140/80 mm Hg. Her abdomen is distended and mildly tender but without rebound or guarding. Initial management should include which of the following?

(A) Ultrasound examination of the abdomen
(B) Nasogastric tube placement
(C) Immediate exploratory laparotomy
(D) Administration of analgesics and antiemetics
(E) Continued observation in the emergency room

49. A 65-year-old man recently diagnosed with renal cell carcinoma presents to the office with complaints of increased abdominal bloating. On physical examination, he is found to have a tense, but nontender abdomen with shifting dullness. The liver edge is also palpable 6 cm below the costal margin. Computed tomography (CT) scan reveals tumor extending through the inferior vena cava to the right atrium. In this patient, which of the following is the most likely cause of ascites and portal hypertension?

(A) Alcoholic cirrhosis
(B) Budd-Chiari syndrome
(C) Schistosomiasis
(D) Cirrhosis secondary to Hepatitis B
(E) Portal vein thrombosis

50. A 65-year-old man presents for an elective total knee replacement. His is otherwise in a good state of health but reports that he remembers being on a ventilator for a long time after a laparoscopic cholecystectomy 5 years prior. A review of his chart reveals that he received succinylcholine and the prolonged paralysis was thought to have been the result of a pseudocholinesterase deficiency. Which of the following agents could potentially result in prolonged muscle relaxation if used in this patient?

(A) Pancuronium
(B) Vecuronium
(C) Atracurium
(D) Rocuronium
(E) Mivacurium

51. A patient who had sustained a severe crush injury to both the lower extremities 2 days prior is noted to have frequent long runs of ventricular tachycardia on the electrocardiogram (ECG) monitor, although his blood pressure is stable at 115/75 mm Hg. A formal ECG reveals deep S waves, peaked T waves, and widening of the QRS complex. Which of the following is the most appropriate initial therapy in the management of this patient?

(A) Administer 1 mg of epinephrine
(B) Administer insulin and 25% dextrose in water
(C) Administer sodium bicarbonate
(D) Administer potassium chloride
(E) Administer calcium gluconate

52. A 33-year-old, intravenous drug abuser presents to the emergency department febrile (40°C) complaining of left upper quadrant abdominal pain. He is tachycardic with a blood pressure of 110/50 mm Hg. Examination reveals a systolic ejection murmur over the right sternal border, several tiny erythematous lesions on the palm of his right hand, and a tender left upper quadrant. Echocardiogram reveals several vegetations on the tricuspid valve. Abdominal ultrasound reveals a fluid-filled mass within the spleen measuring 4×5 cm^2. A peripheral blood smear is notable for gram-positive cocci. Which of the following is the best treatment option for this patient?

(A) Image-guided drainage of the splenic lesion alone
(B) Intravenous (IV) antibiotics alone
(C) IV antibiotics and cardiac catheterization
(D) IV antibiotics and splenectomy
(E) Splenectomy alone

53. An 80-year-old man presents to the office with a history of "abdominal fullness" sensation that has been worsening over the past several months. A computed tomography (CT) scan reveals a 9-cm lesion suggestive of a retroperitoneal sarcoma. Which of the following is the most important prognostic factor in this patient?

(A) Age of the patient
(B) Number of positive lymph nodes
(C) Histologic grade
(D) Aneuploidy
(E) Location of the lesion

54. A 68-year-old man presents to the office after noting a neck mass. On examination, he has a 1.5-cm mass in the left lobe of the thyroid gland. Which of the following characteristics is most suggestive that this thyroid nodule is benign?

(A) The presence of only 1 nodule
(B) The lesion is cystic
(C) History of radiation exposure
(D) Family history of multiple endocrine neoplasia (MEN) II
(E) Dysphagia or hoarseness

55. A 68-year-old woman presents after referral from a primary care physician who noted occult positive stools on routine physical examination. The patient denies any previous history of bleeding from her rectum but has noticed a significant decrease in the caliber of her stools over the past several months. Which of the following is the most appropriate diagnostic method in the evaluation of this patient?

(A) Computed tomography (CT) scan
(B) Colonoscopy
(C) Flexible sigmoidoscopy
(D) Laparoscopy
(E) Exploratory laparotomy

56. A 25-year-old woman with recurrent episodes of headaches, sweating, and hypertension is noted to have elevated vanillylmandelic acid (VMA) and metanephrines. Computed tomography (CT) scan reveals no abnormalities in either adrenal gland. Which of the following is the most likely location of the pheochromocytoma?

(A) Bladder
(B) Bifurcation of the aorta
(C) Paravertebral ganglia
(D) Carotid body
(E) Thorax

57. A 68-year-old man presents to the office with a 7-cm mass in his posterior right thigh. A recent biopsy revealed a high-grade sarcoma. A complete work-up revealed no evidence of metastatic disease. Which of the following is the most appropriate definitive treatment for this patient?

(A) Surgical resection plus combination chemotherapy
(B) External beam radiation alone
(C) Surgical resection plus immunotherapy
(D) Surgical resection plus radiation therapy
(E) Surgical resection alone

58. A 43-year-old woman undergoes elective left thyroid lobectomy and isthmusectomy for follicular cell carcinoma. Mobilization of the lobe was initially difficult but the patient tolerated the procedure well and was transferred to the postoperative recovery room where she was extubated. Twelve hours later, the patient is noted to be developing worsening shortness of breath and stridor with associated anxiety. Which of the following is the most likely cause of her current condition?

(A) Left recurrent laryngeal nerve injury
(B) Hematoma formation
(C) Bilateral recurrent laryngeal nerve injury
(D) Bilateral superior laryngeal nerve injury
(E) Thyroid storm syndrome

59. A 45-year-old woman consults her gynecologist for menorrhagia and during the review of systems she also reports weakness and fatigue. Work-up includes a serum aldosterone level, which is elevated. Which of the following clinical findings would most likely be found in this patient?

(A) Hyperkalemia
(B) Edema
(C) Hypotension
(D) Expanded blood volume
(E) Oliguria

60. A 35-year-old woman is found to have a 2-cm, solid mass in the right lobe of the liver on computed tomography (CT) scan evaluation during a trauma work-up following a motor vehicle accident. Based on the CT scan findings, the lesion is diagnosed as a benign hepatic adenoma. The patient otherwise was found to have no major injuries and was discharged the following day. In the office, the patient denies any symptoms potentially related to the adenoma. Which of the following is an appropriate statement regarding hepatic adenomas?

(A) Administration of oral contraceptive agents may produce regression of the lesion
(B) These lesions are benign and are not associated with malignant transformation
(C) The risk of rupture of these lesions is an appropriate indication for surgical resection in some cases
(D) Further diagnostic studies should be performed because these lesions rarely occur in women of child-bearing age
(E) The patient should be reassured that there is no indication for surgery on this lesion unless it becomes symptomatic

61. A 35-year-old woman presents to your office with the primary complaint of nodular, painful, lumpy breast tissue. She states that her symptoms include mastodynia and sometimes nipple discharge. She has noted that her pain increases just before her menses and seems to diminish after, but rarely is she asymptomatic. She has a history of irregular menses, but was able to have 3 children. She is of a normal body weight and has never been on birth control pills. On physical examination, you discover that she has very tender breasts with no dominant masses. You obtain a mammogram and discover an area of microcalcifications. A needle localized excisional biopsy reveals microscopic and macroscopic cysts with fibrosis, adenosis with lymphocytic infiltration, and regularity of nuclei with an absence of mitoses. Which of the following is the best treatment for this patient?

(A) Modified radical mastectomy
(B) Reassuring the patient that the process is benign with close follow-up
(C) Axillary node dissection with postoperative radiation therapy
(D) Radiation therapy alone
(E) Reassurance in combination with pain control alone

62. A 34-year-old, diabetic man undergoes combined kidney-pancreas transplantation. The pancreatic exocrine drainage is performed using an enteric anastomosis. Close monitoring of which of the following is most effective in monitoring for pancreatic rejection?

(A) Glucose levels
(B) Urinary amylase levels
(C) Fecal amylase levels
(D) Serum amylase levels
(E) Serum creatinine levels

63. A 25-year-old man presents to the emergency department with acute onset of severe abdominal pain. His vital signs are: heart rate, 135 beats/min; blood pressure, 70/20 mm Hg; respiration, 30/min; temperature, 36.0°C. Examination reveals a rigid abdomen. Which of the following is the most appropriate next step in the management of this patient?

(A) Obtain a detailed history
(B) Insert a urinary catheter
(C) Obtain a computed tomography (CT) of the abdomen and pelvis
(D) Provide fluid resuscitation
(E) Perform a barium enema

64. A 45-year-old man presents for evaluation with complaints of epigastric pain and gastroesophageal reflux. He has been treated with proton pump inhibitor therapy for 3 months without relief of his symptoms. Which of he following statements is true regarding further treatment of this patient?

(A) If 24-hour pH probe reveals gastroesophageal reflux, surgery is indicated without further work-up
(B) An additional 3 months of medical therapy is recommended before surgery
(C) The presence of a 5-cm tongue of Barrett's esophagus with dysplasia is an indication for surgery
(D) Manometry is not indicated, because the patient has no difficulty swallowing
(E) Barrett's changes can be cured by Nissen fundoplication

65. A 38-year-old, asymptomatic, human immunodeficiency virus (HIV)-positive woman presents with complaints of a new breast mass in her right breast noted on routine self-examination. She states that she noticed the mass about 1 month before and that it has gradually increased in size. On physical examination, there is a 2-cm, firm mass in the upper outer quadrant of the right breast without any evidence of palpable axillary nodes. Core needle biopsy reveals ductal adenocarcinoma. Which of the following is appropriate regarding the management of this patient?

(A) Treatment should be palliative, given the likelihood of unrecognized metastatic disease
(B) Administration of prophylactic perioperative antibiotics two days before and after any surgery, given the increased risk of wound infections in HIV-positive patients
(C) A modified radical mastectomy is favored over lumpectomy with lymph node dissection and postoperative radiation therapy because of the risk of wound complications with radiation
(D) Breast reconstruction is contraindicated, given the risk of wound healing problems in the HIV-positive patient
(E) Either a modified radical mastectomy or lumpectomy with lymph node dissection and postoperative radiation therapy would be appropriate in an HIV-positive patient

66. A 62-year-old male smoker with a history of peripheral vascular disease presents to the office for a routine visit. On physical examination the patient is noted to have a 2-cm nonhealing ulcer on his right leg at the site of previous skin grafting for a burn injury 15 years previously. The patient states that the ulcer has not bothered him and that he has been taking good care of it with frequent cleansing and dressing changes at home. He states that the ulcer has remained stable in size since he first noticed it 5 months ago. Distal pulses are noted by Doppler. Which of the following is most appropriate in the initial management of this patient?

(A) Continued wound care with subsequent arteriography
(B) Aggressive wound débridement and continued wound care at home
(C) Biopsy of wound
(D) Regrafting of wound with split-thickness skin graft
(E) Recommended cessation of smoking and observation of wound as outpatient

67. A 65-year-old woman with a history of coronary artery disease is admitted to the hospital with a high-output pancreaticocutaneous fistula 6 weeks after a Whipple procedure performed for treatment of pancreatic cancer. She complains of nausea, vomiting, and weakness. Her physician has great difficulty maintaining adequate serum levels of potassium. Which of the following coexisting electrolyte imbalances may be contributing to this patient's condition?

(A) Hyponatremia
(B) Hypomagnesemia
(C) Hypocalcemia
(D) Hypercalcemia
(E) Hypermagnesemia

68. A 45-year-old woman who is a known alcoholic presents to the emergency department in extremis. Foul-smelling, bloody vomit is grossly visible on her dress. Her skin is cold and ashen gray. Her blood pressure is 80/40 mm Hg and her heart rate is 130 beats/min. Her abdomen is cachectic and her stool is guaiac-positive. Initial nasogastric tube placement evacuates 1200 ml of bright red blood. After initial management steps are taken, including administration of 2 L of normal saline and 2 units of packed red blood cells (PRBCs), the patient's heart rate is 109 beats/min with a blood pressure of 98/65 mm Hg. However, nasogastric aspirate still demonstrates significant bright red blood. Which of the following is the most appropriate next step in the management of this patient?

(A) Immediate laparotomy
(B) Vasopressin infusion
(C) Esophagogastroduodenoscopy (EGD)
(D) Placement of Sengstaken-Blakemore tube
(E) Administration of omeprazole, continued intravenous fluids, and observation

69. A 28-year-old man presents to the emergency room with the complaint of recurrent, colicky, midabdominal pain. Physical examination reveals a palpable abdominal mass and several areas of increased pigmentation on his lips, palms, and soles. He states that his mother had a polyp removed from her colon several years ago. Which of the following is the most likely diagnosis?

(A) Familial polyposis with malignant degeneration
(B) Gardner's syndrome with intussusception
(C) Peutz-Jeghers syndrome with intussusception
(D) Symptomatic Crohn's disease
(E) Human immunodeficiency virus (HIV) enteropathy

70. A 38-year-old, previously healthy, white woman presents 1 week after a laparoscopic cholecystectomy at an outside institution. Approximately 3 days after her surgery she developed recurrent high fever associated with abdominal pain. She is placed on broad spectrum antibiotics with some improvement in her clinical course. Abdominal computed tomography (CT) scan reveals a moderately large fluid collection in the gallbladder fossa. Cholangiography demonstrates a leak in the common bile duct. Which of the following statements is appropriate regarding the management of this patient?

(A) There is no role for administration of antibiotics
(B) Proximal biliary decompression and external drainage can be used to control the leak
(C) Immediate surgical intervention is necessary to prevent further spread of infection
(D) Surgical intervention is required in most cases to allow for resolution of the leak
(E) A Roux-en-Y choledochojejunostomy is contraindicated

71. A 45-year-old woman presents to the office with a nontender right groin mass. The patient states she noticed the mass approximately 1 week ago after working in the garden all day. On examination, the mass is approximately 5 cm and is soft. Which of the following is the most likely cause of this mass?

(A) Femoral hernia
(B) Direct inguinal hernia
(C) Indirect inguinal hernia
(D) Obturator hernia
(E) Femoral artery aneurysm

72. After an uneventful laparoscopic cholecystectomy, a 58-year-old woman had the urinary catheter removed and began to ambulate. During routine vital sign checks, she was noted to have had no urine output over the previous 8 hours. An intravenous bolus of normal saline (500 mL) was ordered but did not stimulate voiding. She underwent straight catheterization of her bladder, which revealed 1000 mL of urine. Urine analysis showed a specific gravity of 1.022, a pH of 5, moderate blood, and positive leukocyte esterase and nitrites. There were 23 red blood cells/high power field (hpf) and 212 white blood cells/hpf. What is the most likely explanation for her failure to void?

(A) Bilateral ureteral obstruction
(B) Acute renal failure (ARF)
(C) Urinary tract infection
(D) Hemorrhagic cystitis
(E) Normal urinary retention

73. A 52-year-old man with a history of stage I colon cancer treated with surgical resection 1 year ago develops chronic renal failure due to diabetes. Which of the following is the best recommendation for this patient?

(A) Treatment with hemodialysis without future transplantation
(B) Treatment with continuous ambulatory peritoneal dialysis without future transplantation
(C) Kidney transplantation within the next year
(D) Hemodialysis for 1 year followed by kidney transplantation
(E) Hemodialysis for 3 months followed by kidney transplantation

74. A 50-year-old woman is receiving a lumbar epidural to provide anesthesia for a transabdominal hysterectomy. During administration of local anesthetic (lidocaine) through the epidural catheter, the woman complains of shortness of breath then rapidly becomes unresponsive and apneic. The local anesthetic had been injected in small divided doses and at no point did the catheter aspirate cerebrospinal fluid or blood. She is promptly intubated and given 100% oxygen with positive pressure ventilation. Which of the following is the most likely cause of this patient's symptoms?

(A) Unintentional subdural or subarachnoid injection
(B) Allergic reaction to lidocaine
(C) Narcotic overdose
(D) Pulmonary embolization
(E) Myocardial infarction

75. A 55-year-old, alcoholic man has been receiving parenteral nutrition for the past 4 weeks following a protracted course of critical illness associated with an episode of necrotizing pancreatitis. Over the past 2–3 days he has tolerated oral intake of water and other liquids and some pureed foods. The next morning his parenteral nutrition is stopped and he continues to tolerate oral water. Later that morning, the patient becomes lethargic and confused, and eventually becomes unresponsive. Which of the following is the most appropriate initial management strategy for this patient?

(A) Fluid resuscitation and immediate pulmonary arteriogram
(B) Fluid resuscitation and immediate head computed tomography (CT)
(C) Administration of naloxone and fluid resuscitation
(D) Fluid resuscitation and chest tube placement
(E) Fluid resuscitation and serum glucose analysis

76. A 67-year-old man presents to the office for a routine check-up. His wife states that he has a dark skin lesion on his back that she would like examined. Which of the following factors would most likely suggest that this is a benign lesion?

(A) 6-mm, smooth lesion, with areas of black and purple pigmentation
(B) 6-mm, blue lesion, with irregular borders
(C) 6-mm, blue lesion, increased in size from 3-mm 1 month ago
(D) 6-mm, smooth, dark purple lesion
(E) 8-mm, smooth, blue lesion, with a central ulceration

Directions: Each set of matching questions in this section consists of a list of four to twenty-six lettered options followed by several numbered items. For each numbered item, select the appropriate lettered option(s). Each lettered option may be selected once, more than once, or not at all.

Questions 77–79

(A) Amylase
(B) Alkaline phosphatase
(C) Lactic acid
(D) Hematocrit
(E) Leukocyte esterase
(F) Lactate dehydrogenase
(G) Thyroid hormone
(H) Serum myoglobin

For each clinical scenario, select the laboratory value or values that are likely to be abnormal.

77. A 60-year-old woman with a history of gallstones presents to the emergency room with severe epigastric pain radiating to the back, nausea, vomiting, and anorexia. Her vital signs are: heart rate, 80 beats/min; blood pressure, 120/70 mm Hg. The patient has had good urine output. Ultrasound of the right upper quadrant shows small gallstones throughout the biliary tree. (SELECT 2 LAB VALUES)

78. A 30-year-old, pregnant woman with a gestational age of 30 weeks presents to the emergency room with suprapubic discomfort and dysuria. Her vital signs are: heart rate, 90 beats/min; blood pressure, 125/70 mm Hg; respiration, 24/min; temperature, 38.3°C. Abdominal films are unremarkable. (SELECT 1 LAB VALUE)

79. A 70-year-old woman presents to the emergency room with pain localized to the upper abdomen. Abdominal ultrasound reveals pericholecystic fluid. The patient takes no medications and has no significant past medical history. Her vital signs are: blood pressure, 130/80 mm Hg; heart rate, 88 beats/min; respiration, 18/min; temperature, 38.3°C. (SELECT 1 LAB VALUE)

Questions 80–81

(A) Radical pancreaticoduodenectomy
(B) Radical cholecystectomy
(C) Roux-en-Y hepaticojejunostomy
(D) Roux-en-Y choledochojejunostomy
(E) Cholecystojejunostomy
(F) Percutaneous cholecystostomy
(G) End-to-end primary anastomosis with T-tube placement

For each clinical scenario, select the most appropriate procedure.

80. A 47-year-old, white man with a previous laparoscopic cholecystectomy performed 1 year ago presents with a 6-month history of fluctuating jaundice, pruritus, and abdominal pain. Computed tomography (CT) scan has been performed and reveals no mass lesions but distension of the intrahepatic ducts. A cholangiogram reveals a 3-cm segmental narrowing of the common bile duct near the cystic duct remnant. (SELECT 2 PROCEDURE)

81. A 68-year-old, African-American man with a history of hypertension, coronary artery bypass surgery, and bilateral inguinal hernia repairs presents with a 2-week history of jaundice and pruritus. Laboratory examination is significant for elevated total and conjugated bilirubin. Computed tomography (CT) scan of the abdomen reveals distended intrahepatic and extrahepatic biliary ducts to the level of the common bile duct. No mass lesions or lymphadenopathy are identified. A cholangiogram reveals a stricture of the common bile duct approximately 2 cm from the ampulla of Vater. Cytology on brushings is suggestive of adenocarcinoma. (SELECT 1 PROCEDURE)

Questions 82–86

(A) Gastrinoma
(B) Pituitary adenoma
(C) Vasoactive intestinal peptide tumors (VIPoma)
(D) Insulinoma
(E) Incidentaloma
(F) Glucagonoma
(G) Somatostatinoma

Match each of the following case scenarios with the associated endocrine neoplasm.

82. A 35-year-old man presents with a history of recurrent bleeding gastric ulcers refractory to 1 year of intensive medical therapy. (SELECT 1 NEOPLASM)

83. A thin, 37-year-old, otherwise healthy man was recently diagnosed with diabetes mellitus. In addition, he is noted to have a 3-cm mass in the head of the pancreas. (SELECT 2 NEOPLASMS)

84. A 33-year-old woman presents with recurrent episodes of diaphoresis and palpitations. Her symptoms are often exacerbated by minimal fasting. (SELECT 1 NEOPLASM)

85. A thin, 38-year-old man presents to the office with complaints of a recurring erythematous rash over his chest, abdomen, and thighs. He states that the rash presents as patches that come and go and appear in different areas each time. (SELECT 1 NEOPLASM)

86. A 43-year-old woman presents to the office with complaints of persistent watery diarrhea over the past several months. An abdominal computed tomography (CT) scan reveals a 2-cm mass in the head of the pancreas. (SELECT 2 NEOPLASMS)

Questions 87–89

(A) History of pelvic inflammatory disease
(B) Gallstones
(C) Bedridden state
(D) Chronic steroid use
(E) Atherosclerosis
(F) Atrial fibrillation
(G) History of myocardial infarction
(H) Chronic laxative use
(I) Rheumatic fever

For each clinical scenario, select the most appropriate risk factor(s) for that disease.

87. A 22-year-old woman presents with abdominal pain, vaginal bleeding, and an ultrasound showing a gestational sac in the ampullary part of the fallopian tube. (SELECT 1 RISK FACTOR)

88. A 64-year-old man with progressively increasing abdominal and back pain presents with an 8-cm pulsatile abdominal mass. (SELECT 1 RISK FACTOR)

89. A 70-year-old man with dementia is admitted from a local nursing home with severe left lower quadrant pain, abdominal distention, and constipation. An extremely dilated sigmoid colon is present on abdominal film and appears to taper both proximally and distally. (SELECT 2 RISK FACTORS)

Questions 90–94

(A) Tension pneumothorax
(B) Cardiac tamponade
(C) Massive liver injury
(D) Aortic disruption
(E) Tension hemothorax
(F) Flail chest
(G) Femur fracture
(H) Pelvic fracture
(I) Spinal cord injury
(J) Closed head injury

Match the following cause(s) of hypotension with the clinical scenario listed below.

90. A 19-year-old man is shot from behind, with a gunshot entrance wound below and just medial to the right scapula. The exit wound is visualized 3–4 finger breadths superior to the inferior costal margin along the anterior axillary line. The patient is hypotensive with decreased breath sounds on the right. (SELECT 4 CAUSES OF HYPOTENSION)

91. A 23-year-old man presents to the emergency room with hypotension. He was involved in a head-on, high-speed motor vehicle accident. He was not wearing his seatbelt and the emergency medical technician noted deformation of the steering wheel. The patient has normal breath and heart sounds although he is tachycardic. His chest film reveals normal lung fields bilaterally, however his mediastinum appears to be slightly widened with no visualization of the aortic knob. The patient's abdominal and pelvic computed tomography (CT) scan are normal. (SELECT 1 CAUSE OF HYPOTENSION)

92. The driver in a high-speed motor vehicle accident presents to the emergency room with hypotension and tachycardia. Examination reveals normal breath sounds bilaterally. Heart sounds are muffled with enlarged jugular veins. Chest and pelvis films appear normal. Abdominal examination is unremarkable, with a negative diagnostic peritoneal lavage. (SELECT 1 CAUSE OF HYPOTENSION)

93. A 35-year-old woman presents to the emergency room after being struck in the lower back and buttocks region with a steel beam. She is conscious but confused, hypotensive, and has a heart rate of 90 beats/min. Examination reveals normal reactive pupils, normal chest and abdominal examinations, and no movement of her lower extremities. Her legs and thighs appear normal with no evidence of trauma. Her chest film is normal. Pelvic radiograph reveals a fracture of the superior ramus on the right and a right acetabular fracture. Rectal examination reveals loss of normal tone of the sphincter muscle. (SELECT 2 CAUSES OF HYPOTENSION)

94. A 23-year-old man presents to the emergency room after being hit in his left chest with a baseball bat. He is hypotensive, tachypneic, and has no breath sounds noted on the left side. Heart sounds are normal and his upper airway is open, although the trachea is deviated to the right. (SELECT 2 CAUSES OF HYPOTENSION)

Questions 95–96

(A) Dilutional coagulopathy
(B) Disseminated intravascular coagulation
(C) Heparin-induced coagulopathy
(D) von Willebrand's disease
(E) Hemophilia A
(F) Hypothermia-induced coagulopathy
(G) Primary fibrinolysis
(H) Vitamin K deficiency

For the each of the following clinical scenarios, select the most likely diagnosis(es).

95. A 44-year-old man sustained a gunshot wound to his left chest and left upper quadrant that required emergent exploratory laparotomy, splenectomy, and left hemicolectomy. On postoperative day 3, he was noted to have necrotizing fasciitis at the blast wound. He subsequently developed acute oliguric renal failure that required intermittent hemodialysis. On postoperative day 20, after a hemodynamically stable hemodialysis session, the patient was noted to be bleeding from his central line and hemodialysis catheter sites. Coagulation profile had the following results: prothrombin time (PT) = 14.0 seconds, partial thromboplastin time (PTT) > 200 seconds, platelets = 230,000. (SELECT 1 DIAGNOSIS)

96. A 32-year-old woman was involved in a high-speed motor vehicle accident where she sustained blunt abdominal injury. She was hypotensive at the scene and throughout most of the operation to resect her damaged intestine. Upon presentation to the intensive care unit, however, she remained hypotensive despite administration of 12 L of crystalloid, 12 units of packed red blood cells (PRBCs), and 5 units of fresh frozen plasma. Current vital signs include a blood pressure of 70/40 mm Hg, heart rate of 140 beat/min, and temperature of 34.5°C. Laboratory studies showed prothrombin time (PT) = 16.2, partial thromboplastin time (PTT) = 48.3, and platelets = 18,000. In addition, she was noted to be bleeding from her wound, mucous membranes, and at all catheter sites. (SELECT 3 DIAGNOSES)

Questions 97–100

(A) Packed red blood cells (PRBCs)
(B) Fresh frozen plasma
(C) Cryoprecipitate
(D) Recombinant factor VIII
(E) Single donor platelets
(F) Desmopressin
(G) 5% Albumin
(H) 25% Albumin
(I) Heparin sodium
(J) Warfarin

For each patient description, select the most appropriate treatment.

97. A 38-year-old female diabetic with acute renal failure requires urgent removal of her gallbladder but has an elevated bleeding time after receiving hemodialysis. Prothrombin time (PT) and partial thromboplastin time (PTT) are normal. (SELECT 2 MODES OF TREATMENT)

98. A 29-year-old man presents with a tibial fracture that will require intraoperative fixation. The patient gives a history of "excessive bleeding" with a tonsillectomy as a child. His PT and PTT are normal, although his bleeding time is elevated. Intraoperatively, there is a significant amount of blood loss from oozing, without any obvious sources of arterial or venous bleeding. (SELECT 2 MODES OF TREATMENT)

99. A 78-year-old woman requires urgent replacement of an implanted defibrillator. She has been taking warfarin for an artificial heart valve. Before surgery, the surgeon wishes to reverse the effects of warfarin. (SELECT 1 MODE OF TREATMENT)

100. A 45-year-old woman with protein C deficiency presents with worsening aortic stenosis secondary to a bicuspid aortic valve. The patient undergoes replacement of this valve with an artificial mechanical valve. Postoperatively, the surgeon wishes to provide anticoagulation therapy to prevent thrombus formation on the valve. (SELECT 2 MODES OF TREATMENT)

Answers and Explanations

1–A. This patient is experiencing a classic manifestation of refeeding syndrome. Refeeding syndrome is seen in severely malnourished patients when aggressive calorie support is initiated, particularly when a large percentage of those calories are provided as carbohydrates. The infusion of carbohydrates results in rapid and extensive peripheral uptake and utilization of glucose. The intracellular utilization of glucose requires the use of a significant amount of intracellular PO_4^-, therefore potentially resulting in severe hypophosphatemia. Characteristics include malaise, lethargy, perioral paresthesias, tremors, dysarthrias, coma, and even death. Treatment involves slowing administration of nutritional support and administration of PO_4^- salts. Thiamine would most likely be provided in the vitamin supplementation and would generally not be associated with such a temporal relationship to parenteral nutrition administration. Insulin may help to decrease overall serum glucose levels, however, it would not specifically address the most serious acute issue of severe hypophosphatemia. $MgCl_2$ administration also does not address the primary issue of hypophosphatemia.

2–B. In an adult, satisfactory urine output is 0.5–1.0 mL/kg/hour, and in a patient with a large burn it needs to be measured continuously with a Foley catheter. An appropriate goal for adequate urine output in this patient is 40–80 mL/hr based on his weight of 80 kg. In a patient with severe burns a minimum of two large-bore intravenous (IV) lines are necessary. Burn patients are extremely hypermetabolic, and have numerous reasons to be tachycardic other than hypovolemia. Edema secondary to leaky vascular membranes is common in patients with severe burn injuries and is not a marker of overhydration.

3–E. Ketamine is unique among anesthetic agents in that it provides anesthesia, analgesia, and possibly amnesia. It is also a potent bronchodilator and tends to maintain cardiac output and blood pressure. Unfortunately, emergence reactions are common. Midazolam, a benzodiazepine with reliable anxiolytic and amnestic properties, can greatly attenuate these reactions. Propofol, fentanyl, lidocaine, and etomidate are other anesthetic agents frequently used for cardioversions, however, these agents do not provide the effective amnestic effect provided by midazolam.

4–B. This patient most likely has appendicitis based on his age and presenting symptoms. The psoas sign is pain in the lower abdomen and psoas region that is elicited when the thigh is flexed against resistance. It suggests an intra-abdominal inflammatory process most frequently associated with appendicitis. Crepitus suggests a rapidly spreading gas forming infection and is a rare finding. Murphy's sign suggests acute cholecystitis, while flank and periumbilical ecchymosis suggest retroperitoneal hemorrhage, often caused by hemorrhagic pancreatitis.

5–B. This patient has developed necrotizing fasciitis of the perineal and scrotal region (Fournier's gangrene) probably originating from an intra-abdominal source (e.g., diverticulitis). Management requires early and aggressive surgical débridement of the affected region. Generally, given the differential blood supply between the scrotum and the testicles, as well as the thick dartos fascia surrounding the testicles, superficial infections of the scrotum extending from the perineum do not affect the testicles, thus orchiectomy is generally not necessary. In some circumstances, persistent infections in the perineal region require fecal diversion with a colostomy to avoid persistent fecal contamination and inhibition of healing. Although resection of the affected colon would be considered appropriate, a primary reanastomosis would not provide for fecal diversion. Sitz baths and antibiotics would be inadequate therapy without surgical débridement.

6–C. Although rare, one of the potentially serious complications associated with laparoscopic intraperitoneal hernia repair is the risk of iatrogenic bowel injury. It is unlikely that a strangulated hernia went undiagnosed prior to or during an elective inguinal hernia repair. It is also unlikely that the hernia would recur by postoperative day 1. In addition, wound infections and adhesion formation do not develop this quickly in the postoperative period and would not necessarily be associated with rebound and guarding.

7–C. Acute renal failure (ARF) is defined as an abrupt change in renal function such that plasma creatinine and urea levels are elevated. Oliguria (< 0.5 mL/kg urine output per hour) or anuria are usually present. Prerenal failure suggests inadequate blood flow to the kidney. Causes of intrinsic renal failure include acute tubular necrosis, nephrotoxicity secondary to drugs, hemoglobinuria, and myoglobinuria. Postrenal failure causes usually present with acute anuria caused by any obstruction to urinary flow from the collecting ducts to the urethra. The fractional excretion of sodium (FE_{Na}) and urine specific gravity can help to delineate prerenal causes from other causes of acute renal failure. Urinalysis including cytology may assist in identifying an intrinsic renal injury. Hemodialysis may be necessary as a bridge due to severe hyperkalemia, metabolic acidosis, uremic complications, and volume overload until renal function returns to normal. Most cases of acute renal failure in this setting will resolve.

8–E. A focal bile duct stenosis in the absence of a history of abdominal surgery is highly suggestive of a biliary neoplasm. Furthermore, this patient presented with a history of painless jaundice, which is also suggestive of malignancy. Primary sclerosing cholangitis may also present with a focal stenosis but usually at an earlier age and with a fluctuating clinical course. Cholangitis and Mirizzi's syndrome would be highly unlikely in a patient with a normal white count and no pain.

9–A. Corticosteroids decrease hypertrophic scarring by enhancing collagenase activity. This is related to an increase in collagen degradation within the hypertrophic scar. Injecting corticosteroids directly into a scar prevents acute inflammation in the healing wound. Injecting keloids and hypertrophic scars with corticosteroids has no effect on the number of fibroblasts present. Collagen turnover is not increased in treated scars. Pressure treatment is not necessary after corticosteroid injection. Corticosteroids do not affect intracellular collagen synthesis or extracellular collagen cross-linking. The cross-linking process contributes to the tensile strength in a healing wound. Increased collagen solubility is not caused specifically by cross-linking.

10–C. Fever, chills, back pain, hemoglobinuria, and rapid deterioration of the cardiovascular and respiratory systems are classic signs of a severe immune reaction to transfused blood caused by ABO incompatibility, as seen in this patient. The cause of this reaction is preformed antibodies in the recipient's serum reacting to nonself antigens on the donor's red blood cells (RBCs) [i.e., patients with Type A blood have antibodies to Type B RBCs]. Bacterial contamination of donor blood is rare and generally would not present within the first few minutes of administration. Donor leukocytes can react with recipient cells, but this is not generally associated with a severe transfusion reaction. It may, however, cause fever and chills in a small number of patients. Volume overload secondary to too-rapid administration of blood can be associated with dyspnea and respiratory insufficiency, but is not associated with the other findings. Hypocalcemia rarely occurs, even with massive transfusions, and would not be associated with the findings in this patient.

11–A. Glucocorticoids are used in most multidrug immunosuppression protocols. In addition, they are commonly used as the first line therapy for rejection by administration of boluses over one to several days. If steroids fail, monoclonal or polyclonal antibodies are added to the regimen. Cyclosporine and azathioprine are essential in maintenance therapy but play no role in the treatment of acute rejection. Mycophenolate mofetil decreases the rate of rejection particularly for kidney transplants, but again plays little or no role in the treatment of acute rejection once it has developed. Cyclophosphamide is rarely used in transplant recipients either for maintenance or for treatment of rejection.

12–D. Although hemorrhage in such a patient could originate from many different sources, upper gastrointestinal bleeding is a frequent cause of hemorrhage in critically ill surgical patients generally resulting from acute stress gastritis. The patient's risk factors include hospitalization with a long stay in the intensive care unit and sepsis. Although airway management and volume resuscitation are initial management steps, early placement of a nasogastric tube may confirm that the bleeding is from an upper gastrointestinal source. In addition, checking the stools for blood (i.e., guaiac test) may also provide support for a gastrointestinal source of bleeding in patients with a falling hematocrit. In the absence of other signs of an intra-abdominal process (e.g., acute abdomen), emergent laparotomy or mesenteric angiography are not indicated at this point in the management of this patient.

13–E. Although conservative medical management of esophageal perforation is appropriate for a small, select group of patients, it is generally reserved for those who have no evidence of sepsis or communication of the rupture with the pleural or peritoneal cavities. In theory, these patients have already "defended themselves" against the rupture and should do well with conservative management with antibiotics and drainage. Boerhaave's syndrome ruptures tend to be the most morbid because of the high incidence of pleural or peritoneal contamination and delayed diagnosis. Survival in these patients is 75%–85% and those presenting earlier tend to fare better than those presenting after 72 hours. Patients who present less than 24 hours after the injury are generally candidates for reinforced primary closure of the perforation. Esophageal rupture secondary to Boerhaave's syndrome usually results in a tear on the left lateral wall, just above the diaphragm. Thus, a left pleural effusion is a common finding on chest radiograph.

14–C. Both the benzodiazepines and most barbiturates are excellent anti-epileptics. Propofol and etomidate also likely possess antiseizure properties but it is thought that etomidate in low doses may provoke seizures. Either midazolam or a low dose of thiopental would rapidly terminate this seizure caused by this unintentional intravascular injection of bupivacaine. Succinylcholine would mask the convulsions, and narcotics (such as fentanyl) also do not suppress seizures. Lidocaine is not as toxic as bupivacaine, but can cause seizures if too much is given intravenously.

15–B. Branched-chain amino acids are essential amino acids and include leucine, isoleucine, and valine. These amino acids are preferentially metabolized by the muscle and therefore in the setting of significant liver disease administering these substrates may decrease the overload of total protein and provide for mechanisms of more efficient glucose production. Administration of nutritional supplements with a high percentage of branched-chain amino acids versus other amino acids may decrease the degree of encephalopathy seen in patients with severe liver failure. These amino acids are not preferentially metabolized by the liver and do not act as hepatotoxins.

16–E. Gallstone ileus is the obstruction of the small intestine (usually at the ileocecal valve) caused by a gallstone that has entered the duodenum through a fistula formed between an inflamed gallbladder and the duodenum. The usual signs of intestinal obstruction are found, plus air in the biliary tree. There is usually a history of attacks of cholecystitis or cholelithiasis. While air in the biliary tree may represent cholangitis, this finding in association with a small bowel obstruction (SBO) without other identifiable causes should raise suspicion for gallstone ileus. Superior mesenteric artery syndrome is a rare cause of duodenal obstruction caused by external compression of the third portion of the duodenum by the overlying vessel. It is characteristically seen in patients with rapid weight loss or those in SPICA casts. The obstruction is proximal and is not associated with distension of small bowel as described above. Right-sided colon cancer can mimic distal SBOs but is not associated with air in the biliary tree. Because the patient has not had prior abdominal surgery, adhesive obstructions would be improbable. Uncomplicated sigmoid diverticulitis is generally not associated with air in the biliary tree.

17–C. Even though less than 1% of all breast cancer occurs in men, it is most likely that this patient is suffering from breast cancer. There are approximately 900 new cases of male breast cancer per year and most cases present with an isolated mass or enlargement of a single breast. The mean age of presentation is 60–65 years with a prominent risk factor being a protracted hyperestrogenemic state. These tumors are ductal in origin, and 80% are estrogen receptor-positive. These tumors tend to become systemic early, with axially node metastasis, or involvement with the chest wall or skin. Therefore, they usually present at a late stage, and a lumpectomy and axillary node dissection is inadequate to remove the majority of the tumor burden. Treatment is a radical mastectomy after the diagnosis is confirmed with fine needle aspiration (FNA) or biopsy. Chemotherapy is needed for adjuvant therapy, but is inadequate single therapy.

18–B. The presence of free peritoneal air in the setting of acute diverticulitis is an indication for emergent laparotomy and resection of the affected colon with formation of an end colostomy and performance of a Hartmann's procedure (oversewing of the unaffected rectosigmoid distal to the resection site creating a pouch drained through the anus). Reanastomosis of the colon to the proximal end of this pouch can be performed at a later date. Percutaneous drainage of such an abscess may be appropriate in some cases of diverticulitis, but not in the presence of free peritoneal air. The affected colon needs to be resected emergently in this setting, given the likelihood of a free colonic perforation. Resection of the diseased colon is sufficient in this setting without the need for a total colectomy.

19–A. Metastatic neoplasms most often originating from the colon, breast, or lung are the most common etiology of malignant liver tumors, while hepatocellular carcinoma is the most common primary malignant lesion of the liver. Worldwide, the most common cause of hepatocellular carcinoma is cirrhosis secondary to hepatitis B infection. α-Fetoprotein is a tumor marker for hepatocellular carcinoma, although it is nonspecific, with elevations also noted in patients with liver metastases, teratocarcinomas, yolk sac tumors, and even cirrhosis. Hepatoblastomas are characteristically very sensitive to chemotherapy.

20–A. Hypersplenism will occasionally occur in patients with acquired immunodeficiency syndrome (AIDS). Criteria for splenectomy are the same for patients with human immunodeficiency virus (HIV) as for those without it. Symptomatic splenomegaly (i.e., hypersplenism) caused by a condition which is otherwise not reversible is an indication for splenectomy. Emergent splenectomy, however, is not indicated. Ideally, this patient would be given the appropriate vaccinations against encapsulated organisms 10 days before the splenectomy. Plasmapheresis would be of no benefit in this patient. Intravenous (IV) gamma globulin is a medical therapy given to patients with idiopathic thrombocytopenic purpura (ITP). Splenic artery embolization is not indicated for the treatment of hypersplenism.

21–B. Thyroid storm generally presents in patients with undiagnosed or inadequately treated hyperthyroidism and can be precipitated by manipulation or palpation of the gland. Preventative measures include preoperative administration of β-blockers and propylthiouracil (PTU) until the patient becomes euthyroid. Treatment of an acute presentation of thyroid storm (fever, tachycardia) involves mechanical cooling, administration of oxygen, β-blockers, PTU, and iodide salt solutions (e.g., Lugol's solution or potassium iodide). Administration of a large amount of iodide with uptake into the thyroid effectively inhibits production of triiodothyronine (T_3) and thyroxine (T_4), resulting in a rapid decrease in serum thyroid hormone levels (Wolff-Chaikoff block).

Thyroid storm is not related to calcium metabolism, and T_4 administration is contraindicated in this setting. Dantrolene is used for malignant hyperthermia, which would be unlikely to develop before induction of anesthesia. Administration of blood products is not indicated in this setting.

22–D. An anastomotic leak is a devastating complication. Principles of performing proper anastomoses include ensuring good blood supply to both ends of bowel (colonic anastomoses are at higher risk because of their more tenuous blood supply), creating a tension-free, serosa-to-serosa, watertight apposition with inverted mucosal surfaces, avoiding gross contamination, and avoiding distal obstruction. Some large bowel anastomotic leaks may be well localized with percutaneous drainage of fluid collections or small abscesses serving as appropriate therapy without the need for immediate reoperation. Severe leaks may result in terrible complications, including abscess formation, enterocutaneous fistulas, or diffuse peritonitis, which will require resuscitation and nasogastric aspiration, followed by laparotomy and exteriorization of free bowel ends.

23–A. This patient has choledocholithiasis. She has secondary common duct stones, most likely representing black pigment stones caused by hemolysis from her sickle cell disease. Brown pigment stones are formed from a combination of bile stasis and bacterial deconjugation of bilirubin. Choledocholithiasis commonly presents with a fluctuating history of pain and jaundice. An endoscopic retrograde cholangiopancreatography (ERCP) may be used not only to diagnose a common duct obstruction but also to treat the condition by removing the stone. Because of the multiple stones present in the gallbladder, some surgeons may take such a patient to the operating room for cholecystectomy and intraoperative choledocoscopy with stone extraction.

24–D. All of these complications can occur during placement of a Swan-Ganz (pulmonary artery) catheter. Inappropriate needle placement can result in a pneumothorax or hemothorax. Cardiac perforation and perforation of the pulmonary artery can occur while advancing the catheter through these structures. Although rare, dislodgment of a large venous thrombus during placement can occur, resulting in a pulmonary embolus. However, sudden hypotension and hemoptysis occurring during placement of this catheter suggests rupture or perforation of the pulmonary artery. Immediate recognition of this injury is essential for appropriate treatment because mortality with this injury is high.

25–E. The patient described displays the characteristics of the multiple endocrine neoplasia (MEN) IIA syndrome, which can include medullary thyroid cancer, hyperparathyroidism, and pheochromocytomas. Any patient who presents with medullary thyroid cancer and a history suspicious for the MEN syndrome should be evaluated for a possible pheochromocytoma and parathyroid abnormalities, including urine tests for catecholamines, metanephrines, vanillylmandelic acid, parathyroid hormone, and calcium. Treatment of medullary thyroid cancer involves total thyroidectomy rather than lobectomy because this type of thyroid cancer tends to be multicentric. Patients with the MEN syndrome who present with a pheochromocytoma have a 50% chance of having bilateral adrenal involvement and should thus be approached transabdominally to evaluate both adrenal glands. A laparoscopic approach is not contraindicated in these patients. Parathyroid disease in these patients is almost always diffuse hyperplasia rather than a solitary adenoma.

26–A. For melanomas less than or equal to 1 mm thick, appropriate treatment of the primary lesion involves wide local excision with 1-cm margins. Establishing general guidelines for adequate margins based upon the thickness of the lesion prevents excessive resections that are difficult to close and attempts to prevent local recurrences because of inadequate margins. Mohs' microsurgical technique is contraindicated in the treatment of melanomas because this may not involve en bloc resection of the entire lesion. Cryosurgical ablation is also contraindicated for melanomas because this does not allow for assessment of the depth of invasion of the lesion versus resection.

27–D. The treatment of Hürthle cell tumors of the thyroid is somewhat controversial. In general, like for follicular cell carcinomas, a total thyroidectomy is considered the most appropriate procedure when surgery is performed. Unlike other follicular carcinomas and papillary tumors, the Hürthle cell variant is characteristically resistant to uptake of radioiodine (^{131}I) and thus resistant to ^{131}I ablation therapy. In addition, many advocate formal lymph node dissection when positive nodes are identified. Lobectomy and isthmusectomy is generally considered inadequate resection, particularly for aggressive Hürthle cell tumors.

28–E. Asymptomatic simple liver cysts generally do not require treatment. There is no associated risk of malignant transformation and the small risk of rupture does not necessitate treatment of such cysts. The walls of simple liver cysts often contain islands of biliary ductal epithelium known as von Meyenburg complexes. Indications for resection or unroofing of the cyst with subsequent oversewing of the cyst wall include symptoms (i.e., pain), rupture, hemorrhage, indeterminate diagnosis, and infection. Initial percutaneous drainage of infected cysts is also an appropriate alternative.

29–C. In patients with the multiple endocrine neoplasia (MEN) II syndrome who present with both medullary thyroid cancer and a pheochromocytoma, the pheochromocytoma should be addressed first. Preoperative treatment with α- and β-adrenergic blockade should be followed by surgical resection. The medullary thyroid cancer should be addressed at a later date with total thyroidectomy. In addition, subtotal parathyroidectomy may be performed if hypercalcemia secondary to parathyroid hyperplasia is identified preoperatively.

30–B. Inadvertent placement of a feeding tube within the airway (e.g., trachea, bronchus) is estimated to occur ≈5% of the time when attempting to place nasoenteric tubes in critically ill patients. Although very rare, significant bronchial injury, including perforation with subsequent development of a tension pneumothorax, can occur and must be recognized and treated immediately by removing the feeding tube and placing a chest tube, based on your clinical assessment of the patient. Fluid resuscitation is important but will not address the primary catastrophic event. In this setting, prompt removal of the feeding tube is essential and injection of contrast is foolish. In addition, the initial steps in the management of this patient do not require performing emergent laparotomy or a pulmonary angiogram given the likelihood of the diagnosis based upon the temporal relationship with feeding tube placement.

31–B. Pernicious anemia can result from several pathophysiologic mechanisms. Loss of cells that make intrinsic factor from autoimmune disease results in the inability to absorb the vitamin B_{12}. Loss of the terminal ileum results in malabsorption of vitamin B_{12}, which results in pernicious anemia. Bacterial overgrowth in segments of bowel (e.g., blind loops) may also lead to consumption of the vitamin by the bacteria, with subsequent deficiency. B_{12} deficiency results in defects in blood cell maturation, as well as peripheral nerve metabolism. Dumping syndrome characteristically occurs after gastric surgery, resulting from disruption of pyloric function or bypass of the pylorus. Ileal resections are not a cause of hypercalcemia. The majority of dietary iron is absorbed within the duodenum; thus, iron deficiency anemia is not a characteristic directly related to ileal resection.

32–C. Infectious mastitis is a relatively uncommon disease, representing a bacterial infection of an obstructed milk duct. *Staphylococcus aureus* is by far the most common pathogen. It primarily affects women who are breast-feeding. Most cases begin as skin cellulitis, and if caught early, may be treated with antibiotics alone. If caught late in the course, after abscess formation, surgical incision and drainage are required. There is no need to stop breast-feeding with infant-safe agents during antibiotic therapy for infectious mastitis, and some believe that the continued stimulation and drainage may aid in treatment. It is important to keep in mind that whenever a primary infection of the breast is suspected clinically, inflammatory breast cancer must be considered in the differential diagnosis and ruled out. Treating this patient with reassurance, nonsteroidal anti-inflammatory drugs (NSAIDs), or danazol would be ineffective in relieving the breast infection.

33–A. Because the site of bleeding had been isolated in this patient, a segmental resection is possible and will cause less morbidity than a subtotal colectomy. However, if the site of bleeding had not been identified, a subtotal colectomy would be indicated because it is the only way to ensure a curative resection and prevent future bleeding. Angiography with embolization or vasopressin infusion is associated with a high rate of rebleeding and a low but significant risk of bowel perforation. These techniques can, however, be useful alternatives in high-risk patients.

34–B. Infected wounds of the hand are treated by aggressive surgical débridement, open drainage, and wound exploration. During these procedures, foreign bodies are removed and devitalized tissue is débrided. The most common pathogen in human bite wounds is *Staphylococcus aureus. Eikenella corrodens* is also frequently cultured. Penicillin is generally included in the antibiotic regimen in these wounds, although broad spectrum antibiotics are frequently used initially until culture and sensitivity data are available. Primary closure is never appropriate for treating a human bite wound because of the high risk of wound contamination and subsequent infection. Tendon lacerations are repaired secondarily after a minimum of 5–7 days.

35–A. Percutaneous or transrectal drainage of pelvic abscesses is an appropriate alternative to laparotomy for treating localized abscesses, although inability to provide adequate drainage or signs and symptoms of peritoneal involvement may require operative intervention. Without adequate drainage of such an abscess, antibiotics alone would be insufficient therapy. Although antibiotic coverage should be adjusted based on the culture results, initial empiric therapy should be directed against both aerobes and anaerobes. Empiric therapy with antifungal agents has not been demonstrated to provide additional benefit to such patients.

36–D. For elective surgery of intractable ulcer disease (persistence or recurrence of symptoms despite adequate medical therapy) parietal cell vagotomy is frequently preferred among the options listed because of the relatively low morbidity associated with this procedure. Procedures involving a truncal vagotomy are associated with an increased risk of gastric emptying problems versus parietal cell vagotomy. Antrectomy and total gastric resection require disruption of intestinal continuity with formation of new anastomoses, thus resulting in a higher complication rate as well. Unfortunately, parietal cell vagotomy is reported as having the highest ulcer recurrence rate among these options, although in experienced hands this may not be the case.

37–C. A woman of childbearing age with hypotension, abdominal distension, and acute abdominal pain should be suspected of having a ruptured ectopic pregnancy. Complications of Crohn's disease, such as perforation, would generally not present in such an acute manner without a history of previous symptoms. A perforated duodenal ulcer generally would not present with progressive lower abdominal pain, but rather sudden onset of severe epigastric pain and rigidity. Ovarian torsion does not typically cause hypotension. A ruptured appendix can lead to hypotension, abdominal rigidity, and guarding, but this is unlikely to occur in the first 8 hours of abdominal pain.

38–C. Many donor organs come from young, previously healthy individuals who sustain irreversible brain injury. The presence of brain death must be determined before donation as determined by: (1) deep coma without response to painful stimuli, (2) absence of spontaneous respiration in the presence of elevated CO_2, (3) absence of movement, (4) absence of brain stem reflexes (e.g., gag reflex), (5) absence of hypothermia, and (6) absence of depressant drugs. Supportive findings include an isoelectric electroencephalogram, absence of intracranial blood flow, or massive cerebral tissue destruction.

39–A. There are four groups, or levels, of axillary breast nodes defined by their relation to the pectoralis minor muscle. An axillary node dissection is the removal of level I, II, and III lymph nodes. It is considered a staging procedure because it has never been shown to directly improve patient outcome. Rather, it is used to direct adjuvant therapies and predict survival. When combined with postoperative radiation to the breast, axillary lymph node dissection is as effective as a modified radical mastectomy. Axillary node dissection without radiation therapy to the breast is associated with a higher local recurrence rate. A simple mastectomy, or subcutaneous mastectomy, removes the bulk of the breast tissue, but provides no information about the axillary node status. A radical mastectomy is the en bloc excision of the breast, the overlying skin, pectoralis major and minor muscles, and the level I, II, and III lymph nodes. For a patient with an early stage breast cancer, this operation is considered too aggressive.

40–A. Chemotherapy is generally indicated in the treatment of stage III colon cancers. This corresponds to Dukes stages C1 and C2. Survival is improved with postoperative adjuvant chemotherapy in these patients. An appropriate chemotherapy regimen would include 5-fluorouracil and levamisole. Chemotherapy is not indicated in stage I lesions; however, current studies are examining the potential benefit in advanced stage II lesions. Radiation therapy is not indicated in the treatment of colon cancer, although it is used in treating rectal cancer.

41–D. A rapid sequence intubation is performed by giving a fast-acting induction agent with a fast-acting paralytic when intubating conditions are desired as quickly as possible. The administration of a paralytic is based on the anesthesiologist's belief after examining the patient's airway that the intubation will be successful. If intubation fails, the patient must be mask ventilated. If the patient can't be mask ventilated, an emergent cricothyrotomy should be performed.

The safest management is to keep the patient spontaneously ventilating, topically anesthetize the airway, and perform the intubation while the patient is awake. Propofol and thiopental could produce unwanted hypotension in this patient, while etomidate, in theory, could trigger a seizure.

42–E. Pressure sores, or decubitus ulcers, are the bane of postoperative patient care in critically ill, obese, and incapacitated patients. These populations of patients are unable to move on their own and are at high risk of developing pressure ulcers, usually near their sacrum. Prevention is best with early mobilization or frequent position changes. There are numerous methods to treat these ulcers, including special air mattress beds and protective coverings placed over the involved area. Adequate nutrition and proper hygiene also help to prevent sores or to assist in their healing. Wound care to ulcers is best done by daily mechanical débridement (wet-to-dry dressing changes).

43–A. The presence of significant rebound tenderness and guarding suggests the presence of peritonitis probably secondary to rupture of a necrotic, strangulated portion of the intestine. This requires immediate abdominal exploration even after the hernia was able to be reduced. Local wound exploration would not allow for identification and treatment of necrotic bowel. Discharge and elective repair would be inappropriate in the setting of peritoneal signs. Observation would only delay the inevitable.

44–D. A Schatzki's ring is a submucosal, circumferential ring in the distal esophagus that is covered by columnar epithelium on the lower surface and squamous epithelium on the upper surface. Almost all patients with this benign lesion have an associated sliding (type I) esophageal hernia. Gastroesophageal reflux symptoms may be present secondary to the effects of the type I hernia but they often respond to conservative management. The mere presence of a Schatzki's ring in not an absolute indication for surgical intervention when gastroesophageal reflux symptoms are present. A complete work-up including upper endoscopy, manometry, and 24-hour pH probe is warranted before any surgical intervention is considered.

45–D. Although parenteral nutritional therapy can provide for maintenance fluid requirements in some settings, it should not be considered the sole source of hydration in many other settings. Patients with necrotizing pancreatitis can have large volume deficits secondary to third spacing of fluid and aggressive replacement of these deficits with crystalloid, not total parenteral nutrition, should be performed and closely monitored. The severe metabolic acidosis associated with a blood urea nitrogen/creatinine ratio much greater than 20 is consistent with severe volume depletion from inadequate volume resuscitation. This is the most likely source of this patient's current condition.

46–D. Gunshot wounds to the abdomen require performance of an exploratory laparotomy. Although this patient may have been shot in the lateral chest, it is important to recognize that the diaphragm rises to the level of the fourth intercostal space on expiration. Thus, gun shot wounds at or below this level need to have the abdomen evaluated surgically. A subxiphoid window and a sternotomy are not necessary because the injury does not seem to have traversed the "box." Similarly, an immediate aortogram to evaluate the great vessels is not necessary given the path of injury and the clinical presentation provided.

47–B. Definitive treatment for resectable gastric carcinoma is surgical resection. The generally poor survival associated with gastric adenocarcinoma is due to the advanced stage of most carcinomas at the time of diagnosis. However, surgical resection is curative for lesions confined to the stomach without significant lymph node disease. Currently, radiation and chemotherapy play a minor role in treatment. A gastric bypass procedure is used to treat morbid obesity. In many situations, palliative surgical resection, gastrojejunostomy, or both, may provide temporary relief of symptoms for incurable disease.

48–B. This patient most likely has a small bowel obstruction secondary to adhesions. The first step in the management of this patient should be to insert a nasogastric tube to relieve symptoms and reduce the risk of aspiration of stomach contents. While radiological studies are appropriate, they should not delay the initiation of treatment with a nasogastric tube. Exploratory laparotomy is necessary in a patient with no prior surgical history and no evidence of a paralytic ileus; however, conservative treatment of obstruction caused by adhesions with placement of a nasogastric tube will frequently result in complete resolution of obstructive symptoms. Analgesics and antiemetics do not address the primary cause of this patient's symptoms. Continued observation in the emergency room without intervention is not appropriate.

49–B. Hepatic vein occlusive disease, or Budd-Chiari syndrome, is a rare postsinusoidal cause of portal hypertension resulting from occlusion of hepatic venous outflow from the liver. A frequent cause of Budd-Chiari syndrome is thrombotic occlusion. This can often be idiopathic, although hematologic disorders such as polycythemia vera, paroxysmal nocturnal hemoglobinuria, hypercoagulable states, and myeloproliferative disorders may precipitate thrombosis. Other causes include vena caval web formation, infection, trauma, and various tumors including hepatocellular carcinoma, renal cell carcinoma, and adrenal carcinoma.

50–E. Although mivacurium is a nondepolarizing agent, it is also metabolized by pseudocholinesterase. Therefore, use of mivacurium in the setting of pseudocholinesterase deficiency should be avoided. The other agents listed are not metabolized by pseudocholinesterase and therefore would be acceptable alternatives for this patient.

51–E. The initial management of severe symptomatic hyperkalemia involves early administration of Ca^{2+}, which stabilizes the electrical potential of the myocardium to prevent the development of life-threatening arrhythmias. Ca^{2+} administration does not, however, decrease the K^+ levels in the serum. Subsequent measures to decrease serum K^+ include administering insulin and $NaHCO_3$, which cause an intracellular shift of K^+. Sodium polystyrene sulfonate enemas may also absorb K^+ in the colon, preventing recirculation of this pool of K^+. Early hemodialysis should also be performed to provide rapid removal of K^+ from the serum.

52–D. Intravenous (IV) drug abusers are prone to developing bacterial endocarditis and can subsequently develop splenic abscesses. Gram-positive organisms are most common in these individuals. This patient has several stigmata of endocarditis including the tricuspid systolic ejection murmur and Janeway lesions of the right palm. The abdominal ultrasound demonstrates signs of a splenic abscess. IV antibiotics are absolutely indicated in this patient with bacterial endocarditis. Cardiac catheterization is not indicated with a patient who is hemodynamically stable and has no signs of right-sided cardiac failure. The combination of antibiotics and splenectomy is the most definitive treatment. Occasionally, splenic abscesses can be drained percutaneously, but there should be a relatively low threshold to perform splenectomy. Regardless, percutaneous drainage alone would not be adequate therapy.

53–C. Unlike most other nonsarcomatous lesions, one of the most important prognostic factors for sarcomas is the histologic grade of the tumor. Factors important in grading sarcomas include cellularity, level of differentiation, pleomorphism, necrosis, and number of mitotic figures. Although the age of the patient, lymph node involvement, and location of the lesion all play a role in predicting the rate of recurrence and overall mortality, these factors are generally not as significant as the histologic grade of the lesion.

54–B. Although thyroid nodules are usually benign, all thyroid nodules may potentially represent a malignancy. There are some factors that increase the likelihood of the presence of malignancy in a thyroid nodule. Cystic lesions are almost always benign lesions, though rarely some malignant tumors may develop central necrosis and subsequently appear cystic. The presence of a single nodule is a bigger risk factor for malignancy compared with the presence of multiple nodules, as are seen in benign conditions of the thyroid (e.g., Hashimoto thyroiditis). A history of radiation exposure to the neck significantly increases the risk of malignancy. A family history of multiple endocrine neoplasia (MEN) II syndrome increases the risk of development of medullary thyroid carcinoma. The presence of symptoms associated with a thyroid nodule such as dysphagia or hoarseness is highly suggestive of an invasive malignancy as well.

55–B. This patient's presentation is highly suggestive of a colon cancer that is causing a partial obstruction of the colonic lumen. Among the choices given, the most appropriate initial step in the evaluation of this patient would be a colonoscopy to attempt to identify a potential mass and obtain a tissue diagnosis with biopsy. A barium enema would also be an appropriate test to evaluate the colon with this presentation. Flexible sigmoidoscopy would not allow for visualization of the entire colon and thus would be inadequate in this situation. Laparotomy or laparoscopy could certainly obtain a tissue diagnosis. However, these procedures are unnecessarily invasive in this case, particularly if the lesion is benign or if it is a cancerous lesion amenable to colonoscopic resection.

56–B. Extra-adrenal sites of chromaffin tissue include the bladder, paravertebral ganglia, the carotid body, and the renal hilum. However, the most common site of chromaffin tissue outside of the adrenal gland is in the organ of Zuckerkandl, which is located at the aortic bifurcation. Any of these sites can harbor an extra-adrenal pheochromocytoma, termed a paraganglioma.

57–D. The current recommendation for local treatment of primary extremity sarcomas larger than 5 cm is wide en bloc surgical excision with postoperative local radiation therapy. Radiation therapy alone is inadequate. Surgical resection alone is generally adequate for lesions smaller than 5 cm. Except for some pediatric sarcomas, chemotherapy has not been shown to provide significant benefit in the treatment of sarcomas. Currently, different types of immunotherapy are being studied for their efficacy in the treatment of sarcomas.

58–B. Unilateral recurrent laryngeal nerve injuries do not result in respiratory compromise and often go unrecognized or may cause hoarseness. Patients with superior laryngeal nerve injury classically develop a weakened voice, which may go unnoticed but may have a significant impact on singers. Bilateral recurrent laryngeal nerve injuries can result in paralysis of the vocal cords in the adducted position, causing airway obstruction and respiratory compromise. After bilateral recurrent nerve injuries, stridor and respiratory distress generally present in the immediate postoperative period following extubation in the recovery room. The diagnosis is unlikely to be delayed for 12 hours in this setting. Hematoma formation from persistent postoperative oozing or frank bleeding can result in delayed airway obstruction and respiratory distress, as described. Treatment involves immediate evacuation of the hematoma at the bedside or in the operating room, depending on the status of the patient. Thyroid storm syndrome would generally present intraoperatively during manipulation of the thyroid gland.

59–D. Hyperaldosteronism (i.e., Conn's syndrome) is a rare disorder characterized by autonomous secretion of aldosterone, causing hypokalemia, expanded blood volume, and hypertension. These fluid and electrolyte disturbances can be attributed to the effect of aldosterone on the distal convoluted tubule, which causes sodium reabsorption in exchange for potassium. Potassium depletion generally causes symptoms of polyuria and polydipsia, and edema is characteristically absent. Women may also have menstrual abnormalities.

60–C. Hepatic adenomas are found predominantly in women of child-bearing age with a distinct positive correlation between oral contraceptive use and the development of adenomas. There is also noted to be a slight increase in patients with diabetes. Frequently, even asymptomatic hepatic adenomas require elective resection because of an approximate 10% risk of malignant transformation, and because of the risk of rupture of these tumors leading to hemorrhage and hypotension or even shock. Occasionally these tumors will regress when oral contraceptives are discontinued, although if regression does not occur, surgical resection is indicated.

61–B. The presentation and pathologic presentation of this patient's breast disease is most consistent with sclerosing adenosis, a histologic subtype of fibrocystic disease. The most common presentation is a cluster of microcalcifications on mammogram without an associated palpable mass or pain. It is the benign breast disease that is most likely to be confused with breast cancer histologically and radiographically. The regularity of nuclei and absence of mitosis are the keys to distinguish it from ductal cancer. Once this diagnosis has been made, reassurance is the only required therapy because sclerosing adenosis does not confer an increased risk of cancer. Additionally, in this patient, with her painful lumpy breasts, close follow-up is probably indicated due to the difficulty of performing self-breast examination. Treatment of pain should first focus on the elimination of known causative agents.

62–E. The detection of pancreatic rejection can be difficult. When performed during the same operation, rejection of a renal graft usually precedes pancreatic rejection, and thus monitoring of serum creatinine is effective in identifying potential pancreatic rejection. Glucose levels often increase after irreversible rejection has occurred. Urinary amylase is useful when bladder anastomosis is present but not for enteric drainage. Fecal and serum amylase levels are not reflective of pancreatic rejection.

63–D. Although early identification of the primary cause of abdominal pain is important, initial management of this patient in shock should be aggressive volume resuscitation. Once his condition is stabilized, a secondary assessment including a detailed history and physical examination should be performed to diagnose the nature of the illness. Diagnostic procedures can then be performed based on clinical suspicion.

64–C. All patients with symptoms of gastroesophageal reflux who are being considered for surgical therapy should undergo 24-hour pH probe, endoscopy, and manometry. The pH probe documents acid reflux, endoscopy looks for the pathologic changes of reflux (e.g., Barrett's esophagus, stricture) in the distal esophagus, and manometry evaluates esophageal motility to ensure that the patient can tolerate a fundoplication. This patient has had an adequate trial of medical therapy and has failed. Further attempts at medical therapy are not necessary before proceeding with surgical therapy. Barrett's changes are not cured by surgical intervention but their progression is halted. Foci of adenocarcinoma can still develop within Barrett's mucosa and life-long endoscopic surveillance is needed in these patients.

65–E. Asymptomatic human immunodeficiency virus (HIV)-positive patients undergoing elective operative procedures do not exhibit an increased rate of infection or wound healing complications compared with HIV-negative patients. Appropriate therapy for this patient, as in HIV-negative patients, would include either a modified radical mastectomy or lumpectomy with lymph node dissection and postoperative local radiation therapy, with or without breast reconstruction.

66–C. This lesion may represent the development of a neoplasm (most likely a squamous cell carcinoma) at the site of a previous wound (Marjolin ulcer). The history of a persistent nonhealing ulcer that does not improve with 5 months of local wound care at the site of a previous injury is suggestive of such a lesion. Thus, biopsy of the lesion is essential in the initial management of this patient to rule out malignancy. Cessation of smoking and continued wound care are important in the treatment of this wound, but do not address the issue of a potential malignancy.

67–B. A pancreatic fistula is frequently associated with significant losses of many electrolytes. Pancreatic secretions contain large amounts of Na^+, K^+, and HCO_3^- and significant amounts of Mg^{2+}. Hypokalemia refractory to aggressive replacement therapy should raise suspicion for a coexisting hypomagnesemia, which can also precipitate K^+ losses. Hypermagnesemia is unlikely in the presence of pancreatic fluid losses, as is hypercalcemia. Hypocalcemia would generally not be associated with the described symptoms. Hyponatremia may rarely be associated with the described symptoms, although refractory hypokalemia is more likely associated with low Mg^{2+}.

68–C. Upper endoscopy is the most reliable method for localizing the source of an upper gastrointestinal bleed. This modality allows treatment of many lesions including peptic ulcer disease and variceal bleeding. For variceal bleeds, one may also use a Sengstaken-Blakemore tube, vasopressin infusion, or somatostatin infusion for temporizing control before definitive treatment. Of significant note, at least 20% of patients with esophageal varices and upper gastrointestinal bleeding will have a gastric or duodenal ulcer as the source of bleeding; hence the value of a full endoscopic examination. Omeprazole therapy alone is not primary in the management of acute upper gastrointestinal bleeding.

69–C. Peutz-Jeghers syndrome is an autosomal dominant familial disease characterized by mucocutaneous pigmentation and intestinal polyposis. The polyps are hamartomas that are most frequently located in the jejunum and ileum but can also be found in the stomach, duodenum, colon, and rectum. It is generally believed that their malignant potential is very low. Peutz-Jeghers syndrome can produce abdominal symptoms caused by intussusception or hemorrhage; as many as one third of patients present with abdominal pain and a palpable abdominal mass as a result of the intussusception. An operation is indicated for abdominal pain or bleeding; it should be limited to conservative resection of involved bowel rather than be an attempt to resect all polyps detected during exploration. While familial polyposis, Gardner's syndrome, and Crohn's disease can cause obstruction, the physical findings of mucocutaneous pigmentation make Peutz-Jeghers syndrome the most likely diagnosis. Human immunodeficiency virus (HIV) enteropathy characteristically presents with malabsorption and diarrhea rather than intussusception.

70–B. Initial management of common duct injuries not detected during surgery is generally conservative. The patient is placed on broad spectrum antibiotics and a combination of external drains and endoscopically or percutaneously placed stents are used to decompress the biliary system. Surgery is delayed because the intense inflammation caused by the leak can make repair extremely difficult. Many leaks will resolve with conservative management, but if not, a biliary bypass procedure may be necessary.

71–C. The most common primary hernia in women is an indirect inguinal hernia. Inguinal hernias occur much more frequently in men than in women. Femoral hernias occur more commonly in women than in men, although femoral hernias are not as common in women as are indirect and direct inguinal hernias. Obturator hernias are very rare and do not generally present with a groin mass. Femoral artery aneurysms are also quite rare.

72–C. Urinary tract infections are among the most common nosocomial infections seen and are a frequent cause of postoperative complications. Hesitancy, dysuria, and inability to void are commons symptoms. Positive leukocyte esterase and nitrites as well as cytologic evidence of leukocytes provides strong evidence for an infection. Treatment involves appropriate antibiotic administration. Bilateral ureteral obstruction is rare in this situation and would generally not be associated with such a large amount of urine in the bladder. Infection may contribute to urinary retention and would not be considered "normal" retention. The findings are not consistent with acute renal failure (ARF) or hemorrhagic cystitis.

73–D. Transplant immunosuppression is associated with rapid tumor growth. Patients who undergo curative resection of malignancies should wait at least 2 years (without evidence of recurrence) before undergoing transplantation. Kidney transplantation has been demonstrated to have a better quality of life and decreased mortality compared with continuous ambulatory peritoneal dialysis and hemodialysis.

74–A. This patient suffered either an unintentional subdural or subarachnoid injection with anesthesia above the level of the cervical spine into the central nervous system. Epidural anesthesia requires much larger doses and volumes of local anesthetic to provide the same sensory level of anesthesia as with spinal anesthesia. Therefore, for an epidural, the anesthetic is given in divided doses when bolused in case the catheter migrates out of the epidural space. Subdural cannulation can occur despite correct epidural placement and is only recognized after an unusually high block after a modest amount of local anesthetic. Hypotension and bradycardia secondary to block of the sympathetic chain are likely to result in this setting and must be aggressively treated.

75–E. Hypoglycemia is a frequent complication of acute cessation of parenteral nutritional therapy because the intravenous carbohydrate load is suddenly discontinued. The patient's symptoms and temporal relationship to discontinuation of the parenteral nutrition therapy is consistent with a hypoglycemic event and initial evaluation should involve checking serum glucose before other major steps are taken. All of the other choices may be reasonable management steps in a patient who abruptly becomes unresponsive; however, in the scenario described, serum glucose analysis is the most prudent step in the initial evaluation.

76–D. It is important to note that any skin lesion of this sort can be malignant. However, there are some findings that may provide additional clues to the malignant potential of some lesions. The classic mnemonic (ABCD) of evaluation of skin lesions is a useful initial tool. Findings suggestive of malignancy include *A*symmetry in color (multiple shades), *B*order irregularity, *C*olor variation (multiple colors in same lesion), and *D*iameter of the lesion (larger lesions are more likely to be malignant). Other factors suggestive of malignancy include nodularity of the lesion, ulceration, itching, bleeding, or lesions that change rapidly over time. Therefore, among the choices, a smooth lesion with consistent coloring throughout is more likely to be benign than the other lesions listed.

77–A, B. Severe epigastric pain radiating to the back, nausea, vomiting, and anorexia are all signs of pancreatitis, although similar symptoms may also be present with cholecystitis or choledocholithiasis. An elevated amylase is commonly found in patients with pancreatitis, while alkaline phosphatase may be elevated in patients with cholecystitis or choledocholithiasis. Identification of multiple gallstones throughout the biliary tree may be associated with pancreatitis or cholecystitis. Other ultrasound findings consistent with cholecystitis include gallbladder wall thickening, pericholecystic fluid, and distension of the gallbladder.

78–E. Suprapubic pain and dysuria are classic signs of urinary tract infection. Leukocyte esterase, nitrates, white blood cells, red blood cells, and bacteria on urinalysis are all signs of infection.

79–B. Ultrasound findings associated with cholecystitis include a distended gallbladder, gallbladder wall thickening, pericholecystic fluid, gallstones, and a sonographic Murphy's sign. Alkaline phosphatase is commonly elevated in patients with cholecystitis. Pancreatitis would typically present with pain in the epigastric region; however, pericholecystic fluid would not be a typical finding.

80–C, D. This patient has a biliary stricture caused by previous biliary surgery. Surgical bypass is indicated and a choledochojejunostomy or hepaticojejunostomy may be performed. In these procedures a portion of the jejunum is anastomosed to the common bile duct to permit drainage of bile around the stricture. A ductal anastomosis above the cystic duct is considered a hepaticojejunostomy, while an anastomosis below the cystic duct is considered a choledochojejunostomy. Thus the choice between these two procedures depends on the location and extent of the lesion. Primary reanastomosis of the remaining bile duct is sometimes possible in these situations but biliary enteric bypass procedures are currently preferred in most settings.

81–A. This patient has a lesion in the lower third of the common bile duct, which is highly suspicious for cholangiocarcinoma. Also high on the differential is pancreatic carcinoma. Regardless, the procedure of choice for treating resectable carcinomas in this area is radical pancreaticoduodenectomy (Whipple's operation). This involves resecting the gallbladder, common bile duct, head of the pancreas, duodenum, and perhaps the distal stomach.

82–A. Gastrinomas cause the Zollinger-Ellison syndrome with intractable peptic ulcers and very high serum gastrin levels. Although these tumors are uncommon, this diagnosis should be considered in any patient with refractory peptic ulcer disease.

83–F, G. Both glucagonomas and somatostatinomas may be associated with the development of glucose intolerance and diabetes mellitus. Glucagonomas may also be associated with a characteristic rash called necrolytic migratory erythema. Somatostatinomas may also be associated with steatorrhea and gallstone development.

84–D. Insulinomas are characterized by a marked catecholamine surge because of a profound insulin-induced hypoglycemia. The hypoglycemia frequently worsens with periods of fasting. The catecholamine surge results in diaphoresis, palpitations, and anxiety.

85–F. Glucagonomas are generally characterized by new onset of glucose intolerance or diabetes mellitus and a characteristic rash called necrolytic migratory erythema.

86–A, C. Vasoactive intestinal peptide tumors (VIPomas) are tumors that are associated with the development of profuse watery diarrhea. VIPomas cause the Verner-Morrison, or WDHA syndrome, with watery diarrhea, hypokalemia, and achlorhydria. In addition, although gastrinomas are generally associated with refractory peptic ulcer disease, these tumors frequently present with persistent chronic diarrhea. Approximately 10%–20% of gastrinomas may present with diarrhea as the only symptom.

87–A. This patient most likely has an ectopic pregnancy. Of the choices listed, pelvic inflammatory disease is the most significant risk factor for ectopic pregnancy. Previous ectopic pregnancy and prior tubal manipulation are also significant risk factors.

88–E. This patient has an abdominal aortic aneurysm that is possibly expanding and is at risk for rupture based on the size and the symptoms described. Among the choices listed, only atherosclerosis is a significant risk factor for abdominal aortic aneurysms.

89–C, H. This patient most likely has a sigmoid volvulus. These patients classically present with left lower quadrant pain, distention, and constipation. Plain films usually show closed loop of bowel and may have the classic "bird's beak" abnormality, which is a tapering of the colon where it is twisted. Significant risk factors for sigmoid volvulus include a chronic bedridden state, pregnancy, laxative use, prior surgery, and residence in psychiatric or nursing home facilities.

90–A, B, C, E. A patient with a right-sided chest wound with decreased breath sounds could have either a tension hemothorax or a tension pneumothorax leading to hypotension. It is also important to recognize the potential risk for liver injury, given the location of the gunshot wounds. Any penetrating injury below the fourth intercostal space warrants exploratory laparotomy to rule out possible abdominal injury. Furthermore, with injuries to this area, cardiac tamponade should be considered as a potential source of hypotension.

91–D. Aortic injury should be suspected in all patients involved in high-speed motor vehicle accidents. A widened mediastinum and loss of the aortic knob are signs of possible aortic arch injury. Other signs on chest radiograph include capping of the left lung or a left sided pleural effusion.

92–B. This patient has all three classic signs of cardiac tamponade—hypotension, muffled heart sounds, and jugular venous distension, or Beck's triad. The presence of all three signs is unusual but often in the presence of hypotension without other obvious causes and with blunt chest trauma, cardiac tamponade should be suspected.

93–H, I. This patient has a documented pelvic fracture confirmed radiographically, which can lead to significant hemorrhage within the pelvis. The patient also has signs of a spinal cord injury, with no movement of her lower extremities and loss of anal sphincter tone characteristic of such an injury.

94–A, E. A hypotensive patient with a chest injury and unilateral decreased breath sounds warrants concern for either a tension hemothorax or a tension pneumothorax as a cause of shock. Tracheal deviation is a characteristic sign that the intrapleural pressure is significantly increased and probably causing impaired venous return to the heart, leading to hypotension. Emergent decompression with chest tube placement should be performed in either case.

95–C. Iatrogenic sources of abnormal bleeding are usually secondary to excess anticoagulation by either heparin or warfarin. Prolonged prothrombin time (PT) is suggestive of over-coumadinization, while a prolonged partial thromboplastin time (PTT) is indicative of excess heparinization. Correction of both may be done acutely with fresh frozen plasma, while vitamin K may also be used to correct an abnormal PT. This patient was relatively stable at the time of the bleeding and this episode followed a session of hemodialysis. Heparin is often used both during hemodialysis to prevent blood clotting in the dialysis machine and to maintain the patency of dialysis catheters while not in use. The only coagulation abnormality noted was a prolonged PTT, indicative of over-heparinization.

96–A, B, F. Disseminated intravascular coagulation is a severe sequelae of trauma, sepsis, or severe hypoxia. Generalized activation of the intrinsic and extrinsic coagulation systems can be caused by many factors including severe trauma and hypotension. Coagulation system activation consumes the available endogenous clotting factors and stimulates the fibrinolytic system. Severe hypothermia can also inhibit coagulation. Rapid administration of fluids and packed red blood cells (PRBCs) with severe blood loss without adequate replacement of platelets and coagulation factors can also lead to significant dilution of coagulation factors and platelets, contributing to such a coagulopathy. Treatment involves early recognition and elimination of the underlying condition, prevention and aggressive treatment of hypothermia, intensive supportive care, as well as rapid administration of fresh frozen plasma, cryoprecipitate, vitamin K, and platelets. Prognosis in this setting is poor.

97–E, F. Renal failure is frequently associated with impairment of platelet function leading to an increased bleeding time even without alterations in prothrombin time (PT) and partial thromboplastin time (PTT). Spontaneous bleeding occurs infrequently with this disorder, although it can lead to significant bleeding intraoperatively. When treatment is indicated, administration of platelets can alleviate symptomatic bleeding. In addition, administering desmopressin can improve function of the patient's platelets in this setting.

98–B, C. Given the normal prothrombin time (PT) and partial thromboplastin time (PTT) with an abnormal bleeding time in a patient with a history of bleeding abnormalities, this patient most likely has a deficiency in von Willebrand factor. This is rarely associated with spontaneous bleeding, although it can be associated with abnormal bleeding after severe injury or surgery.

The most appropriate treatment of von Willebrand factor deficiency would be cryoprecipitate, which could be given in this situation. Fresh frozen plasma contains a small amount of this factor and could also be used, although in the presence of von Willebrand factor deficiency, cryoprecipitate is preferred.

99–B. Reversing the effects of warfarin therapy requires replacement or regeneration of the anticoagulation factors affected by this therapy (i.e., factors II, VII, IX, and X). Administering vitamin K can reverse the effects of warfarin, although this generally takes 6–12 hours before adequate improvement in coagulation occurs. Fresh frozen plasma is a good source of these key coagulation factors and can be administered in situations in which rapid reversal of the effects of warfarin is necessary.

100–I, J. Patients receiving artificial mechanical valves generally require anticoagulation therapy to prevent thrombus formation on the valve. In this situation, both heparin and warfarin therapy may play a role in such therapy. Initially, heparin therapy can be started to provide rapid anticoagulation until the effects of warfarin become therapeutic, at which time the heparin can be discontinued and the warfarin continued chronically. In patients without protein C deficiency, starting heparin therapy before administering warfarin is essential because warfarin therapy can initially cause an acute increase in protein C function with a procoagulant effect. Thus, heparin provides an anticoagulation effect during this transient period.

Index

Page numbers in *italics* denote illustrations; those followed by *t* denote tables; those followed by Q denote questions; those followed by E denote explanations.